MANUAL OF NEPHROLOGY

Ninth Edition

MANUAL OF NEPHROLOGY

Ninth Edition

Edited by

Edgar V. Lerma, MD
Clinical Professor of Medicine
Department of Medicine
Section of Nephrology
University of Illinois at Chicago
Chicago, Illinois

Educational Coordinator
Section of Nephrology
Advocate Christ Medical Center
Oak Lawn, Illinois

Associates in Nephrology
Chicago, Illinois

Seth Furgeson, MD
Associate Professor of Medicine
Renal Med Disease/Hypertension
University of Colorado-Anschutz Medical Campus
University of Colorado Hospital
Aurora, Colorado

Denver Health
Denver, Colorado

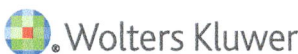

Philadelphia · Baltimore · New York · London
Buenos Aires · Hong Kong · Sydney · Tokyo

Acquisitions Editor: James Sherman
Product Development Editor: Ariel S. Winter
Marketing Manager: Kirsten Watrud
Production Project Manager: Frances M. Gunning
Editorial Coordinator: Thirupura Sundari
Manager, Graphic Arts & Design: Stephen Druding
Manufacturing Coordinator: Bernard Tomboc
Prepress Vendor: Aptara, Inc.

Ninth Edition

Copyright © 2025 Wolters Kluwer

Copyright © 2015 by Wolters Kluwer Health; © 2009 by LIPPINCOTT WILLIAMS & WILKINS, a Wolters Kluwer business; © 2005 Lippincott Williams & Wilkins; © 1999 Lippincott Williams & Wilkins; © 1995 Little, Brown & Co. All rights reserved. This book is protected by copyright. No part of this book may be reproduced or transmitted in any form or by any means, including as photocopies or scanned-in or other electronic copies, or utilized by any information storage and retrieval system without written permission from the copyright owner, except for brief quotations embodied in critical articles and reviews. Materials appearing in this book prepared by individuals as part of their official duties as U.S. government employees are not covered by the above-mentioned copyright. To request permission, please contact Wolters Kluwer at Two Commerce Square, 2001 Market Street, Philadelphia, PA 19103, via email at permissions@lww.com, or via our website at shop.lww.com (products and services).

9 8 7 6 5 4 3 2 1

Printed in The United States of America

978-19752-1891-1

Library of Congress Cataloging-in-Publication data available upon request

Care has been taken to confirm the accuracy of the information presented and to describe generally accepted practices. However, the authors, editors, and publisher are not responsible for errors or omissions or for any consequences from application of the information in this book and make no warranty, expressed or implied, with respect to the currency, completeness, or accuracy of the contents of the publication. Application of the information in a particular situation remains the professional responsibility of the practitioner.

The authors, editors, and publisher have exerted every effort to ensure that drug selection and dosage set forth in this text are in accordance with current recommendations and practice at the time of publication. However, in view of ongoing research, changes in government regulations, and the constant flow of information relating to drug therapy and drug reactions, the reader is urged to check the package insert for each drug for any change in indications and dosage and for added warnings and precautions. This is particularly important when the recommended agent is a new or infrequently employed drug.

Some drugs and medical devices presented in the publication have Food and Drug Administration (FDA) clearance for limited use in restricted research settings. It is the responsibility of the health care provider to ascertain the FDA status of each drug or device planned for use in their clinical practice.

shop.lww.com

Dedication

I dedicate this book to my wife Michelle, and my two daughters Anastasia and Isabella, all of whom have been always exceedingly patient and immensely supportive of all my endeavors ... truly, they continue to serve as my daily inspiration

Edgar V. Lerma, MD

I dedicate this book to my wife Shaila and my two children, Jatin and Leela. I truly appreciate their support throughout this project.

Seth Furgeson, MD

Contributors

Anip Bansal, MD
Associate Professor
Division of Renal Diseases and Hypertension
University of Colorado Anschutz Medical Campus
Aurora, Colorado

Natalie Beck, MD
Assistant Clinical Professor
Department of Nephrology
University of California Davis
Sacramento, California

Ruth Campbell, DO
Assistant Professor
Division of Renal Diseases and Hypertension
University of Colorado-Anschutz Medical Campus
Aurora, Colorado

Michel Chonchol, MD
Professor of Medicine
Division of Renal Diseases and Hypertension
University of Colorado Anschutz Medical Campus
Aurora, Colorado

Gates Colbert, MD
Assistant Professor of Medicine
Department of Internal Medicine
Baylor University Medical Center
Dallas, Texas

James Cooper, MD
Professor of Medicine
Department of Medicine/Renal/Transplant Center
University of Colorado-Anschutz Medical Campus
Aurora, Colorado

Charles Edelstein, MD, PhD
Professor of Medicine
Division of Renal Diseases and Hypertension
University of Colorado Anschutz Medical Campus
Aurora, Colorado

David Ellison, MD
Professor
Director of Oregon Clinical & Translational Institute
Oregon Health & Science University Hospital
Portland, Oregon

Sarah Faubel, MD
Professor of Medicine
Department of Internal Medicine, Nephrology
University of Colorado-Anschutz Medical Campus
Denver, Colorado

Seth Furgeson, MD
Associate Professor of Medicine
Renal Med Disease/Hypertension
University of Colorado-Anschutz Medical Campus
University of Colorado Hospital
Aurora, Colorado

Denver Health
Denver, Colorado

Sixto Giusti, MD
Assistant Professor of Medicine
Division of Renal Diseases and Hypertension
Renal Transplant Section
University of Colorado School of Medicine
Aurora, Colorado

L. Parker Gregg, MD, MSCS
Assistant Professor
Department of Medicine, Section of Nephrology
Baylor College of Medicine, Michael E. DeBakey Veterans Affairs Medical Center, and Veterans Affairs Health Services Research & Development Center for Innovations in Quality, Effectiveness and Safety
Houston, Texas

Maitreyee Gupta, MD
Assistant Professor
Department of Medicine
Thomas Jefferson University Hospitals
Philadelphia, Pennsylvania

Contributors

Mohamed Hassanein, MD
Assistant Professor of Medicine
Department of Medicine
Division of Nephrology and
  Hypertension
University of Mississippi Medical Center
Jackson, Mississippi

Alexander Hlepas, MD
Nephrology Fellow
Department of Nephrology
University of Chicago
Chicago, Illinois

Jessica Kendrick, MD, MPH
Professor of Medicine
Department of Medicine
University of Colorado-Anschutz
  Medical Campus
Aurora, Colorado

Edgar V. Lerma, MD
Clinical Professor of Medicine
Department of Medicine
Section of Nephrology
University of Illinois at Chicago
Chicago, Illinois

Educational Coordinator
Section of Nephrology
Advocate Christ Medical Center
Oak Lawn, Illinois

Associates in Nephrology
Chicago, Illinois

Stuart Linas, MD
Professor of Medicine
Department of Medicine
University of Colorado-Anschutz
  Medical Campus
Aurora, Colorado

Denver Health
Denver, Colorado

Muner M. B. Mohamed, MD
Assistant Professor of Medicine
Ochsner Clinical School/The University
  of Queensland
New Orleans, Louisiana

Sankar Navaneethan, MD, MS, MPH
Garabed Eknoyan MD Endowed
  Professor in Nephrology
Medicine-Nephrology
Baylor College of Medicine
Houston, Texas

Chief, Renal Section
Michael E. DeBakey VA Medical Center
Houston, Texas

Ali Olyaei, Pharm D
Professor of Medicine
Department of Nephrology and
  Hypertension
Oregon Health & Science University
Portland, Oregon

Shehzad Rehman, MD
Associate Professor of Medicine
Department of Internal Medicine,
  Division of Nephrology & Hypertension
Oregon Health & Science University
Portland, Oregon

Amanda DeMauro Renaghan, MD
Professor of Medicine
Department of Medicine
University of Virginia Health System
Charlottesville, Virginia

Katherine Rizzolo, MD
Instructor in Nephrology
Section of Nephrology
Boston University Chobanian &
  Avedisian School of Medicine
Boston Medical Center
Boston, Massachusetts

Helbert Rondon-Berrios, MD, MS
Associate Professor of Medicine
Renal-Electrolyte Division
University of Pittsburgh School
  of Medicine
Pittsburgh, Pennsylvania

Robert Rope, MD
Assistant Professor
Department of Internal Medicine
Oregon Health & Science University
Portland, Oregon

Mitchell H. Rosner, MD
Henry B. Mulholland Professor of
  Medicine
Chairman, Department of Medicine
University of Virginia Health System
Charlottesville, Virginia

Silvi Shah, MD, MS
Associate Professor
Department of Nephrology and Hypertension
University of Cincinnati College of Medicine
Cincinnati, Ohio

Erik Stites, MD
Associate Professor
Department of Medicine
University of Colorado
Aurora, Colorado

Abdul-Rehman Syed, DO
Renal Fellow
Department of Medicine, Division of Renal Diseases and Hypertension
University of Colorado-Anschutz Medical Campus
Aurora, Colorado

Jie Tang, MD, MPH
Associate Professor of Medicine
Department of Medicine/Nephrology
Alpert Medical School of Brown University
Providence, Rhode Island

Joshua Thurman, MD
Professor of Medicine
Division of Renal Diseases and Hypertension
University of Colorado-Anschutz Medical Campus
Aurora, Colorado

Joel Topf, MD
Assistant Clinical Professor of Medicine
Department of Medicine
Oakland University William Beaumont School of Medicine
Rochester, Michigan

Neil Samuel Umles, MD
Nephrology Fellow
Department of Medicine
Ascension St. John Hospital
Detroit, Michigan

Juan Carlos Q. Velez, MD
Professor of Medicine
Ochsner Clinical School/The University of Queensland
System Chair, Department of Nephrology
Ochsner Heath
New Orleans, Louisiana

Prasoon Verma, MD
Assistant Professor in Pediatrics
Department of Neonatology
Cincinnati Children's Hospital Medical Center
Cincinnati, Ohio

Russell S. Whelan, MD, PhD
Assistant Professor
Department of Pediatrics
University of Colorado
Aurora, Colorado

Raghav Wusirika, MD
Associate Professor
Division of Nephrology and Hypertension
Oregon Health & Science University
Portland, Oregon

Anna Zisman, MD
Associate Professor of Medicine
Department of Medicine
Section of Nephrology
University of Chicago
Chicago, Illinois

Preface

This ninth edition comes a decade later since the previous edition, and highlights the latest developments in the field of nephrology, hypertension and kidney transplantation.

In 2023 we gathered a select group of highly motivated individuals who were authoritative figures in the field of nephrology, and who had exemplary reputations with regard to the profession of teaching medicine. In keeping with the design of the original *Manual of Nephrology*, we have reorganized some of the previous chapters and added new ones, as well as new authors.

As in the previous editions of *Manual of Nephrology*, the ninth edition continues to focus on the practical clinical aspects of the diagnosis and management of patients with electrolyte and acid–base disorders, urinary tract infections, kidney stones, glomerulonephritis and vasculitis, acute kidney injury, chronic kidney disease, hypertension, hypertension and kidney disease in pregnancy, and drug dosing with kidney impairment. There are also separate chapters on kidney replacement therapy and kidney transplantation. In addition, in recognition of new developments in certain areas of nephrology, this new edition presents new chapters on diabetic kidney disease and cancer and kidney involvement.

From personal experience, we know that very few people read a textbook from cover to cover. For a variety of reasons, the majority would read only one or a few chapters at any given time. Therefore, we tried to ensure that each chapter would be complete in itself. As a consequence, there is unavoidable overlap among some of the information provided in some chapters; we, however, feel that this was truly necessary, at least from an information-retrieving standpoint, and in this way it will not be necessary for readers to read bits of information between one or more chapters just to get complete information regarding a particular subject.

We hope that this book will be used not only by nephrologists and nephrology fellows, medical residents and interns, and medical students, but also by primary care providers and other subspecialists (outside of nephrology) with particular interest in this very exciting field of medicine.

Certainly this book would not have been possible were it not for so many people. First, we would like to thank the contributing authors, who have spent countless hours in producing high-quality, up-to-the-last-minute information. We spent a significant amount of time communicating via telephone and e-mail as we reviewed the chapters and discussed recommendations, most of which were agreed upon, but, on occasion, disputed. We express our sincere gratitude for their openness to this very collegial collaboration, which has been a truly rewarding learning experience for us.

In particular, we appreciate the help and support of all the staff of Wolters Kluwer, most especially James Sherman (Senior Content Editor), Ariel S. Winter (Senior Development Editor), Thirupura Sundari (Editorial Coordinator), and Dinesh Pokhriyal (Project Manager), all of whom have been very patient with our procrastinations and stubbornness at times.

In the eighth edition, Dr Schrier dedicated the book to Professor Hugh de Wardener who is recognized as having made enormous contributions to the fields of hypertension and nephrology as a clinician, scientist, and educator for over 60 years.

As new editors, we are humbled and honored to continue what Dr Robert Schrier has started over four decades ago, when the first edition of this book was published in 1981, and we dedicate this to him. Dr Schrier served as the head of the Department of Medicine and Division of Renal Diseases at the University of Colorado for over 20 years. During his tenure, he transformed the institution into a renowned research institution. He also served as the president of both the American Society of Nephrology and the International Society of Nephrology. One of his greatest legacies is related to his career as a medical educator. Dr Schrier was a world-class teacher who trained countless medical students, medical residents, and nephrology fellows. Those of us who trained under him will forever remember his discussions of water disorders, acute kidney injury, and congestive heart failure. His former trainees now practice throughout the world and continue his legacy.

Last and most importantly, we thank our teachers and mentors, who themselves, have devoted their own time to educate and train us to become who we are. We thank all the medical students, residents, and fellows who in one way or another have given us inspiration to persevere in the teaching profession. Mostly, we thank all of our patients, who have been truly instrumental in our learning and devotion to medicine. On behalf of all the contributors to this book, we fervently hope that all our efforts will contribute to relieving your suffering and perhaps lead to your recovery.

Edgar V. Lerma, MD
Seth Furgeson, MD

Contents

Dedication v
Contributors vii
Preface xi

1 The Nephrology Consult (Urine Examination, Urine Studies Interpretation, Imaging) 1
Muner M. B. Mohamed, Juan Carlos Q. Velez

2 The Edematous Patient: Cardiac Failure, Cirrhosis, and Nephrotic Syndrome 9
Robert Rope, David Ellison, Raghav Wusirika

3 The Patient With Hyponatremia and Hypernatremia 33
Helbert Rondon-Berrios

4 The Patient With Hypokalemia or Hyperkalemia 52
Jie Tang, Stuart Linas

5 The Patient With an Acid–Base Disorder 65
Anip Bansal

6 The Patient With Hypocalcemia or Hypercalcemia 77
Mohamed Hassanein, Edgar V. Lerma

7 The Patient With Hypophosphatemia or Hyperphosphatemia 100
Gates Colbert, Edgar V. Lerma

8 The Patient With Hypomagnesemia or Hypermagnesemia 109
Neil Samuel Umles, Joel Topf

9 The Patient With Urinary Tract Obstruction (Emphasis on Kidney Stones) 125
Alexander Hlepas, Anna Zisman

10 The Patient With Urinary Tract Infection 144
Abdul-Rehman Syed, Jessica Kendrick

11 The Patient With Glomerular Disease or Vasculitis 172
Russell S. Whelan, Joshua Thurman

12 The Patient with Acute Kidney Injury 194
Sarah Faubel, Charles Edelstein

13 The Patient With Chronic Kidney Disease 228
Katherine Rizzolo, Michel Chonchol

14 The Patient Receiving Chronic Kidney Replacement With Dialysis 239
Natalie Beck, Seth Furgeson

15 The Patient With a Kidney Transplant 248
Sixto Giusti, James Cooper, Erik Stites

16 The Patient With Kidney Disease and Hypertension in Pregnancy 267
Maitreyee Gupta, Prasoon Verma, Silvi Shah

17 The Patient With Hypertension 294
Ruth Campbell, Seth Furgeson

18 The Patient With Diabetes and Chronic Kidney Disease 322
L. Parker Gregg, Sankar Navaneethan

19 The Patient With Cancer and Kidney Involvement 338
Mitchell H. Rosner, Amanda DeMauro Renaghan

20 Practical Guidelines for Drug Dosing in Patients With Impaired Kidney Function 370
Shehzad Rehman, Ali Olyaei

Index 429

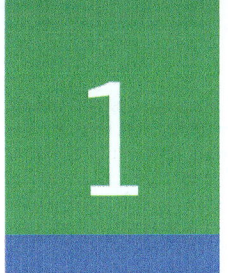

The Nephrology Consult (Urine Examination, Urine Studies Interpretation, Imaging)

Muner M. B. Mohamed, Juan Carlos Q. Velez

Acute kidney injury (AKI) (see *Chapter 12: The Patient with Acute Kidney Injury*) is defined by a rise in the serum creatinine concentration or a decrease in urine output that develops over hours to days. Its clinical presentation varies from case to case. Patients can present to an emergency department with symptoms and signs related to the AKI such as deceased urine output, hematuria, elevated blood pressure, edema, and/or signs of uremia. Other patients can be asymptomatic and present with an elevated serum creatinine found incidentally during laboratory testing. Herein, we discuss how to approach a consultation prompted by a case of AKI.

Steps for Evaluating a Consult for AKI (*See Chapter 12: The Patient with Acute Kidney Injury*)

STEP 1: Carefully Review the History and Perform Physical Examination

Taking good history is the first step to diagnose the cause of AKI. The history should focus on the onset of AKI (if there is a frequent measurement of serum creatinine or accurate urine output), which will help to identify the possible etiology. Reviewing systems is important, for example, vomiting and diarrhea make volume depletion the most likely reason for prerenal AKI. History of other comorbidities such as liver cirrhosis or heart failure, toxic ingestion, and home medications review are very important elements of the history.

Physical examination may reveal signs associated with many diseases causing AKI. As an example, volume depletion in prerenal, volume overload in cardiorenal syndrome, skin rash in interstitial nephritis or vasculitis, and ascites and jaundice in hepatorenal syndrome. Some patients show symptoms and signs of uremia such as flapping tremor and uremic encephalopathy. For more details about the history and physical exam in AKI, see Chapter 12: The Patient with Acute Kidney Injury.

STEP 2: Start Your Investigation by Obtaining History and Reviewing the Patient Chart

This step can be taken before or after obtaining history and performing physical examination. Before going further with investigating the cause of AKI, the acuity and the need for emergent treatment need to take the priority in the assessment. As an example, if the patient presents with severe volume overload with respiratory distress or life-threatening hyperkalemia not responding to medical treatment, the emergent need for renal replacement therapy should take priority before further investigation for the etiology of AKI.

Once the need for emergent treatment has been addressed, the next step in the investigation is to search for prior medical records to determine if the rise in serum creatinine is indeed an acute event. That entails looking for available laboratory results to detect the onset of AKI by determining the first elevated serum creatinine and comparing it to the baseline value, if available. By looking at the trend of serum creatinine rise, the rapidity of the progression in kidney function decline can be determined.

In patients who present with AKI, emphasis must be placed on obtaining a thorough history and physical in an effort to identify the potential culprit. Preexisting diagnoses and associated outpatient medications may be important in determining the risk of AKI. In addition, interview should include inquiring about recent acute illnesses that might have led to prescription of new medications.

In hospitalized patients in whom the AKI was acquired during the hospitalization, attention must be paid to specific factors that could elicit an AKI event. First, review of vital signs: searching for evidence of hemodynamic changes that could cause or contribute to the development of AKI. Such changes include hypotension, tachycardia, and unstable arrythmias such as rapid atrial fibrillation. If an episode of hemodynamic instability occurs, ischemic acute tubular injury (ATI) would be a likely cause of AKI.

Second, records of intake and output must be reviewed to determine whether the patient may be in negative fluid balance potentially leading to a prerenal state which could have evolved into ischemic ATI. Importantly, when output is reviewed, urinary retention must be ruled out. Accordingly, a permanent or intermittent bladder catheter is often required. Communication with nursing personnel is essential to fully address this factor.

Third, intraoperative hypotension is a common precipitant of AKI. Therefore, it is necessary to review all anesthesia records of surgeries or other invasive procedures that were performed prior to the onset of AKI. In those records, identification of hypotension and tachycardia could be informative, as well as the use of vasopressors, such as vasopressin or phenylephrine, since their use implies that the blood pressure tended to fall during the surgical intervention.

Fourth, contrast-enhanced imaging studies could have introduced a risk for contrast-induced AKI, therefore radiologic and cardiovascular (CV) interventional reports 24 to 96 hours prior to the AKI must be reviewed.

Finally, a thorough review of medication exposure must be conducted. Importantly, actual drug administration should be reviewed rather than ordered drugs, to correctly ascertain drug exposure. Multiple drug classes have the potential for being nephrotoxic, but the most common ones to consider in hospital-acquired AKI include nonsteroidal anti-inflammatory drugs (NSAIDs), diuretics, laxatives, antibacterials (e.g., vancomycin, aminoglycosides, colistin, penicillins), antivirals (e.g., IV acyclovir), chemotherapeutic agents (e.g., cisplatin, IV methotrexate, checkpoint inhibitors), among others.

Regarding laboratory data, certain findings may be associated with certain etiologies of AKI. For instance, in serum chemistry, hypernatremia reflects dehydration, so, when present, prerenal AKI must be suspected. On the other hand, hyponatremia can be associated with serious underlying disorders such as heart failure and liver cirrhosis. Presence of hyperkalemia may point to specific types of AKI (see ***Chapter 12: The Patient with Acute Kidney Injury***): those involving cell lysis (rhabdomyolysis, tumor lysis syndrome, hemoglobinuric AKI), obstructive uropathy, or tubulointerstitial nephritis. Hyperglycemia as in diabetic ketoacidosis can be associated with prerenal AKI from osmotic diuresis. Urine dipstick may be positive for heme (as in rhabdomyolysis) or protein (as in glomerular disease). Urine sodium, urine urea nitrogen, and osmolality, as well as fractional excretion of sodium (FENa) and fractional excretion of urea nitrogen (FEUN) can be helpful in differentiating prerenal azotemia from ATI, but those urinary indices generally have limited diagnostic utility. Certain laboratory abnormalities may direct the diagnosis, such as anemia and hypercalcemia in patients with plasma dyscrasias. Urinalysis may point to a kidney parenchymal disease when hematuria, leukocyturia, and/or proteinuria are present. However, urinalysis must be accompanied by urinary sediment microscopy (see below).

Finally, imaging studies are needed to rule out obstructive uropathy. In most instances, a renal ultrasound is sufficient, although in some cases, computed tomography or nuclear medicine scan is required.

STEP 3: Enhance Your Workup to Find the AKI Cause: Urinary Sediment Microscopy

In cases when prerenal AKI is strongly suspected, intravenous volume resuscitation should be instituted. If the kidney function improves, one could ascertain the diagnosis of prerenal AKI. But if volume administration does not resolve the AKI, and obstructive uropathy has been ruled out, a search for a parenchymal cause of AKI must ensue.

Urinary sediment microscopy is useful to identify elements suggestive of tubular, interstitial, or glomerular injury as a potential cause of AKI. It is critical to perform urinary sediment microscopy in a systematic and comprehensive fashion to be able to extract clinically useful information. Here are the elements necessary for optimal urinary sediment microscopy:

1. *Required equipment:*
    - Microscope equipped with bright field illumination, phase contrast, and polarized light
    - Centrifuge calibrated to 600 g
    - Disposable plastic centrifuge tubes
    - Microscope slides and coverslips
    - Pasteur pipettes
    - Sternheimer–Malbin stain
2. *Specimen collection:*
    - Random urine specimen, preferably clean catch. In females, collect "midstream urine" to avoid contamination from vaginal elements
    - Ideally 10 to 12 mL, but OK to perform with 5 mL if oligoanuria collections from bladder catheters are acceptable (from catheter, not from bag)
    - Collect sample in a clean container
    - Specimen containers must be labeled with the patient's full name and date of birth or medical record number.
3. *Procedure:* See Figure 1-1.

STEP 4: Enhance Your Workup to Find the AKI Cause: Additional Testing

After completion of the first three steps, a primary suspicion should be entertained. In addition to serum chemistry, complete urinalysis, urine sediment microscopy (see Figs. 1-2 and 1-3), and a complete blood count, further workup should be appropriate for the suspected etiology:

- If *prerenal azotemia (see Chapter 12: The Patient with Acute Kidney Injury)* suspected: check blood urea nitrogen:creatinine ratio (elevated in prerenal, poor sensitivity), serum uric acid (elevated in prerenal). When safe, IV volume expansion should be used as both diagnostic and therapeutic intervention.
- If *ischemic ATI (see Chapter 12: The Patient with Acute Kidney Injury)* suspected: check fractional excretion of urinary sodium (>2% very specific in ATI).
- If *toxic ATI (see Chapter 12: The Patient with Acute Kidney Injury)* suspected: check creatinine phosphokinase (CPK) level, serum uric acid, serum phosphorus (elevated in rhabdomyolysis, tumor lysis syndrome, acute phosphate nephropathy).
- If *nephritic syndrome (glomerulonephritis, see Chapter 11: The Patient with Glomerular Disease or Vasculitis)* suspected: check serum complements (C3 and C4), antinuclear antibodies (ANA), anti–double-stranded DNA (anti-dsDNA) titers, proteinase 3 (PR3-ANCA antibody), myeloperoxidase (MPO-ANCA antibody), c/p-ANCA, anti-GBM antibodies, serum cryoglobulin, rheumatoid factor, serology for hepatitis B and C virus, serum IgA.
- If *nephrotic (glomerulopathy, podocytopathy, see Chapter 11: The Patient with Glomerular Disease or Vasculitis)* suspected: serum protein electrophoresis (SPEP), free light chains, check serum complements (C3 and C4), ANA, anti-dsDNA titers, anti-GBM antibodies, serum cryoglobulin, rheumatoid factor, serology for hepatitis B and C virus, HIV, phospholipase A2 receptor antibodies.
- If *microangiopathic hemolytic anemia* (MAHA) suspected *(thrombotic microangiopathy [TMA] syndromes, see Chapter 11: The Patient with Glomerular Disease or Vasculitis):* check CBC for anemia and thrombocytopenia, haptoglobin, LDH level and peripheral blood smear for schistocytes. Stool culture for enterohemorrhagic *Escherichia coli* for Shiga toxin–mediated hemolytic uremic syndrome.

Step 3.1: Pour the volume of approximately 10 mL of urine into centrifuge tube.

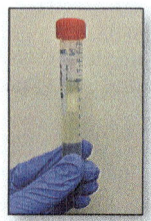

Step 3.2: Centrifuge for 5 minutes at 600 g. Balance the centrifuge with a tube with the same volume.

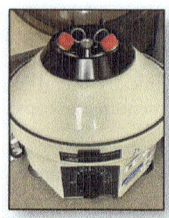

Step 3.3: Pour off approximately 9.5 mL of the remaining liquid and re-suspend the sediment in the remaining 0.5 mL, tap on the end of the tube to detach the pellet from the tube.

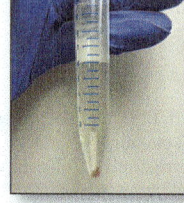 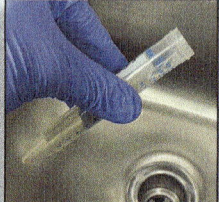 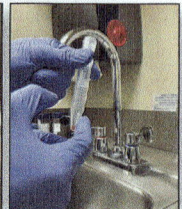

Step 3.4: Place one drop of this concentrated sediment on a slide, apply a coverslip and examine microscopically.

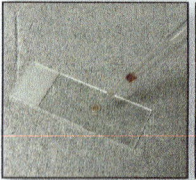 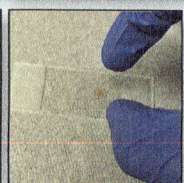

Step 3.4: Sternheimer-Malbin (SM) stain greatly facilitates identification of white blood cells (WBCs), acanthocytes, epithelial cells, and casts. It is quite simple to use and requires no fixation or special steps: during the usual specimen preparation process, after centrifugation and pouring off the supernatant, resuspend the sediment and add one drop of stain. Mix gently and allow 1–2 minutes for uptake of stain before preparing the slide.

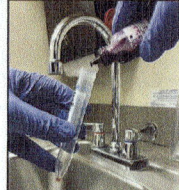 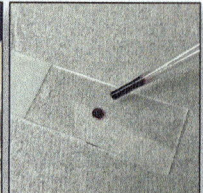

Step 3.5: Slide inspection should begin under low power (10x objective). Adjust illumination to lowest possible level for optimal contrast. Further inspection of specific structures should be done under high power (40x objective). Further magnification with 100x objective and oil immersion may be needed to assess cellular casts. Polarized light should be applied to search for crystals and lipids. Phase contrast is helpful to identify cast matrix and to inspect erythrocyte morphology.

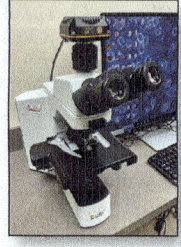

Figure 1-1. Guide for the performance of urinary sediment microscopy by the practicing clinician.

- If *interstitial nephritis* (see Chapter 12: The Patient with Acute Kidney Injury) suspected: check urine culture to determine if leukocyturia is sterile.
- If *obstructive uropathy* (see Chapter 9: Obstruction [Emphasis on Kidney Stones]) suspected: kidney ultrasound, computed tomography of abdomen/pelvis (nephrolithiasis), diuretic renal scintigraphy (verification if anatomical hydronephrosis represents current obstruction).

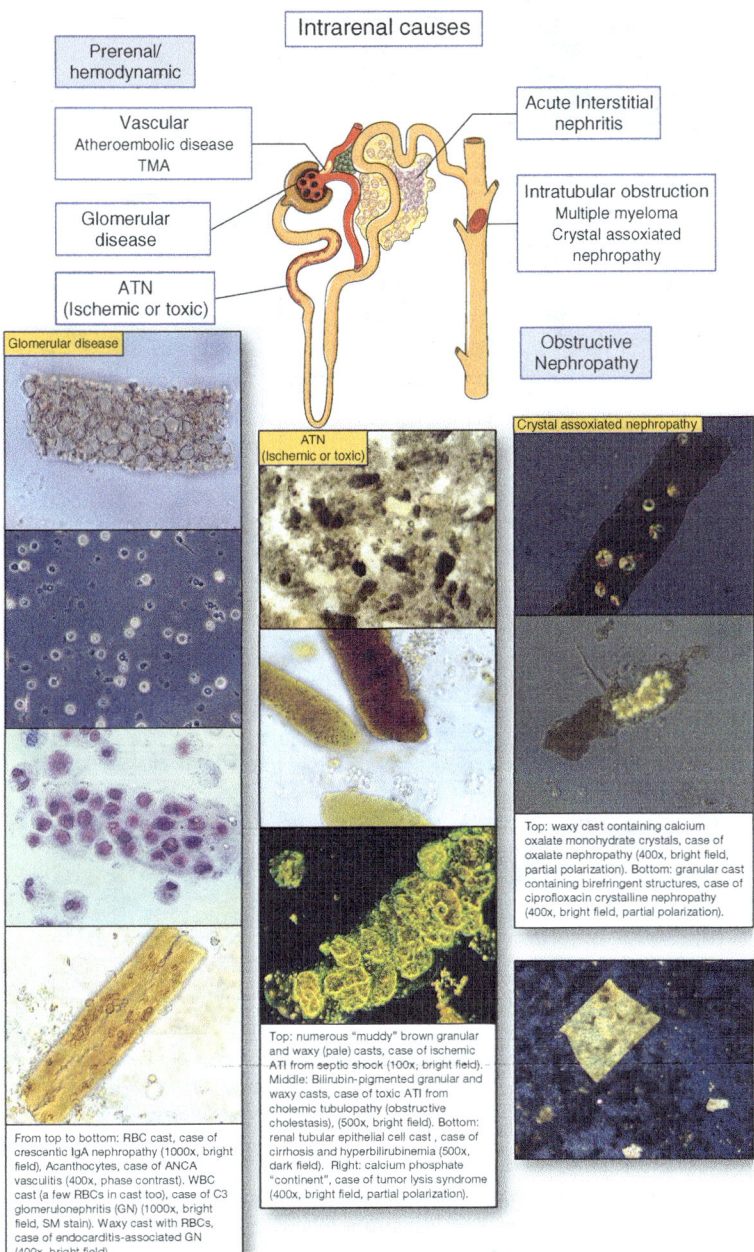

Figure 1-2. Differential diagnosis of AKI and examples of associated urinary sediment microscopy findings.

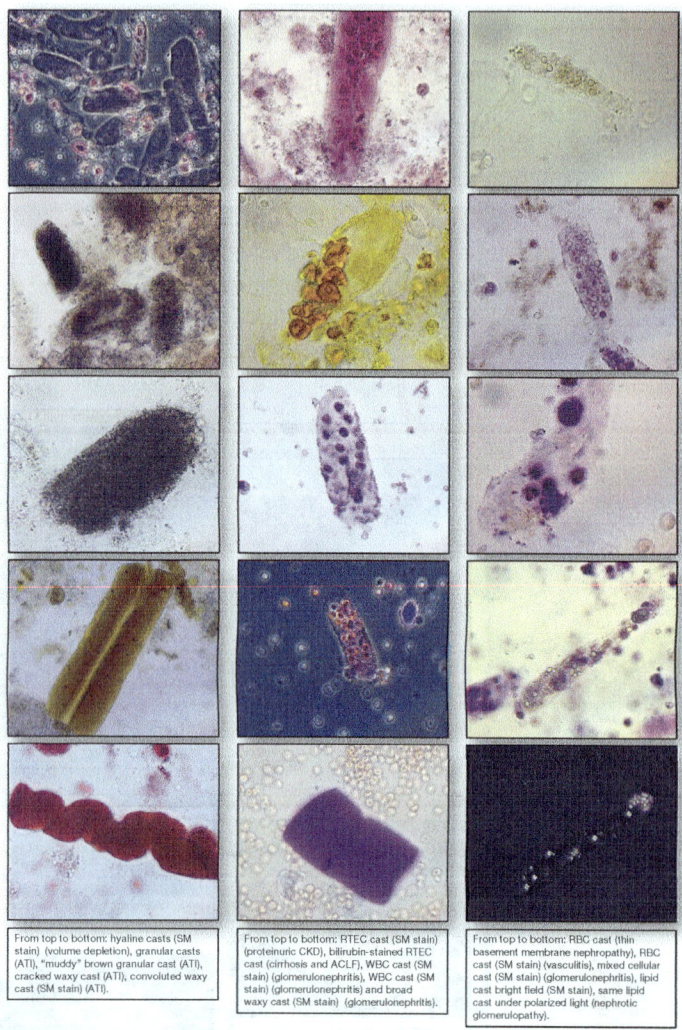

From top to bottom: hyaline casts (SM stain) (volume depletion), granular casts (ATI), "muddy" brown granular cast (ATI), cracked waxy cast (ATI), convoluted waxy cast (SM stain) (ATI).

From top to bottom: RTEC cast (SM stain) (proteinuric CKD), bilirubin-stained RTEC cast (cirrhosis and ACLF), WBC cast (SM stain) (glomerulonephritis), WBC cast (SM stain) (glomerulonephritis) and broad waxy cast (SM stain) (glomerulonephritis).

From top to bottom: RBC cast (thin basement membrane nephropathy), RBC cast (SM stain) (vasculitis), mixed cellular cast (SM stain) (glomerulonephritis), lipid cast bright field (SM stain), same lipid cast under polarized light (nephrotic glomerulopathy).

Figure 1-3. Examples of urinary sediment microscopy findings in various cases of AKI.

STEP 5: Enhance Your Workup to Find the AKI Cause: Kidney Biopsy
When all the above steps do not reach a clear diagnosis, and establishing a diagnosis may lead to change in management, a percutaneous kidney biopsy must be considered.

Step 6: Evaluate Need for Urgent Kidney Replacement Therapy (KRT)
When you assess your patient, keep in mind the following indications of renal replacement therapy in patients with AKI:

1. Life-threatening hyperkalemia
2. Volume overload with pulmonary edema

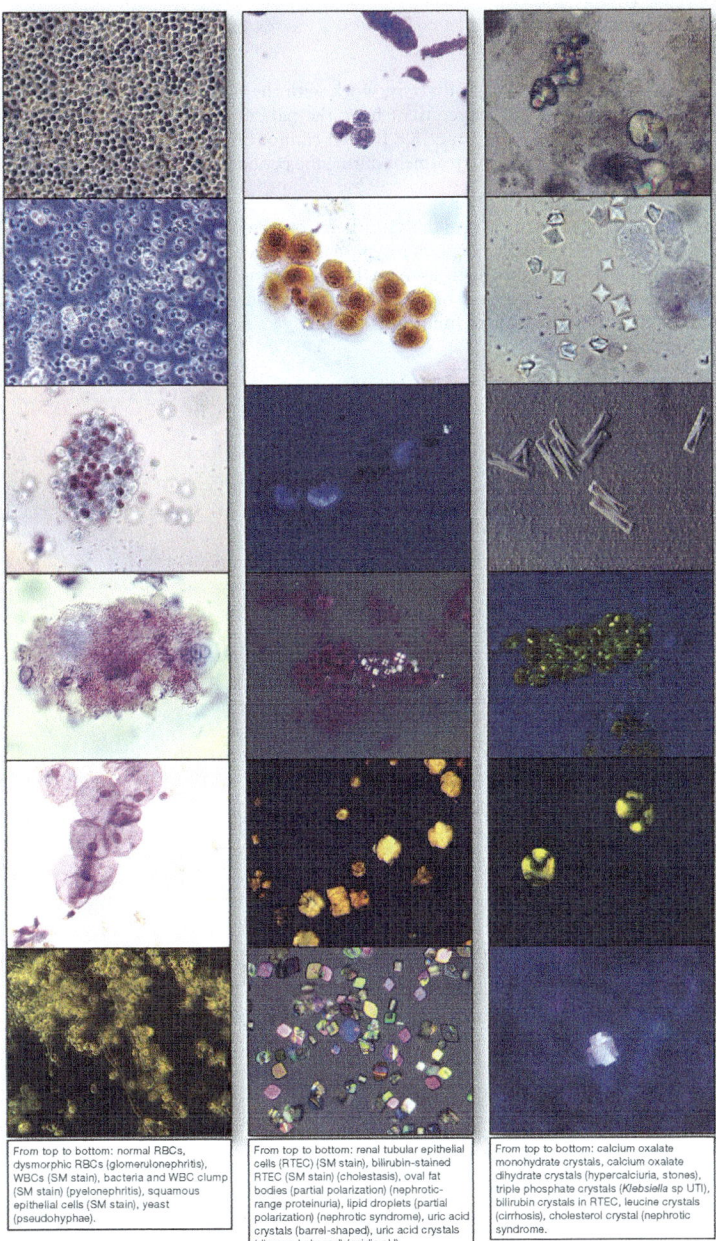

From top to bottom: normal RBCs, dysmorphic RBCs (glomerulonephritis), WBCs (SM stain), bacteria and WBC clump (SM stain) (pyelonephritis), squamous epithelial cells (SM stain), yeast (pseudohyphae).

From top to bottom: renal tubular epithelial cells (RTEC) (SM stain), bilirubin-stained RTEC (SM stain) (cholestasis), oval fat bodies (partial polarization) (nephrotic-range proteinuria), lipid droplets (partial polarization) (nephrotic syndrome), uric acid crystals (barrel-shaped), uric acid crystals (diamond-shaped) (acidic pH).

From top to bottom: calcium oxalate monohydrate crystals, calcium oxalate dihydrate crystals (hypercalciuria, stones), triple phosphate crystals (*Klebsiella* sp UTI), bilirubin crystals in RTEC (cirrhosis), leucine crystals (cirrhosis), cholesterol crystal (nephrotic syndrome).

Figure 1-3. (*Continued*)

3. Uremic complications
4. Severe metabolic acidosis
5. Toxic ingestion

If your patient needs urgent dialysis, work with the primary team to facilitate the initiation of dialysis by getting consent from the patient and securing dialysis access as soon as possible. However, since KRT often cannot be immediately provided, such patients usually require medical treatment during the period prior to the initiation of KRT.

Step 7: Initial Management of AKI

If there is no indication for urgent dialysis, the priority will be to eliminate the possible causes of AKI, for example, treat the hypotension, avoid iodinated contrast agents, or discontinue medications such as NSAIDs, angiotensin-converting enzyme (ACE) inhibitors, angiotensin receptor blockers (ARBs), and nephrotoxins. See Chapter 12: The Patient with Acute Kidney Injury for details.

The Edematous Patient: Cardiac Failure, Cirrhosis, and Nephrotic Syndrome

Robert Rope, David Ellison, Raghav Wusirika

I. Body Fluid Distribution

Of the total fluid in the human body, two-thirds reside inside the cells (i.e., intracellular fluid) and one-third resides outside the cells (i.e., extracellular fluid [ECF]). A patient with generalized edema has an excess of ECF. The ECF resides in two locations: in the vascular compartment (plasma fluid) and between cells, but outside of the vascular compartment (interstitial fluid). In the vascular compartment, approximately 85% is venous and 15% arterial (Table 2-1). An excess of interstitial fluid constitutes edema. With pressure, the interstitial fluid can generally be moved from the area, leaving an indentation; this is *pitting* edema. This demonstrates that the excess interstitial fluid can move freely within its space between the body's cells. If pressure does not cause pitting in the edematous patient, then interstitial fluid cannot move freely. Nonpitting edema can occur with lymphatic obstruction (i.e., lymphedema) or fibrosis of subcutaneous tissue, which may occur with chronic venous stasis.

Although generalized edema always signifies an excess of ECF in the *interstitial* compartment, the *intravascular* volume may be decreased, normal, or increased. For example, because two-thirds of ECF reside in the interstitial space and only one-third resides in the vessels, a rise in total ECF volume may occur due to excess interstitial fluid (i.e., chronic generalized edema from heart failure) even with decreased intravascular volume (i.e., acute intravascular hypovolemia from gastroenteritis or hemorrhage).

A. **Starling's law** states that the rate of fluid movement across a capillary wall is proportional to the hydraulic permeability of the capillary, the transcapillary hydrostatic pressure difference, and the transcapillary oncotic pressure difference. The classical understanding of Starling's forces noted that fluid leaves the capillary at the arterial end because the hydrostatic pressure difference favoring transudation exceeds the oncotic pressure difference favoring resorption. In contrast, fluid returns to the capillary at the venous end as this relationship reverses. This approach minimized the importance of lymphatic absorption. However, current evidence suggests that transudation happens along the entire length of the capillary with the lymphatic system then absorbing excess fluid from the intersition to return to the circulation via lymphatic ducts that generally parallel the venous system (Fig. 2-1).

Because serum albumin is the major determinant of capillary oncotic pressure, which acts to maintain fluid in the capillary, hypoalbuminemia can lead to excess transudation of fluid from the vascular to the interstitial compartment. However, several factors buffer the effects of hypoalbuminemia on fluid transudation and edema formation. First, an increase in transudation tends to dilute interstitial fluid, thereby reducing the interstitial protein concentration and oncotic force. Second, increases in interstitial fluid volume increase interstitial hydrostatic pressure. Third, lymphatic flow into the jugular veins increases, returning more transudated fluid to the circulation. In cirrhosis, where hepatic fibrosis causes high capillary hydrostatic pressures and hypoalbuminemia is common, the lymphatic flow can increase 20-fold to 20 L/d, attenuating the

TABLE 2-1 Body Fluid Distribution

Compartment	Amount	Volume (L) in 70-kg Person
Total-body fluid (TBF)	60% of body weight	42.0
Intracellular fluid	40% of body weight 2/3 of TBF	28.0
Extracellular fluid (ECF)	20% of body weight 1/3 of TBF	14.0
Interstitial fluid	2/3 of ECF	9.4
Plasma fluid	1/3 of ECF	4.6
Venous fluid	85% of plasma fluid	3.9
Arterial fluid	15% of plasma fluid	0.7

collection of interstitial fluid. When these buffering factors are overwhelmed, interstitial fluid accumulation can lead to edema. This generally occurs when serum albumin concentration (<2.0 g/L), and thus oncotic pressure, is quite low. An increase in the fluid permeability (hydraulic conductivity) of the capillary wall can also cause edema. This is seen with capillary leak syndromes, hypersensitivity reactions, and angioneurotic edema (e.g., ACEi-induced angioedema), and it may be a factor in edema associated with diabetes mellitus and idiopathic cyclic edema.

B. These comments refer to **generalized edema** (i.e., an increase in total-body interstitial fluid), though this edema may still have a **predilection for specific**

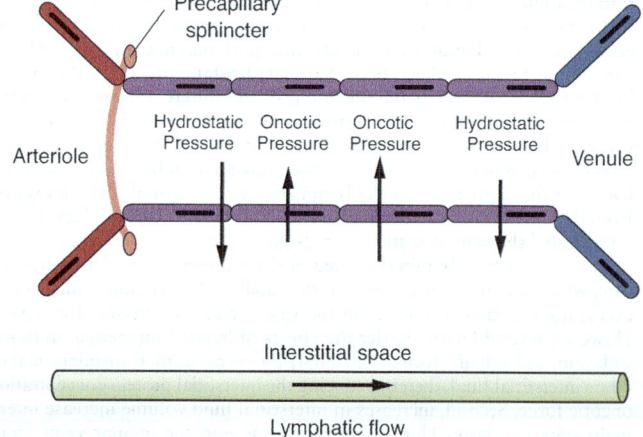

Figure 2-1. Effect of Starling forces on fluid movement across capillary walls. Modified from Rennke HG, Denker BM. *Renal Pathophysiology The Essentials*. 5th ed. Wolters Kluwer, 2020.

areas. With cirrhosis, edema collects in the abdominal cavity due to portal hypertension. With upright activity, an accumulation of edema in the lower extremities is expected, whereas supine rest predisposes to edema in the sacral and periorbital areas.

C. Although generalized edema may have a predilection for certain body sites, it is nevertheless a **total-body phenomenon** of excess interstitial fluid, unlike localized edema caused by local factors. Tissue responses to trauma, burns, inflammation, and cellulitis can cause localized edema. Venous obstruction, as with thrombophlebitis, may cause edema of one lower extremity. Lymphatic obstruction (e.g., from malignancy) can cause an excessive accumulation of interstitial fluid and, therefore, localized edema. The physical examination of a patient with ankle edema should include a search for venous incompetence (e.g., varicose veins) and evidence of lymphatic disease. Deep venous disease may not be detectable on physical examination and ultrasonography, or other imaging may be of assistance. Rarely, venous or lymphatic disease may be bilateral (e.g., a proximal venous thrombosis or pelvic lymphatic obstruction from malignancy) and must be considered when evaluations for the more common causes of generalized edema (e.g., cardiac failure, cirrhosis, and nephrotic syndrome) are not fruitful.

II. Body Fluid Volume Regulation

The edematous patient presents a challenge in the understanding of volume regulation. In the healthy subject, if ECF is expanded with isotonic saline, the kidney will excrete the excess sodium and water, returning ECF volume to normal. Why unhealthy patients continue to retain sodium and water despite excessive ECF volume expansion is less clear. It is understandable that when kidney function is markedly impaired (i.e., acute or chronic kidney failure), the kidney continues to retain sodium and water even to a degree causing hypertension and pulmonary edema. Much more perplexing are those circumstances in which the kidneys are known to be normal and yet continue to retain sodium and water in spite of the expansion of ECF and edema formation (e.g., cirrhosis and congestive heart failure [CHF]). For example, if the kidneys from a cirrhotic patient are transplanted to a patient with end-stage kidney disease but without liver disease, excessive renal sodium, and water retention no longer occur. Neither total ECF nor its interstitial component, both of which are expanded in the patient with generalized edema, modulates renal sodium and water excretion. Rather, as Peters suggested in the 1950s, some body fluid compartment other than total ECF or interstitial fluid volume must regulate renal sodium and water excretion. The term *effective blood volume* describes this undefined, enigmatic body fluid compartment that signals the kidney to regulate sodium and water retention. If effective blood volume is reduced, even in spite of an expansion of total ECF, sodium and water retention ensues through multiple neurohormonal pathways (discussed below). Identifying the physiologic drivers of reduced effective blood volume was a critical step in understanding the common sodium-retentive states of cirrhosis and heart failure.

A. **Low cardiac output states,** seen in some patients with heart failure, clearly drive sodium and water retention. However, many patients with heart failure and decompensated cirrhosis avidly retain sodium and water with normal or elevated cardiac outputs.

B. Expanded total plasma and blood volumes are frequently present in CHF and cirrhosis and cannot, therefore, drive reduced effective arterial volume. Elevated left atrial pressure (as seen with increased plasma volume) causes natriuresis, in part by suppression of vasopressin and a decrease in neutrally mediated renal vascular resistance. Another stimulus for natriuresis is increased right and left atrial pressure via increased atrial natriuretic peptide. However, despite these effects, renal sodium and water retention

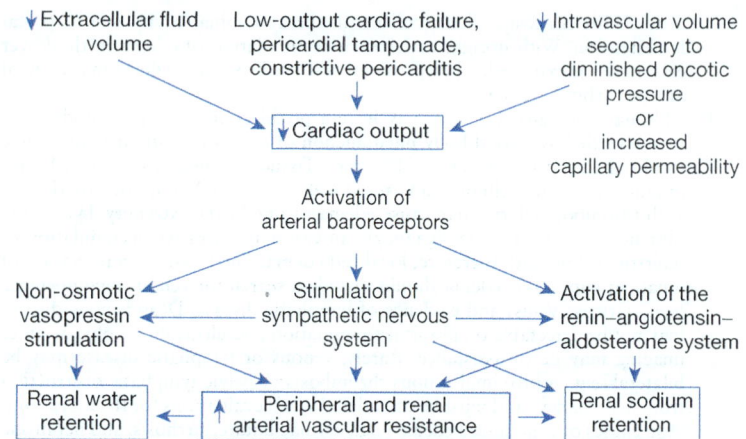

Figure 2-2. Decreased cardiac output as the initiator of arterial underfilling. (Adapted from Schrier RW. A unifying hypothesis of body fluid volume regulation. *J R Coll Physicians Lond.* 1992;26:296. Reprinted with permission.)

are hallmarks of CHF, a situation in which pressures in the atria and venous component of the circulation are routinely increased. These mild atrial responses to excess plasma volume are likely more important in healthy subjects responding to volume expansion from daily activities (e.g., eating a salty meal).

C. The **arterial portion of body fluids** (see Table 2-1) is the critical component in the regulation of renal sodium and water excretion. The relationship between cardiac output and systemic arterial resistance constitutes the effective arterial blood volume (EABV), which is the predominant regulator of renal sodium and water reabsorption. This relationship establishes the "fullness" of the arterial vascular tree. In this context, a primary decrease in cardiac output or systemic arterial vasodilation, or a combination thereof, causes arterial underfilling driving a renal sodium- and water-retaining state, which leads to generalized edema. Pressure sensors in the renal afferent arterioles as well as the aortic arch and carotid sinus detect arterial underfilling and increase renin and sympathetic signaling, respectively. The sodium- and water-retaining states that are initiated by a decline in cardiac output are shown in Figure 2-2 and include (a) ECF volume depletion (e.g., diarrhea, vomiting, hemorrhage); (b) low-output cardiac failure, pericardial tamponade, and constrictive pericarditis; (c) intravascular volume depletion secondary to protein loss and hypoalbuminemia (e.g., nephrotic syndrome, burns or other protein-losing dermopathies, protein-losing enteropathy); and (d) increased capillary permeability (capillary leak syndrome).

The causes of increased renal sodium and water retention leading to generalized edema that are initiated by primary systemic arterial vasodilation are equally numerous and are shown in Figure 2-3. Severe anemia, beriberi, Paget disease, and thyrotoxicosis are causes of high-output cardiac failure that may lead to sodium and water retention by the normal kidney. A high-flow arteriovenous fistula, hepatic cirrhosis, sepsis, pregnancy, and vasodilating drugs (e.g., minoxidil, hydralazine, doxazosin) also cause systemic arterial vasodilation leading to arterial underfilling and decreased renal sodium and water excretion. Unfortunately for patients with reduced

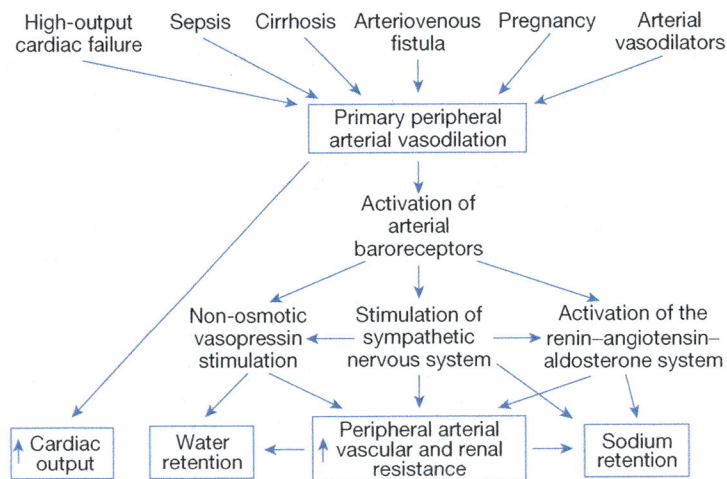

Figure 2-3. Systemic arterial vasodilation as the initiator of arterial underfilling. (Adapted from Schrier RW. A unifying hypothesis of body fluid volume regulation. *J R Coll Physicians Lond.* 1992;26:296. Reprinted with permission.)

EABV, our kidneys cannot distinguish between states where sodium retention is acutely therapeutic (e.g., true ECF volume depletion from gastroenteritis or hemorrhage) and where it is ultimately harmful (e.g., cirrhosis and heart failure).

D. Two major **compensatory processes** protect against arterial underfilling. One process is rapid and consists of a neurohumoral and systemic hemodynamic response. The other is slower and involves renal sodium and water retention. In the edematous patient, these compensatory responses have occurred to varying degrees depending on the clinical course. Due to the rapid hemodynamic compensatory responses, mean arterial pressure is a poor index of the integrity of the arterial circulation. Whether a primary fall in cardiac output or systemic arterial vasodilation is the initiator of arterial underfilling, the compensatory responses are similar. As depicted in Figures 2-2 and 2-3, the common neurohormonal response to a decreased EABV involves the stimulation of three vasoconstrictor pathways, the sympathetic nervous system, angiotensin, and vasopressin (ADH). In addition to its direct vasoconstrictive and chronotropic effects, the sympathetic nervous system also increases angiotensin, through increased kidney β-adrenergic–mediated release of renin, and vasopressin, through neurally mediated nonosmotic release from the pituitary. With a primary fall in cardiac output or systemic arterial vasodilation, secondary increases in systemic arterial vascular resistance or cardiac output occur, respectively, to acutely maintain arterial pressure. This rapid compensation, driven by these vasoconstrictor and chronotropic pathways, allows time for the slower renal sodium and water retention to occur to attempt to attenuate arterial circulatory underfilling. With a decrease in ECF volume, such as occurs with acute gastrointestinal losses, sufficient sodium, and water retention can occur to restore cardiac output to normal and therefore terminate renal sodium and water retention before edema forms. This is often not the case with cardiac failure or cirrhosis, because even these compensatory responses may not restore EABV to normal. The presence of excess ECF (e.g., ascites, edema) in these disorders generally speaks to a "decompensated" state with reduced EABV.

1. Therefore, the **neurohumoral** and **renal sodium- and water-retaining mechanisms** persist as important compensatory processes in maintaining EABV. However, neither the acute nor the chronic compensatory mechanisms are successful in restoring cardiac contractility or reversing cardiac tamponade or constrictive pericarditis. Compensatory renal sodium and water retention lead to an expansion of the venous side of the circulation as arterial vascular filling improves but does not return to normal. The resultant rise in venous pressure enhances capillary hydrostatic pressure and thereby transudation of fluid into the interstitial fluid, creating edema. In hypoalbuminemia and capillary leak syndromes, excessive transudation of fluid occurs across the capillary bed and also prevents the restoration of cardiac output; therefore, continuous renal sodium and water retention occur exacerbating edema.

2. **Systemic arterial vasodilation**, the other major initiator of arterial underfilling, also generally cannot be completely reversed by the compensatory mechanisms and therefore may lead to edema formation. Systemic arterial vasodilation results in dilation of precapillary arteriolar sphincters, increasing capillary hydrostatic pressure and probably capillary surface area. A larger proportion of retained sodium and water is therefore transudated across the capillary bed into the interstitium in these edematous disorders (see Fig. 2-3). Similarly, dihydropyridine calcium-channel blockers (dCCBs), common antihypertensives, dilate arterioles without affecting venules, causing edema. Combining dCCBs with renin–angiotensin system inhibitors, which dilate both arterioles and venules, can reduce edema by decreasing capillary hydrostatic pressure.

E. Another reason why low cardiac output or systemic arterial vasodilation may lead to edema formation is the inability of these patients, as compared with healthy subjects, to escape the **sodium-retaining effect of aldosterone** (Fig. 2-4). In the healthy subject receiving large exogenous doses of aldosterone or another mineralocorticoid hormone, ECF expansion is associated with a rise in the glomerular filtration rate (GFR) and a decrease in proximal tubular sodium and water reabsorption, which leads to an increase in sodium and water delivery to the distal nephron site of aldosterone action. This increase in distal sodium delivery is the major mediator of escape from the sodium-retaining effect of mineralocorticoids in healthy subjects, thereby avoiding edema formation. In contrast, in patients with cirrhosis or cardiac failure, the renal vasoconstriction–mediated reduction in GFR and proximal tubule sodium retention that accompanies the compensatory neurohumoral response to arterial underfilling (from increased sympathetic and angiotensin effect) leads to a decrease in sodium and water delivery to the distal nephron site of aldosterone action. This diminution in distal sodium delivery makes it easier for the elevated aldosterone levels seen in heart failure and cirrhosis to drive further sodium retention and edema.

The importance of kidney hemodynamics, particularly the GFR, in the aldosterone escape phenomena is emphasized by the observation that in pregnancy, a state of primary arterial vasodilation and elevated serum aldosterone levels, aldosterone escape occurs despite arterial underfilling because of an associated 30% to 50% increase in the GFR with increased sodium filtration. It is unclear why pregnancy is associated with this large increase in the GFR, which occurs within 2 to 4 weeks of conception. However, there is evidence that an increase in relaxin may be involved. The increase in the filtration rate cannot be due to plasma volume expansion, because this does not occur until several weeks after conception. The occurrence of aldosterone escape in pregnancy attenuates edema formation when compared with other edematous disorders.

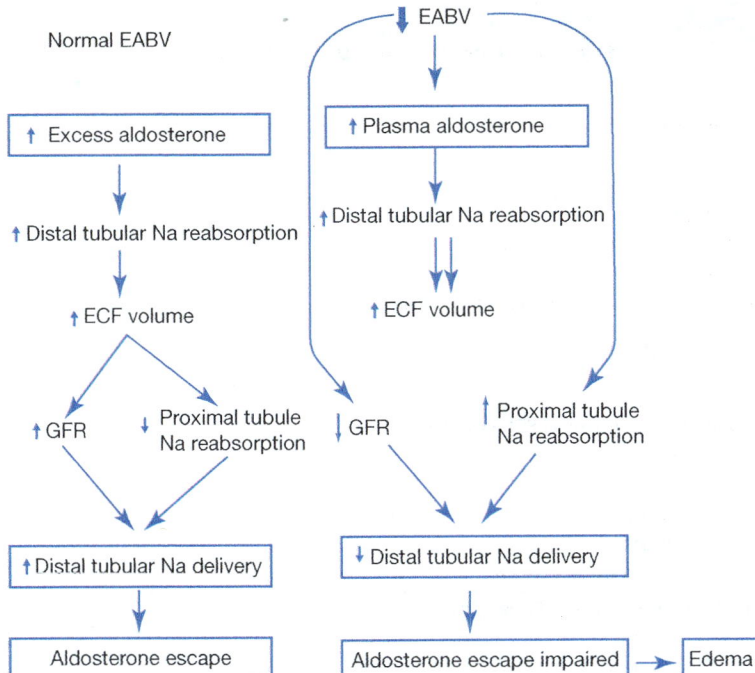

Figure 2-4. Aldosterone escape in a healthy subject (**left side**) and failure of aldosterone escape in patients with arterial underfilling (**right side**). EABV, effective arterial blood volume; ECF, extracellular fluid; GFR, glomerular filtration rate. (Used with permission of American College of Physicians, from Schrier RW. Body fluid regulation in health and disease: a unifying hypothesis. *Ann Intern Med*. 1990;113:155–159; permission conveyed through Copyright Clearance Center, Inc.)

III. Dietary and Diuretic Treatment of Edema: General Principles

The daily sodium intake in the United States is typically 3 to 4 g (1 g of sodium contains 43 mEq; 1 g of sodium chloride [NaCl] contains 17 mEq of sodium). A typical "low-salt" diet contains 2 g (86 mEq). Diets that are even lower in NaCl content can be prescribed to limit ECF expansion or reduce blood pressure, but many individuals find them unpalatable. If salt substitutes are used, it is important to remember that these contain potassium chloride, so caution is needed with kidney disease or those using potassium-sparing diuretics (i.e., spironolactone, eplerenone, triamterene, and amiloride). Other drugs that increase serum potassium concentration must also be used with caution in the presence of salt substitute intake (i.e., angiotensin-converting enzyme inhibitors [ACEis], angiotensin receptor blockers [ARBs], β-blockers, and nonsteroidal antiinflammatory drugs [NSAIDs]). For edematous patients, it is important to emphasize that sodium restriction is required, even when using diuretics, as the therapeutic potency of diuretic drugs varies inversely with salt intake.

Diuretic drugs act by increasing urinary sodium excretion. They are divided into five classes based on their predominant site of action along the nephron (Table 2-2). Osmotic diuretics (e.g., mannitol, urea) and proximal diuretics (e.g., acetazolamide, empagliflozin) are not used as the sole agent to treat edematous

TABLE 2-2	Physiologic Classification of Diuretic Drugs
Osmotic Diuretics	
Mannitol	
Urea	
Proximal Diuretics	
Carbonic anhydrase inhibitors	
Acetazolamide	
Sodium-glucose cotransporter type 2 inhibitors	
Canagliflozin	
Empagliflozin	
Dapagliflozen	
Loop Diuretics (Maximal FENa = 30%)	
Na-K-2Cl inhibitors	
Furosemide	
Bumetanide	
Torsemide	
Ethacrynic acid	
DCT Diuretics (Maximal FENa = 9%)	
NaCl inhibitors	
Chlorothiazide	
Hydrochlorothiazide	
Metolazone	
Chlorthalidone	
Indapamide	
Collecting Duct Diuretics (Maximal FENa = 3%)	
Na channel blockers	
Amiloride	
Triamterene	
Steroidal mineralocorticoid (aldosterone) receptor antagonists	
Spironolactone	
Eplerenone	
Nonsteroidal mineralocorticoid (aldosterone) receptor antagonists	
Finerenone	

DCT, distal convoluted tubule; FENa, fractional excretion of sodium.

disorders. Loop diuretics (e.g., furosemide, torsemide, bumetanide), distal convoluted tubule (DCT) diuretics (e.g., hydrochlorothiazide, chlorthalidone, metolazone), and collecting duct diuretics (e.g., spironolactone, eplerenone, amiloride), however, all play important but distinct roles in treating edematous patients.

The goal is to reduce excess ECF volume and then maintain the ECF volume at a normal level. This requires an initial natriuresis, but, at steady state, urinary sodium excretion returns close to baseline despite continued diuretic administration. Importantly, an increase in sodium and water excretion does *not* indicate therapeutic efficacy if ECF volume does not decline. Conversely, a return to "basal" levels of urinary sodium excretion does not indicate diuretic resistance if ECF volume is controlled. A rapid return to ECF volume expansion after stopping a diuretic indicates its efficacy.

A. When starting a loop diuretic for edema in the setting of heart failure or cirrhosis, it is important to establish a therapeutic goal, usually a target body weight. Identifying additional specific clinical concerns to address (e.g., pulmonary edema, ascites, jugular venous distension [JVD]) also helps guide treatment. If a certain dose does not lead to natriuresis, it can be doubled repeatedly until the maximum recommended dose is reached (Table 2-3). When a **diuretic drug is administered by mouth**, the magnitude of the natriuretic response is determined by the intrinsic potency of the drug, the dose, the bioavailability, the amount delivered to the kidney, the amount that enters the tubule fluid (most diuretics act from the luminal side), and the physiologic state of the individual. Except for proximal diuretics, the maximal natriuretic potency of a diuretic relates to its site of action. As noted in Table 2-2, loop diuretics can maximally increase fractional sodium excretion to 30%, DCT diuretics can increase it to 9%, and sodium channel blockers can increase it to 3% of the filtered load.

The intrinsic diuretic potency of a diuretic is defined by its dose–response curve, which is generally sigmoid. The steep sigmoid relation is the reason that loop diuretic drugs are described as *threshold drugs*. When starting loop diuretic treatment, providers must ensure that each dose reaches the steep part of the dose–response curve before increasing the dose frequency. Because loop diuretics are rapid acting, many patients note an increase in urine output within several hours of taking the drug; this can be helpful in establishing that an adequate dose has been reached. Directly measuring urine sodium excretion 2 hours after a dose can also demonstrate an appropriate natriuretic effect. Because most loop diuretics are short acting, they should be administered at least twice daily. For inpatient management, targeting a urine output of 3 to 5 L/d can help ensure appropriate diuresis.

B. The **bioavailability of diuretic drugs** varies widely among classes, within classes, and even between patients for some drugs (e.g., furosemide). The bioavailability of loop diuretics varies ranging from 10% to 100% (mean, 50%

TABLE 2-3 Typical Doses of Loop Diuretics

Kidney Insufficiency	Furosemide (mg)		Bumetanide (mg)		Torsemide (mg)	
	IV	PO	IV	PO	IV	PO
GFR 20–50 mL/min	80	80–160	2–3	2–3	50	50
GFR <20 mL/min	200	240	8–10	8–10	100	100
Severe acute kidney failure	500	NA	12	NA	–	–
Nephrotic syndrome	120	240	3	3	50	50
Cirrhosis	40–80	80–160	1	1–2	10–20	10–20
Congestive heart failure	40–80	160–240	2–3	2–3	20–50	50

GFR, glomerular filtration rate; IV, intravenous; NA, not available.

for furosemide; 80% to 100% for bumetanide and torsemide). Limited bioavailability can usually be overcome by appropriate dosing, but some drugs, such as furosemide, are variably absorbed by the same patient on different days, making precise titration difficult. Doubling the furosemide dose when changing from intravenous to oral therapy is customary, but the relation between intravenous and oral dose may vary. For example, the amount of sodium excreted during 24 hours is similar whether furosemide is administered to a healthy individual by mouth or by vein, despite its 50% bioavailability. This paradox results from the fact that oral furosemide absorption is slower than its clearance, leading to "absorption-limited" kinetics. Therefore, effective serum furosemide concentrations persist longer when the drug is given by mouth because a reservoir in the gastrointestinal tract continues to supply furosemide to the body. This relation holds for a healthy individual but not all sick patients. Predicting the precise relation between oral and intravenous doses, therefore, is difficult. However, providers can closely follow urine output, urine sodium, and changes in patient symptoms to determine the diuretic effect and adjust therapy as appropriate.

IV. Diuretic Resistance

Patients are considered to be **diuretic resistant** when an inadequate reduction in ECF volume is observed despite near-maximal doses of loop diuretics. Several causes of resistance can be determined by considering factors that affect diuretic efficacy, as discussed earlier.

A. Causes of Diuretic Resistance
1. **Excessive Dietary NaCl Intake Is One Cause of Diuretic Resistance.** When sodium intake is high, renal sodium retention can occur between diuretic-induced natriuretic periods, thereby maintaining the ECF volume expansion. Measuring the sodium excreted during 24 hours can be useful in diagnosing excessive intake. If the patient is at steady state (the weight is stable), then the urinary sodium excreted during 24 hours is equal to dietary NaCl intake. If sodium excretion exceeds 100 to 120 mM (approximately 2 to 3 g sodium/d), then dietary NaCl consumption is too high, and dietary counseling should be undertaken.
2. **Impaired diuretic delivery to its active site** in the kidney tubule is another cause of diuretic resistance. Most diuretics, including the loop diuretics, DCT diuretics, and amiloride, act from the luminal surface. Although diuretics are small molecules, most circulate tightly bound to protein and reach the tubular fluid primarily by tubular secretion. Loop and DCT diuretics bind albumin and are secreted through the organic anion pathway in the proximal tubule. Although experimental data suggest that diuretic resistance results when serum albumin concentrations are very low, because the volume of diuretic distribution increases, most studies suggest that this effect is only marginally significant clinically and is observed only when serum albumin concentration declines below 2 g/L. However, a variety of endogenous and exogenous substances that compete with diuretics for secretion into tubule fluid are more probable causes of diuretic resistance. Uremic anions, NSAIDs, bile acids, organic acids, free fatty acids, probenecid, and penicillin all inhibit loop and DCT diuretic secretion into the tubular fluid. Under some conditions, this may predispose to diuretic resistance, because the concentration of drug achieved in tubular fluid does not exceed the diuretic threshold. For example, chronic kidney failure shifts the loop diuretic dose–response curve to the right, therefore requiring a higher dose to achieve maximal effect.
3. **The presence of significant proteinuria, as seen in nephrotic syndrome,** may also influence diuretic effectiveness. Initial investigations suggested proteinuria may reduce diuretic effectiveness by directly binding diuretic

drugs and preventing their interaction with target receptors. However, more recent data suggest that heavy proteinuria may directly stimulate sodium retention in the kidney. Increasing diuretic dosing can generally overcome this potential concern.
4. **Enhanced sodium retention in the kidney,** due to the neurohormonal adaptations (renin–angiotensin–aldosterone activation and increased sympathetic drive) driven by reduced EABV also directly combat diuretic-induced sodium excretion. Furthermore, the chronic increases in distal sodium delivery generated by loop diuretics can stimulate hypertrophy of the distal tubule leading to sodium retention and blunting of the loop diuretic effect.

B. Treatment of Diuretic Resistance. Several strategies are available to achieve effective control of ECF volume in patients who do not respond to full doses of loop diuretics (Fig. 2-5).
1. **A diuretic of another class may be added** to a regimen that includes a loop diuretic (Table 2-4). This strategy produces synergy; the combination of agents is more effective than the *sum* of the responses to each agent alone. DCT diuretics are most commonly combined with loop diuretics. DCT diuretics inhibit the adaptive changes in the distal nephron that increase the reabsorptive capacity of the tubule and limit the potency of loop diuretics. Because DCT diuretics have longer half-lives than loop diuretics, they attenuate sodium retention during the periods between doses of loop diuretics, thereby increasing their net effect. Metolazone is frequently combined with loop diuretics because its half-life is relatively long. Other thiazide and thiazide-like diuretics, however, appear to be equally effective, even in severe kidney failure.

   The dramatic effectiveness of combination diuretic therapy is accompanied by complications in a significant number of patients. Massive fluid and electrolyte losses (i.e., sodium, potassium, and magnesium) have led to circulatory collapse and arrhythmia during combination therapy, and patients must be followed up carefully. The lowest effective dose of DCT diuretic should be added to the loop diuretic regimen. Patients are frequently treated with combination therapy for only a few days and then can be placed back on a single-drug regimen. When continuous combination therapy is needed, low doses of DCT diuretics (2.5 mg metolazone or 25 mg chlorthalidone) administered only two or three times per week may be sufficient. Historically, chronic DCT diuretic use was considered ineffective with advanced chronic kidney disease (CKD) (GFR <30 mL/min), however clinical experience and recent trial data do not support this. Chlorthalidone has demonstrated efficacy for hypertension in patients with GFR <30 and most CHF diuresis protocols include DCT diuretics even with severely reduced kidney function.

   Other classes of diuretics have shown benefits for heart failure in randomized trials. **Sodium-glucose cotransporter-2 inhibitors** (SGLT2is, e.g., empagliflozin, dapagliflozin) reduce symptom burden and mortality in systolic heart failure. **Acetazolamide** reduces congestion in patients with acute decompensated heart failure. Both acetazolamide and SGLT2is block sodium reabsorption in the proximal tubule and are combined with concomitant loop diuretic use.
2. For hospitalized patients who are resistant to diuretic therapy, the continuous infusion of loop diuretics is an alternative approach. **Continuous diuretic infusions** (Table 2-5) have several advantages over bolus diuretic administration. First, because they avoid peaks and troughs of diuretic concentration, continuous infusions prevent periods of positive NaCl balance (postdiuretic NaCl retention) from occurring. Second, continuous infusions

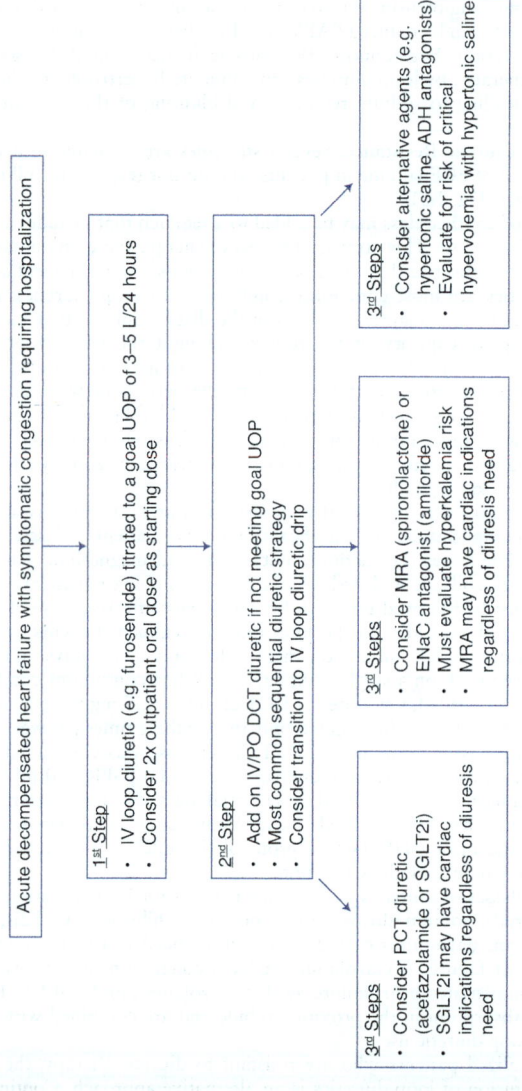

Figure 2-5. Flowsheet for the potential escalation of diuretics in patients with refractory hypervolemia. ADH, antidiuretic hormone; ENaC, epithelial sodium channel; DCT, distal convoluted tubule; MRA, mineralocorticoid receptor antagonist; PCT, proximal convoluted tubule; UOP, urine output.

TABLE 2-4 Combination Diuretic Therapy (to Add to a Loop Diuretic)

Distal Convoluted Tubule Diuretics
- Metolazone 2.5–10 mg p.o. daily[a]
- Hydrochlorothiazide (or equivalent) 25–100 mg p.o. daily
- Chlorothiazide 500–1,000 mg i.v. daily-b.i.d.

Proximal Tubule Diuretics
- Acetazolamide 500 mg i.v. daily
- Empagliflozin 10–25 mg p.o. daily
- Dapagliflozin 5–10 mg p.o. daily

Collecting Duct Diuretics
- Spironolactone 25–400 mg p.o. daily
- Amiloride 5–10 mg p.o. daily

[a]Metolazone is generally best given for a limited period (3 to 5 d) or should be reduced in frequency to three times per week once extracellular fluid volume has declined to the target level. Long-term combination therapy is only needed for persistent volume expansion.

Dosing varies based on GFR and indication (e.g., heart failure vs. cirrhosis).

may be more efficient than bolus therapy (the amount of NaCl excreted per milligram of drug administered is greater). Third, some patients who are resistant to large doses of diuretics given by bolus respond to continuous infusion. Fourth, diuretic response can be titrated; in the intensive care unit, where obligate fluid administration must be balanced by fluid excretion. Finally, complications associated with high doses of loop diuretics, such as ototoxicity, appear to be less common when large doses are administered as a continuous infusion. Total daily furosemide doses exceeding 1 g have been tolerated well when administered over 24 hours.

One approach is to administer a loading dose of 20 to 200 mg of furosemide followed by a continuous infusion at 4 to 40 mg/h. The actual dosing required will depend on the patient's level of kidney function and diuretic resistance as discussed above. When kidney failure is present, higher doses are generally needed, but patients should be monitored carefully for side effects, such as ECF volume depletion from excessive diuretic use.

TABLE 2-5 Continuous Infusion of Loop Diuretics

Diuretic	Starting Bolus (mg)	Infusion Rate (mg/h)		
		GFR <25 mL/min	GFR 25–75 mL/min	GFR >75 mL/min
Furosemide	40	20, then 40	10, then 20	10
Bumetanide	1	1, then 2	0.5, then 1	05
Torsemide	20	10, then 20	5, then 10	—

GFR, glomerular filtration rate.

The randomized double-blind controlled DOSE trial (Diuretic Optimization Strategies Evaluation) examined the mode and dose of loop diuretics in decompensated heart failure patients. There was no difference in global symptom relief or change in kidney function at 72 hours between intermittent bolus versus continuous infusion of furosemide or between low dose (outpatient dose) and high dose (2.5 times outpatient dose). However, body weight loss was better with the continuous infusion. There was no difference in outcomes between the groups at 60 days follow-up. Therefore, the use of continuous infusions is primarily driven by individual clinical circumstances (e.g., failure of standard IV bolus approaches).

3. After the optimization of loop, distal tubule, and proximal tubule diuretics, alternative agents could be considered. Small boluses of **hypertonic saline** (HS, 3% normal saline) combined with high-dose loop diuretic therapy may augment diuresis in some patients with refractory congestion unresponsive to the measures described above. HS boluses may generate an osmotic force to mobilize water into the arterial tree from the intracellular and interstitial spaces, improve kidney blood flow, and allow for a greater response to diuretic therapy. Studies to date are very limited and providers must ensure their patients can accommodate the salt load that happens before the diuretic effect. **Tolvaptan**, an ADH antagonist, can improve cardiac symptoms and aid in decongestion, however has not yet been shown to improve cardiovascular outcomes. There are ongoing studies on the use of tolvaptan for diuresis in CHF. **Dopamine**, which can reduce proximal tubule sodium reabsorption, has not shown consistent efficacy in small trials and is not commonly used.

4. **Mechanical ultrafiltration**, which removes excess sodium and water through a dialysis unit or similar machine in the absence of total kidney failure, has not been shown to improve outcomes. The multicenter Ultrafiltration in Decompensated Heart Failure with Cardiorenal Syndrome (CARRESS-HF) trial compared stepwise pharmacologic treatment versus ultrafiltration in 188 patients with persistent congestion and rising serum creatinine. Both groups had the same weight loss and dyspnea score, but only the ultrafiltration group had an increase in serum creatinine. There was no difference in 60 days follow-up for mortality or rehospitalization. Ultrafiltration is now reserved only for patients with advanced kidney failure who are unable to manage their ECF volume with maximal diuretic strategies.

V. Congestive Heart Failure

A. Early **clinical symptoms** of cardiac failure occur before overt physical findings of pedal edema and pulmonary congestion. These symptoms relate to the inadequate cardiac function the patient has as well as the compensatory renal sodium and water retention that accompany arterial underfilling. The patient may present with a history of weight gain, weakness, dyspnea on exertion, decreased exercise tolerance, paroxysmal nocturnal dyspnea, or orthopnea. Nocturia may occur because cardiac output, and therefore renal perfusion, may be enhanced by the supine position. Patients with CHF may lose considerable weight during the first few days of hospitalization because of the supine position of bed rest, even without the administration of diuretics. Although overt edema is not detectable early in the course of CHF, the patient may complain of swollen eyes on awakening and tight rings and shoes, particularly at the end of the day. As much as 3 to 4 L of fluid can be retained before the occurrence of overt edema.

The period of incipient edema is then followed by more overt symptoms and physical findings: basilar pulmonary rales, ankle edema, JVD, tachycardia, or a gallop rhythm with a third heart sound. Although the chest x-ray may only show cephalization of pulmonary markings early in cardiac failure, increased hilar markings, Kerley B lines, and pleural effusions occur later, generally accompanied by an enlarged heart size. Point-of-care ultrasound, increasingly used in conjunction with the clinical examination, may allow earlier and more sensitive detection of pulmonary edema, JVD, or cardiac dysfunction.

B. Etiology. Two mechanisms that reduce cardiac output are recognized to cause CHF: systolic dysfunction (with reduced ejection fraction) and diastolic dysfunction (with preserved ejection fraction). Because more specific and life-saving therapy is available for systolic dysfunction, it is essential to determine whether systolic dysfunction is present when a patient presents with symptoms and signs of heart failure. Although physical examination, chest x-ray, and electrocardiogram are useful in this regard, additional diagnostic tests are usually indicated. An echocardiogram (cardiac ultrasound) provides information about cardiac structure, systolic and diastolic function, and valvular disease. Rare causes of heart failure exist (e.g., thyroid dysfunction, alcoholic cardiomyopathy, thiamine deficiency), however, coronary artery disease is the most common cause and must be excluded in all cases. Uncontrolled chronic hypertension commonly contributes to left ventricular hypertrophy and the eventual development of CHF as well. Cardiac angiography or noninvasive stress testing to evaluate for coronary artery disease is indicated in virtually all patients who present with new-onset CHF. In patients with preexisting cardiac disease, a cardiac arrhythmia, progression of ischemic disease, pulmonary emboli, cessation of medicines, severe anemia or fever, dietary sodium indiscretion, and worsening of chronic obstructive lung disease with infection and resultant hypoxia are examples of potentially treatable precipitants of worsening CHF.

C. Treatment. Specific primary or precipitating causes of CHF should be identified and treated.

Patients with systolic dysfunction should be treated with an **ACEi or ARB**. ACEis and ARBs are unique agents that reduce blood pressure (reduce afterload), shift the renal function curve to the left (promote continued sodium losses), and block maladaptive neuroregulatory hormones (Fig. 2-6). If neither class of drug can be employed safely, then therapy with hydralazine and isosorbide dihydrate or monohydrate should be used. **Combining ARBs with neprilysin inhibition** (e.g., valsartan/sacubitril) provides additional diuretic effect and potential mortality benefit in heart failure, however, may cause intolerable hypotension.

β-**Blockers** improve symptoms and mortality in patients with systolic dysfunction. Both selective β-blockers (metoprolol, bisoprolol) and nonselective β-blockers with α-blocking properties (carvedilol) are approved for the treatment of CHF. Because β-blockers can lead to symptomatic exacerbations of heart failure, these drugs are initiated in low doses only when patients are clinically stable.

If symptomatic pulmonary congestion or peripheral edema is present, **diuretic therapy** is indicated. A loop diuretic is usually employed as first-line therapy, although some patients may be managed using a thiazide. In patients with CHF, diuretic therapy must be instituted with full knowledge of the Starling–Frank curve of myocardial contractility (Fig. 2-7). The patient with CHF who responds to a diuretic will have reduced symptoms as end-diastolic volume and pulmonary congestion decrease. However, because the Starling–Frank curve is usually either flat or upsloping even in failing hearts, an improvement in cardiac output may not occur. If, during diuretic treatment of a patient with CHF, the serum creatinine and blood urea nitrogen levels begin to rise, cardiac output may have fallen. This situation is especially pronounced in patients who are receiving ACEi or ARB therapy. ACEis/ARBs impair renal autoregulation and make patients prone to prerenal azotemia. When mild azotemia develops in a patient treated with diuretics and an ACEi, it is usually

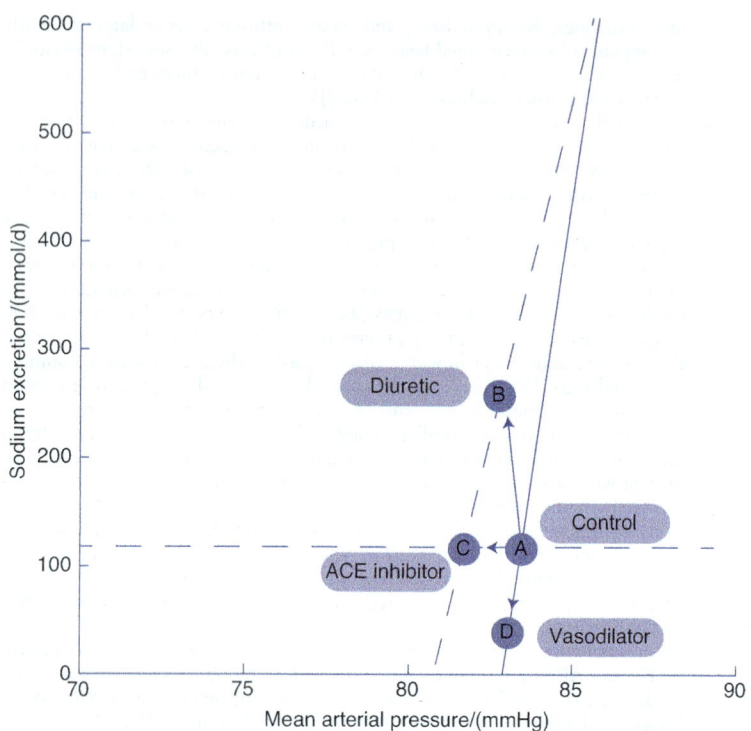

Figure 2-6. Comparison of diuretic, angiotensin-converting enzyme (ACE) inhibitor, and vasodilator effects on mean arterial pressure and natriuresis. The normal renal function curve is shown (*solid line*, starting point A). Adding a vasodilator (*D*) reduces mean arterial pressure but also reduces natriuresis because blood pressure declines. A diuretic (*B*) moves the individual to a new renal function curve (*dashed line*), thereby increasing natriuresis, but has little effect on blood pressure. An ACE inhibitor (*C*) moves the individual to a new renal function curve, maintaining natriuresis at a lower blood pressure.

advisable to reduce the diuretic dose or liberalize dietary salt intake, if the patient is mildly hypovolemic by examination. This approach has been shown to permit the continued administration of ACEi in many patients.

Continuously evaluating the patient's physical examination, treatment goals, and potential medication interactions are key and increases in serum creatinine are permitted if needed to achieve clinical euvolemia. Patients with CHF are especially sensitive to kidney function deterioration if NSAIDs are used together with diuretics and ACEis or ARBs. Therefore, NSAIDs should be diligently avoided in this patient population.

Both CHF and treatment with loop diuretics stimulate the renin–angiotensin–aldosterone axis. Two large studies have provided evidence that **blocking mineralocorticoid (aldosterone) receptors** can improve mortality in heart failure with reduced ejection fraction. In one trial, adding spironolactone (25 mg/d) to a regimen that included an ACEi and a diuretic (with or without digoxin) reduced all-cause mortality by 30%. This effect was independent of a negative sodium balance, but rather due to inhibition of cardiac fibrosis, inflammation,

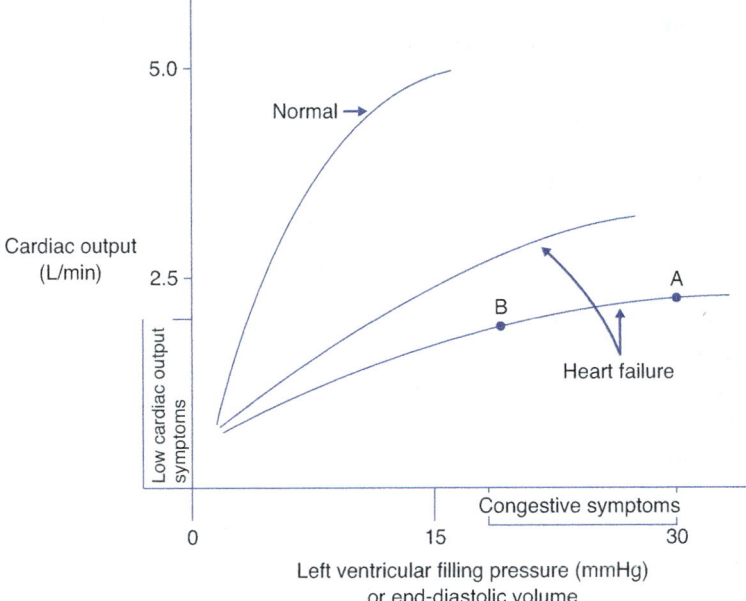

Figure 2-7. Relationship between cardiac output and left ventricular filling pressure under normal circumstances (*upper curve*) and low-output congestive heart failure (*lower curve*). Reduction of afterload (e.g., angiotensin-converting enzyme [ACE] inhibitor or a vasodilator) or improved contractility (inotropic agents) may shift the lower curve to the *middle curve*. Diuretic-induced preload reduction or other causes of volume depletion may decrease cardiac output (e.g., shift from point A to point B on the *lower curve*). (From Brenner BM, ed. *The Kidney*. Saunders Elsevier; 2008, with permission.)

and apoptosis. Gynecomastia, menstrual irregularities, and reduced libido are potential side effects as spironolactone also blocks androgen and progesterone receptors. Eplerenone, also effective in heart failure, is a more specific aldosterone blocker that mitigates these concerns. Eplerenone use is, however, limited by its cost, need for b.i.d. dosing, and increased drug interactions compared to spironolactone.

Spironolactone and eplerenone are steroidal aldosterone antagonists. Nonsteroidal antagonists (e.g., finerenone) offer the potential of aldosterone blockade without androgen or progesterone receptor blockade. They also may offer more cardiovascular-specific activity relative to kidney effects, which may reduce the risk of hyperkalemia, however, their true clinical benefit compared to steroidal mineralocorticoid receptor antagonist (MRA) is unclear.

Hyperkalemia is of concern when any aldosterone blockade is instituted, and serum potassium should be monitored closely (e.g., every 1 to 2 weeks when initiating/changing doses). An increase in serum potassium greater than 5.5 mEq/L should prompt an evaluation of dietary potassium intake and for medications such as potassium supplements or NSAIDs that might be contributing to hyperkalemia. If such factors are not detected, the dose of aldosterone blocker should be reduced. It is prudent to avoid aldosterone blockers in patients with an eGFR of less than 30 mL/min and use caution in those with

TABLE 2-6	Complications of Diuretics
Intravascular volume depletion	
Orthostatic hypotension (from volume depletion)	
Hypokalemia (loop and DCT diuretics)	
Hyperkalemia (spironolactone, eplerenone, triamterene, and amiloride)	
Gynecomastia (spironolactone)	
Hyperuricemia	
Hypercalcemia (thiazides)	
Hypercholesterolemia	
Hyponatremia (especially with DCT diuretics)	
Metabolic alkalosis	
Gastrointestinal upset	
Hyperglycemia	
Pancreatitis (DCT diuretics)	
Allergic interstitial nephritis	

DCT, distal convoluted tubule.

eGFR between 30 and 50 mL/min. Oral potassium binders (e.g., patiromer, sodium zirconium cyclosilicate) may reduce serum potassium levels and preserve the use of MRAs in some patients with advanced kidney disease.

Complications of diuretic therapy are shown in Table 2-6. Although hyponatremia may be a complication of diuretic treatment, furosemide, when combined with ACEi, may ameliorate hyponatremia in some patients with CHF, possibly by improving cardiac output and water excretion. In patients with heart failure, hypokalemia and hypomagnesemia are frequent complications of diuretic treatment because of secondary hyperaldosteronism, which increases sodium delivery to the distal sites at which aldosterone stimulates potassium and hydrogen ion secretion. Severe renal magnesium wasting may also occur in the setting of secondary hyperaldosteronism and loop diuretic administration. Because both magnesium and potassium depletion cause similar deleterious effects on the heart, and potassium repletion is very difficult in the presence of magnesium depletion, supplemental replacement of both these cations is frequently necessary for patients with cardiac failure. The need for frequent potassium repletion can be a trigger to add aldosterone blockade in patients with heart failure. While avoidance of hyperkalemia is critical, providers must recognize that chronic hypokalemia can not only predispose to cardiac arrhythmias but can also worsen CKD progression, generate polyuria through ADH resistance, and increase sodium retention in the DCT by activating the apical sodium-chloride transporter.

SGLT2is (e.g., empagliflozin, dapagliflozin) have shown mortality benefit in heart failure, primarily with reduced ejection fraction, even in the absence of symptomatic pulmonary congestion or edema. They can increase kaliuresis and improve hyperkalemia control (similar to potassium binders) and preserve the use of ACEis, ARBs, or MRAs for some patients. SGLT2is do affect renal tubuloglomerular feedback and reduce GFR. However, this loss of GFR acutely is limited and reduces the risk of CKD progression over time. Therefore, SLGT2i are now standard of care alongside ACEis, ARBs, and beta-blockers in heart failure.

The treatment of patients with CHF and preserved systolic function is less clearly defined. Hypertension control is paramount in these patients, as hypertension is a frequent cause of cardiac hypertrophy and diastolic dysfunction, as well as a strong cardiovascular risk factor. Diuretics are usually necessary to control symptoms of dyspnea and orthopnea. β-Blockers, ACEis, ARBs, and SGLT2is, may be beneficial in some patients with preserved ejection fraction. Notably, trials showing potential benefits of specific classes of medications in HFpEF (e.g., SGLT2is, spironolactone, ARBs/ARNis) have often included patients with mildly reduced ejection fractions between 40% and 55%, which limits their application to patients with CHF and truly preserved ejection fraction of >55%.

VI. Hepatic Cirrhosis

The pathogenesis of renal sodium and water retention is similar in all varieties of cirrhosis, including alcoholic, viral, and biliary cirrhosis. Studies in both humans and animals indicate that renal sodium and water retention precede the formation of ascites in cirrhosis. To explain this phenomenon, the systemic arterial vasodilation theory has been proposed. This theory, summarized in Table 2-7, is compatible with observations in patients during the various stages of cirrhosis. **Cirrhosis causes systemic arterial vasodilation** with activation of the neurohumoral axes (e.g., renin–angiotensin, sympathetic drive, and nonosmotic vasopressin release). The cause of the initial arterial vasodilation is not clear, but it is known to present early and primarily in the splanchnic circulation. The inherent hepatic dysfunction in cirrhosis likely leads to either increased production or reduced clearance of vasoactive substances. Several mediators, including nitric oxide, substance P, vasoactive intestinal peptide, endotoxin, and glucagon, have been proposed to play a role in splanchnic arterial vasodilation. In addition, the opening of existing splanchnic arteriovenous shunts may account for some early arterial vasodilation. Later, anatomically new portosystemic and arteriovenous shunting secondary to portal hypertension may also occur.

TABLE 2-7 Systemic Arterial Vasodilation Hypothesis. Stages of Progression of Cirrhosis

	Compensated Cirrhosis (no ascites)	Decompensated Cirrhosis (ascites)	Hepatorenal Syndrome
Peripheral arterial vasodilation	↑	↑↑	↑↑↑
Plasma hormones (AVP, renin, aldosterone, NE)	Normal[a]	↑	↑↑
Plasma volume[b]	↑	↑↑	↑↑↑

AVP, arginine vasopressin; NE, norepinephrine.

[a]Given the positive sodium and water balance that has occurred, these plasma hormones would be suppressed in healthy subjects without liver disease. Instead in compensated cirrhosis, they are inappropriately normal or mildly elevated.

[b]The progressive renal sodium and water retention increase extracellular fluid, interstitial fluid, and plasma volume, but are inadequate to correct the arterial underfilling. The concomitant occurrence of hypoalbuminemia in decompensated cirrhosis and hepatorenal syndrome may attenuate the degree of volume expansion.

A. Options for treating cirrhotic ascites and edema include dietary sodium restriction, diuretic drugs, large-volume paracenteses, peritoneovenous shunting, portosystemic shunting (usually transjugular intrahepatic portosystemic shunting [TIPS]), and liver transplantation. Each of these approaches has a role in the treatment of cirrhotic ascites, but most patients can be treated successfully with dietary sodium restriction, diuretics, and intermittent large-volume paracenteses. Ascites in the decompensated cirrhotic patient is associated with substantial complications including (a) spontaneous bacterial peritonitis (SBP), which does not occur in the absence of ascites; (b) impaired mobility, decreased appetite, and back and abdominal pain; (c) an elevated diaphragm with decreased ventilation predisposing to hypoventilation, atelectasis, and pulmonary infections; (d) the development of pleural effusions (e.g., hepatic hydrothorax) which can further compromise respiratory function; and (e) negative cosmetic and psychological effects.

The **initial therapy of cirrhotic ascites** is supportive, including dietary sodium restriction and cessation of any alcohol use, regardless of the primary cause of cirrhosis. When these measures prove inadequate, diuretic treatment should begin with spironolactone. Spironolactone has several advantages. First, a controlled trial showed that spironolactone is more effective than furosemide alone in reducing ascites in cirrhotic patients. Second, spironolactone is a long-acting diuretic that can be given once per day in doses ranging from 25 to 400 mg. Third, unlike most other diuretics, hypokalemia does not occur when spironolactone is administered. This is important because hypokalemia increases kidney ammonia production and can precipitate encephalopathy. The most common side effect of spironolactone is painful gynecomastia. As noted in the treatment of heart failure, gynecomastia is much less common with eplerenone however drug interactions can be a concern. Despite the latter concerns, eplerenone can be used safely and effectively in many patients with cirrhosis. Although amiloride, another K-sparing diuretic, can be used as an alternative, spironolactone is more effective than amiloride in reducing ascites.

In patients who do not respond to a low dose of spironolactone, it can be combined with furosemide. Commonly a ratio of 100 mg spironolactone to 40 mg furosemide is used, to a daily maximum of 400 mg spironolactone and 160 mg furosemide. The exact ratio is based on limited evidence however may offer the advantage of once per day dosing and minimal hypokalemia. Diuretic resistance in cirrhosis has been defined as the absence of a natriuretic response to 400 mg spironolactone and 160 mg furosemide. As with heart failure, patients with advanced CKD may require higher doses and the risk of hyperkalemia from spironolactone must be reassessed over time.

B. The appropriate **rate of diuresis** depends on the presence or absence of peripheral edema. Because mobilizing ascitic fluid into the vascular compartment is slow (approximately 500 mL/d), the rate of daily diuresis should be limited to 0.5 kg/d if peripheral edema is absent. In the presence of peripheral edema, most patients can tolerate up to 1.0 kg/d of fluid removal. Diuresis that exceeds the mobilization rate of ascites or edema into the vascular tree can cause hypovolemia leading to orthostatic hypotension, AKI, and potentially hepatic encephalopathy.

An alternative approach to diuretics is **large-volume paracentesis** in patients with advanced cirrhosis and ascites. Total paracentesis has been shown to have few complications; in some studies, paracentesis appears to have a lower incidence of complications than diuretic treatment. IV albumin is given after procedures to preserve the intravascular volume and reduce hemodynamic compromise and the activity of vasoregulatory hormones. While patients often favor paracenteses because of the rapid improvement in symptoms and decreased hospitalizations, diuretics and salt restriction are still critical between paracenteses.

TABLE 2-8	Potential Contraindications to Transjugular Intrahepatic Portosystemic Shunt (TIPS)

Advanced cirrhosis (MELD >18, Child–Pugh Class C)
Hepatic encephalopathy
Advanced cardiopulmonary disease (e.g., CHF, severe tricuspid regurgitation, pulmonary hypertension)
Structural hepatic disease (e.g., hepatic/portal vein thrombosis, tumors, polycystic liver disease, biliary obstruction)
Systemic infection

MELD, Model for end-stage liver disease; CHF, congestive heart failure.

When diuretics and paracenteses are not sufficient, portosystemic shunting via TIPS can be done in some patients. In two uncontrolled trials, TIPS led to an increase in urine output, a reduction in ascites, and a reduction in diuretic usage. Kidney function also improved. Yet in a controlled trial, mortality increased in patients who received TIPS as compared with controls, and TIPS can precipitate hepatic encephalopathy, especially in patients with more advanced cirrhosis (e.g., Model for End-stage Liver disease [MELD] score >18 or Child–Pugh Class C). TIPS also cannot be done in patients with significant cardiac disease as the patient's cardiac function may not tolerate the increased venous return shunting around the liver. Given its contraindications (Table 2-8) and complication rate, TIPS is best reserved for truly refractory patients who are often not eligible for a liver transplant.

Similar considerations apply to peritoneovenous shunting. In controlled trials, peritoneovenous shunting was shown to reduce ascites more effectively than paracentesis or diuretics, but was associated with a high rate of complications (e.g., shunt clotting); and there was no survival advantage.

The development or worsening of ascites in a patient with previously compensated or stable cirrhosis may be an indication for liver transplantation if reversible hepatic insults (e.g., hepatocellular carcinoma, portal vein thrombosis), excess sodium intake, or sodium-retaining drugs (e.g., NSAIDs). Given the morbidity and mortality associated with diuretic-resistant decompensated cirrhosis, liver transplantation is the primary treatment if available. Worsening of ascites in a previously stable individual is most often caused by progressive liver disease but should also compel a search for hepatocellular carcinoma and portal vein thrombosis.

C. **Treatment aimed at the systemic arterial vasodilation** of cirrhosis was originally used in patients with portal hypertension and acutely bleeding esophageal varices. Portal venous hypertension is caused not only by intrahepatic capillary fibrosis that increases resistance to flow but also by increased splanchnic flow. Therefore, the administration of vasopressin, which selectively constricts the splanchnic vasculature, has been shown to decrease portal venous pressure and thereby diminish acute esophageal variceal bleeding.

The use of vasoconstrictors in association with albumin administration has emerged as a treatment for hepatorenal syndrome (HRS). HRS can be divided into HRS-AKI (e.g., HRS type 1) and HRS-CKD (e.g., HRS type 2), however, the clinical distinctions are often challenging. Both entities demonstrate inappropriate renal sodium retention despite a lack of intravascular volume depletion. There is no evidence of glomerular or tubular damage (e.g., proteinuria, hematuria, cellular casts) nor urinary obstruction in isolated HRS. HRS-AKI is common in patients with advanced cirrhosis and has a high mortality risk. If untreated it is often rapidly progressive and precipitating events (e.g., infection, gastrointestinal bleeding) are often found. Midodrine, an α-agonist, and octreotide, a splanchnic vasoconstrictor, as well as norepinephrine, an intravenous vasoconstrictor, have been used with albumin to treat HRS-AKI. The V_1 (vascular) vasopressin receptor agonist, terlipressin, has also been approved for use in HRS-AKI (e.g., HRS type 1). IV albumin to help preserve intravascular volume is often added. However, especially with aggressive vasoconstrictor use and/or significant kidney disease, providers must avoid excessive volume expansion which could precipitate pulmonary edema.

Vasoconstrictor therapy may take several days to fully reverse the neurohormonal activation in HRS if it can, and an increase in mean arterial pressure of 10 to 15 mmHg over baseline may be a critical target when titrating medications. These treatments can alleviate AKI but have not improved mortality. Therefore, the advantage of this approach is to allow time for the improvement of any acute hepatic insult or for liver transplantation. HRS-CKD presents with a slower deterioration of kidney function, inappropriate renal sodium retention despite refractory ascites and volume expansion, and a similar lack of hematuria or proteinuria. HRS-CKD may improve with liver transplantation though the reversibility of GFR loss is less clear and simultaneous kidney–liver transplantation may be required.

SBP is probably the most frequent trigger of HRS-AKI, which frequently occurs on a background of HRS-CKD. In a prospective, randomized trial of cirrhotic patients with SBP, the combination of albumin and cefotaxime decreased the occurrence of kidney failure (33% vs. 11%, $p < .002$) and hospital mortality (18% vs. 10%, $p < .01$) compared with cefotaxime. A diagnostic peritoneal tap, therefore, should be done in all cirrhotic patients with ascites and AKI, even without classic infectious signs (e.g., fever, leukocytosis, abdominal pain).

VII. Nephrotic Syndrome

Another major cause of edema is nephrotic syndrome, the clinical hallmarks of which include proteinuria (>3.5 g/d), hypoalbuminemia, hypercholesterolemia, and edema. Patients with severe nephrotic syndrome are also at higher risk of venous thromboemboli and infection. The edema may range from pedal edema to total-body anasarca, including ascites and pleural effusions. The lower the plasma albumin concentration, the more likely the occurrence of anasarca; the degree of sodium intake is, however, also a determinant of the degree of edema. Compared to nephritic syndromes, patients are less likely to present with hematuria, worsening AKI, and accelerated hypertension. However, some patients do show a reduction in GFR and hypertension as discussed below. Nephrotic syndrome has many causes (see Chapter 8). Systemic causes of nephrotic syndrome include diabetes mellitus, autoimmune diseases (e.g., lupus), chronic infections (e.g., HIV, HCV, HBV, recurrent skin and soft tissue infections), drugs (e.g., alpha-lipoic acid, phenytoin, heavy metals, NSAIDs, heroin), malignancies (e.g., multiple myeloma, paraneoplastic syndromes from solid tumors), and primary kidney diseases (e.g., minimal-change nephropathy, membranous nephropathy, focal segmental glomerulosclerosis).

A. The **pathogenesis** of ECF volume expansion in nephrotic syndrome appears to be more variable than the pathogenesis of edema in patients with CHF or cirrhotic ascites. Traditionally, ECF volume expansion in nephrotic syndrome was believed to depend on hypoalbuminemia and underfilling of the arterial circulation. Several observations, however, have raised questions about this hypothesis. First, transudation of fluid during ECF volume expansion reduces the interstitial oncotic pressure, thereby minimizing the change in transcapillary oncotic pressure. Second, patients recovering from minimal-change nephropathy frequently begin to excrete sodium before their serum albumin concentration rises. Third, the circulating concentrations of volume-regulatory hormones are not as high in nephrotic syndrome compared to severe cirrhosis or CHF. These and other observations have **suggested a role for primary renal sodium retention (overfill hypothesis) in the pathogenesis of nephrotic edema.**

B. **Likely primary renal sodium retention, hypoalbuminemia, and some element of arterial underfilling with neurohormonal activation contribute to volume expansion in most patients, particularly in patients with serum albumin concentrations below 2.0 g/L.** Primary renal sodium retention alone may not lead to edema in the absence of another contributing factor, such as a decrease in cardiac output, systemic arterial vasodilation, or a loss of GFR. As noted in Figure 2-4, "aldosterone escape" prevents the development of edema if GFR is preserved and proximal tubule sodium reabsorption is appropriately reduced. Importantly, while neurohormonal activation is less than in cirrhosis and CHF, it is greater than expected given the presence of ECF expansion. Nephrotic syndrome may reflect a combination of primary renal sodium retention and/or relative arterial underfilling. A preponderance of one or the other mechanism may be observed in nephrotic syndromes from different causes. In general, a normal or near-normal GFR is associated with hypovolemic, vasoconstrictor nephrotic syndrome, whereas a diminution in GFR, primary renal sodium retention, and evidence of intravascular volume expansion (e.g., decreased plasma renin activity) are characteristic of hypervolemic nephrotic syndrome (Table 2-9).

C. **Treatment.** As most patients have an identifiable secondary cause of their nephrotic syndrome, the primary therapy is directed at that cause. The treatment of primary renal nephrotic syndromes is described in Chapter 11.

The treatment of edema in nephrotic patients involves **dietary sodium restriction and diuretics.** In general, loop diuretics and mineralocorticoid antagonists are used as initial therapy. Some nephrotic patients may be relatively resistant to these drugs. Although low serum albumin concentrations may increase the volume of diuretic distribution, and filtered albumin may bind to diuretics in the tubule lumen, these factors do not appear to be the predominant causes of diuretic resistance. Rather, diuretic resistance may reflect a combination of

TABLE 2-9 Comparison of Overfill Versus Underfill Edema in the Setting of Nephrotic Syndrome

Overfill Edema

Loss of GFR (acute kidney injury [AKI] and/or CKD)

Modest hypoalbuminemia (e.g., >2 g/dL)

Various nephrotic pathologies (may be complicated by acute tubular necrosis)

Hypertension

Decreased renin/angiotensin activity (volume expansive nephrotic syndrome)

Underfill Edema

Preserved GFR

Severe hypoalbuminemia (e.g., <2 g/dL)

Classically minimal change disease (may be seen with other nephrotic syndromes)

Normotensive/hypotensive

Increased renin/angiotensin activity (vasoconstrictive nephrotic syndrome)

GFR, glomerular filtration rate.

reduced GFR and intense renal sodium retention. When the GFR is reduced, endogenous organic anions impair diuretic secretion into the tubule lumen. Therefore, higher doses of loop diuretics are often required to achieve natriuresis.

For severely hypoalbuminemic patients, <2 mg/dL, administering albumin with a loop diuretic may improve diuresis, though there is a risk of increasing pulmonary edema. This approach should be limited to those with severe hypoalbuminemia where dual or triple nephron diuretic blockade is unsuccessful.

SUGGESTED READINGS

Bansal S, Lindenfeld JA, Schrier RW. Sodium retention in heart failure and cirrhosis: potential role of natriuretic doses of mineralocorticoid antagonist? *Circ Heart Fail.* 2009;2(4):370–376.

Bart BA, Goldsmith SR, Lee KL, et al; Heart Failure Clinical Research Network. Ultrafiltration in decompensated HF with CRS. *N Engl J Med.* 2012;367(24):2296–2304.

Brater DC. Update in diuretic therapy: clinical pharmacology. *Semin Nephrol.* 2011;31(6):483–494.

Cadnapaphornchai MA, Tkancheko O, Shchekochikhin D, Schrier RW. The nephrotic syndrome: pathogenesis and treatment of edema formation and other complications. *Pediatr Nephrol J.* 2014;29(7):1159–1167.

Constanzo MR, Guglin ME, Saltzberg MT, et al; UNLOAD Trial Investigators. Ultrafiltration versus intravenous diuretics for patients hospitalized for acute decompensated HF. *J Am Coll Cardiol.* 2007;49(6):675–683.

Deegen JKJ, Schrier RW, Wetzel JF. The nephrotic syndrome, Chapter 69. In: Schrier RW, ed. *Schrier's Diseases of the Kidney.* 9th ed. Lippincott Williams & Wilkins; 2013:1997–2011.

Ellison DH, Hoorn EJ, Schrier RW. Mechanisms of diuretic action, Chapter 66. In: Schrier RW, ed. *Schrier's Diseases of the kidney.* 9th ed. Lippincott Williams & Wilkins; 2013:1906–1937.

Ellison DH. Diuretic therapy and resistance in congestive heart failure. *Cardiology.* 2001; 96(3-4):132–143.

Felker GM, Lee KL, Bull DA, et al; NHLBI Heart Failure Clinical Research Network. Diuretic strategies in patients with acute decompensated HF. *N Engl J Med.* 2011;364(9):797–805.

Fliser D, Zurbruggen I, Mutschler E, et al. Coadministration of albumin and furosemide in patients with the nephrotic syndrome. *Kidney Int.* 1999;55(2):629–634.

Mullens W, Dauw J, Martens P, et al. Acetazolamide in decompensated heart failure with volume overload trial (ADVOR): baseline characteristics. *Eur J of Heart Fail.* 2022;24(9):1601–1610.

Nadim M, Garcia-Tsao G. Acute kidney injury in patients with cirrhosis. *N Engl J Med.* 2023; 388(8):733–745.

Okusa MD, Ellison DH. Physiology and pathophysiology of diuretic action, Chapter 37. In: Alpern RJ, Hebert SC, eds. *The Kidney: Physiology and Pathophysiology.* 4th ed. Elsevier Science; 2008:1051–1094.

Packer M, Anker S, Butler J, et al; EMPEROR-Reduced Trial Investigators. Cardiovascular and renal outcomes with empagliflozin in heart failure. *N Engl J Med.* 2020;383(15):1413–1424.

Pitt B, Filippatos G, Agarwal R, et al; FIGARO-DKD Investigators. Cardiovascular events with finerenone in kidney disease and type 2 diabetes. *N Engl J Med.* 2021;385(24):2252–2263.

Schrier RW. A unifying hypothesis of body fluid volume regulation. *J R Coll Physicians Lond.* 1992; 26(3):295–306.

Schrier RW. Role of diminished renal function in cardiovascular mortality: marker or pathogenetic factor? *J Am Coll Cardiol.* 2006;47(1):1–8.

Schrier RW. Use of diuretics in heart failure and cirrhosis. *Semin Nephrol.* 2011;31(6):503–512.

Schrier RW, Abraham WT. Hormones and hemodynamics in heart failure. *N Engl J Med.* 1999; 341(8):577–585.

Schrier RW, Arroyo V, Bernardi M, Epstein M, Henriksen JH, Rodés J. Systemic arterial vasodilation hypothesis: a proposal for the initiation of renal sodium and water retention in cirrhosis. *Hepatology.* 1998;8(5):1151–1157.

Schrier RW, Fassett RG. A critique of the overfill hypothesis of sodium and water retention in the nephrotic syndrome. *Kidney Int.* 1998;53(3):1111–1117.

Zinman B, Wanner C, Lachin J, et al; EMPA-REG OUTCOME Investigators. Empagliflozin, cardiovascular outcomes, and mortality in type 2 diabetes. *N Engl J Med.* 2015;373(22):2117–2128.

The Patient With Hyponatremia and Hypernatremia

Helbert Rondon-Berrios

Hyponatremia. *Hyponatremia*, defined as a plasma sodium less than 135 mEq/L is considered the most common electrolyte disorder in clinical practice with an estimated prevalence of up to 30% in hospitalized patients.

I. Physiologic Principles

Homeostasis is the capacity of life forms to maintain constant composition and parameters in the ECF which is required for survival. Plasma or ECF tonicity is one of those important parameters that needs to be maintained constant as it is primarily responsible for cell volume. Under conditions of hypotonicity, cells swell, while under conditions of hypertonicity, cells shrink.

A. Plasma Tonicity and Plasma Osmolality. Plasma osmolality (POsm) denotes the number of milliosmoles of solute in 1 kg of plasma water. The main solutes present in plasma are sodium, glucose, and urea. POsm can be approximated using the following equation:

$$POsm(mOsm/kg) = 2 \times PNa(mEq/L) + \frac{Glucose(mg/dL)}{18} + \frac{BUN(mg/dL)}{2.8}$$

where PNa is plasma sodium, glucose is plasma glucose, and BUN is blood urea nitrogen. In contrast, plasma tonicity refers only to those solutes that are effective osmoles, that is, solutes that do not cross cell membranes and cause water to move out of the cells into the ECF when their plasma concentration is elevated. While both effective and ineffective osmoles contribute to POsm, only effective osmoles contribute to plasma tonicity (Table 3-1).

Therefore, when estimating plasma tonicity, the effect of urea should be disregarded since urea crosses cell membranes and is considered an ineffective osmole. Plasma tonicity can be calculated using the following equation:

$$Plasma\ tonicity(mOsm/kg) = 2 \times PNa(mEq/L) + \frac{Glucose(mg/dL)}{18}$$

Under normal conditions plasma glucose concentration is about 90 mg/dL contributing to only 5 mOsm/kg to plasma tonicity. Therefore, **plasma sodium is the main determinant of plasma tonicity** as represented below:

$$Plasma\ tonicity(mOsm/kg) \approx 2 \times PNa(mEq/L)$$

B. Plasma Sodium Concentration. In 1956, Edelman provided empirical evidence that plasma sodium concentration (PNa) is determined by the ratio of total body exchangeable sodium (Na_E) and total body exchangeable potassium (K_E), and total body water (TBW). This relationship is expressed by the simplified **Edelman equation** as follows:

$$PNa = \frac{Na_E + K_E}{TBW}$$

TABLE 3-1 Effective and Ineffective Osmoles

Characteristic	Ineffective Osmoles	Effective Osmoles
Distribution	Total body water (ECF and ICF)	ECF
Effect on plasma osmolality	↑	↑
Effect on plasma tonicity	↔	↑
Examples	Urea Ethanol Toxic alcohols (e.g., ethylene glycol, methanol)	Glucose (in the absence of insulin) Mannitol

ECF, extracellular fluid; ICF, intracellular fluid; ↑, increase; ↔, no change.

While the effects of total body exchangeable sodium and TBW on plasma sodium are readily apparent, the effect of total body exchangeable potassium is counterintuitive. While sodium is the main solute and the primary determinant of ECF and plasma tonicity, potassium constitutes the most abundant solute in the ICF playing a major role in ICF tonicity. Hence, changes in potassium balance can affect plasma sodium, with potassium losses leading to reduced plasma sodium and potassium supplementation leading to increase in plasma sodium.

C. Electrolyte-Free Water Balance. Isotonic fluid gain/loss, that is, adding/subtracting to the numerator ($Na_E + K_E$) of the simplified Edelman equation in the same proportion as to the denominator (TBW) will not impact plasma sodium, only hypotonic or hypertonic fluid gain/loss will affect plasma sodium. Hence, this concept can be more precisely defined as the balance of electrolyte-free water, encompassing the nonisotonic components of fluid intake and output.

Thirst is the primary regulator of electrolyte-free water intake although cognitive beliefs can override lack of thirst (e.g., drinking because one believes water is a "detoxifying" agent). In contrast, the kidneys regulate electrolyte-free water excretion and have a key role in maintaining electrolyte-free water balance by matching rates of excretion to rates of intake.

D. Handling of Electrolyte-Free Water by Kidney. Kidney's electrolyte-free water handling depends on the following factors:
1. **Glomerular filtration:** This is the first step in allowing a proper amount of filtrate to be delivered to the diluting segments of the nephron.
2. **Proximal tubular fluid reabsorption:** the proximal tubule reabsorbs 65% to 80% of glomerular filtrate. As fluid absorption decreases in this segment, a larger quantity will be delivered to the diluting segments of the nephron.
3. **Tubular dilution:** Dilution of tubular fluid by transporting sodium chloride (in the absence of water) mainly via the Na^+-K^+-$2Cl^-$ cotransporter (NKCC2) in the thick ascending limb of the loop of Henle, and to a lesser extent via the Na^+-Cl^- cotransporter (NCC) in the distal convoluted tubule, generates electrolyte-free water.
4. **Osmolar excretion rate:** This is the daily urine solute excretion which matches dietary solute intake under balance conditions (solute input = solute output). Only protein (urea) and salt are considered solutes. An adequate solute intake (i.e., 600 to 900 mOsm/d) will ensure a proper solute

concentration in the cortical collecting duct creating a lower osmotic gradient for recently generated electrolyte-free water to be reabsorbed into the renal interstitium, and hence, maximizing its excretion.
5. **Arginine vasopressin:** Arginine vasopressin (AVP), also known as antidiuretic hormone (ADH), is synthesized as prohormone in the magnocellular neuron bodies of the supraoptic and paraventricular nuclei located in the hypothalamus. From here AVP travels down their neurons axons toward the posterior pituitary while simultaneously undergoing enzymatic cleavage generating two other peptides: neurophysin II and copeptin. AVP is secreted into the circulation in equimolar amounts to copeptin and neurophysin II. Physiologic stimuli for AVP release include plasma hypertonicity (POsm >280 to 285 mOsm/kg) and decreased effective arterial blood volume (EABV). AVP works in three distinctive receptors: V1, located in smooth muscle of blood vessels resulting in vasoconstriction; V2, located in the basolateral membrane of collecting duct principal cells resulting in insertion of aquaporin 2 water channels in their apical membrane and subsequent water reabsorption; and V3 located in pituitary corticotropes resulting in adrenocorticotropin (ACTH) release.

II. Pathogenesis and Etiology of Hyponatremia

Since plasma sodium is the main determinant of plasma tonicity, most hyponatremias are associated with hypotonicity, although in some cases, hyponatremia can be associated with hypertonicity and isotonicity.

A. Hypertonic Hyponatremia. Hyponatremia associated with hypertonicity is caused by accumulation of effective osmoles in plasma such as glucose or mannitol leading to translocation of water from the ICF causing dilution of plasma sodium. Hypertonic hyponatremias are true dilutional hyponatremias. The expected plasma sodium when glucose returns to normal can be estimated by the following formula:

$$\text{Corrected PNa}(mEq/L) = \text{PNa}(mEq/L) + \mathbf{1.6} \times \frac{[\text{Glucose}(mg/dL) - 100]}{100}$$

B. Isotonic Hyponatremia. Hyponatremia associated with isotonicity is due to pseudohyponatremia, a laboratory artifact. This phenomenon occurs in the setting of hyperproteinemia (e.g., multiple myeloma, IVIG), hypertriglyceridemia, and cholestasis (caused by lipoprotein X which is measured as LDL cholesterol). The diagnosis can be confirmed by obtaining a normal plasma sodium using the direct ion-selective electrode (ISE) method (e.g., whole blood sodium in a blood gas analyzer).

C. Hypotonic Hyponatremia. From the simplified Edelman equation, it can be inferred that hypotonic hyponatremia occurs in clinical practice in four distinct scenarios (Table 3-2). All of the above scenarios share in common a reduction in the ratio of $\frac{Na_E + K_E}{TBW}$ where total body water (TBW) is always proportionally greater than the sum of total body exchangeable cations ($Na_E + K_E$), that is, electrolyte-free water excess. Hence, hypotonic hyponatremia is always characterized by an electrolyte-free water excess and it is therefore considered a water disorder, rather than a sodium disorder.

Electrolyte-free water excess in hypotonic hyponatremia occurs because of an increased in intake and/or a decreased in kidney excretion (Fig. 3-1):

1. **Increased electrolyte-free water intake:** The kidneys have an extraordinary capacity to excrete large water loads, but there is a limit after which hyponatremia develops. Primary polydipsia is the prototypical example of this. Theoretically, the limit of water one can drink without developing

TABLE 3-2 Edelman Equation Scenarios for Hypotonic Hyponatremia

Scenario	$Na_E + K_E$	TBW	$\dfrac{Na_E + K_E}{TBW}$	Clinical Example
1	↔	↑	↓	Primary polydipsia
2	↓↓	↓	↓	Hypovolemia
3	↑	↑↑	↓	Heart failure, cirrhosis
4	↓	↑	↓	SIAD

Na_E, total body exchangeable sodium; K_E, total body exchangeable potassium; TBW, total body water; SIAD, syndrome of inappropriate antidiuresis; ↔, normal; ↑, increased; ↓, decreased.

hyponatremia is close to 18 L/d but due to other coexisting factors present that increase AVP (e.g., drugs), most patients develop hyponatremia by ingesting just above 8 L/d.

2. **Decreased electrolyte-free water excretion:** Multiple mechanisms account for decreased electrolyte-free water excretion leading to hypotonic hyponatremia:
   a. **Decreased glomerular filtration rate (GFR):** as occurs in acute kidney injury or chronic kidney disease with GFR <20 to 25 mL/min.
   b. **Enhanced proximal tubular fluid reabsorption:** as occurs in states of reduced EABV such as hypovolemia, heart failure, and cirrhosis contributing to hyponatremia.
   c. **Impairment of tubular dilution:** due to diuretic use. This occurs more commonly with thiazide diuretics. In contrast, loop diuretics are rarely responsible for hyponatremia because they also interfere with urinary concentration resulting in a diluted urine.
   d. **Decreased dietary solute intake:** as observed in patients with beer potomania or "tea-and-toast" diets.

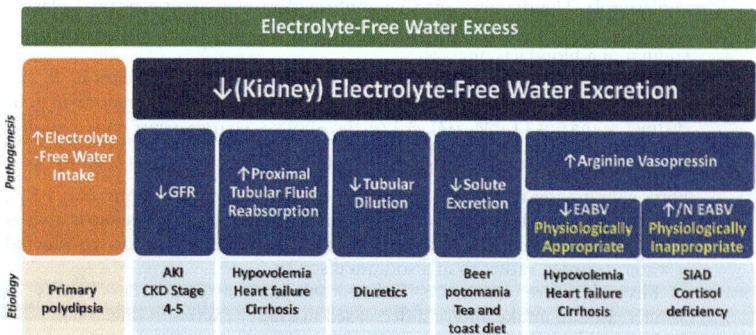

Figure 3-1. Pathogenesis of hypotonic hyponatremia. ↑, increased; ↓, decreased; N, normal; GFR, glomerular filtration rate; EABV, effective arterial blood volume; AKI, acute kidney injury; CKD, chronic kidney disease; SIAD, syndrome of inappropriate antidiuresis.

e. **Increased AVP secretion:** This could be physiologically appropriate (as in states of reduced EABV) or inappropriate (e.g., syndrome of inappropriate antidiuresis [SIAD]). This is undoubtedly the most common mechanism underlying hypotonic hyponatremia.

More often than not, more than one mechanism is responsible for hyponatremia.

III. Clinical Manifestations

A. Brain Adaptation to Plasma Hypotonicity. Plasma hypotonicity mainly affects the central nervous system and leads to the generation of an osmotic gradient between the ICF and ECF resulting in water translocation into brain cells resulting in cerebral edema. Due to limited space within the skull, the brain's water content cannot exceed a 10% increase, as larger increases are not compatible with life. Protective mechanisms are then put into place to decrease intracranial pressure and minimize cell swelling:

1. **Within minutes:** When then brain swells, it causes an increase in hydrostatic pressure within its interstitial space. This elevated pressure compels the interstitial fluid to exit the brain and enter the cerebrospinal fluid (CSF). Subsequently, the excess CSF enters the systemic circulation.
2. **Within the first 3 hours:** Movement of solutes from ICF to ECF to equalize tonicities and stop water entry into the cell. The first solutes that are extruded are sodium, chloride, and potassium ions out of brain cells.
3. **Within 48 hours:** The movement of solutes continues but after 3 hours these are mainly organic osmolytes such as glutamate, taurine, glycine, and myoinositol, which restore cellular volume closer to normal.

   When a reduction in plasma tonicity occurs acutely, in less than 48 hours (i.e., acute hyponatremia), there is very little time for full adaptation to take place and significant cerebral edema occurs. In contrast, when the reduction in plasma tonicity occurs gradually over 48 hours (i.e., chronic hyponatremia), full adaptation occurs, and cerebral edema is minimal.

B. Classification of Hyponatremia. Hyponatremia can be classified based on symptoms, duration, or biochemical severity.

1. **Symptoms:** These are mostly localized to the central nervous system. Hyponatremic encephalopathy is the clinical entity that encompasses symptomatic hyponatremia due to cerebral edema which puts the patient at risk for brain herniation. Symptoms of hyponatremia have been arbitrarily classified as mild, moderate, or severe. Severity of symptoms of hyponatremia correlates with degree of cerebral edema.
   a. **Severe symptoms** (cerebral edema +++): seizures, coma, and cardiorespiratory arrest.
   b. **Moderate symptoms** (cerebral edema ++): nausea, vomiting, and headaches are considered by some in this category, however, these symptoms are only foreboding indications of cerebral edema in patients with self-inflicted water intoxication (primary polydipsia, ecstasy, exercise-induced hyponatremia).
   c. **Mild symptoms** (cerebral edema +): less severe than moderate
   d. **No apparent symptoms** (cerebral edema +/−): recent data suggest that even mild chronic and apparently "asymptomatic" hyponatremia is actually associated with subtle attention deficits and gait impairment that can only be detected with specialized testing.
2. **Duration:** hyponatremia can be classified as:
   a. **Acute:** onset less than 48 hours
   b. **Chronic:** onset 48 hours or greater

      While acute hyponatremia usually presents with moderate to severe symptoms, chronic hyponatremia often presents with mild or no apparent symptoms.

3. **Biochemical severity:** Hyponatremia can be classified based on plasma sodium values in:
   a. **Mild:** plasma sodium 130 to 134 mEq/L
   b. **Moderate:** plasma sodium 120 to 129 mEq/L
   c. **Severe:** plasma sodium <120 mEq/L

IV. Diagnostic Approach to the Hyponatremic Patient (Fig. 3-2)

A. Is the hyponatremia hypotonic?
1. Use plasma osmolality as a surrogate for plasma tonicity
2. If POsm is less than 275 mOsm/kg, then this is a hypotonic hyponatremia.
3. If POsm is 275 mOsm/kg or greater, then hyponatremia could be hypertonic (increased effective osmoles), isotonic (laboratory artifact) or even hypotonic (any hypotonic hyponatremia with concomitant presence of ineffective osmoles).

B. Is the hypotonic hyponatremia mediated by AVP?
1. Use urine osmolality (UOsm) as a surrogate for AVP activity.
2. If UOsm is less than 100 mOsm/kg, then urine is maximally diluted, that is an appropriate response to a hypotonic plasma, that is, AVP is absent. Differential diagnosis of AVP-independent hypotonic hyponatremia includes primary polydipsia, low solute intake, and decreased GFR.
3. If UOsm is 100 mOsm/kg or greater, then urine is not maximally diluted, that is an inappropriate response to a hypotonic plasma, that is, AVP is present. Differential diagnosis includes reduced EABV states, SIAD, and low cortisol.

C. Is the secretion of AVP physiologically appropriate?
1. Use urine sodium as a surrogate for renin–angiotensin–aldosterone system (RAAS) activation, and hence the state of EABV.
2. If urine sodium is less than 20 mEq/L, that means kidneys are sodium avid, RAAS is active, and therefore, EABV is reduced. **AVP secretion when EABV is reduced is considered physiologically appropriate.** Differential diagnosis of hyponatremia with reduced EABV includes hypovolemia, heart failure, and cirrhosis.
3. If urine sodium is 30 mEq/L or more, that means kidneys are not sodium avid, RAAS is inactive, and EABV is either normal or elevated. **AVP secretion when EABV is normal or elevated is considered physiologically inappropriate.** Differential diagnosis includes SIAD and low cortisol. Under normal conditions, cortisol inhibits AVP. Hence, AVP is uninhibited when cortisol is reduced (adrenal insufficiency).
4. Certain conditions associated with reduced EABV can be accompanied by a urine sodium of 30 mEq/L or more. These include hypovolemia due to diuretics, primary adrenal insufficiency, and salt wasting nephropathies (e.g., cisplatin).

D. Syndrome of Inappropriate Antidiuresis
1. The syndrome of inappropriate antidiuresis (SIAD), formerly known as SIADH, is the most common cause of hyponatremia.
2. The diagnosis of SIAD requires meeting the 1967 Bartter and Schwartz criteria:
   a. Hyponatremia
   b. POsm <275 mOsm/kg
   c. UOsm >100 mOsm/kg
   d. Urine sodium >30 mEq/L
   e. Clinical euvolemia (absence of symptoms/signs of hypovolemia and hypervolemia)
   f. Normal thyroid, adrenal and kidney function
   g. Absence of diuretics within 1 week
3. Hypouricemia (plasma uric acid <4 mg/dL), although not part of the diagnostic criteria, also supports the diagnosis of SIAD.

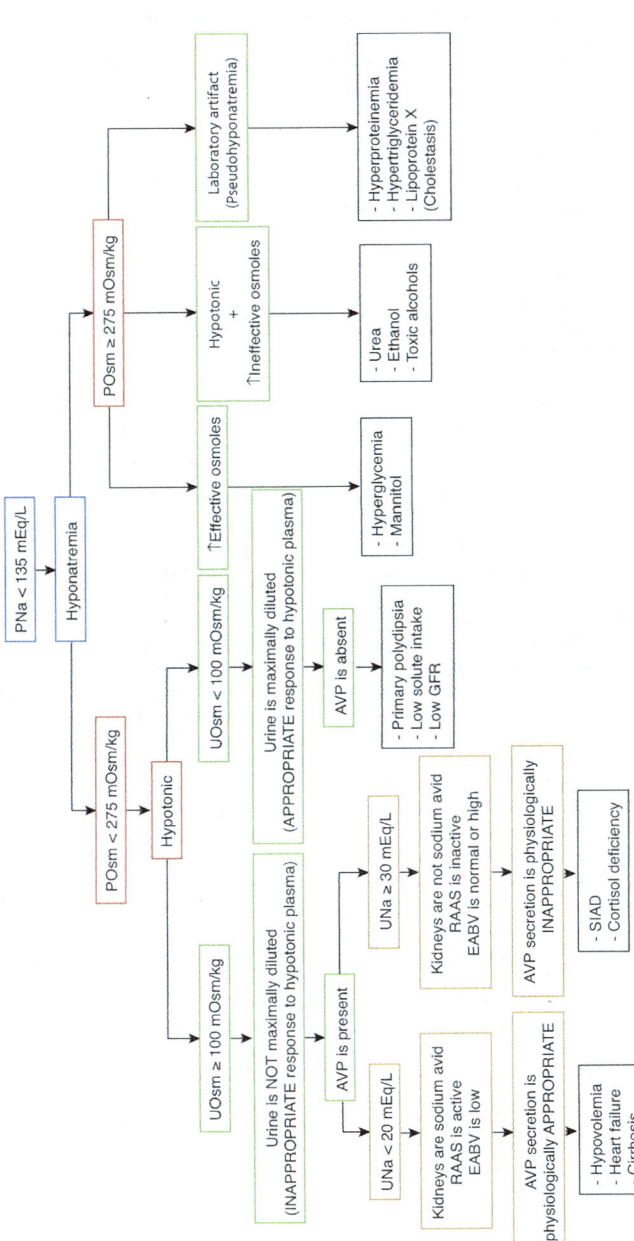

Figure 3-2. Diagnostic approach to hyponatremia. PNa, plasma sodium; POsm, plasma osmolality; UOsm, urine osmolality; ↑, increased; AVP, arginine vasopressin; UNa, urine sodium; RAAS, renin–angiotensin–aldosterone system; EABV, effective arterial blood volume; GFR, glomerular filtration rate; SIAD, syndrome of inappropriate antidiuresis.

4. Although TSH measurement has been traditionally recommended, **it is unusual for hypothyroidism to cause clinically significant hyponatremia**.
5. In contrast, it is important to rule out adrenal insufficiency since this can mimic SIAD. At a minimum, an early morning cortisol should be measured.
6. SIAD is a syndrome with multiple etiologies. However, it is helpful to group them into following categories:
    a. **Malignancy:** small cell lung cancer, head and neck cancer, etc.
    b. **Drugs:** antidepressants, antiepileptics, antipsychotics, etc.
    c. **Lung disorders:** pneumonia, pleural effusion, pneumothorax, etc.
    d. **Central nervous system disorders:** subarachnoid hemorrhage, meningitis, encephalitis, etc.
    e. **Miscellanea:** Nausea and pain
    f. **Idiopathic**
7. When no apparent cause of SIAD is present, extensive routine workup (e.g., MRI brain, CT chest, CT abdomen/pelvis) looking for the etiology of SIAD is low yield.

V. Therapy
A. Therapeutic Principles
1. **Severity of symptoms of hyponatremia dictates urgency:** Severely and moderately symptomatic hyponatremia indicate a greater degree of cerebral edema and risk for brain herniation. Hence, this constitutes a medical emergency requiring prompt therapy. On the other side, mildly symptomatic or apparently asymptomatic hyponatremia does not require emergent treatment and therapy should focus on the underlying pathogenesis of hyponatremia (e.g., volume expansion for hypovolemic hyponatremia, glucocorticoid replacement for adrenal insufficiency, etc.)
2. **Goals and Limits of Correction of Plasma Sodium**
    a. **Goals of correction:** This is the plasma sodium correction rate we aim to in order to decrease the risk of brain herniation. An increase in plasma sodium of 4 to 6 mEq/L in any 24-hour period is sufficient to alleviate even the most extreme manifestations of hyponatremia. Goals of correction are similar for acute and chronic hyponatremia with the caveat that this goal should be reached within the first few hours in acute hyponatremia, but gradually over 24 hours in chronic hyponatremia.
    b. **Limits of correction:** It is the plasma sodium correction rate that when exceeded can lead to neurologic complications. Rapid correction rates are well tolerated in patients with acute hyponatremia while they can lead to neurologic complications in patients with chronic hyponatremia, especially when certain risk factors are present (see Complications of Therapy). Published guidelines suggest a correction limit of no more than 8 mEq/L in any 24-hour period in patients at risk. When duration of hyponatremia is not known, it is best to be cautious and correct as chronic hyponatremia.

B. Complications of Therapy
1. **Overcorrection of hyponatremia:** This is an increase in plasma sodium that exceeds correction limits. Overcorrection occurs when factors impairing kidneys' water excretory capacity suddenly wane and a water diuresis emerge (Table 3-3). Overcorrection of hyponatremia is usually preceded by a large volume of diluted urine. Overcorrection of hyponatremia is a medical emergency and requires relowering of plasma sodium just below correction limits to avoid neurologic sequelae.
2. **Osmotic demyelination syndrome (ODS):** This is triggered by excessive brain dehydration due to overcorrection of plasma sodium during treatment of chronic hyponatremia although it can also be observed with other osmotic insults (e.g., hypernatremia and severe hyperglycemia). Some conditions place patients at higher risk for ODS (Table 3-4). Pathologically,

TABLE 3-3	Risk Factors for Overcorrection of Hyponatremia
Volume expansion in hypovolemia	
Glucocorticoid replacement in adrenal insufficiency	
Resolution of transient SIAD	
Discontinuation of thiazide diuretics or desmopressin	
Initiation of vasopressin antagonists	
Increase dietary solute intake or volume expansion in low solute intake states	

SIAD, syndrome of inappropriate antidiuresis.

demarcated areas of demyelination with very little to no inflammation and sparing of axons appear in the pons (central pontine myelinolysis or CPM) and/or outside the pons (extrapontine myelinolysis or EPM). It is important to note that ODS is not synonymous with CPM/EPM; rather ODS represents a distinctive subgroup within CPM/EPM. It is worth mentioning that CPM/EPM lesions can occur, for reasons that are not yet fully understood, even in the absence of any osmotic insult (e.g., malignancy, thiamine deficiency, and hyperammonemia). The clinical symptoms of ODS usually exhibit a biphasic pattern, wherein the initial phase involves an improvement in hyponatremic symptoms as plasma sodium level rise followed 2 to 6 days later by the onset of dysarthria, dysphagia, altered mental status, and quadriparesis although other symptoms can occur (e.g., ataxia and parkinsonism). Diagnosis is made on clinical grounds. MRI brain can be used as an aid in the diagnosis, but lesions are often absent at symptom onset and may take up to 4 weeks to appear, if at all. The treatment of established ODS is supportive care although a few case reports document success with plasma sodium relowering, glucocorticoids, IVIG, and plasma exchange. Historically, the prognosis of these patients has been considered poor but recent literature suggests that the majority of patients with ODS survive and recuperate without notable consequences.

C. **Treatment of Hyponatremia With Moderate or Severe Symptoms**
  1. **This is a medical emergency** and requires immediate treatment with hypertonic saline 3% to prevent brain herniation.

TABLE 3-4	Risk Factors for Osmotic Demyelination Syndrome
Overcorrection of chronic hyponatremia	
Plasma sodium ≤105 mEq/L	
Advanced liver disease	
Alcohol use disorder	
Malnutrition	
Hypokalemia	

TABLE 3-5	Strategies to Prevent and Treat Overly Rapid Correction of Hyponatremia Using Desmopressin	
Strategy	Indications	Description
Proactive	Start immediately when PNa <120 mEq/L AND: • High risk for rapid correction,[a] AND/OR • High risk for ODS[b]	• Desmopressin 2–4 mcg IV/SC every 6–8 h, AND • NaCl 3% 100 mL bolus for seizures, coma, or rapidly falling PNa,[c] OR • NaCl 3% 1–1.5 mL/kg IV over 6 h (to increase PNa by ≈ 1 mEq/L every 6 h)
Reactive	Worrisome PNa trajectory: • PNa goal of 6 mEq/L in a 24-h period has been achieved, AND/OR • UOP >1 mL/kg/h	• Desmopressin 2–4 mcg IV/SC every 6–8 h
Rescue	Overly rapid correction of hyponatremia has already occurred: • Increase in PNa ≥8 mEq/L in any 24-h period	• Desmopressin 2–4 mcg IV/SC every 6–8 h, AND • Dextrose 5% in water 3 mL/kg IV (to decrease PNa by ≈ 1 mEq/L)

PNa, plasma sodium; UOP, urine output; IV, intravenously; SC, subcutaneously.
[a]Low solute intake, hypovolemia, adrenal insufficiency, transient SIAD, thiazide diuretics, desmopressin, vasopressin antagonists.
[b]Alcohol use disorder, hypokalemia, liver disease, malnutrition, PNa ≤105 mEq/L
[c]Self-induced water intoxication or acute post-operative hyponatremia (risk that PNa will fall due to delayed absorption of ingested water or excretion of hypertonic urine)
Reproduced with permission from Rondon-Berrios H, Sterns RH. Hypertonic saline for hyponatremia: Meeting goals and avoiding harm. *Am J Kidney Dis*. 2022;79(6):890–896.

2. Hypertonic saline 3% contains 513 mEq of sodium per liter.
3. Hypertonic saline 3% is administered as 100 mL IV bolus up to three times as needed to alleviate moderate or severe symptoms.
4. Hypertonic saline 3% can be safely administered via peripheral intravenous line.
5. Once plasma sodium goal is achieved, further correction should be postponed for the next day.

D. Treatment of Severe Hyponatremia (Plasma Sodium <120 mEq/L) With Mild or No Apparent Symptoms
1. **This is not a medical emergency** and the main concern here is rapid correction of plasma sodium leading to neurologic sequelae.
2. Given the heightened risk of ODS in patients with plasma sodium <120 mEq/L, we recommend the use of the proactive approach combining hypertonic saline with desmopressin as described in Table 3-5 which can be discontinued when plasma sodium reaches a safe level of 125 to 130 mEq/L.
3. **Use of hypertonic saline:**
   a. Hypertonic saline can be used in these patients either as rapid intermittent bolus or slow continuous infusion.
   b. For slow continuous infusion, formulas have developed to calculate the rate of administration based on estimated plasma sodium change. However, these **formulas are notably inaccurate** and are not substitute for frequent plasma sodium measurements.

c. A simple weight-based calculation (1 to 1.5 mL/kg) can be used to estimate the volume of hypertonic saline 3% to be administered as slow continuous infusion over 6 hours. For instance, for an 80-kg man, we can estimate a volume of hypertonic saline equivalent to 1.5 mL/kg × 80 kg or 120 mL to be administered over 6 hours at a rate of 120 mL/6 hours or 20 mL/h. The rate can be then adjusted based on subsequent plasma sodium measurements.
   d. Since **sodium and potassium are osmotically equivalent**, if potassium replacement is given, rate of hypertonic saline 3% needs to be decreased or temporarily held to account for potassium supplementation. As a rule, **1 mEq of hypertonic KCl is equivalent to 2 mL of hypertonic saline 3%**.
4. **Use of Desmopressin**
   a. Desmopressin, an AVP analog, is used in hyponatremia to suppress water diuresis responsible for rapid correction of plasma sodium.
   b. Desmopressin in hyponatremia can be used in three different strategies (see Table 3-5).
   c. When using desmopressin, patients should be on a fluid restriction (i.e., ≤800 mL/d) to prevent hyponatremia from worsening.
5. **Plasma Sodium Monitoring**
   a. Frequent plasma sodium measurements are recommended (e.g., every 2 hours).
   b. Plasma sodium values measured using the direct ISE method are on average 2 mEq/L lower than values obtained via indirect ISE method. Therefore, to prevent confusion, adhering to a single method of plasma sodium measurement is crucial. Whole blood sodium measurement using blood gas analyzer (direct ISE method) is convenient for this purpose as the turnaround time tends to be shorter.

E. **Treatment of Nonsevere Hyponatremia (Plasma Sodium ≥120 mEq/L) With Mild or No Apparent Symptoms.** The treatment targets the underlying pathogenesis of hyponatremia (e.g., volume expansion for hypovolemia, glucocorticoid replacement for adrenal insufficiency, etc.). Our emphasis in this section will be on the management of SIAD.
   1. **Fluid Restriction**
      a. The aim of fluid restriction is to elicit a state of negative electrolyte-free water balance.
      b. Only 30% to 40% of patients with SIAD will respond to fluid restriction.
      c. The urine-to-plasma electrolyte ratio $\left(\dfrac{UNa + UK}{PNa}\right)$ can identify which patients will respond to fluid restriction (Table 3-6).

TABLE 3-6	The Urine-to-Plasma Electrolyte Ratio Guides Fluid Restriction in Hyponatremia	
$\dfrac{UNa + UK}{PNa}$	C_eH_2O	Likely to Respond to Fluid Restriction
<1	Positive	Yes
1	Zero	No
>1	Negative	No

UNa, urine sodium; UK, urine potassium; PNa, plasma sodium; C_eH_2O, electrolyte-free water clearance.

d. Even in patients who respond to fluid restriction, the benefit is modest and long-term adherence is difficult.
2. **Oral Urea**
   a. Oral urea works as an osmotic diuretic providing a significant solute load necessary to force electrolyte-free water excretion.
   b. Initial dose is usually 15 g BID (equivalent to 500 mOsm of solute/d)
   c. BUN is expected to increase with oral urea but this does not mean the onset of renal failure or uremia.
   d. Main side effects of urea include distaste and nausea.
3. **Loop Diuretics and Salt Tablets**
   a. Loop diuretics interfere with urinary concentration by blocking the NKCC2 in the thick ascending limb of the loop of Henle. This transporter delivers sodium chloride into the kidney medulla contributing to the hypertonic gradient essential for osmotic water reabsorption at the level of the collecting duct. NKCC2 inhibition decreases medullary gradient for water reabsorption resulting in the formation of a hypotonic urine.
   b. In contrast to urea, salt tablets at usual doses (e.g., 6 g/d) provide a very small solute load (equivalent to 205 mOsm of solute) and hence are mainly used to replete sodium losses from loop diuretics.
4. **Vasopressin antagonists ("Vaptans")**
   a. Vaptans antagonize AVP by blocking the V2 receptor in principal cells of collecting duct leading to the formation of a diluted urine
   b. Only two drugs are available in this category: tolvaptan (oral) and conivaptan (intravenous)
   c. Vaptans need to be started in the hospital
   d. Main side effects include polydipsia, polyuria, risk of liver injury, and overcorrection of hyponatremia

Hypernatremia. *Hypernatremia* is defined as a plasma sodium greater than 145 mEq/L.

I. Pathogenesis and Etiology

From the Edelman equation, it can be inferred that hypernatremia occurs in clinical practice in three distinct scenarios (Table 3-7). All of these scenarios share in common an increase in the ratio $\frac{Na_E + K_E}{TBW}$ where total body water (TBW) is always proportionally smaller than the sum of total body exchangeable cations

TABLE 3-7   Edelman Equation Scenarios for Hypernatremia

Scenario	$Na_E + K_E$	TBW	$\frac{Na_E + K_E}{TBW}$	Clinical Example
1	↔	↓	↑	Obligatory and insensible water loss AVP deficiency AVP resistance
2	↓	↓↓	↑	Gastrointestinal and skin water loss
3	↑↑	↑	↑	Hypertonic fluid administration

Na_E, total body exchangeable sodium; K_E, total body exchangeable potassium; TBW, total body water; AVP, arginine vasopressin; ↔, normal; ↑, increased; ↓, decreased.

($Na_E + K_E$), that is, electrolyte-free water deficit. This electrolyte-free water deficit can be due to different factors:

A. Inability to drink water: This is a requirement for the development of hypernatremia. In contrast to hyponatremia, **hypernatremia is always associated with hypertonicity** which stimulates thirst, driving water drinking behavior. Therefore, even if a significant net water loss (or less commonly net sodium gain) occurs, if patient is able to drink water then hypernatremia will not occur.

Inability to drink water is the result of:
1. **Water is unreachable:** for example, being lost in a desert, bedbound
2. **Altered mental status:** for example, patient is intubated and sedated
3. **Decreased thirst sensation:** for example, elderly, adipsia

B. Electrolyte-Free Water Loss. This is usually the result of hypotonic fluid loss. Sources of hypotonic fluid loss include:
1. Normal hypotonic fluid loss
   a. Obligatory water loss: stool and sweat
   b. Insensible loss from skin: trans epidermal water loss, that is, water that passively evaporates through skin. Insensible loss from respiratory tract is not considered as it matches metabolic water production resulting in net zero water loss.
2. Abnormal hypotonic fluid loss
   a. Extrarenal: gastrointestinal (e.g., vomiting, nasogastric suction, diarrhea, gastrointestinal fistulas, or ostomies) or skin (e.g., excessive sweat, burns)
   b. Kidney: this could be due to solute diuresis (high urine concentrations of a solute obligating water excretion) or water diuresis (AVP deficiency or AVP resistance). Solutes that lead to polyuria include **glucose** (hyperglycemia), **mannitol** (treatment of increased intraocular or intracranial pressure), **urea** (high protein diet, post ATN diuresis, postobstructive diuresis), or **electrolytes** (IV fluids). **AVP deficiency** (formerly known as central diabetes insipidus) is most commonly **idiopathic** thought to be caused by autoimmune destruction of AVP-producing hypothalamic cells. Other less common causes include neurosurgery, head trauma, malignancy, and infiltrative disorders (e.g., sarcoidosis). **AVP resistance** (formerly known as nephrogenic diabetes insipidus) is most commonly due to **lithium** and **hypercalcemia**. Other less common causes include hypokalemia, kidney disease (e.g., obstructive uropathy, sickle cell nephropathy, autosomal dominant kidney disease), drugs (e.g., amphotericin B, foscarnet, demeclocycline). Gestational diabetes insipidus, an unusual form of AVP resistance can occur in the third trimester of pregnancy when placenta produces large amounts of vasopressinase, an enzyme which degrades AVP.

C. Net Sodium Gain. Usually the result of hypertonic fluid gain due to excessive administration of normal saline or hypertonic solutions such as sodium bicarbonate 8.4% for metabolic acidosis.

II. Clinical Manifestations
A. Brain Adaptation to Plasma Hypertonicity
1. Hypertonicity leads to brain volume reduction from cell shrinking.
2. Brain cell activates defense mechanisms to preserve normal cell volume including accumulation of intracellular solutes to increase ICF tonicity and prevent water from leaving cells. During the first 3 hours, there is accumulation of sodium and chloride ions. This is followed by accumulation of organic osmolytes (e.g., myoinositol) that reach a steady state by 48 hours.
3. Similar to the process of adaptation to acute and chronic hyponatremia, acute hypernatremia (duration of onset <48 hours) tends to cause greater

degrees of brain volume reduction compared to chronic hypernatremia (duration of onset ≥48 hours).
  B. Symptoms
    1. Similar to acute hyponatremia, acute hypernatremia usually presents with more severe neurologic manifestations (e.g., seizures and coma) reflecting incomplete brain adaptation to hypertonicity. In contrast, chronic hypernatremia is better tolerated and tends to present with milder neurologic symptoms.
    2. Most hypernatremias are chronic in duration.
III. **Diagnostic Approach to the Hypernatremic Patient**
  A. **Determine why patient is unable to drink water**
    1. Water is unreachable
    2. Altered mental status
    3. Decreased thirst sensation
  B. **Determine source of electrolyte-free water loss (or net sodium gain)** (Fig. 3-3)
    1. If UOsm ≥800 mOsm/kg then urine is appropriately concentrated for hypertonic plasma and AVP system is intact. This suggests extrarenal electrolyte-free water loss or net sodium gain.
    2. If UOsm is <800 mOsm/kg, then urine is not appropriately concentrated for hypertonic plasma and AVP system is impaired. This suggests kidney electrolyte-free water loss (polyuria).
IV. **Diagnostic Approach to the Polyuric Patient (Fig. 3-4)**
  A. Polyuria is defined as a urine output greater than 3 L/d or 50 mL/kg/d.
  B. Calculate the osmolar excretion rate (OER).
    1. OER = V × UOsm, where V is 24-hour urine volume in L/d and UOsm is urine osmolality in mOsm/L. Normal OER is 600 to 900 mOsm/d.
    2. OER ≥1,000 mOsm/d suggests a solute or osmotic diuresis.
    3. OER <1,000 mOsm/d suggests water diuresis.
  C. **Solute diuresis:** Identify the solute responsible for diuresis
    1. Glucose: hyperglycemia
    2. Mannitol
    3. Urea: high protein diet, post ATN diuresis, postobstructive diuresis
    4. Electrolytes: IV fluids
  D. Water Diuresis
    1. The traditional **indirect water deprivation test (Fig. 3-5) has a poor diagnostic accuracy in the diagnosis of polyuria due to water diuresis** and it has been replaced by the determination of plasma copeptin.
    2. AVP is synthesized as a pro-hormone which undergoes enzymatic cleavage resulting in the release of equimolar amounts of three peptides: AVP, neurophysin II, and copeptin.
    3. In contrast to AVP, copeptin is easy to measure and it has been shown to have a very good correlation with AVP concentration and POsm.
    4. In patients with water diuresis, a random plasma copeptin level should be checked.
    5. If plasma copeptin ≥21.4 pmol/L then patient has AVP resistance (formerly known as nephrogenic diabetes insipidus).
    6. If plasma copeptin <21.4 pmol/L then proceed to stimulated plasma copeptin (preferably with arginine, although hypertonic saline can also be used).
    7. If arginine-stimulated plasma copeptin ≥3.8 pmol/L then this suggests primary polydipsia.
    8. If arginine-stimulated plasma copeptin <3.8 pmol/L then this suggests AVP deficiency (formerly known as central diabetes insipidus).
V. **Therapy**
  A. Therapeutic Principles
    1. Most hypernatremias encountered in clinical practice are chronic
    2. Rates of correction

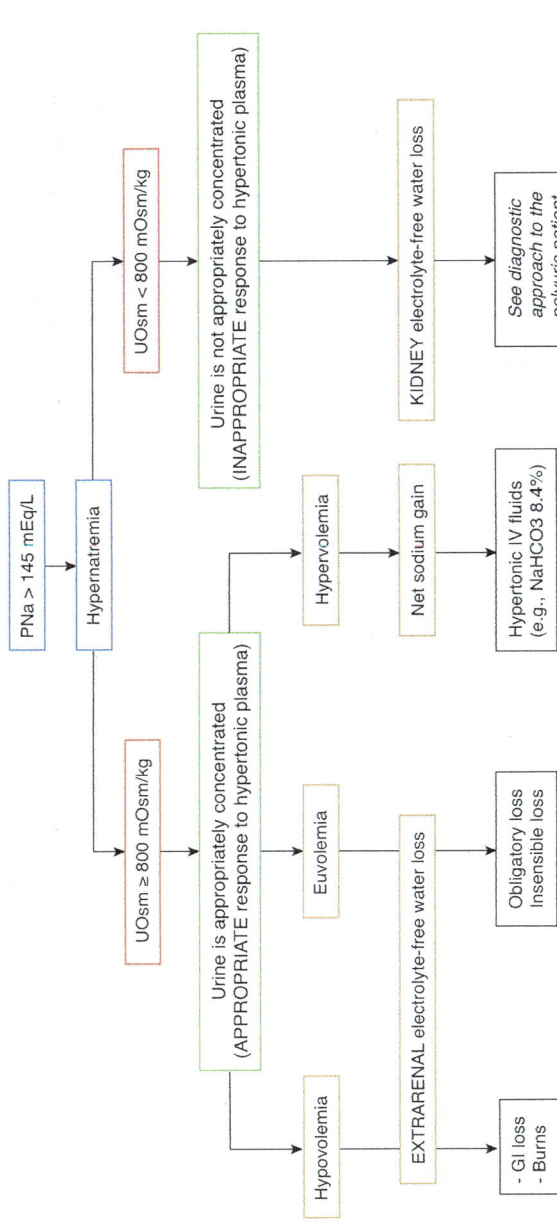

Figure 3-3. Diagnostic approach to hypernatremia. PNa, plasma sodium; UOsm, urine osmolality; GI, gastrointestinal; IV, intravenous.

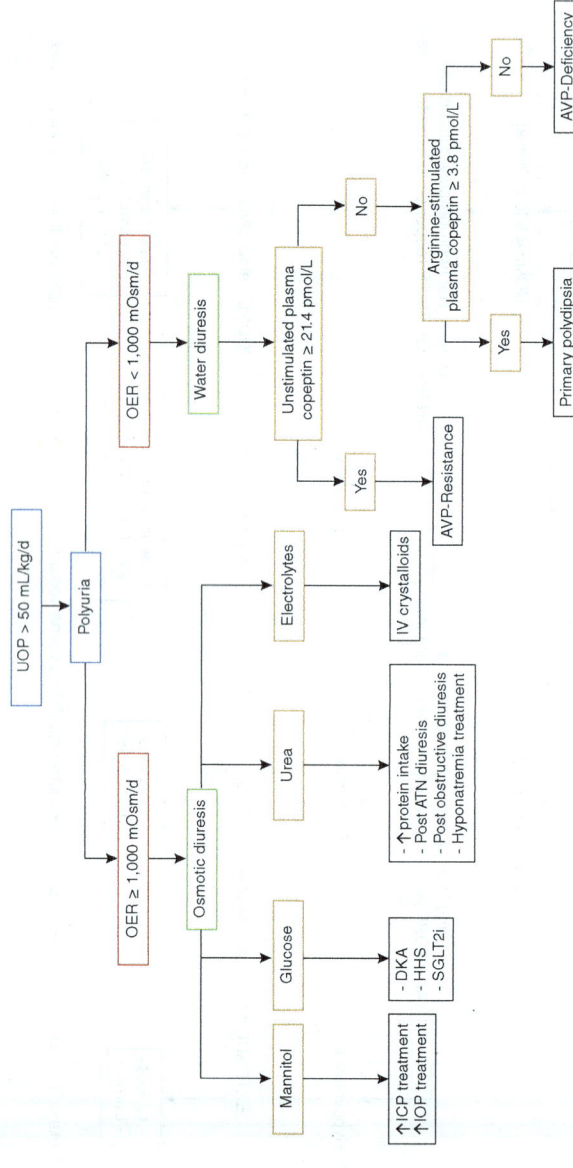

Figure 3-4. Diagnostic approach to polyuria. UOP, urine output; OER, osmolar excretion rate; ↑, increased; ICP, intracranial pressure; IOP, intraocular pressure; DKA, diabetic ketoacidosis; HHS, hyperosmolar hyperglycemic state; SGLT2i, sodium-glucose cotransporter 2 inhibitors; ATN, acute tubular necrosis; IV, intravenous; AVP, arginine vasopressin.

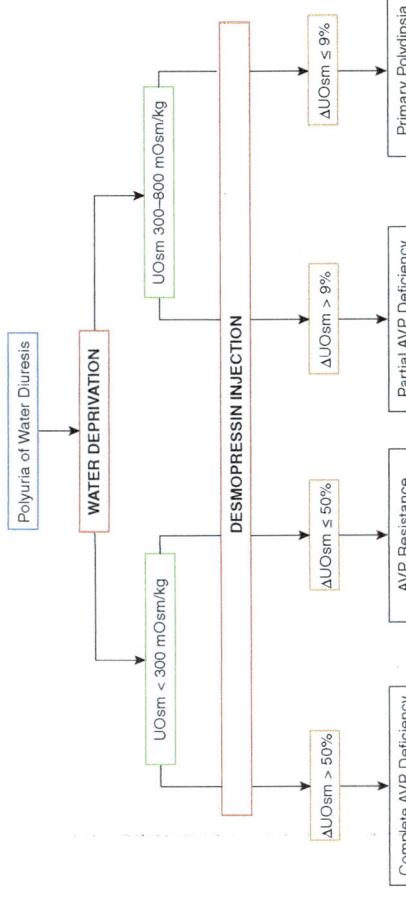

Figure 3-5. Indirect water deprivation test. The traditional water deprivation test. The dehydration phase and the desmopressin phase: During the dehydration phase, patients are placed NPO for 8 hours. Vital signs, weight, urine output, plasma sodium, plasma and urine osmolalities are measured at baseline and every 2 hours. There are circumstances where the dehydration phase maybe terminated prematurely including: plasma sodium >145 mEq/L and plasma osmolality >295 mOsm/kg, two consecutive urine osmolalities that do not differ by >10% and loss of 2% body weight, >3% loss of body weight, orthostatic hypotension, or intractable thirst. In addition, the dehydration phase can be obviated if initial plasma sodium ≥148 mEq/L. Once the dehydration phase is completed, we proceed to the desmopressin phase where desmopressin 2 mcg is administered intravenously once. Patients can now eat and drink. Plasma sodium, plasma and urine osmolalities are measured every hour for 2 hours. In patients with a urine osmolality of <300 mOsm/kg after dehydration phase, an increase in urine osmolality >50% after desmopressin administration suggests complete AVP deficiency while an increase of ≤50% suggests AVP resistance. In contrast, in patients with urine osmolality between 300 and 800 mOsm/kg after the dehydration phase, an increase in urine osmolality >9% after desmopressin administration suggests partial AVP deficiency while an increase of ≤9% suggests primary polydipsia. UOsm, urine osmolality; Δ, change; AVP, arginine vasopressin.

a. In contrast to hyponatremia, rapid correction of hypernatremia has not been associated with poor neurologic outcomes.
b. Suggested goal of correction: 10 to 15 mEq/L per any 24-hour period

B. Water Replacement. We will illustrate how to provide water replacement with an example. A 65-year-old man with a history of bipolar disorder previously on lithium is admitted with septic shock due to pneumonia. Patient is intubated and sedated. He has a feeding tube in place, weight = 70 kg, urine output = 4 L/d, plasma sodium = 164 mEq/L, urine osmolality = 150 mOsm/kg, urine sodium = 25 mEq/L, and urine potassium = 35 mEq/L.

1. **Calculating free water deficit (FWD)**
   a. $FWD = TBW \times \left(\dfrac{PNa\ current}{PNa\ goal} - 1 \right)$

   where TBW is total body water and PNa is plasma sodium.

   b. We aim to correct plasma sodium by 10 to 15 mEq/L in 24 hours, so arbitrarily we will set our plasma sodium goal to 150 mEq/L (correction of 14 mEq/L in 24 hours).

   c. $FWD = 70 \times 0.6 \times \left(\dfrac{164}{150} - 1 \right) = 3.92\ L$

2. **Calculating daily ongoing water losses**
   a. Urine water loss

   $$C_e H_2 O = V \times \left(1 - \dfrac{UNa + UK}{PNa} \right)$$

   Where $C_e H_2 O$ is electrolyte-free water clearance, V is the daily urine volume, UNa is urine sodium, UK is urine potassium, and PNa is plasma sodium.

   b. $C_e H_2 O = 4 \times \left(1 - \dfrac{25 + 35}{164} \right) = 2.53\ L/d$

   c. Obligatory and insensible water loss: ≈0.8 L/d

3. Total water replacement: 3.92 + 2.53 + 0.8 = 7.25 L

4. Initial prescription:
   a. Enteral water 300 mL every 2 hours per GI (total of 3.6 L), AND
   b. Dextrose 5% at 150 mL/h for 24 hours (total of 3.6 L)

5. Follow-up:
   a. The next day when PNa is down to 150 mEq/L, recalculate FWD as

   $$FWD = 70 \times 0.6 \times \left(\dfrac{150}{140} - 1 \right)$$

C. Other therapies:
1. **AVP deficiency:**
   a. **Desmopressin**, either intranasal or oral.
   b. Oral formulation has 1/10 of the potency of intranasal formulation.
2. **AVP resistance:**
   a. **All patients:** Most patients with AVP resistance have partial rather than complete resistance to AVP, so **desmopressin can still be used**. **Thiazide diuretics** can also be used as they cause mild hypovolemia, increasing proximal tubular fluid reabsorption, decreasing distal delivery of water and attenuating polyuria. In addition, **low solute intake** is also recommended to decreased electrolyte-free water excretion.
   b. **Patient currently on lithium without severe concentration defect:** lithium exerts its nephrotoxic effects by entering principal cells of the collecting duct via the epithelial sodium channel (ENaC) and interfering with different cellular pathways. **Amiloride** blocks ENaC, prevents intracellular lithium accumulation, and can be effective in patients with mild to moderate concentrating defect.

SUGGESTED READINGS

Arima H, Cheetham T, Christ-Crain M, et al; Working Group for Renaming Diabetes Insipidus. Changing the name of diabetes insipidus: A position statement of the working group for renaming diabetes insipidus. *J Clin Endocrinol Metab*. 2022;108(1):1–3.

Christ-Crain M, Bichet DG, Fenske WK, et al. Diabetes insipidus. *Nat Rev Dis Primers*. 2019;5(1):54.

Christ-Crain M, Winzeler B, Refardt J. Diagnosis and management of diabetes insipidus for the internist: an update. *J Intern Med*. 2021;290(1):73–87.

Rondon-Berrios H. Mild chronic hyponatremia in the ambulatory setting: Significance and management. *Clin J Am Soc Nephrol*. 2015;10(12):2268–2278.

Rondon-Berrios H, Sterns RH. Hypertonic saline for hyponatremia: Meeting goals and avoiding harm. *Am J Kidney Dis*. 2022;79(6):890–896.

Rondon-Berrios H. Urea for chronic hyponatremia. *Blood Purif*. 2020;49(1–2):212–218.

Spasovski G, Vanholder R, Allolio B, et al; Hyponatraemia Guideline Development Group. Clinical practice guideline on diagnosis and treatment of hyponatraemia. *Nephrol Dial Transplant*. 2014;29(Suppl 2):i1–i39.

Sterns RH. Disorders of plasma sodium–causes, consequences, and correction. *N Engl J Med*. 2015;372(1):55–65.

Sterns RH. Treatment of severe hyponatremia. *Clin J Am Soc Nephrol*. 2018;13(4):641–649.

Verbalis JG, Goldsmith SR, Greenberg A, et al. Diagnosis, evaluation, and treatment of hyponatremia: expert panel recommendations. *Am J Med*. 2013;126(10 Suppl 1):S1–S42.

Workeneh BT, Meena P, Christ-Crain M, et al. Hyponatremia demystified: integrating physiology to shape clinical practice. *Adv Kidney Dis Health*. 2023;30(2):85–101.

4. The Patient With Hypokalemia or Hyperkalemia

Jie Tang, Stuart Linas

Potassium (K) is the most abundant cation in the human body. It regulates intracellular enzyme function and helps determine neuromuscular and cardiovascular tissue excitability. Over 98% of total body K is located in the intracellular fluid (ICF; primarily in muscles), less than 2% in the extracellular fluid (ECF). The ratio of extracellular K to intracellular K determines membrane potential. The acuity of changes in serum K concentration and membrane potential determines the severity of clinical symptoms and underlies the clinical findings caused by disorders of K metabolism.

I. Overview of Potassium Physiology
The typical Western diet contains 40 to 120 mEq of K a day. Tight control of the serum K between 3.5 and 5.5 mEq/d is primarily accomplished by the kidney where secretion varies between 40 and 120 mEq/d. K losses in stool and sweat are small (5 to 10 mEq). In addition, the interplay of several hormonal systems and the internal acid–base environment contribute to the exchange of K between the ECF and ICF, which helps keep the serum K concentration tightly controlled. Although total body K declines with aging, and the rate of decline appears to be influenced by sex and race, the clinical significance of these observations is not clear.

A. Internal Balance

Under certain physiologic conditions, K is rapidly redistributed between the intracellular and extracellular compartments. Several hormones and physiologic factors interact to regulate the transcellular movement of K.

1. **Insulin.** High serum K increases insulin levels. The binding of the insulin hormone to insulin receptors causes a hyperpolarization of cell membranes that facilitates K uptake in liver, fat, cardiac and skeletal muscles. Insulin also activates sodium (Na)–K–adenosine triphosphatase (ATPase) pumps and causes the cellular uptake of K.

2. **Catecholamines.** Activation of the β_2-adrenoreceptor results in cellular K uptake in the liver and muscle. In addition to the activation of inwardly directed Na^+-K^+-2Cl^- (NKCC) cotransporters, the effect is also transduced by cyclic adenosine monophosphate (cAMP) activation of Na–K–ATPase pumps, causing an influx of K in exchange for Na. Therapeutic agents such as theophylline potentiate β_2-adrenoreceptor–mediated K uptake by inhibiting the degradation of cAMP. Activation of α_1-adrenoreceptors prevents K movement into cells and accounts for increases in serum K observed in patients treated with α_1-receptor agonists such as norepinephrine.

3. **Acid–Base.** Inorganic acidosis such as renal tubular acidosis or diarrhea increases in extracellular proton (H^+) concentrations and prevent cellular extrusion of H^+ through Na^+/H^+ exchangers resulting in decreases in intracellular Na. This decrease in cellular Na inhibits cellular uptake of K through Na–K–ATPase to counteract passive K^+ efflux through K^+ channels. Bolus administration of bicarbonate as given during cardiac resuscitation reduces extracellular H^+ and enhances K uptake into cells. Organic acidosis such as lactic acidosis has a less effect on serum K due to the inward flux of lactate and H^+ through the monocarboxylate transporter,

resulting in a reduction in intracellular pH and subsequent stimulations of Na^+/H^+ exchanger and Na^+/HCO_3^- cotransporter, leading to an enhanced Na–K–ATPase activity. Furthermore, ischemic or injured cells may not have functional transporters, making the change in serum K less predictable.
   4. **Tonicity.** Hyperglycemia causes K-rich fluid to leave the cell, thereby increasing ECF K. Under most conditions, increases in insulin modulate and reverse the effect of increased extracellular tonicity. However, when insulin cannot be increased (e.g., type 1 diabetes mellitus) or hyperglycemia occurs rapidly (as with the administration of 50% glucose), hyperkalemia occurs. Rapid infusions of mannitol also may cause hyperkalemia.
B. **External Balance**
   1. Kidney
      Urinary K excretion is the result of a difference between the K secreted and K reabsorbed in the distal nephron. K is freely filtered at the glomerulus. More than 50% of filtered K is reabsorbed in the proximal convoluted tubule through paracellular pathways. In the descending limb of Henle loop, especially in deep nephrons, K concentration increases. In the medullary thick ascending limb of the loop of Henle, the Na–K–2Cl–cotransporter leads to the reabsorption of K. When the tubular fluid reaches the early distal convoluted tubule, only 10% to 15% of filtered K remains. K is secreted by the principal cells of the connecting tubule and cortical collecting duct. K is reabsorbed in the outer medullary collecting duct, an effect mediated by intercalated cells. A fall in glomerular filtration rate (GFR) is not generally associated with decreased K excretion and hyperkalemia until the GFR is less than 20 mL/min. It is due to an adaptive increase in K excretion in the remaining functioning nephrons. The major factors regulating K excretion follow.
      a. **K Switch via With-No-Lysine Kinases (WNKs) and Their Regulation of the Na–Cl Cotransporter (NCC).** WNK kinases, specifically, WNK1 and WNK4, have been shown to regulate the balance between Na and K excretions in the distal nephron. The NCC co transporter control distal Na delivery and therefore downstream cortical collecting tubule-mediated K secretion. WNK activation results in phosphorylation and activation of NCC causing decreased Na delivery to the distal nephron and reduced K excretion. This process requires Kir4.1, expressed at the basolateral side of the distal nephron. When complexed with Kir5.1, the resulting Kir4.1/Kir5.1 heterotetrameric channel serves as a "K-sensor." The K switch refers to the regulatory effect of K on NCC. Low K is sensed on NCC resulting in activation of WNK and NCC with subsequent K retention. Mutations in WNK1 or WNK4 lead to type II pseudohypoaldosteronism (Gordon syndrome) with enhanced NCC activity and reduced K excretion.
      b. **Distal Nephron Flow Rate and Na Delivery at the Epithelial Sodium Channels (ENaC) Acting Site.** Under normal conditions, Na delivered to the cortical collecting tubule is reabsorbed through amiloride-sensitive ENaCs in the principal cells. The resulting negative potential in the tubular lumen results in increased K excretion through apical K channels (renal outer medullary K [ROMK] channel). This system requires Na delivery to the distal tubule. In addition, increases in tubular flow rate help maintain a low urinary K concentration, which favors the movement of K from cells into tubular fluid.
      c. **Mineralocorticoids.** Aldosterone is the major mineralocorticoid; it increases K secretion into the tubular fluid by the following:
         i. Increasing the number and activity of apical ENaCs in the connecting tubule and cortical collecting duct in the distal tubule. This

increases Na reabsorption, thereby creating a negative lumen and driving force for K excretion into the tubular lumen.
    ii. Increasing basolateral Na–K–ATPase activity.
   d. **Changes in Dietary K.** In addition to the regulatory effect of K switch, renal adaptation to high K intake is mediated by a potassium-induced increase in aldosterone secretion and by an increase in distal nephron Na–K–ATPase activity. In response to K restriction, mineralocorticoid activity decreases, thereby causing a decline in K secretion.
   e. Increases in relatively nonresorbable anions (e.g., bicarbonate, penicillin) trap secreted K in the tubular lumen and limit K reabsorption in the medullary collecting duct. The resulting renal K losses may lead to severe K depletion.
  2. **Extrarenal**
   a. **Gastrointestinal (GI) Tract**
    Adaptive changes for K secretion in the colon can occur when there is a significant loss of nephron mass, indicating that the GI tract may play a critical role in handling the extra K load when the kidney function is compromised. The relative contribution of GI K excretion may be different in people with different racial backgrounds.
   b. **Others**
    Both salivary and sweat glands are involved in K excretion regulated by aldosterone. However, its clinical significance in K homeostasis is not clear.

II. Hypokalemia

  A. Diagnosis. The initial approach to hypokalemia is to determine whether it is spurious, secondary to a shift of K from the extracellular to intracellular compartments, or a result of a true decrease in total body K (Fig. 4-1).
  1. Spurious hypokalemia occurs in the setting of extreme leukocytosis (in vitro white blood cells uptake K in the test tube) and is not associated with changes in either internal or external K balance.
  2. K shifts into cells may occur acutely in conditions associated with increases in endogenous insulin or catecholamines. For example, catecholamine release

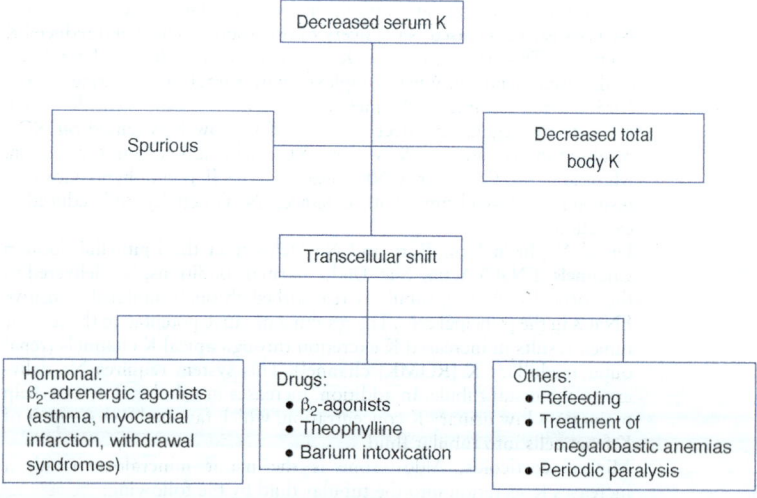

Figure 4-1. Diagnostic approach to hypokalemia, part 1. K, potassium; MI, myocardial infarction.

associated with shortness of breath (asthma, chronic obstructive pulmonary disease exacerbations, heart failure, and chest pain syndromes including myocardial infarction or angina) or catecholamine release from certain drug withdrawals (alcohol, narcotics, or barbiturates) shifts K into cells, thereby decreasing the serum K concentration. Hypokalemia may also be caused by insulin administration (correction of diabetic ketoacidosis, postresuscitation for hyperkalemia) or β_2-adrenoreceptor agonist (β_2-agonists, theophylline). Other common causes of decreases in serum K without decreases in total body K include hypokalemic periodic paralysis (familial and hyperthyroid types), treatment of megaloblastic anemias, and refeeding syndromes (probably insulin mediated). The refeeding syndrome, in which severely malnourished patients are started on nasogastric feeding, is also seen in older adults in whom the clinical manifestations of malnutrition are less clinically apparent.

3. Decreases in total body K (Fig. 4-2) are caused by either inadequate K intake or by excessive renal or extrarenal K losses. The measurement of urinary K excretion (by 24-hour measurements or "spot" K concentrations) is used to distinguish renal versus extrarenal K loss. Urinary K concentrations less than 20 mEq/L suggest poor K intake and/or extrarenal K loss. Serum acid–base status is helpful in evaluating hypokalemia with low urinary K excretion. Metabolic acidosis may suggest lower GI losses (diarrhea of any cause, e.g., infectious, toxic, and laxative abuse). A normal serum pH is less helpful because hypokalemia can be secondary to both decreases in intake and GI losses. Metabolic alkalosis with urinary K of less than 20 mEq/L, although rare, is associated with laxative abuse, villous adenoma, or congenital chloride-losing diarrhea. Hypokalemia with a urinary K excretion of greater than 20 mEq/L suggests renal K wasting. The serum pH again is helpful to further evaluate etiologies. Metabolic acidosis suggests renal tubular acidosis (type 1 or type 2), diabetic ketoacidosis (osmotic diuresis), ureterosigmoidostomy, or carbonic anhydrase inhibitor use. More commonly, renal K losses are associated with metabolic alkalosis. In this clinical setting, the urinary chloride concentration is helpful. A low urinary chloride concentration (less than 20 mEq/L) suggests upper GI K losses, recent (but not current) diuretic use, or a posthypercapnic syndrome. Hypokalemia with a high urinary chloride concentration is further distinguished on the basis of the presence or absence of hypertension. In normotensive individuals, hypokalemia with metabolic alkalosis and a high urinary chloride occurs with diuretic use (loop or distal convoluted tubule–acting diuretics), in Bartter and Gitelman syndromes, and with severe decreases in total body magnesium or K. Hypokalemia with renal K wasting, renal chloride wasting, and hypertension is further evaluated by urinary aldosterone concentrations. An elevated aldosterone level suggests either primary aldosteronism (adenoma, hyperplasia, glucocorticoid remedial) or secondary aldosteronism (renovascular or accelerated hypertension, diuretic use, renin-secreting tumor). Conversely, normal aldosterone levels with increases in serum cortisol suggest Cushing syndrome or exogenous steroid use. Normal cortisol and aldosterone levels indicate Liddle syndrome (caused by increases in the activity of the cortical collecting tubule Na channel) or apparent mineralocorticoid excess syndrome (decreases in 11-β-hydroxysteroid dehydrogenase activity in kidney tissue [congenital, licorice ingestion] causing the mineralocorticoid receptor to respond to glucocorticoid). Increases in urinary K excretion without a significant acid–base disorder are seen during the recovery phase of acute tubular necrosis, postobstructive diuresis, and magnesium depletion associated with drugs such as aminoglycosides and cisplatin, or in myelomonocytic leukemia (secondary to lysozymuria).

Of note, hypokalemia is frequently associated with chronic heavy alcohol use. The mechanism behind this electrolyte abnormality is not well

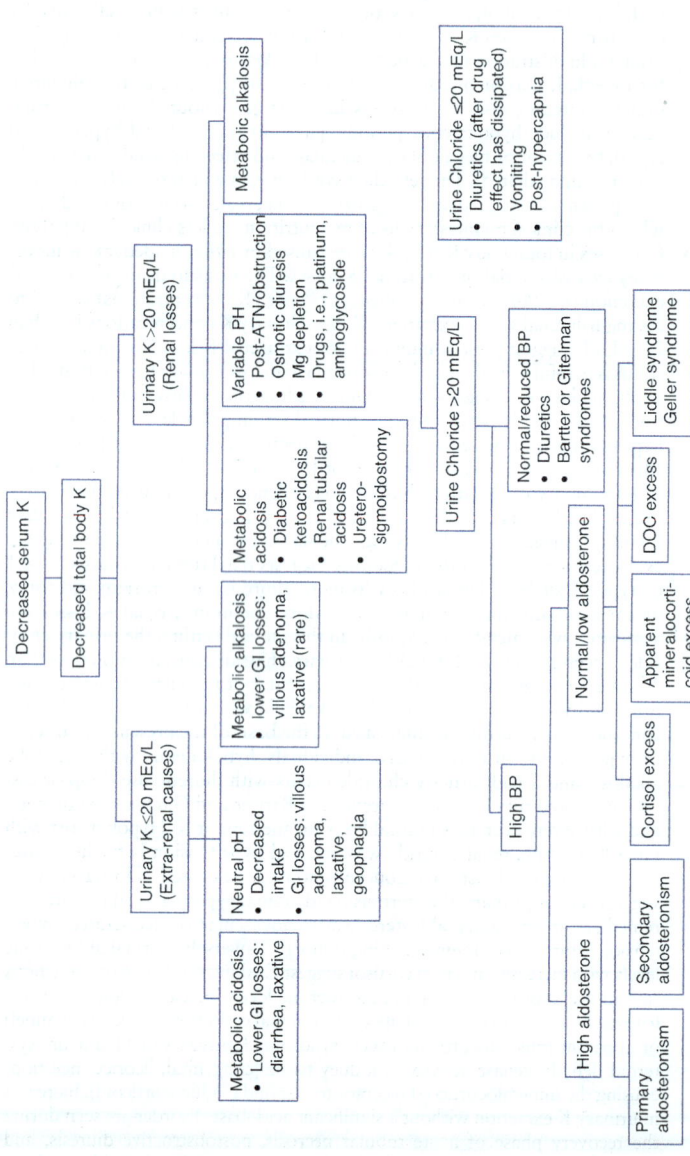

Figure 4-2. Diagnostic approach to hypokalemia, part 2. ATN, acute tubular necrosis; BP, blood pressure; DOC, deoxycorticosterone; GI, gastrointestinal tract; K, potassium; Mg, magnesium.

defined but is probably multifactorial secondary to poor intake, diarrhea, alcohol withdrawal with respiratory alkalosis, and kaliuresis associated with hypomagnesemia.

4. Genetic disorders associated with hypokalemia: These disorders, mentioned earlier, are characterized by either excess mineralocorticoid production/activity or abnormal renal K excretion independent of mineralocorticoid activity.

Disorders associated with increased aldosterone production include glucocorticoid-remediable aldosteronism and congenital adrenal hyperplasia. Bartter and Gitelman syndromes are characterized by abnormalities in renal epithelial K metabolism. There are six variants of Bartter syndrome. The phenotypes vary but all are associated with hypokalemia and normotension. Mutations have been identified in the genes coding for bumetanide-sensitive Na^+–K^+–$2Cl^-$–cotransporter (NKCC2), melanoma-associated antigen D2 (MAGE-D2), ROMK channel in the ascending loop of Henle, Barttin (β-subunit for ClC-Ka and ClC-Kb chloride channels), ClC-KB, and calcium-sensing receptor. Gitelman syndrome is a hypokalemia tubulopathy associated with a mutation in the thiazide-sensitive NaCl cotransporter (NCC). Liddle syndrome is an autosomal recessive disorder caused by a gain-of-function mutation in the ENaC. As a result, extracellular volume is expanded with hypertension. However, as the ROMK channel is secondarily activated, K excretion is increased and hypokalemia results.

Although cell-shift hypokalemia and decreases in total body K do occur as isolated problems, they frequently occur simultaneously. Decreases in total body K potentiate the effects of drugs and hormones to shift K into cells. For example, small changes in K during insulin therapy may not cause hypokalemia if total body K is normal, but in the setting of total body K depletion (e.g., during the treatment of diabetic ketoacidosis or with diuretic use), cellular shifts of K during insulin therapy can result in profound hypokalemia.

B. The manifestations of hypokalemia are mainly cardiac and neuromuscular (Table 4-1). The most dramatic neuromuscular symptoms are paresis, paralysis, and respiratory failure. K depletion causes supraventricular and ventricular arrhythmias, especially in patients on digitalis therapy. Although severe hypokalemia is more likely to cause complications, even minimal decreases in serum or total body K can be arrhythmogenic in patients with underlying heart disease or who are receiving digitalis therapy.

C. The treatment of hypokalemia depends on the underlying cause, the degree of K depletion, and the risk of K depletion to the patient. In general, hypokalemia secondary to cell shift is managed by treating the underlying conditions. For example, hypokalemia in the setting of catecholamine increases, as in chest pain syndromes, is managed with appropriate treatments for the pain. However, when cell-shift hypokalemia is associated with life-threatening conditions such as paresis, paralysis, or hypokalemia in the setting of myocardial infarction, the administration of K is indicated. With K depletion, replacement therapy depends on the estimated degree of decreases in total body K. For example, decreases in total body K accompanied by a fall in serum K from 3.5 to 3.0 mEq/L are associated with a K deficit of 150 to 200 mEq. Decreases in serum K from 3 to 2 mEq/L are associated with 200- to 400-mEq additional decreases in total body K. K can be administered intravenously, but in limited quantities (10 mEq/h into a peripheral vein; 15 to 20 mEq/h into a central vein). Larger K requirements can only be accomplished by oral therapy or with dialysis.

III. Hyperkalemia

A. The approach to hyperkalemia (Fig. 4-3) is to determine whether increases in serum K are spurious, caused by shifts of K from cellular to extracellular spaces, or represent a true increase in total body K. Spurious hyperkalemia is caused by

TABLE 4-1 Clinical Manifestations of Hypokalemia

Cardiovascular

Electrocardiographic abnormalities: U waves, QT prolongation, ST depression
- Predisposition to digitalis toxicity
- Atrial/ventricular arrhythmias

Neuromuscular

Skeletal muscle
- Weakness
- Cramps
- Tetany
- Paralysis—flaccid
- Rhabdomyolysis

Smooth muscle
- Constipation
- Ileus
- Urinary retention

Endocrine
- Carbohydrate intolerance
- Diabetes mellitus
- Decreased aldosterone
- Growth retardation

Renal/electrolyte
- Decreased renal blood flow, glomerular filtration rate
- Nephrogenic diabetes insipidus
- Increased ammoniagenesis (hepatic encephalopathy)
- Chloride wasting/metabolic alkalosis
- Cyst formation
- Interstitial nephritis
- Tubular vacuolization

---

red blood cell hemolysis in vitro, ischemic blood draws, extreme thrombocytosis (greater than 1 million/µL), or leukocytosis (greater than 50,000/µL). Spurious hyperkalemia is distinguished from true hyperkalemia by the absence of electrocardiographic (ECG) abnormalities. Hyperkalemia caused by cell shifts of K occurs acutely and results from decreased K transfer into cells (with decreases in insulin or β-adrenergic blocker therapy), increased K movement from cells to the extracellular space (with metabolic acidosis), hypertonicity (with hyperglycemia or the administration of mannitol), exercise, muscle breakdown (with rhabdomyolysis), or drug intoxications from digitalis or succinylcholine.

Sustained hyperkalemia is caused by decreases in renal K excretion. This usually is not seen until the GFR is less than 20 mL/min. However, it may be seen with less severe decreases in GFR when the kidney is challenged with a K load from K ingestion (e.g., diet, salt substitutes, or drugs, including potassium chloride and potassium citrate) and from increases in endogenous K production (e.g.,

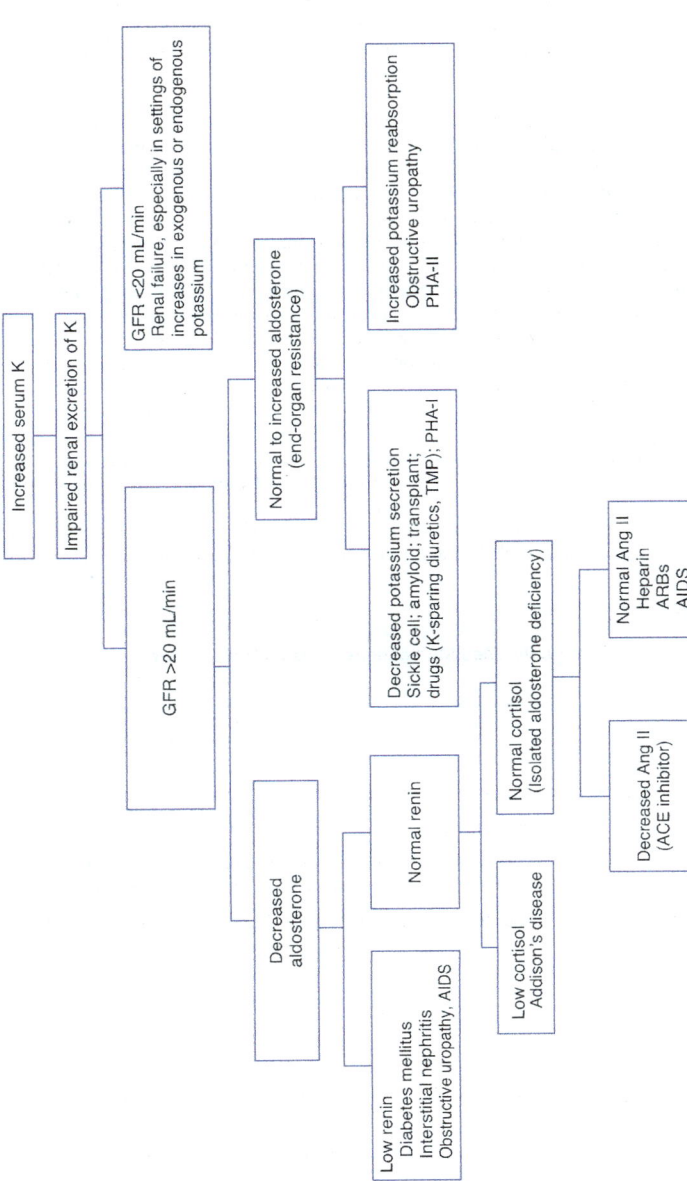

Figure 4-3. Diagnostic approach to hyperkalemia. ACE, angiotensin-converting enzyme; AIDS, acquired immunodeficiency syndrome; ARB, angiotensin receptor blocker; GFR, glomerular filtration rate; PHA, pseudohypoaldosteronism.

GI bleed, resolving hematoma, rhabdomyolysis, catabolic states, and tumor lysis). Hyperkalemia with less severe decreases in renal function is also associated with reductions in the distal nephron flow rate or low serum aldosterone levels as, for example, with hyporenin hypoaldosteronism. Last, hyperkalemia is also associated with less severe decreases in GFR when drugs that alter K physiology are administered. Hyperkalemia occurs in the setting of drugs that inhibit renin secretion (β-adrenergic blockers), renin activity (direct renin inhibition), angiotensin II generation (angiotensin-converting enzyme inhibitors), and the angiotensin receptor (AT1). Hyperkalemia also occurs when drugs that block activation of the mineralocorticoid receptor (spironolactone, eplerenone) or inhibit the rate-limiting step in aldosterone synthesis (heparin) are administered. Drugs that directly inhibit ENaC such as amiloride, trimethoprim, and pentamidine cause hyperkalemia. The protease inhibitor, nafamostat, indirectly inhibits ENaC through inhibition of membrane-associated proteases. Nonsteroidal antiinflammatory drugs (NSAIDs) may cause hyperkalemia by blocking prostaglandin production. As 70% of renin production is prostaglandin dependent, blocking the latter indirectly results in hyporeninemia. Cyclosporine, tacrolimus, and digoxin inhibit Na^+–K^+–ATPase, the enzyme responsible for K excretion in the collecting duct and this can cause hyperkalemia. Succinylcholine causes hyperkalemia by depolarizing skeletal muscle.

Clinical studies also suggest that older adults are at increased risk for hyperkalemia. Although no clear explanation exists for this observation, it may be related to an age-associated decline in aldosterone synthesis or possibly a decline in tubular sensitivity to its action. Commonly used medications causing hyperkalemia are shown in Table 4-2.

Hyperkalemia also occurs in the setting of a relatively well-preserved GFR. The causes of hyperkalemia in this setting are distinguished on the basis of

TABLE 4-2 Commonly Used Medications Causing Hyperkalemia

Medication	Mechanism
Digitalis overdose	Inhibition of the NA-K-ATPase pump
Angiotensin II inhibitors	Decreased aldosterone excretion
NSAIDs	Blocks prostaglandin stimulation of renin
Trimethoprim	A cationic agent that decreases the number of open sodium channels in the luminal membrane of cortical collection ducts
Pentamidine	Same mechanism as trimethoprim—blocks distal potassium excretion
Spironolactone	Competes for aldosterone receptor in collecting tubule
Amiloride	Blocks sodium channel
Heparin	Decrease aldosterone
Salt substitutes	Contain potassium
Succinylcholine	Moves potassium from intracellular to extracellular fluid
Cyclosporine	Multifactorial, including hyporenin hypoaldosteronism and interference with aldosterone action in the potassium-secreting cells of the cortical collecting duct
Pentamidine	Blocks distal potassium secretion

ATPase, adenosine triphosphatase; NSAIDs, nonsteroidal antiinflammatory drugs.

plasma or urinary aldosterone levels. Decreases in aldosterone occur in the setting of normal, increased, or decreased plasma renin activity. Decreased plasma renin activity (hyporeninemic hypoaldosteronism) tends to occur in older adults and is associated with a number of renal diseases, including diabetes, interstitial nephritis (e.g., sickle cell anemia, analgesic use, and heavy metal toxicity), obstructive uropathy, systemic lupus erythematosus, and amyloidosis. Decreases in plasma renin activity are also associated with acquired immunodeficiency syndrome–associated nephropathy, transplantation, and medications including cyclosporine and NSAIDs. Hyper-reninemic hypoaldosteronism also occurs both with decreases in cortisol production (Addison disease) and with normal cortisol production when medications such as angiotensin-converting enzyme inhibitors, angiotensin receptor blockers, and heparin are used. Finally, increases in serum K can be associated with normal to high levels of aldosterone and end-organ resistance to aldosterone. Aldosterone resistance is caused by drugs (such as K-sparing diuretics, trimethoprim, and pentamidine), interstitial renal diseases (systemic lupus erythematosus, sickle cell anemia), obstructive uropathy, or transplantation. It also occurs in an unusual hereditary disease called pseudohypoaldosteronism type 1, in which the etiology is either a decrease in aldosterone receptor number or decreased activity of the ENaC in the distal convoluted tubule. Gordon syndrome is associated with hyperkalemia in the setting of a normal GFR, decreased renal K excretion, and metabolic acidosis. Its mode of heritance is autosomal dominant. It is caused by a WNK4 gene mutation causing a gain-of-function mutation in NCC with an increase in ECF and as a result, suppression of plasma renin, decreased aldosterone, and hyperkalemia. Hyperkalemia in association with normal K secretion and increased K reabsorption occurs with obstructive uropathy.

B. Diagnosis. The urinary K excretion rate or transtubular K gradient (TTKG) ([urine K/serum K]/[urine osmolarity/serum osmolarity]) is used to distinguish aldosterone deficiency/resistance from extrarenal causes of hyperkalemia. This test measures the amount of K secreted by the distal tubule corrected by water absorption in the medullary collecting tubules. Although recent evidence suggested that the assumption inherent in the calculation of the TTKG lacked validity, we still find it useful in the initial assessment. A normal value for TTKG is 6 to 12. In the setting of hyperkalemia, a value greater than 10 suggests normal aldosterone levels and activity and points to an extrarenal cause of hyperkalemia. In contrast, renal causes of hyperkalemia (hypoaldosteronism) are associated with decreases in urinary K excretion (less than 20 mEq/d) and TTKG less than 5 to 7. In this setting, the administration of a mineralocorticoid (0.05 mg fludrocortisone) results in increases in urinary K excretion (greater than 40 mEq/d) and TTKG greater than 10 in patients with aldosterone deficiency. However, no increase in urinary K excretion or in TTKG suggests aldosterone resistance (e.g., sickle cell anemia).

C. The clinical manifestations of hyperkalemia are predominantly cardiac and neuromuscular. It is important to note that patients with hyperkalemia often present with vague GI complaints and nonspecific unwell feelings. ECG abnormalities associated with mild hyperkalemia include peaked T waves. With moderate hyperkalemia there is prolongation of the PR interval, decrease in amplitude of P waves, and widening of the QRS complex. With severe hyperkalemia, the P wave is absent, there is progressive widening of the QRS complex, and if left untreated, sine waves develop with asystole. Neuromuscular abnormalities include weakness, constipation, and paralysis.

D. The treatment of hyperkalemia (Fig. 4-4) depends on the presence or absence of ECG and neuromuscular abnormalities. In the absence of symptoms or ECG abnormalities, hyperkalemia is treated conservatively—for example, by decreasing dietary K or withdrawing offending drugs. In the presence of ECG abnormalities

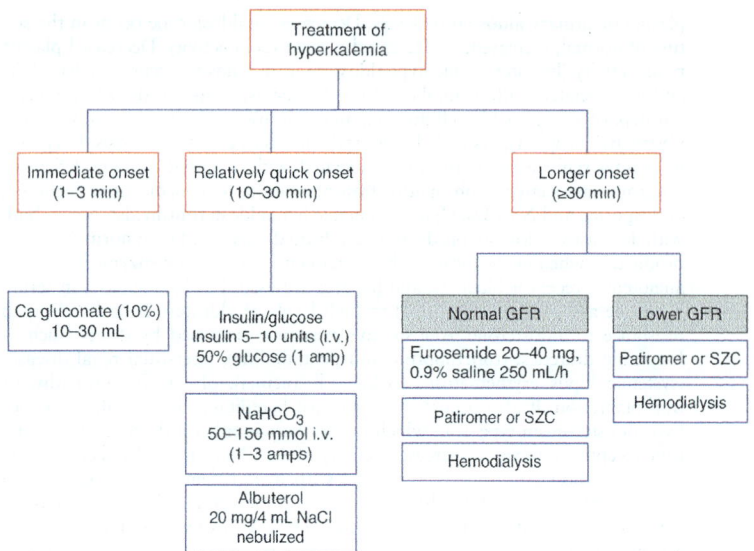

Figure 4-4. Treatment of hyperkalemia. Ca, calcium; GFR, glomerular filtration rate; K, potassium; SZC, sodium zirconium cyclosilicate.

or symptoms, the goal of therapy is to stabilize cell membranes. First-line therapy includes calcium gluconate, 10 to 30 mL as a 10% solution (onset of action 1 or 2 minutes). Although the mechanism remains undefined, calcium "stabilizes" the cardiac membranes. Other therapies include sodium bicarbonate, 50 to 150 mEq (onset 15 to 30 minutes) and insulin 5 to 10 units intravenously (onset 5 to 10 minutes). Insulin increases the activity of the Na–K–ATPase pump in skeletal muscle and drives K into cells. Glucose, 25 g intravenously, is given simultaneously to prevent hypoglycemia. Blood sugars should be monitored for approximately 6 hours to identify and treat hypoglycemia from insulin. Albuterol nebulizer, 20 mg in 4 mL normal saline (onset 15 to 30 minutes), also activates the Na–K–ATPase and drives K into cells. K driven intracellularly generally begins to move extracellularly again after approximately 6 hours, increasing the serum K concentration. Therefore, therapy to remove K from the body should be started simultaneously. Reductions in total body K may be achieved through a K exchange resin. Sodium polystyrene sulfonate (SPS) is an old exchange resin that had been used extensively in the past. One gram of this medication binds approximately 1 mEq of K and releases 1 to 2 mEq of Na back into the circulation. This medication may be given orally (onset 2 hours) or by enema with sorbitol to induce diarrhea (onset 30 to 60 minutes). However, SPS/sorbitol-associated colonic necrosis is a major concern, especially in patients with preexisting bowel injury/dysfunction or recent abdominal surgery. Seventy percent sorbitol administered with SPS is likely the main culprit for this devastating complication. In 2015, patiromer (Veltassa) was approved by FDA for the management of hyperkalemia. Later in 2018, sodium zirconium cyclosilicate (SZC, Lokelma) was also approved. The starting dose for patiromer is 8.4 g daily with a titration up to 25.2 g daily. For SZC, the initial loading dose is 10 g TID for ≤48 hours, then the maintenance dose ranges from 5 g every other day to 15 g daily. Both patiromer and SZC are highly effective in reducing total body K stores, and have been used

TABLE 4-3	Important Features of Patiromer and SZC	
	Patiromer	**SZC**
Mechanism of action	K^+ binding in exchange for Ca^{2+}	K^+ binding in exchange for Na^+ and H^+
Site of action	Large intestine	Small and large intestines
Onset of action	7 h	1 h
Na+ content	None	400 mg per 5 g dose
Ca2+ content	1.6 g per 8.4 g dose	None
Sorbitol content	4 g per 8.4 g dose	None
Common AEs	Nonspecific GI symptoms Hypomagnesemia Hypercalcemia (rare)	Nonspecific GI symptoms Edema (mild–moderate)

AE, adverse effect; GI, gastrointestinal.

extensively in both in-patient and out-patient settings. Table 4-3 summarized the characteristics of these two new exchange resins. Thus far, there have been no serious adverse effects reported. Finally, hemodialysis is very effective in removing excess K, and is considered the last resort for the control of life-threatening hyperkalemia.

SUGGESTED READINGS

Allon M. Hyperkalemia in end stage renal disease: mechanisms and management. *J Am Soc Nephrol.* 1995;6:1134–1142.
Aronson PS, Giebisch G. Effects of pH on potassium: new explanations for old observations. *J Am Soc Nephrol.* 2011;22(11):1981–1989.
Bakris GL, Pitt B, Weir MR, et al; AMETHYST-DN Investigators. Effect of patiromer on serum potassium level in patients with hyperkalemia and diabetic kidney disease: The AMETHYST-DN randomized clinical trial. *JAMA.* 2015;2:151–161.
Bushinsky DA, Williams GH, Pitt B, et al. Patiromer induces rapid and sustained potassium lowering in patients with chronic kidney disease and hyperkalemia. *Kidney Int.* 2015;88(6):1427–1433.
Ethier JH, Kanel KS, Magner PO, Lemann J Jr, Halperin ML. The transtubular potassium concentration in patients with hypokalemia and hyperkalemia. *Am J Kidney Dis.* 1990;15(4):309–315.
Flynn MA, Nolph GB, Baker AS, Martin WM, Krause G. Total body potassium in aging humans: a longitudinal study. *Am J Clin Nutr.* 1989;50(4):713–717.
Gennari FJ. Hypokalemia. *N Engl J Med.* 1998;339:451–458.
Halperin ML, Kamel SK. Electrolyte quintet: potassium. *Lancet.* 1998;352:135–140.
Kahle KT, Ring AM, Lifton RP. Molecular physiology of the WNK kinases. *Annu Rev Physiol* 2008;70:329–355.
Kahle KT, Wilson FH, Lalioti M, Toka H, Qin H, Lifton RP. WNK kinases: molecular regulators of integrated epithelial cell transport. *Curr Opin Nephrol Hypertens.* 2004;13(5):557–562.
Kamel KS, Halperin ML. Treatment of hypokalemia and hyperkalemia. In: Brad HR, Wilcox CS, eds. *Therapy in Nephrology and Hypertension.* WB Saunders; 1999:270–278.
Kellerman PS, Linas SL. Disorders of potassium metabolism. In: Feehally J, Johnson R, eds. *Comprehensive Clinical Nephrology.* Mosby; 1999:10.0–10.10.
Kosiborod M, Peacock WF, Packham DK. Sodium zirconium cyclosilicate for urgent therapy of severe hyperkalemia. *N Engl J Med.* 2015;372(16):1577–1578.
Kosiborod M, Rasmussen HS, Lavin P, et al. Effect of sodium zirconium cyclosilicate on potassium lowering for 28 days among outpatients with hyperkalemia: the HARMONIZE randomized clinical trial. *JAMA.* 2014;312(21):2223–2233.

Landua D. Potassium-related inherited tubulopathies. *Cell Mol Life Sci.* 2006;63(17):1962–1968.

Moonseong QH, Heshka S, Wang J, et al. Total body potassium differs by sex and age across the adult life span. *Am J Clin Nutr.* 2003;78(1):72–77.

Musso C, Liakopoulos V, Miguel RD, Imperiali N, Algranati N. Transtubular potassium concentration gradient: comparison between healthy old people and chronic renal failure patients. *Int Urol Nephrol.* 2006;38(2):387–390.

Osorio FV, Linas SL. Disorders of potassium metabolism. In: Schrier RW, ed. *Atlas of Diseases of the Kidney.* Vol. 1, Sec. 1. Blackwell Science; 1998:2–17.

Oster JR, Singer I, Fishman LM. Heparin-induced aldosterone suppression and hyperkalemia. *Am J Med.* 1995;98(6):575–586.

Packham DK, Rasmussen HS, Lavin PT, et al. Sodium zirconium cyclosilicate in hyperkalemia. *N Engl J Med.* 2015;372(3):222–231.

Perazella M, Asghar R. Disorders of potassium and acid-base metabolism in association with renal disease. In: Schrier RW, ed. *Diseases of the Kidney and Urinary Tract.* 7th ed. Lippincott Williams & Wilkins; 2001:2577–2606.

Perazella MA, Mahnensmith RL. Hyperkalemia in the elderly: drugs exacerbate impaired potassium homeostasis. *J Gen Intern Med.* 1997;12(10):646–656.

Peterson L, Levi M. Disorders of potassium metabolism. In: Schrier RW, ed. *Renal and Electrolyte Disorders.* 6th ed. Lippincott Williams & Wilkins; 2003:171–215.

Proctor G, Linas S. Type 2 pseudohypoaldosteronism: new insights into renal potassium, sodium, and chloride handling. *Am J Kidney Dis* 2006;48(4):674–693.

Wang MX, Gallardo CC, Su XT, et al. Potassium (K^+) intake modulates NCC activity via the K^+ channel, Kir4.1. *Kidney Int.* 2018;93(4):893–902.

Weiner ID, Linas SL, Wingo CS. Disorders of potassium metabolism. In: Johnson RJ, Feehally JF, eds. *Comprehensive Clinical Nephrology.* 2nd ed. Mosby; 2003;109–121.

Weiner ID, Wingo CS. Hyperkalemia: a potential silent killer. *J Am Soc Nephrol.* 1998;9(8):1535–1543.

Weiner ID, Wingo CS. Hypokalemia–consequences, causes, and correction. *J Am Soc Nephrol.* 1997;8(7):1179–1188.

Yang CL, Angell J, Mitchell R, Ellison DH. WNK kinases regulate thiazide-sensitive Na-Cl cotransport. *J Clin Invest.* 2003;111(7):1039–1045.

5. The Patient With an Acid–Base Disorder

Anip Bansal

I. Introduction

The relative acidity of the extracellular fluid (ECF) is usually measured by pH and is normally in the range of 7.35 to 7.45. This range represents a 25% difference in hydrogen ion concentration [H^+], thus the regulation of [H^+] must be tightly regulated by various homeostatic mechanisms. A normal pH is essential for optimal operation of practically all biochemical processes involving proteins and membrane function. Varied pathologic conditions can lead to alterations of the determinants of a normal pH and hence detection of these laboratory alterations can be an essential diagnostic tool in several clinical scenarios.

II. Physiology of Acid–Base Homeostasis

Normally metabolism leads to addition of acid to the ECF, and this would lead to a rapid change in pH if homeostatic mechanisms didn't exist. Acid is first immediately buffered by various buffering systems in the body which includes ECF proteins like albumin, immunoglobulins, histidines, amines, bone, etc. The bicarbonate buffer system is the major buffering system that regulates [H^+] as exemplified by the following formula:

$$H^+ + HCO_3^- \rightleftharpoons H_2CO_3 \rightleftharpoons H_2O + CO_2$$

When the pH is low (i.e., serum H^+ is high), HCO_3^- binds the excess H^+ driving the above reaction to the right toward production of $H_2O + CO_2$ thus lowering the H^+ concentration and returning pH toward normal.

$$\uparrow H^+ + HCO_3^- \rightarrow H_2CO_3 \rightarrow H_2O + CO_2$$

While buffering of acid leads to maintenance of pH, it does not lead to elimination of the obligate acid load from the body. Depending on the type of acid, the lungs and kidneys play key roles in this as below.

There are two main mechanisms that lead to addition of acid to the body:

1. Volatile acid—this is produced from glucose and fat metabolism. It leads to production of carbonic acid and neutral end products of metabolism like water and carbon dioxide (CO_2). The CO_2 thus produced is normally eliminated effectively by the lungs.
2. Nonvolatile acid—this is produced from metabolism of proteins and nucleic acid. This acid must be eliminated by the kidneys. In an adult on a usual diet, this leads to production of roughly 1 mmol/kg of [H^+] per day.

III. Definitions Essential to Understanding Acid–Base Disorders

1. Acidemia—usually refers to a pH <7.35 which reflects an increase in blood [H^+]
2. Alkalemia—usually refers to a pH >7.45 which reflects a decrease in blood [H^+]
3. Acidosis—refers to a process resulting in accumulation of [H^+] in the body causing acidemia. It can be either respiratory or metabolic in origin.
4. Alkalosis—refers to a process resulting in reduction of [H^+] in the body causing alkalemia. It can be either respiratory or metabolic in origin.

The Henderson–Hasselbach equation is a chemistry principle that defines the relationship between the pH of acids (in aqueous solutions) and their pKa (acid dissociation constant). Serum pH is mainly determined by the ratio of serum bicarbonate concentration [HCO_3^-] to partial pressure of CO_2 [PCO_2] as shown in the following relationship which is a modified version of the Henderson–Hasselbach equation:

$$pH = pK + \log \frac{[HCO_3^-]}{[PCO_2]}$$

Therefore, a change in pH can occur if there is a change in HCO_3^- or CO_2. Depending on these alterations, the physiologic approach to identification of acid–base disorders identifies four main types of acid–base disturbances:
1. Respiratory alkalosis (decrease in PCO_2 resulting in an increase in pH)
2. Respiratory acidosis (increase in PCO_2 resulting in a decrease in pH)
3. Metabolic alkalosis (increase in HCO_3^- resulting in an increase in pH)
4. Metabolic acidosis (decrease in HCO_3^- resulting in a decrease in pH)

IV. Laboratory Evaluation of Acid–Base Disorders

Whenever an acid–base disorder is suspected ideally an arterial blood gas (ABG) should be obtained (in addition to a basic metabolic panel to assess the serum anion gap [AG] as below). An arterial puncture required to obtain a sample for an ABG can be associated with some potential complications like pain, infection, nerve injury, bleeding, arterial injury leading to distal ischemia due to thrombosis, or dissection. This has led to an increased use of venous blood gas (VBG) sampling as an alternative to ABGs. Venous and arterial pH and bicarbonate agree reasonably in multiple studies. However, peripheral venous CO_2 cannot be relied upon as an absolute representation of arterial CO_2 ($PaCO_2$). The peripheral venous pH is approximately 0.03 to 0.04 pH units lower than in arterial blood, the HCO_3^- concentration is approximately 2 to 3 mEq/L higher, and the PCO_2 is approximately 3 to 8 mmHg higher in venous blood. Normal $PaCO_2$ is 35 to 45 mmHg whereas normal serum HCO_3^- concentration is 22 to 26 mEq/L.

A. HCO_3^- **from ABG Measurement Versus Serum Total** CO_2 **(tCO_2).** The HCO_3^- in blood can be estimated reasonably by measuring the tCO_2 in venous serum. The serum tCO_2 is 1 to 3 mmol/L greater than the arterial HCO_3^- because it is from venous blood, which has more HCO_3^-, and it includes dissolved CO_2 and trivial amounts of other substances. Normal sea level serum tCO_2 levels average 26 to 27 mmol/L. A value below 24 or above 30 likely marks a clinical acid–base disorder.

In contrast, the ABG reported HCO_3^- is a calculated value and not a directly measured test. Hence, in case of marked discrepancy between the two, the tests might need to be repeated.

The **serum AG** is calculated from the venous serum sodium, chloride, and [HCO_3^-]/tCO_2 as follows:

$$\text{Serum Anion gap} = [Na^+] - ([Cl^-] + [HCO_3^-])$$

The units are in mEq/L, because this calculation estimates the difference between the so-called unmeasured anions (serum total anions represented by Cl^- and HCO_3^-) and unmeasured cations (serum total cations represented by Na^+). The average normal value is 10 ± 2 mEq/L, but varies in different laboratories. Since albumin is the main determinant of the normal AG, a fall in serum albumin of 1 g/dL decreases the AG by 2.5 mEq/L. Thus, in conditions associated with hypoalbuminemia, the corrected serum AG is calculated using this adjustment (add 2.5 mEq/L to the calculated AG for every decrease in serum albumin below normal; i.e., ~4 g/dL).

V. Approach to Simple Acid–Base Disorders

The first step in assessment of an acid–base disorder is a careful clinical evaluation. The underlying medical problems, active medications, preceding symptoms, vital signs, and examination findings may all provide important clues to the etiology of the laboratory abnormality.

Using the underlying clinical context, the interpretation of the ABG (or VBG) and other laboratory parameters should then proceed in a systematic fashion. The following section focuses on the approach to the interpretation of the ABG results.

The identification of an acid–base disorder requires progression through simple steps as below.

1. Look at the measured pH. This identifies acidemia or alkalemia. The change in $[HCO_3^-]$ and PCO_2 then indicates whether the primary process is metabolic or respiratory. For example, in acidemia, a low $[HCO_3^-]$ is suggestive of a primary metabolic acidosis whereas a high PCO_2 is suggestive of a primary respiratory acidosis. The changes in the $[HCO_3^-]$, PCO_2, and pH in the four simple acid–base disorders are listed in Table 5-1.
2. Check if the expected compensatory response to the primary acid–base disorder is appropriate (see below).
3. Calculate the serum AG to identify if a high AG metabolic acidosis is present.
4. Determine the cause of the acid–base disorder from the clinical setting and additional laboratory tests.

A. Understanding the Concept of Compensation for Primary Acid–Base Disorders. Both metabolic and respiratory acid–base disorders are compensated by homeostatic responses to normalize the pH.

The kidneys compensate for respiratory acid–base disorders by adjusting the excretion or retention of $[H^+]$ and $[HCO_3^-]$ in the urine. In respiratory acidosis, the kidneys respond by increasing the reabsorption of $[HCO_3^-]$ and excreting $[H^+]$ into the urine. In contrast in respiratory alkalosis, the kidneys compensate by decreasing the reabsorption of $[HCO_3^-]$ (allowing it to be excreted in the urine) and decreasing the excretion of $[H^+]$. In general, compensation by the kidneys is slower than respiratory compensation and happens over a few days.

In metabolic acidosis, the lungs compensate for the decreased systemic pH by increasing minute ventilation to expel more CO_2 from the body. A decrease in $PaCO_2$ helps to raise the blood pH back toward normal levels (as per the modified Henderson–Hasselbach equation). In contrast, metabolic alkalosis is compensated for by the lungs by a reduction in minute ventilation to retain CO_2, effectively increasing the concentration of carbonic acid in the blood. This increase in the PCO_2 helps to raise the blood pH back toward normal levels (as per the modified Henderson–Hasselbach equation). This respiratory compensation occurs quickly, within minutes, as the central nervous system can rapidly alter the breathing rate and depth.

TABLE 5-1 Relationship of $[HCO_3^-]$, PCO_2, and pH in Simple Acid–Base Disorders

	Initial Change	pH	Compensation	pH
Respiratory alkalosis	↓ $PaCO_2$	↑↑	↓ $[HCO_3^-]$	↑
Respiratory acidosis	↑ $PaCO_2$	↓↓	↑ $[HCO_3^-]$	↓
Metabolic alkalosis	↑ $[HCO_3^-]$	↑↑	↑ $PaCO_2$	↑
Metabolic acidosis	↓ $[HCO_3^-]$	↓↓	↓ $PaCO_2$	↓

TABLE 5-2	Expected Compensatory Response to Simple Acid–Base Disorders (Rules of Compensation)		
Primary Acid–Base Disorder	Primary Change in Laboratory Parameter	Compensatory Acid–Base Disorder	Expected Compensatory Response
Respiratory alkalosis[a]	↓ $PaCO_2$	Metabolic acidosis	↓ HCO_3^- (Acute: 2 mEq/L for each 10 mmHg ↓ in $PaCO_2$; Chronic: 5 mEq/L for each 10 mmHg ↓ in $PaCO_2$)
Respiratory acidosis[a]	↑ $PaCO_2$	Metabolic alkalosis	↑ HCO_3^- (Acute: 1 mEq/L for each 10 mmHg ↑ in $PaCO_2$; Chronic: 4 mEq/L for each 10 mmHg ↑ in $PaCO_2$)
Metabolic alkalosis	↑ $[HCO_3^-]$	Respiratory acidosis	↑ $PaCO_2$ (0.6–0.7 mmHg for each mEq/L increase in HCO_3^-)
Metabolic acidosis	↓ $[HCO_3^-]$	Respiratory alkalosis	↓ $PaCO_2$ (1–1.5 mmHg for each mEq/L decrease in HCO_3^-) Or Expected $PaCO_2 = 1.5 \times [HCO_3^-] + 8 \pm 2$

[a]Expected compensatory response is different for acute disorders versus chronic disorders. In general, the pH will change by 0.08 for every 10 mmHg change in $PaCO_2$ in acute situations and 0.03 for every 10 mmHg change in $PaCO_2$ in chronic conditions.

While analyzing compensatory response to a primary acid–base disorder, the following two principles must be followed:
1. Normally the acid–base buffer pair changes from normal in the same direction in all simple acid–base disorders, for example, in a metabolic acidosis with a decrease in $[HCO_3^-]$ a decrease in PCO_2 is the expected compensatory response. If $[HCO_3^-]$ and PCO_2 change in opposite directions, the disorder must be mixed.
2. Compare the magnitude of the expected compensation of the PCO_2 or HCO_3^- with the measured change in the HCO_3^- or PCO_2. In metabolic disorders, the primary change occurs in the HCO_3^-, with the compensation occurring in the PCO_2. The opposite is true in the respiratory disorders. The expected compensatory responses to simple acid–base disorders are listed in Table 5-2 and can be used to estimate whether compensation is appropriate. The respiratory disorders have two stages of compensation: acute, when only tissue buffering slightly changes the HCO_3^-, and chronic (usually after 24 hours) when the kidneys cause major changes in the HCO_3^- concentration. If the measured change in the compensating factor does not approximate the change predicted, a mixed disorder is likely.

VI. Identification of Mixed Acid–Base Disorders

The occurrence of multiple acid–base disorders simultaneously is referred to as mixed acid–base disorders. A mixed acid–base disorder should not be confused with the normal compensatory responses to primary acid–base imbalances. The detection of mixed acid–base disorders first requires the calculation of the expected

TABLE 5-3	Identification of Mixed Acid–Base Disorders		
Primary Acid–Base Disorder	**Compensatory Acid–Base Disorder**	**Is the Expected Compensation Appropriate?**	
		Yes	**No**
Respiratory alkalosis	Metabolic acidosis	Isolated respiratory alkalosis	Combined respiratory alkalosis and metabolic disorder[a]
Respiratory acidosis	Metabolic alkalosis	Isolated respiratory acidosis	Combined respiratory acidosis and metabolic disorder[a]
Metabolic alkalosis	Respiratory acidosis	Isolated metabolic alkalosis	Combined metabolic alkalosis and respiratory disorder[b]
Metabolic acidosis	Respiratory alkalosis	Isolated metabolic acidosis	Combined metabolic acidosis and respiratory disorder[b]

[a]If the measured HCO_3^- is lower than expected, then an additional metabolic acidosis is present and if the measured HCO_3^- is higher than expected, then an additional metabolic alkalosis is present.

[b]If the measured PCO_2 is lower than expected, then an additional respiratory acidosis is present and if the measured PCO_2 is higher than expected, then an additional respiratory alkalosis is present.

compensatory response using the rules in Table 5-2. Depending on the whether the expected compensatory response is significantly different from the measured levels of HCO_3^- and PCO_2, a mixed acid–base disorder can be suspected as summarized in Table 5-3. The complete step-wise approach to interpretation of acid–base disorders is outlined in Table 5-4.

In a primary metabolic disorder, an additional respiratory acidosis or alkalosis may be diagnosed if the calculated PCO_2 is greater or less than predicted, respectively. Similarly, in a primary respiratory disorder, an additional metabolic alkalosis or acidosis may be diagnosed if the calculated $[HCO_3^-]$ is greater or less than predicted, respectively. In cases with a high AG metabolic acidosis, additional evaluation for the possible presence of either a concomitant normal AG acidosis or metabolic alkalosis should be done (see legend of Table 5-4). This could lead to the detection of three simultaneous acid–base disorders aka "triple" acid–base disorders.

The impact of mixed disorders on systemic pH may intensify or counteract pH fluctuations; for instance, concurrent metabolic and respiratory acidosis will cause severe systemic acidosis, while concurrent metabolic acidosis and respiratory alkalosis might not cause any appreciable change in the systemic pH. Two examples of mixed acid–base disorders are described below.

- **A. Metabolic Acidosis and Respiratory Acidosis.** In the presence of a metabolic acidosis, if the measured PCO_2 is more than the expected PCO_2 by 5 mmHg (as calculated using the rules of compensation defined in Table 5-2), it indicates the presence of a concomitant respiratory acidosis. This can be seen in various clinical scenarios like cardiopulmonary arrest, shock-causing lactic acidosis in a patient who also has respiratory failure, severe acute kidney injury in patients with hypercapnic respiratory failure, etc.
- **B. Metabolic Acidosis and Respiratory Alkalosis.** In the presence of a metabolic acidosis, if the measured PCO_2 is lower than the expected PCO_2 by 5 mmHg, it indicates the presence of a concomitant respiratory alkalosis. Due to the opposing effects on systemic pH, this mixed disorder can lead to minimal alteration of the pH. An example of a clinical scenario leading to this mixed disorder is salicylate intoxication which leads to a high AG metabolic acidosis

TABLE 5-4	Step-Wise Approach to Clinical Identification of Acid–Base Disorders	
Step	Question	Action
1	Is the patient acidemic or alkalemic?	Determine blood pH.
2	Is the disturbance respiratory or metabolic?	Assess $PaCO_2$ and serum bicarbonate levels.
3	If a respiratory disturbance is present, is it acute or chronic? Is the metabolic compensation appropriate?	Compare measured pH with expected change in pH.
4	If a metabolic disturbance is present, is there an increased anion gap? If the serum anion gap is normal, consider calculating the urine anion gap.	Measure serum sodium, chloride, and bicarbonate levels to assess anion gap.
5	If a metabolic disturbance is present, is the respiratory system compensating adequately?	Compare measured $PaCO_2$ with expected $PaCO_2$ to assess whether an additional respiratory acidosis or alkalosis is also present.
6	If an increased anion gap metabolic acidosis is present, is there an additional metabolic disorder?	Determine the change in bicarbonate level and compare with change in serum anion gap.[a]

[a]Step 6 refers to the "delta/delta" rule. This is only used once a high AG metabolic acidosis is present to uncover whether an additional metabolic acid–base disorder is present. This requires comparing the "delta HCO_3^-" (or change in HCO_3^- from normal) with the "delta serum anion gap" (or change in AG from normal).

If a low serum bicarbonate is the result of a high AG acidosis alone, then the change in AG should be approximately the same as the change in serum HCO_3^-. If ΔHCO_3^- is greater than the ΔAG, then something else is also causing HCO_3^- consumption and there is an additional normal AG metabolic acidosis. If the ΔHCO_3^- is less than ΔAG, then there is an additional metabolic alkalosis (in addition to a high AG metabolic acidosis).

with hyperventilation causing a respiratory alkalosis. Often patients who present with this emergency are unable to give a history of excessive intake of salicylates and, hence, identification of the acid–base disorder is an important clinical clue to its presence. Critically ill patients with metabolic acidosis due to lactic acidosis or severe acute kidney injury in combination with hyperventilation often also have this mixed disorder.

VII. Identification of the Underlying Cause of an Acid–Base Disorder

A. Metabolic Acidosis. If the serum AG is normal, metabolic acidosis is due to a loss in HCO_3^- but if the serum AG is increased, metabolic acidosis is due to the addition of acid, thus, the differential diagnosis of metabolic acidosis is first based on identification of whether it is a high AG metabolic acidosis or a normal AG metabolic acidosis (normal serum AG). The overall approach to metabolic acidosis is shown in Figure 5-1.

B. High Anion Gap Metabolic Acidosis (HAGMA). The AG (a measure of unmeasured anions) can increase either due to increased production of acid or due to decreased excretion of acid. The mnemonic "GOLD MARK" provides a structured approach to identify the diverse causes of HAGMA, and includes Glycols, Oxoproline, L-lactate, D-lactate, Methanol, Aspirin, Renal failure, and Ketoacidosis (Table 5-5). Several of these disorders are considered medical emergencies and prompt identification of the cause of a HAGMA is an essential first step in the management of patients with these disorders.

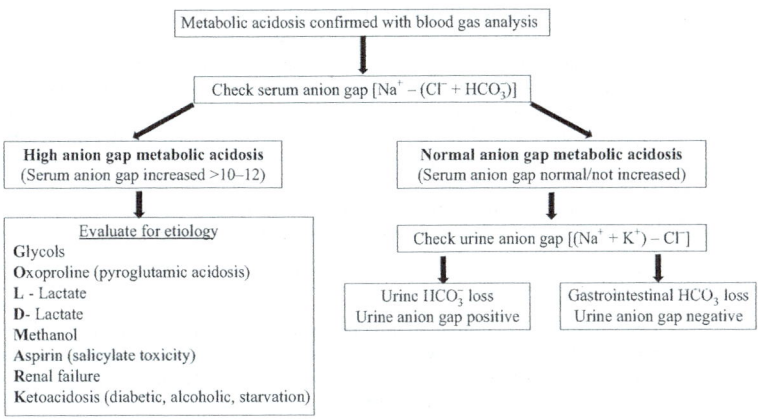

Figure 5-1. Approach to metabolic acidosis.

TABLE 5-5	Causes of Metabolic Acidosis

High Anion Gap Type
  Glycols (ethylene glycol or propylene glycol)
  Oxoproline (pyroglutamic acidosis)
  L-Lactate
  D-Lactate
  Methanol
  Aspirin (salicylate toxicity)
  Renal failure
  Ketoacidosis (diabetic, alcoholic, starvation)

Normal Anion Gap Type
  Gastrointestinal HCO_3 loss
    Diarrhea
    Urinary diversions (ureterosigmoidostomy, ureteroileostomy)
    Pancreatic or biliary fistulae
  Renal HCO_3 loss
    Carbonic anhydrase inhibitors, e.g., acetazolamide, topiramate
    Proximal renal tubular acidosis (RTA)
    Distal RTA
    Hyperkalemic RTA
  Miscellaneous
    NH_4Cl ingestion
    Hyperalimentation
    Toluene inhalation
    Large volume saline

1. **Glycols (Ethylene and Propylene Glycol):** Ethylene glycol, commonly found in antifreeze, leads to HAGMA through its metabolism to oxalic acid and other organic acids. Propylene glycol, found in certain intravenous medications, can also be metabolized into lactic acid, contributing to the AG. Laboratory confirmation of such toxic alcohol ingestion is generally not rapidly available, and additional testing of the serum osmolality can be used to suspect their presence in the setting of a HAGMA. The osmolal gap is the difference between measured serum osmolality and calculated serum osmolality as below. A higher-than-expected osmolal gap (>10 mmol/L) provides an important clue to the presence of toxicity due to glycols and methanol.

$$\text{Calculated serum osmolality} = 2 \times [Na^+] \text{ in mmol/L} + [(\text{glucose in mg/dL}) \div 18] + [(\text{BUN in mg/dL}) \div 2.8]$$

2. **Oxoproline (Pyroglutamic Acid):** This is an uncommon cause of HAGMA and is often associated with chronic acetaminophen use. It involves the accumulation of pyroglutamic acid, an intermediate in the gamma-glutamyl cycle, which can build up in certain metabolic conditions or with glutathione depletion.
3. **L-Lactate:** Lactic acidosis is one of the most common causes of HAGMA and can result from various conditions that cause hypoperfusion or hypoxia, leading to anaerobic metabolism and subsequent lactic acid production. The clinical causes of lactic acidosis are often subclassified into those associated with tissue hypoxia (type A), and those in which there is no apparent tissue hypoxia (type B). Some causes of type B lactic acidosis include thiamine deficiency, seizures, various malignancies, and numerous medications.
4. **D-Lactate:** A less common form of lactic acidosis, D-lactate acidosis, occurs due to bacterial overgrowth in the intestines or short bowel syndrome.
5. **Methanol:** Ingestion of methanol, found in some solvents and windshield wiper fluids, leads to HAGMA through its metabolism to formaldehyde and formic acid, which are toxic and can also cause visual disturbances and neurologic depression.
6. **Aspirin (Salicylate Toxicity):** Overdose of aspirin or salicylates initially causes respiratory alkalosis due to direct stimulation of the respiratory center in the brain but later leads to HAGMA by interfering with oxidative phosphorylation, resulting in the accumulation of organic acids.
7. **Renal Failure:** In severe acute kidney injury or chronic kidney disease, the kidneys are unable to excrete acid and reabsorb bicarbonate efficiently. Accumulation of sulfates, phosphates, urate, and other organic acids contributes to the high AG (advanced kidney disease is usually associated with a combined high AG and normal AG metabolic acidosis).
8. **Ketoacidosis:** This includes diabetic ketoacidosis (DKA), alcoholic ketoacidosis, and starvation ketoacidosis. These conditions involve the accumulation of ketoacids due to alteration in rates of lipolysis and ketogenesis.

   If the etiology of a HAGMA is unclear, testing for one or all of the above causes can be pursued. Treatment involves both supportive cares to correct the acid–base imbalance and specific interventions to address the underlying etiology, which may include hemodialysis (to treat severe acute kidney injury or advanced CKD or to remove toxic alcohols), antidotes (e.g., fomepizole for glycol poisonings), or insulin therapy in the case of DKA. The use of supplementation bicarbonate in the setting of a HAGMA is usually not useful by itself but can be used in life-threatening situations to maintain pH >7.1 while addressing the underlying cause.

C. **Normal Anion Gap Metabolic Acidosis.** Normal anion gap metabolic acidosis (NAGMA), or hyperchloremic acidosis, is an acid–base disorder caused by a primary deficit of HCO_3^-, typically with a compensatory increase in chloride (Cl^-), thus maintaining a normal AG. The mnemonic "HARDUPS" can be used to remember some of the common causes (Table 5-5):

1. **Hyperalimentation:** Excessive total parenteral nutrition especially which includes certain amino acid supplements (lysine, histidine, or arginine hydrochloride) can lead to acidosis.
2. **Addison Disease:** Adrenal insufficiency causes NAGMA due to decreased aldosterone levels leading to sodium loss and retention of hydrogen and potassium ions.
3. **Renal Tubular Acidosis (RTA):** RTA refers to conditions that lead to renal loss of bicarbonate due to a defect in renal bicarbonate or H^+ handling. There are three major forms of RTAs: (a) proximal—due to defect in bicarbonate reabsorption in the proximal tubule; (b) distal—due to defect in H^+ secretion in the distal tubule; and (c) hyperkalemic. Each of these subtypes has a list of etiologies and hence identification of an RTA should lead to a search for possible etiology of the RTA.
4. **Diarrhea:** Loss of HCO_3^- in stool more than the body's ability to compensate, resulting in NAGMA due to HCO_3^- deficit.
5. **Ureteral Diversion:** Surgical procedures like urostomies (ureterosigmoidstomy or uretero-ileostomy) or malfunctional ileal conduits can cause HCO_3^- loss due to urine contact with the bowel.
6. **Pancreatic Fistula or Drainage:** Loss of HCO_3^--rich fluids from the pancreas.
7. **Spironolactone:** This aldosterone antagonist can impair the kidney's ability to handle acids and bases.

The **urine anion gap (UAG)** is a useful tool in the evaluation of NAGMA. It is calculated using the following formula: $UAG = [Na^+] + [K^+] - [Cl^-]$, using spot measurements of these electrolytes in the urine. The UAG is an indirect estimate of ammonium (NH_4^+) concentration in the urine and helps to determine whether the kidneys are appropriately excreting acid. A positive UAG suggests that the kidneys are not appropriately excreting NH_4^+ and points toward a kidney-specific cause of acidosis, such as RTA. A negative UAG suggests nonkidney causes, such as HCO_3^- loss. Due to limitations with the UAG, there has been a push toward the adoption of direct NH_4^+ measurement in the urine but this is not widely available.

Management of NAGMA involves treating the underlying cause while carefully correcting the acid–base and electrolyte imbalances. For RTA, this may involve alkali therapy with bicarbonate or citrate salts. For adrenal insufficiency, glucocorticoid and mineralocorticoid replacement is essential.

D. Metabolic Alkalosis. Metabolic alkalosis is a metabolic process that causes a primary increase in the HCO_3. A primary increase in plasma bicarbonate leading to metabolic alkalosis is classically considered to be two-step process that requires generation and maintenance.

Generation of metabolic alkalosis can occur in several ways: (1) addition of HCO_3^-; (2) loss of H^+; (3) loss of chloride rich fluids (previously known as contraction alkalosis); (4) posthypercapnia; and (5) hypokalemia. Maintenance of metabolic alkalosis is usually due to factors that impair the ability of the kidney to excrete the excess HCO_3^- (e.g., chloride depletion or potassium depletion).

Clinically, metabolic alkalosis is divided into two categories:
- chloride responsive (also known as saline responsive)
- chloride unresponsive or chloride replete (also known as saline resistant)

To differentiate between the two categories, urine $[Cl^-]$ is measured. If the urine $[Cl^-]$ is <20 mEq/L, metabolic alkalosis is categorized as chloride responsive (aka saline responsive). If the urine $[Cl^-]$ is >20 mEq/L, metabolic alkalosis

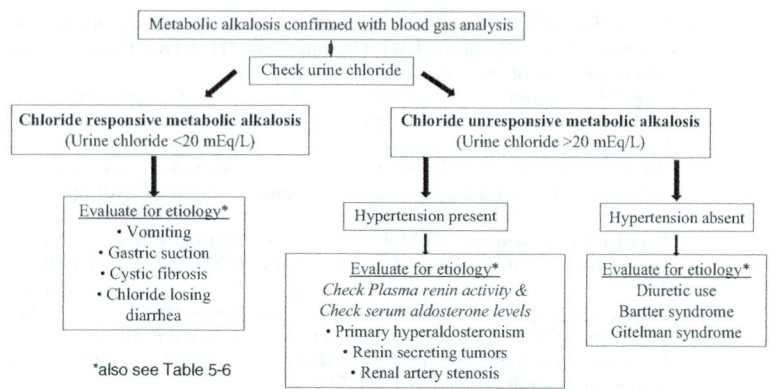

Figure 5-2. Approach to metabolic alkalosis.

is categorized as chloride resistant (aka saline resistant). The overall approach to metabolic alkalosis is shown in Figure 5-2 and the common causes of metabolic alkalosis are listed in Table 5-6.

There are two main reasons to consider urgent treatment of a metabolic alkalosis:

1. Cardiac arrhythmias—Alkalosis increases sensitivity to catecholamines and may precipitate life-threatening arrhythmias.

TABLE 5-6	Causes of Metabolic Alkalosis
Chloride-Depletion Type	
Gastric acid loss	
Vomiting	
Nasogastric suction	
Renal chloride loss	
Remote diuretic use	
Posthypercapnia	
Cystic fibrosis	
Chloride-Repletion Type	
With hypertension	
Primary hyperaldosteronism	
Renal artery stenosis	
Cushing syndrome	
Licorice excess (apparent mineralocorticoid excess)	
Without hypertension	
Bartter syndrome	
Gitelman syndrome	
Severe hypokalemia	

2. **Hypocalcemia**—Calcium circulates in two forms: free and active ionized calcium and "bound" which refers primarily to calcium bound to albumin. Alkalosis increases the binding of free calcium to albumin, thereby lowering plasma ionized calcium concentration. This may increase neuromuscular irritability.

In these scenarios, options for treatment include adjustment of mechanical ventilation to decrease the pH and use of acetazolamide in certain patients to increase renal excretion of bicarbonate. However, in most scenarios, the treatment of metabolic alkalosis involves treatment of the underlying cause alone. In chloride-responsive metabolic alkalosis, use of chloride-rich fluids like normal saline usually corrects the acid–base disorder. The treatment of chloride-resistant metabolic alkalosis requires identification of the specific etiology. Use of a mineralocorticoid receptor antagonist for primary hyperaldosteronism or surgical removal of aldosterone-secreting adenomas is an example of such treatment. Since metabolic alkalosis is often associated with hypokalemia, potassium supplementation may be needed.

E. Respiratory Acidosis. Respiratory acidosis can occur due to problems in any of the following: (1) decreased respiratory drive—due to sedatives, obesity, hypoventilation syndrome; (2) respiratory muscle weakness for example, due to severe hypokalemia or hypophosphatemia, Guillain–Barré syndrome; (3) airway obstruction; (4) impaired gas exchange—pneumonia, acute lung injury; and (5) chest wall disorders causing a restriction in respiratory drive. Increased CO_2 production by itself (e.g., due to fever, increased metabolic production) can be compensated by increased respiratory drive and doesn't lead to clinical consequences in the absence of one of the above problems. If the respiratory acidosis is severe, it can manifest as headaches, decreased arousal/sleepiness (aka CO_2 narcosis), and can lead to high intracranial pressure, cardiac arrhythmias, and hypotension from peripheral vasodilatation.

Acute respiratory acidosis leads to buffering of the hydrogen ions by nonbicarbonate buffers, for example, proteins in the blood. However, if the respiratory acidosis persists, the kidneys respond by increasing their excretion of hydrogen ions causing a compensatory metabolic alkalosis. This compensation is limited by the increased filtered load of bicarbonate that results in and leads to a partial renal compensation with elevated serum bicarbonate. Complete renal adaptation takes 3 to 5 days.

The treatment of respiratory acidosis usually requires identification and treatment of the underlying cause. Evaluation of the partial pressure of arterial oxygen (PaO_2) relative to ventilation, with the alveolar–arterial oxygen-tension difference may distinguish pulmonary from extrapulmonary diseases. In some situations, noninvasive or invasive mechanical ventilation may be needed till the underlying pathology improves.

F. Respiratory Alkalosis. Primary respiratory alkalosis is usually due to hyperventilation (breathing too fast or too deep or both). Hyperventilation can occur due to pulmonary diseases, hypoxemia, voluntary, mechanical ventilation, and miscellaneous causes that directly simulate the respiratory center such as fever, liver disease, pregnancy, head injuries, and salicylate toxicity. Respiratory alkalosis is usually associated with a small decrease in serum potassium and in serum phosphorus (latter may be large). It can manifest as paresthesias, carpopedal spasms, and can lead to decreased intracranial pressure, and cardiac arrhythmias.

Chronic respiratory alkalosis is compensated by the kidneys by the development of a metabolic acidosis to attempt to normalize the pH. This involves a decrease in hydrogen ion secretion by the kidneys in the distal tubule and the full compensatory effect takes 3 to 5 days also.

The treatment of respiratory alkalosis usually involves treatment of the underlying cause. If alkalemia is severe (pH >7.55), then depressing ventilation with a sedative could be considered to prevent arrhythmias or tetany.

In summary, a careful approach to identification of an acid–base disorder can be used to identify and characterize a variety of clinical disorders. It is an essential tool in both the diagnosis and management of patients with these disorders.

SUGGESTED READINGS

Achanti A, Szerlip HM. Acid-base disorders in the critically ill patient. *Clin J Am Soc Nephrol.* 2023;18(1):102–112.

Batlle DC, Hizon M, Cohen E, Gupta R. The use of the urinary anion gap in the diagnosis of hyperchloremic metabolic acidosis. *N Engl J Med.* 1988;318:594–599.

Berend K, de Vries AP, Gans RO. Physiological approach to assessment of acid-base disturbances. *N Engl J Med.* 2014;371(15):1434–1445.

Emmett M. Metabolic alkalosis: a brief pathophysiologic review. *Clin J Am Soc Nephrol.* 2020;15(12):1848–1856.

Fenves AZ, Emmett M. Approach to patients with high anion gap metabolic acidosis: core curriculum 2021. *Am J Kidney Dis.* 2021;78(4):590–600.

Hamm LL, Nakhoul N, Hering-Smith KS. Acid-base homeostasis. *Clin J Am Soc Nephrol.* 2015;10(12):2232–2242.

Kraut JA, Kurtz I. Toxic alcohol ingestions: clinical features, diagnosis, and management. *Clin J Am Soc Nephrol.* 2008;3:208–225.

Luke RG, Galla JH. It is chloride depletion alkalosis, not contraction alkalosis. *J Am Soc Nephrol.* 2012;23:204–207.

Palmer BF, Clegg DJ. Electrolyte and acid-base disturbances in patients with diabetes mellitus. *N Engl J Med.* 2015;373(6):548–559.

Palmer BF, Clegg DJ. Respiratory acidosis and respiratory alkalosis: core curriculum 2023. *Am J Kidney Dis.* 2023;82(3):347–359.

Rastegar A. Use of the DeltaAG/Delta HCO_3^- in the diagnosis of mixed acid–base disorders. *J Am Soc Nephrol.* 2007;18:2429–2431.

Uribarri J, Goldfarb DS, Raphael KL, Rein JL, Asplin JR. Beyond the urine anion gap: in support of the direct measurement of urinary ammonium. *Am J Kidney Dis.* 2022;80(5):667–676.

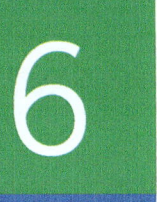

The Patient With Hypocalcemia or Hypercalcemia

Mohamed Hassanein, Edgar V. Lerma

I. Background

Calcium is an important, divalent cation (Ca^{+2}) that is essential for many vital functions of the body, including bone mineralization, blood coagulation, intracellular signaling, neuromuscular conduction, and muscle contraction. Most calcium in the body is in the form of hydroxyapatite in bone (99%). Although a small fraction of total body calcium is contained in the extracellular fluid (ECF), only the concentration of ionized calcium (~50%) in the ECF is physiologically active and regulated. Approximately 60% of calcium in the ECF is ultrafilterable by the kidney and exists either free in solution as biologically active ionized calcium (50%) or complexed to anions such as citrate, phosphate, sulfate, and bicarbonate (10%). The remaining 40% is bound to proteins (primarily albumin). Serum or plasma calcium concentration is measured as either total or ionized calcium (Fig. 6-1).

Total calcium varies with albumin level and blood pH. Since 40% of calcium is primarily albumin-bound, total calcium should be adjusted for the serum albumin level using the equation below:

$$\text{Adjusted (Corrected) total } Ca^{+2} \text{ (mg/dL)} = \text{Measured serum } Ca^{+2} \text{ (mg/dL)} + 0.8 \times (4 - \text{serum albumin in g/dL})$$

For example, if the measured serum Ca^{+2} is 7.2 and the serum albumin is 2 g/dL, the adjusted (corrected) total $Ca^{+2} = 7.2 + 0.8 (4 - 2) = 8.8$ mg/dL which is normal. When in doubt, one must always measure ionized calcium to confirm the diagnosis of hypercalcemia or hypocalcemia.

The formula above, known as "Payne formula," was developed using the bromocresol green (BCG) method for albumin measurement. BCG binds to other proteins besides albumin, thus overestimating the albumin level. Nowadays, laboratories use the bromocresol purple (BCP) method to measure albumin, which yields less accurate results when incorporated into Payne formula. Additionally, Payne formula assumes a steady relationship between albumin and calcium binding, which does not always occur. Thus, the albumin-corrected calcium using this formula might not be reflective of the true calcium level, especially in critically ill patients, those with kidney failure, or those with primary hyperparathyroidism.

Measuring the free ionized calcium is more accurate than the albumin-corrected calcium as it reflects the concentration of biologically active calcium. Free ionized calcium is regulated by pH. In an alkaline environment, proteins including albumin become more negatively charged, facilitating the binding of ionized calcium with proteins, leading to decreased ionized calcium. On the contrary, acidemia leads to decreased protein binding, increasing ionized calcium levels.

Total calcium concentration normally ranges between 8.8 and 10.4 mg/dL (4.4 to 5.2 mEq/L or 2.2 to 2.6 mmol/L). Ionized calcium is roughly half the total calcium. Total calcium is measured with a colorimetric assay and includes ionized, complexed, and bound calcium. Ionized calcium concentration is measured with a calcium-specific electrode and represents physiologically regulated calcium. Both total and ionized calcium can be expressed in conventional units of mg per dL or

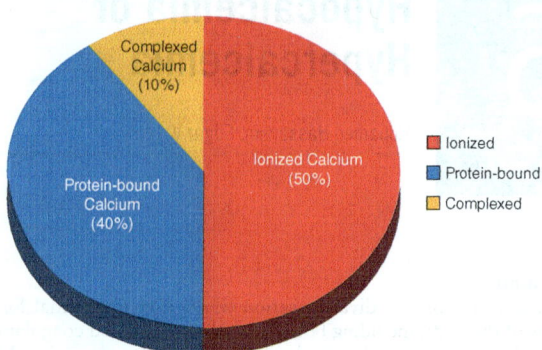

Figure 6-1. Pie chart depicting the distribution of calcium in the blood. Fifty percent of calcium exists as free or "ionized" calcium. This portion plays an important role in calcium homeostasis through feedback mechanisms. Forty percent of calcium is protein bound (primarily albumin) and is pH dependent. Ten percent of calcium is complexed with anions such as sulfate, bicarbonate, citrate, and phosphate. Serum calcium is measured as total or ionized calcium.

mEq per L or in International System (SI) of units of mmol per L. SI units (mmol per L) can be converted to mg per dL by multiplying by 4 (multiplying by 40—the atomic weight of calcium—and dividing by 10). Measuring total calcium levels is inexpensive and convenient. A determination of the ionized calcium concentration requires that the sample be placed on ice and measured within 2 hours, making it difficult for routine use, especially in the outpatient setting.

The total body calcium ranges between 1,000 and 1,200 g, with 99% residing in the bone and 1% residing in the intracellular and extracellular space. About 1% of calcium is freely exchangeable between the bone and extracellular space. Figure 6-2 illustrates the calcium fluxes between the ECF, intestine, kidney, and bone. Net intestinal calcium absorption amounts to approximately 200 mg of the normal dietary intake of 800 to 1,000 mg. In the steady state, this net intestinal absorption is matched by urinary excretion. As a result, 10,600 mg of the approximately 10,800 mg (98%) of calcium that is filtered by the glomerulus daily is reabsorbed by the kidney tubules.

II. Calcium regulation

Plasma-ionized calcium is regulated through a complex and coordinated interplay of parathyroid hormone (PTH) and $1,25(OH)_2$ vitamin D_3 (calcitriol) in the intestine, bone, and kidney. The parathyroid gland senses ECF-ionized calcium concentration through a calcium-sensing receptor (CaSR). High concentrations of ECF calcium stimulate the receptor and activate second messenger pathways that, in turn, inhibit PTH release. Low ECF calcium concentration stimulates PTH secretion and production and increases parathyroid gland mass. The parathyroid gland responds quickly (within minutes) to alterations in ionized calcium concentration. An inverse sigmoid relationship exists between ECF calcium concentration and PTH secretion, with a nonsuppressible component present even at high plasma calcium concentrations. The amount of hormone stored is enough to support basal secretion for 6 hours and stimulated secretion for 2 hours.

In bone, PTH in the presence of permissive amounts of calcitriol stimulates reabsorption by increasing osteoclast number and activity. In the intestine, PTH enhances calcium and phosphate absorption indirectly by promoting the formation of calcitriol. In the kidney, PTH augments distal tubular calcium reabsorption, stimulates calcitriol formation in the proximal tubule, and decreases proximal tubular phosphate and bicarbonate reabsorption.

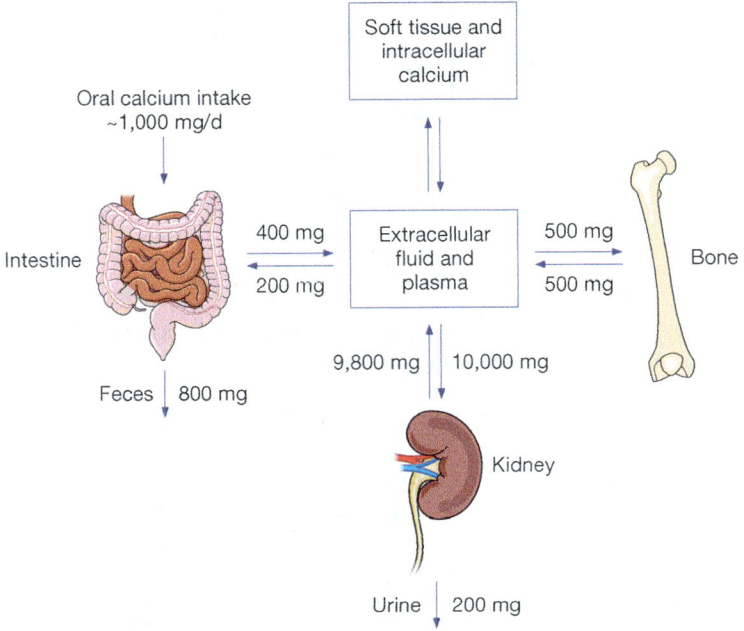

Figure 6-2. Calcium homeostasis between the intestine, extracellular fluid, bone, and kidneys. Adapted with permission from Blaine J, Chonchol M, Levi M. Renal control of calcium, phosphate, and magnesium homeostasis [published correction appears in *Clin J Am Soc Nephrol*. 2015;10(10):1886–1887. doi:10.2215/CJN.08840815]. *Clin J Am Soc Nephrol*. 2015;10(7):1257–1272. doi:10.2215/CJN.09750913

Vitamin D, known as calciferol, is a fat-soluble vitamin that can be produced by the skin. Vitamin D_2 (ergocalciferol) and Vitamin D_3 (cholecalciferol) are synthesized commercially as plant-based and animal-based calciferols, respectively, and are used to supplement vitamin D in humans. Once absorbed, vitamin D is activated in the liver by the 25-hydroxylase enzyme forming 25-hydroxy vitamin D (25-OH vitamin D) which is also known as calcidiol. Calcitriol is produced in the proximal tubule through 1α-hydroxylation of 25-OH vitamin D_3 (calcidiol). The calcitriol biosynthetic pathway is illustrated in Figure 6-3. Principal stimulators of 1α-hydroxylase are PTH and hypophosphatemia. The major function of calcitriol is to enhance calcium and phosphate availability for new bone formation and prevention of symptomatic hypocalcemia and hypophosphatemia. In the intestine and kidney, calcitriol increases the production of calcium-binding proteins (calbindins) that aid in transcellular calcium movement. In bone, calcitriol potentiates PTH actions, stimulates osteoclastic reabsorption, and induces differentiation of monocytes into osteoclasts.

In the parathyroid gland, calcitriol binds to its receptor, leading to a decrease in PTH production. The *PTH* gene promoter contains regions that bind the calcitriol receptor. Binding results in a dramatic decrease in PTH expression. Calcitriol is the most potent suppressor of *PTH* gene transcription.

Approximately 10 g of calcium is filtered through the kidney with only 1% to 2% (<200 mg) excreted daily. Kidney regulation of calcium varies by nephron segment. Up to 70% of filtered calcium is reabsorbed in the proximal convoluted

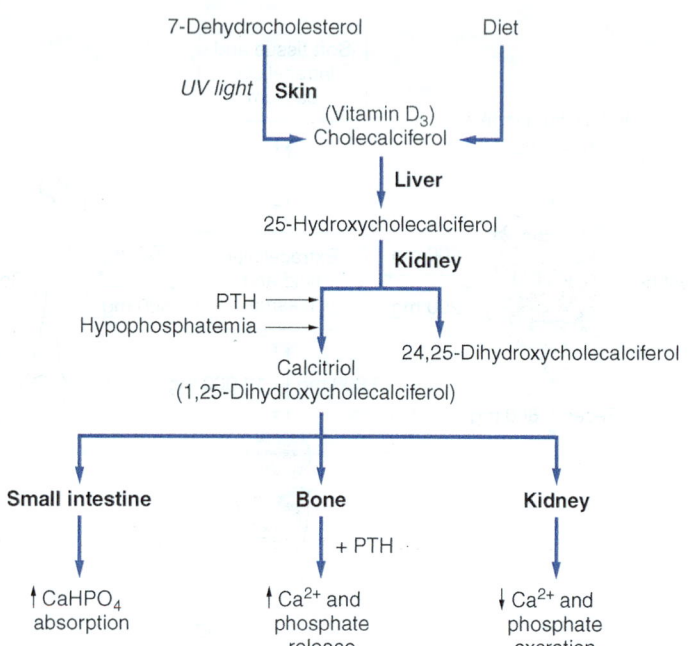

Figure 6-3. Vitamin D metabolism. Adapted with permission from Rennke HG, Denker BM. *Renal Pathophysiology The Essentials*. 5th ed. Wolters Kluwer, 2020.

tubules, followed by 20% in the loop of Henle, 10% in the distal tubule, and 5% in the collecting duct.

In the proximal tubule, most of the calcium is reabsorbed by passive, paracellular diffusion following sodium and water reabsorption. A small portion is absorbed intracellularly through an active transport process regulated by PTH and calcitonin. In the thick ascending limb of the loop of Henle, 20% of filtered calcium is reabsorbed by both paracellular and intracellular routes. Paracellular transport is stimulated by the driving force generated by the $Na^+-K^+-2Cl^-$ apical cotransporter and renal outer medullary potassium (ROMK) channels. CaSRs also exist on the basolateral membrane of the thick ascending limb of the loop of Henle. Activation of CaSR, as with the calcimimetic cinacalcet decreases the paracellular permeability of calcium in the ascending loop of Henle leading to calcium loss. The remainder of calcium reabsorption occurs in the distal tubule solely via a transcellular route using an active transport process powered by basolateral calcium and sodium-potassium ATPases. Inhibition of the luminal sodium chloride (NaCl) cotransporter as with thiazide use indirectly increases calcium reabsorption in the distal tubule. Figure 6-4 outlines the reabsorption of calcium in the nephrons.

III. Hypocalcemia
  A. **Etiology.** True hypocalcemia is the result of decreased calcium absorption from the gastrointestinal tract or decreased calcium resorption from bone. Given that 98% of total body calcium is contained within the skeleton, sustained hypocalcemia cannot occur without an abnormality of either PTH or calcitriol action in bone.

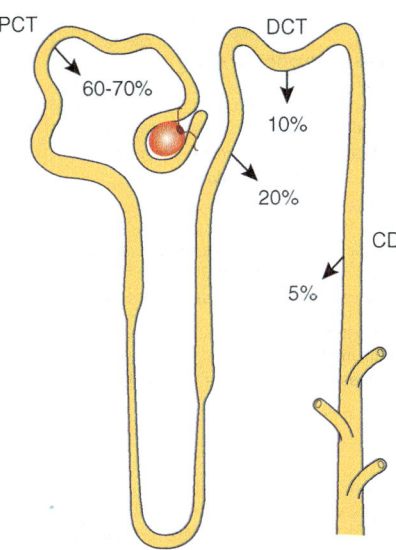

Figure 6-4. Reabsorption of calcium along different segments of the nephron. Ca, calcium; DCT, distal convoluted tubule; PCT, proximal convoluted tubule; TAL, thick ascending limb of loop of Henle. (Adapted with permission from Blaine J, Chonchol M, Levi M. Renal control of calcium, phosphate, and magnesium homeostasis [published correction appears in *Clin J Am Soc Nephrol*. 2015;10(10):1886–1887. doi:10.2215/CJN.08840815]. *Clin J Am Soc Nephrol*. 2015;10(7):1257–1272. doi:10.2215/CJN.09750913)

As noted earlier, total plasma calcium is composed of three components: ionized calcium (50%); complexed calcium (10%); and protein-bound calcium (40%). True hypocalcemia is present only when ionized calcium concentration is reduced. The reference range for ionized calcium concentration is 4.2 to 5.0 mg/dL (1.05 to 1.25 mmol/L). Therefore, whenever a low total serum calcium concentration is observed, this value must be compared with the serum albumin concentration. For every decrease of 1 g/dL in serum albumin concentration from its normal concentration of 4 g/dL, a decrease of 0.8 mg/dL in total serum calcium concentration can be expected. Therefore, for each fall of 1 g/dL in serum albumin concentration, 0.8 mg/dL must be added to total serum calcium concentration. This correction factor was shown to be unreliable in patients with critical illness as indicated previously. It is also unreliable in patients with CKD due to errors in albumin measurement using the BCG or BCP methods. If clinical suspicion warrants, ionized calcium concentration should be measured. Calcium binding to albumin is affected by ECF pH. Acidemia increases and alkalemia decreases ionized calcium concentration. Ionized calcium concentration increases by approximately 0.2 mg/dL for each 0.1 decrease in pH. These correction factors are only general guidelines and should not be used as a substitute for the direct measurement of serum ionized calcium concentration if clinical suspicion warrants.

True hypocalcemia is caused by decreased PTH secretion, end-organ resistance to PTH, or disorders of vitamin D metabolism. Occasionally, hypocalcemia occurs acutely as a result of either extravascular calcium deposition or intravascular calcium binding. The most common etiologies of true hypocalcemia are illustrated in Table 6-1.

TABLE 6-1	Causes of Hypocalcemia

I. Hypoparathyroidism (Decreased PTH production)
- Autoimmune (Polyglandular autoimmune syndrome type I)
- **Surgical excision of parathyroid glands ± HBS**
- Neck irradiation
- Thyroid surgery
- Infiltrative disorders: Hemochromatosis, HIV, Wilson disease
- Parathyroid hypoplasia (developmental abnormality), for example, DiGeorge syndrome
- ^aSevere hypomagnesemia (can decrease PTH secretion)

II. End-organ resistance to PTH (PTH elevated)
- Pseudohypoparathyroidism
- ^aSevere hypomagnesemia (can induce PTH resistance)

III. Vitamin D deficiency or defects in metabolism
- Vitamin D deficiency
- Malabsorption
- Drugs such as phenytoin (inactivates vitamin D)
- Liver disease (decreases 25-hydroxylation of vitamin D)
- Chronic kidney disease (decreases 1 alpha hydroxylation of 25-hydroxy vitamin D)
- Vitamin D–dependent rickets (VDRR) due to genetic mutations
  - Type 1 (genetic inability to 1-alpha hydroxylase calcidiol)
  - Type 2 (end-organ resistance to vitamin D)

IV. Calcium depletion due to increased calcium uptake or binding
- Acute pancreatitis (binding of calcium during saponification)
- Hyperphosphatemia (binding of calcium to phosphorus)
  - Tumor lysis syndrome
  - Chronic kidney disease
  - Sepsis
  - Toxic shock syndrome
- Osteoblastic metastasis (increased uptake of calcium by bone)
- Calcium chelators
  - Citrate
  - EDTA
- Gadolinium-based contrasts such as gadopentetate dimeglumine and gadodiamide)
- Other drugs: Foscarnet (binds to ionized calcium)

EDTA, ethylenediaminetetraacetic acid; HBS, hungry bone syndrome; HIV, human immunodeficiency virus; PTH, parathyroid hormone.
^aCisplatin can cause hypomagnesemia.

1. **Hypoparathyroidism** is caused by a wide variety of acquired and inherited diseases that result from impaired PTH synthesis and release or from peripheral tissue resistance to PTH.
    a. The most common autoimmune cause of hypoparathyroidism is **polyglandular autoimmune syndrome type I,** characterized by chronic mucocutaneous candidiasis and primary adrenal insufficiency. Other conditions that have been described to be associated with it include pernicious anemia, diabetes mellitus, vitiligo and autoimmune thyroid disease. Mucocutaneous candidiasis often presents first in early childhood and is followed several years later by hypoparathyroidism. Adrenal insufficiency appears in adolescence. The combination of

hypoparathyroidism, adrenal insufficiency, and mucocutaneous candidiasis was previously referred to as *hypoparathyroidism, adrenal insufficiency, and mucocutaneous candidiasis (HAM) syndrome*. Mutations in the autoimmune regulator (AIRE) gene, a transcription factor, were shown to cause the disease.
  b. **Familial hypocalcemia** results from activating mutations in the CaSR that increase its sensitivity to calcium.
  c. **Parathyroid and radical neck surgery or irradiation** can result in a loss of glandular tissue. In a small percentage of patients, hypocalcemia is permanent. Risk factors for the development of permanent hypocalcemia include removal of three or more parathyroid glands; postoperative PTH concentration ≤12 pg/mL; total serum calcium concentration ≤8 mg/dL after 1 week of oral calcium supplementation; and serum phosphorus concentration ≤4 mg/dL after 1 week of calcium supplementation. Surgical removal of parathyroid tissue in secondary or tertiary hyperparathyroidism in patients on dialysis is often complicated by severe hypocalcemia due to remineralization of bone, the so-called **hungry bone syndrome (HBS)**.

  HBS results from parathyroid or thyroid surgery in patients with primary, secondary, or tertiary hyperparathyroidism who have been exposed to prolonged PTH-induced bone resorption and turnover states. Following parathyroidectomy, bones suddenly shift to a marked osteoblastic activity leading to severe life-threatening hypocalcemia. Risk factors for HBS include elevated PTH, alkaline phosphatase, elevated body mass index, large volume of parathyroid excision, and radiologic evidence of bone disease. Patients usually require hospitalization for intravenous calcium infusion after the parathyroidectomy. After discharge, they may require high doses of calcitriol and oral calcium supplements. Remnant parathyroid tissue is usually left in the neck or autotransplanted in the sternocleidomastoid or a forearm muscle. If inadequate tissue is left behind or the transplanted parathyroid tissue does not survive, the patient may be left with permanent hypoparathyroidism and hypocalcemia.
  d. Hypocalcemia also occurs after **thyroid surgery** (5% of cases).
  e. Transient hypoparathyroidism may occur after the **removal of a parathyroid adenoma** due to suppression of remaining parathyroid tissue.
  f. **Infiltrative disorders** such as hemochromatosis, Wilson disease, and infection with human immunodeficiency virus (HIV) can also decrease PTH secretion.
  g. **Severe hypomagnesemia** can result in end-organ resistance to PTH and a decrease in PTH secretion. Patients with hypocalcemia as a result of hypomagnesemia do not respond to calcium or vitamin D replacement until the magnesium deficit is replaced.
  h. **Poor development of the parathyroid glands** can result from genetic defects and congenital syndromes associated with parathyroid hypoplasia such as DiGeorge syndrome.
2. A variety of rare genetic disorders cause **end-organ resistance to PTH**, including pseudohypoparathyroidism types I and II. Patients with pseudohypoparathyroidism are classified based on the response of nephrogenous cyclic adenosine monophosphate to PTH administration. A decreased response is indicative of type I and a normal response is indicative of type II.
3. **Defects in vitamin D metabolism** also cause hypocalcemia. Etiologies include decreased intake of vitamin D, malabsorption, drugs, liver disease, CKD, and vitamin D–dependent rickets. Nutritional vitamin D deficiency is uncommon in the United States as a result of the supplementation of milk and other food products. It can occur, however, in poorly nourished

patients with little sun exposure. Groups that were shown to be at high risk include the institutionalized elderly, postmenopausal women, and adolescents. Because vitamin D is fat-soluble, vitamin D deficiency can be seen in gastrointestinal malabsorption from any cause. Patients with chronic biliary drainage from a cholecystostomy are at risk for developing deficiencies of vitamins D, A, E, and K. Anticonvulsants such as **Phenytoin** induce hypocalcemia through a variety of mechanisms including induction of the P-450 system with increased metabolism of vitamin D, inhibition of bone resorption, impaired calcium absorption from the gastrointestinal tract, and peripheral resistance to PTH action. This generally occurs in patients with additional predisposing factors, such as poor nutrition and decreased sun exposure. **Phenobarbital** enhances the hepatic metabolism of vitamin D and calcidiol. Vitamin D deficiency can result from hepatocellular disease if the disease is severe enough to impair 25-hydroxylation of vitamin D to calcidiol. CKD impairs the 1α-hydroxylation of calcidiol to calcitriol. **Vitamin D–dependent rickets** is a result of either impaired hydroxylation of calcidiol to calcitriol (type I) or end-organ resistance to calcitriol (type II). Patients with type 1 respond to physiologic calcitriol doses. Patients with type II disease have dramatically increased calcitriol concentrations, respond poorly to calcitriol therapy, and have mutations in the vitamin D receptor.

4. **Less common causes** of hypocalcemia include **tumor lysis syndrome, osteoblastic metastases, acute pancreatitis, toxic shock syndrome, and sepsis**. The acute addition or release of phosphate into the extracellular space may cause hypocalcemia through a variety of mechanisms. Calcium and phosphate may precipitate in tissues, although the exact tissue in which the deposition occurs has never been identified. In addition, phosphate infusion increases the rate of bone formation and inhibits PTH-induced bone resorption; both of these processes act to decrease serum calcium concentration.

5. **Drugs and contrast agents** can also cause hypocalcemia and include calcium chelators such as citrate anticoagulation during continuous kidney replacement therapy and ethylenediaminetetraacetic acid (EDTA) added to specimen tubes which bind calcium and cause hypocalcemia. Other drugs that cause hypocalcemia include bisphosphonates and denosumab (decrease bone resorption), cinacalcet (downregulates PTH production), chemotherapeutic agents such as cisplatin (can cause hypomagnesemia), and foscarnet (binds to ionized calcium).

Gadolinium-containing chelates (gadopentetate dimeglumine and gadodiamide) used as contrast agents for magnetic resonance imaging may falsely lower serum calcium concentration. The effect persists for only 3 to 6 hours in those with normal kidney function but can result in the spurious lowering of serum calcium concentration by up to 3 mg/dL or more. However, in patients with severe kidney dysfunction, serum calcium concentration may remain low for up to 4 days. This is an important entity to be aware of because in many reported cases patients were treated with intravenous calcium for the spuriously low serum calcium concentration.

B. **Signs and symptoms** of hypocalcemia depend not only on the degree of hypocalcemia but also on the rate of decline of serum calcium concentration. The threshold at which symptoms develop also depends on serum pH and whether concomitant hypomagnesemia, hypokalemia, or hyponatremia is present. Symptoms of neuromuscular excitability predominate. The patient may complain of circumoral and distal extremity paresthesias or carpopedal spasm. Central nervous system manifestations include mental status changes, irritability, and seizures. On physical examination, hypotension, bradycardia, laryngeal spasm, and bronchospasm may be present. Chvostek and Trousseau signs should be checked. Chvostek sign is a facial twitch elicited by tapping

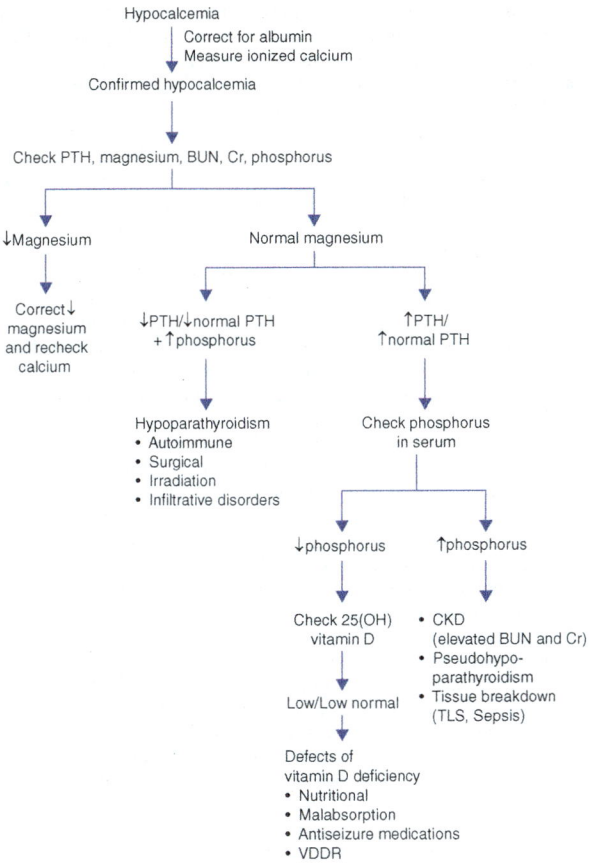

Figure 6-5. Algorithm for workup of hypocalcemia. 25-(OH) vitamin D, 25-hydroxy vitamin D; BUN, blood urea nitrogen; CKD, chronic kidney disease; Cr, creatinine; PTH, parathyroid hormone; TLS, tumor lysis syndrome; VDDR, vitamin D–dependent rickets.

on the facial nerve just below the zygomatic arch with the mouth slightly open. A positive sign is occasionally observed in normal patients. Trousseau sign is the development of wrist flexion, metacarpophalangeal joint flexion, hyperextended fingers, and thumb flexion after a sphygmomanometer cuff is inflated around the arm to 20 mmHg above systolic pressure for 3 minutes. Hypocalcemia can also prolong the QT interval and cause ventricular and atrial arrhythmias and impair myocardial contractility.

C. Diagnosis. The differential diagnosis of true hypocalcemia is often straightforward, and a diagnostic algorithm is shown in Figure 6-5. The most common causes are magnesium deficiency, CKD, and complications of parathyroid surgery. Initial evaluation includes a history and physical examination and thorough clinical assessment. Medications should be reviewed.

1. The first step in the evaluation of the patient with a decreased total serum calcium concentration is to **examine the serum albumin concentration** and,

if necessary, measure ionized serum calcium concentration. If true hypocalcemia is documented, then blood analysis should be obtained for PTH, magnesium, blood urea nitrogen (BUN), creatinine, and phosphorus concentration.
   a. If magnesium is low, then a diagnosis of hypomagnesemia is confirmed. Hypomagnesemia is the most common cause of hypocalcemia in hospitalized patients. A high index of suspicion should be present in patients with a history of steatorrhea, diarrhea, or chronic alcoholism. These patients generally have severe hypomagnesemia, and hypocalcemia will not correct until magnesium losses are replaced. It frequently requires several days for serum calcium concentration to correct after magnesium deficiency is reversed.
   b. **In the setting of normal magnesium, intact PTH concentration is used to guide diagnosis.** A reduced or low normal PTH in the setting of high phosphorus is suggestive of hypoparathyroidism. Differential diagnosis includes autoimmune hypoparathyroidism, postoperative hypoparathyroidism due to surgical removal (with or without HBS depending on risk factors and severity of hypocalcemia), or infiltrative disorders. If PTH is elevated or high normal with low phosphorus, check 25-hydroxy vitamin D levels. If low, then replace vitamin D and recheck calcium. If calcium and vitamin D do not normalize, further workup is warranted for malabsorption or vitamin D–dependent rickets.
   c. Hyperphosphatemia in the absence of CKD suggests a diagnosis of either hypoparathyroidism or pseudohypoparathyroidism. Measuring PTH concentration can differentiate these disorders. In primary hypoparathyroidism, PTH is low; in pseudohypoparathyroidism, PTH is increased. A decrease in serum phosphorus concentration indicates a defect in vitamin D metabolism. Hypocalcemia results in secondary hyperparathyroidism that, in turn, reduces proximal tubular phosphate reabsorption and results in phosphate wasting. Therefore, the fractional excretion (FE) of phosphate is expected to be high (more than 5%). In hypophosphatemia, the kidney has an extraordinary ability to conserve phosphate, and, in extrarenal disorders, the FE of phosphate is below 1%. If phosphaturia is noted, then calcidiol and calcitriol concentration should be measured. Calcidiol concentration is reduced with malabsorption, liver disease, and phenobarbital use. Calcitriol concentration is reduced in CKD and increased in type II vitamin D–dependent rickets.
D. Management of hypocalcemia is dependent on its severity and cause.

In an emergency situation in which hypocalcemia is suspected and seizures, tetany, hypotension, or cardiac arrhythmias are present, intravenous calcium should be administered (100 to 300 mg over 10 to 15 minutes) before results of the serum calcium concentration return from the clinical laboratory. Patients with symptomatic hypocalcemia or a total serum calcium concentration corrected for albumin of ≤7.5 mg/dL should be initially managed with parenteral calcium. Chronic, mild hypocalcemia, as seen in the outpatient setting, can be treated with oral calcium supplements, to which a vitamin D preparation may be added if necessary. Table 6-2 highlights the commonly used oral and intravenous calcium formulations in the United States.
   1. **Acute symptomatic hypocalcemia** is treated with intravenous calcium. In the absence of seizures, tetany, or cardiac arrhythmias, an infusion of 1.5 mg/kg of elemental calcium given over 4 to 6 hours raises the total serum calcium by 2 to 3 mg/dL. Calcium gluconate (10%) is supplied in 10 mL ampules and contains 94 mg of elemental calcium. The first ampule can be administered over several minutes, followed by a constant infusion begun at a rate of 0.5 to 1.0 mg/kg/hour, with rate adjustments based on serial determinations of serum calcium concentration. Treatment of

TABLE 6-2 Oral and Intravenous Calcium Formulations

Preparation	Elemental Calcium (mg)	Dose	Comments
Oral Calcium Formulations			
Calcium carbonate 500 mg tablets	200	1–2 g of elemental calcium divided into 2–3 daily doses. Up titrate to maintain low normal calcium.	H2 receptor blockers and PPI decrease absorption of calcium carbonate.
Calcium citrate 950 mg	200	1–2 g of elemental calcium divided into 2–3 daily doses. Up titrate to maintain low normal calcium.	Use in patients with achlorhydria, malabsorption, IBD, and those on PPI or H2 receptor blockers.
Calcium acetate	169	Mainly used as a phosphate binder in patients with kidney failure.	May bind to tetracyclines or fluoroquinolones thus decreasing their bioavailability.
IV Calcium Formulations			
Calcium gluconate 1,000 mg	93	Initial bolus: 1–2 g in 50 mL NS/D5W. Infuse over 10–20 min. Continuous infusion: 11 g (110 mL of 10% solution) in 890 mL NS or D5W infused at 50 mL/h.	Mainly used IV in repleting calcium inpatient. Preferred over calcium chloride as it is less irritant if extravasated.
IV Calcium chloride 1,000 mg	273	Initial bolus: 1 g in 100 mL NS or D5W, infuse into **a central or large vein** over 10–20 min. Continuous infusion: 4 g (40 mL of a 10% solution) in 960 mL NS or D5W. Infuse at 50 mL/h **into a central or large vein.**	Causes tissue necrosis if extravasated, thus must be given into a central or large vein.

H2 receptor blockers, histamine 2 receptor blockers; D5W, dextrose 5% in water; IBD, inflammatory bowel disease; IV, intravenous; NS, normal saline; PPI, proton pump inhibitors.

hypocalcemia is ineffective in the presence of hypomagnesemia. In the setting of metabolic acidosis, hypocalcemia should be corrected before acidosis is reversed because excess protons in acidemia bind albumin in place of calcium, increasing ionized calcium concentration.

Patients with **hypoparathyroidism** are managed with calcium and vitamin D supplements. Serum calcium concentration should be maintained at the lower limit of normal. Oral elemental calcium, 1 to 2 g/d, is usually sufficient. A variety of oral calcium preparations are available, some of which are shown in Table 6-2. Calcium is best absorbed when taken between meals because an acidic environment improves calcium absorption. Proton pump inhibitors (PPIs) are associated with decreased calcium absorption and osteoporosis. Calcium citrate is more soluble than calcium carbonate, especially in patients who require H_2 blockers or PPIs. In the presence of severe hyperphosphatemia, calcium supplementation should be delayed, if possible, until the serum phosphorus concentration is reduced below 6 mg/dL using non–calcium-containing phosphate binders. Severe hypocalcemia, however, may need to be treated despite hyperphosphatemia and clinical judgment must be used.

2. Calcitriol is the most potent of the **vitamin D preparations** and has the fastest onset and shortest duration of action, but is also the most expensive. A dose of 0.5 to 1.0 µg/d is usually required. As one moves back up the metabolic pathway to calcidiol, cholecalciferol, and ergocalciferol, cost decreases and duration of action increases. These agents, however, may be less efficacious in the presence of kidney or liver disease. Patients with hypoparathyroidism have decreased distal tubular calcium reabsorption as a result of a lack of PTH. Therefore, the increase in filtered calcium load that results from calcium and vitamin D replacement can lead to hypercalciuria, nephrolithiasis, and nephrocalcinosis. If urinary calcium excretion exceeds 350 mg/d despite a low serum calcium concentration, sodium intake should be restricted; if this is not effective, a thiazide diuretic should be added. The primary goal of treatment should be the elimination of symptoms and not necessarily the normalization of serum calcium concentration.

3. **Active vitamin D analogs** are currently being used in the US for the management of secondary hyperparathyroidism in patients on dialysis. **Doxercalciferol or paricalcitol** can be given both orally and intravenously three times weekly at the end of dialysis. Currently, there is no evidence to support their use in patients with CKD who are not on dialysis.

IV. Hypercalcemia
   A. **Etiology.** Hypercalcemia is generally divided into PTH-mediated and non–PTH-mediated hypercalcemia (Table 6-3).
   1. PTH-Mediated Hypercalcemia.
      a. Hyperparathyroidism
         i. Primary
            Primary hyperparathyroidism is a common cause of hypercalcemia. The estimated incidence ranges from 0.4 to 26 per 100,000 patient-years. The underlying pathology is most often a solitary adenoma (80%). Among the remainder, 15% to 20% have diffuse hyperplasia, and approximately one-half of these have a familial syndrome (multiple endocrine neoplasia [MEN] type 1, associated with pituitary adenomas and islet cell tumors, or MEN type II, associated with medullary carcinoma of the thyroid and pheochromocytoma). Multiple adenomas are uncommon, and parathyroid carcinoma is rare (occurring in less than 1%). Hypercalcemia results from increased calcium resorption from bone, increased intestinal calcium absorption mediated by calcitriol, and increased distal tubular kidney calcium reabsorption. In primary hyperparathyroidism, hypercalcemia is often mild, asymptomatic, and identified on routine blood chemistries in the outpatient setting.
         ii. **Secondary**
            Secondary hyperparathyroidism is seen in patients with CKD or patients with end-stage kidney disease (ESKD) on dialysis. Uremia causes PTH resistance and requires a higher PTH level than normal. Decreased production of $1,25(OH)_2$ vitamin D_3 by the kidney results in less PTH suppression, as well as hypocalcemia that

TABLE 6-3	Causes of Hypercalcemia

I. Parathyroid Hormone Mediated
- Primary and tertiary hyperparathyroidism
- FHH
- Jansen-type metaphyseal chondroplasia
- Lithium use

II. Nonparathyroid Hormone Mediated
  A. Increased absorption by the GIT
  - Milk-alkali syndrome
  - Vitamin D intoxication
  - CKD with increased ingestion of calcium
  - Increased 1,25-OH vitamin D production (granulomatous diseases such as sarcoidosis, TB, histoplasmosis, Crohn's disease, or hematologic malignancies such as lymphomas)

  B. Increased bone resorption
  - Malignancy including multiple myeloma and pheochromocytoma (HHM, PTHrP-mediated hypercalcemia)
  - Immobilization
  - Hyperthyroidism
  - Hypervitaminosis A

  C. Decreased excretion by the kidney
  - Thiazides
  - Adrenal insufficiency
  - Acute kidney injury
  - Bartter syndrome

FHH, familial hypocalcuric hypercalcemia; GIT, gastrointestinal tract; HHM, humoral hypercalcemia of malignancy; PTHrP, parathyroid hormone–related peptide; TB, Tuberculosis.

increases the half-life of PTH mRNA. Reduced phosphorus excretion by the kidneys results in hyperphosphatemia and also increases the half-life of PTH mRNA.

iii. **Tertiary**

Tertiary hyperparathyroidism is a result of prolonged stimulation of the parathyroid gland from secondary hyperparathyroidism in ESKD. The patient will have hypercalcemia instead of hypocalcemia as a result of parathyroid gland hyperplasia. It can also be seen after kidney transplantation when plasma phosphorus concentration, vitamin D metabolism, and kidney function improve, but PTH secretion remains high, secondary to increased parathyroid mass. In most patients, PTH levels drop, and hypercalcemia resolves during the first year following transplantation.

b. **Familial Hypocalcuric Hypercalcemia.** Familial hypocalcuric hypercalcemia (FHH) is an autosomal dominant disorder most commonly caused by a heterozygous inactivating mutation in the CaSR. It is rare with a prevalence of 1 in 78,000 in one study. Recently, mutations in two additional genes were reported to cause FHH, the G-protein subunit α_{11} and the S1 subunit of adaptor protein 2. The syndrome presents with mild hypercalcemia early in life, hypocalciuria, and a normal or slightly increased PTH concentration in the absence of signs or symptoms of hypercalcemia. As a result of the mutations, the CaSR is less sensitive to plasma calcium concentration, and a higher-than-normal calcium concentration is required to suppress PTH. One should be aware of FHH, because this condition is often misdiagnosed as primary hyperparathyroidism, and patients may be inappropriately subjected to neck exploration. FHH may account for a small percentage of patients who undergo surgery for primary hyperparathyroidism in whom no adenoma is found.

c. **Jansen-Type Metaphyseal Chondroplasia (Activating PTH1R Variant).** A rare genetic cause of hypercalcemia due to continuous activation of PTH—parathyroid hormone–related peptide (PTHrP) receptors with lower or normal levels of PTH due to a mutation affecting the receptor gene.

d. **Lithium.** Lithium causes parathyroid hyperplasia by increasing the threshold for hypercalcemia-induced PTH suppression.

2. **Non–PTH-Mediated Hypercalcemia.** Three basic pathophysiologic mechanisms contribute to non–PTH-mediated hypercalcemia: increased calcium absorption from the gastrointestinal tract, decreased kidney calcium excretion, and increased bone calcium resorption.

   a. **Increased calcium absorption from the gastrointestinal tract** plays a primary role in the hypercalcemia of the milk-alkali syndrome, vitamin D intoxication, and granulomatous disorders.

      i. **Milk-alkali syndrome** is the result of ingestion of excess calcium and alkali. In the past, peptic ulcer disease was treated with milk and sodium bicarbonate. This calcium and alkali source used to be the most common cause of the milk-alkali syndrome. This regimen was replaced with histamine antagonists and PPIs so that milk and sodium bicarbonate are now rare causes of this syndrome. Currently, this syndrome most often occurs in elderly women consuming excess calcium carbonate or calcium citrate for the treatment of osteoporosis. As a result, many now refer to this as the calcium-alkali syndrome rather than the milk-alkali syndrome. Alkalosis decreases kidney calcium excretion and the resultant hypercalcemia, nephrocalcinosis, and subsequent kidney dysfunction prevent correction of the alkalosis. Many of these patients are also receiving vitamin D supplements that increase intestinal calcium absorption. Patients present with the classic triad of hypercalcemia, metabolic alkalosis, and elevated serum creatinine concentration. Treatment is volume replacement with normal saline and avoidance of calcium and alkali supplements. The kidney injury may persist and result in CKD. Bisphosphonates should be avoided because these agents prevent bone calcium release, which is not a contributing factor in this syndrome and can also result in hypocalcemia. Treatment of hypercalcemia in these patients is often complicated by hypocalcemia resulting from sustained PTH suppression.

      ii. **Hypercalcemia in CKD** is uncommon, except in patients treated with calcium and vitamin D supplements. This disorder and the milk-alkali syndrome illustrate the important concept that hypercalcemia from excessive dietary calcium ingestion alone does not occur in the absence of kidney impairment.

      iii. **Vitamin D intoxication** or increased ingestion of vitamin D analogs such as calcitriol and paracalcitol also results in hypercalcemia. Calcium is absorbed primarily in the small intestine, and this process is stimulated by calcitriol.

      iv. **Increased 1,25-dihydroxy vitamin D production:** Hypercalcemia may also be secondary to **hematologic malignancies such as lymphomas and granulomatous disorders**, such as sarcoidosis, tuberculosis, histoplasmosis, and Crohn's disease. Activated macrophages

produce 1-alpha hydroxylase which increases calcitriol production, leading to increased intestinal absorption of dietary calcium. Hypercalciuria is seen more commonly than hypercalcemia.
b. **Increased calcium resorption from bone** plays a primary role in hypercalcemia resulting from primary, secondary, and tertiary hyperparathyroidism, malignancy, hyperthyroidism, immobilization, Paget disease, and hypervitaminosis A.
  i. **Malignancy** is a common cause of hypercalcemia. Hypercalcemia of malignancy results from several pathophysiologic mechanisms: overproduction of PTHrP, local bone reabsorption around sites of tumor infiltration (mediated through a variety of cytokines and osteolytic prostaglandins), and calcitriol production (e.g., with lymphomas). Patients with squamous cell lung cancer, breast cancer, multiple myeloma, and renal cell carcinoma are at highest risk. Hypercalcemia due to tumoral PTHrP production is often referred to as *humoral hypercalcemia of malignancy* (HHM). PTHrP has 70% amino acid identity to the first 13 amino acids of PTH and binds to the PTH receptor. It normally functions as a regulator of chondrocyte growth and differentiation in developing long bones; calcium mobilization from bones and into breast milk during lactation; calcium transport across the placenta to the developing fetus; and uterine blood flow. It is usually produced in the placenta during pregnancy and by mammary glands during lactation. In certain cancers, the gene for PTHrP is inappropriately activated. HHM often presents with severe hypercalcemia (calcium concentration greater than 14 mg/dL) in a patient with either a known history of malignancy or evidence of malignancy at initial presentation. PTHrP is immunologically distinct from PTH and is not detected by standard PTH assays, but specific assays for PTHrP are commercially available. The normal range for PTHrP is less than 2.0 pmol/L because in normal health its functions are autocrine or paracrine and higher circulating levels are not required. Median survival from the onset of hypercalcemia with HHM is only 3 months. Squamous cell tumors, renal cell carcinomas, and most breast neoplasms produce PTHrP. The diagnoses of primary hyperparathyroidism and malignancy are not mutually exclusive. An increased incidence of primary hyperparathyroidism was reported in patients with malignancy.

  Multiple myeloma is associated with hypercalcemia and localized osteolytic skeletal lesions. Approximately 30% of patients with myeloma experience hypercalcemia at some time during the course of their disease. Bone destruction occurs as a consequence of interleukin-6, interleukin-1, and tumor necrosis factor-beta release by malignant plasma cells. Bony lesions demonstrate a marked increase in osteoclastic resorption without manifestations of increased bone formation, in contrast to metastatic lesions of breast and prostate cancer, which generally show some increase in bone formation and radionuclide uptake at sites of increased osteoblastic activity. Because of excessive bone resorption, multiple myeloma can cause severe osteoporosis in addition to hypercalcemia. Bisphosphonates are frequently used to treat these complications. Bisphosphonates can cause acute kidney injury if given at high doses for a prolonged period of time. This risk is higher if the patient has CKD. Unfortunately, patients with multiple myeloma frequently develop CKD, and standard- or low-dose bisphosphonates might not be as effective in treating hypercalcemia and osteoporosis.

Pheochromocytoma can be associated with hyperparathyroidism in MEN syndrome, or produce ectopic PTHrP; with both mechanisms leading to hypercalcemia.

ii. **Hyperthyroidism** results in mild hypercalcemia in 10% to 20% of patients as a result of increased bone turnover. There is also an increased prevalence of hyperparathyroidism in patients with hyperthyroidism.

iii. **Paget disease** is a disease of bone with focal areas of disrupted bone turnover, disorganized and structurally weak bone, and increased vascularity. There are both hereditary and environmental factors that cause Paget disease. The most common mode of inheritance is autosomal dominant. Immobilization with Paget disease can cause hypercalcemia, although this is more likely in children. In adults, hypercalciuria is more common than hypercalcemia.

iv. **Immobilization**: Immobilization leads to increased bone resorption and hypercalcemia.

v. **Hypervitaminosis A**: Hypervitaminosis A leads to increased interleukin 6 release which stimulates bone resorption and hypercalcemia.

c. **Decreased calcium excretion by the kidney**: Thiazides, adrenal insufficiency, acute kidney injury, and Bartter syndrome are all associated with decreased calcium excretion by the kidney, which leads to hypercalcemia.

B. **Signs and symptoms** of hypercalcemia are related to the severity and rate of rise in plasma-ionized calcium concentration. Mild hypercalcemia is generally asymptomatic and often incidentally discovered on routine blood chemistries, as is the case in many patients with primary hyperparathyroidism. In contrast, severe hypercalcemia is often associated with neurologic and gastrointestinal symptoms. The patient may present with a wide range of central nervous system symptoms, from mild mental status changes to stupor and coma. Gastrointestinal symptoms include constipation, anorexia, nausea, and vomiting. Abdominal pain may result from hypercalcemia-induced peptic ulcer disease or pancreatitis. Hypercalcemia results in polyuria and secondary polydipsia and can lead to hypernatremia, ECF volume contraction, a reduction in the glomerular filtration rate (GFR), and an elevation in BUN and creatinine concentrations. Hypercalcemia also potentiates the cardiac effects of digitalis toxicity.

C. **Diagnosis.** The most common causes of hypercalcemia are primary hyperparathyroidism and malignancy. These two disorders make up more than 90% of all cases. Initial evaluation includes a history and physical examination and thorough clinical assessment. Medications should be reviewed, particularly the use of calcium supplements, antacids, vitamin preparations, over-the-counter medications, and thiazide diuretics. Figure 6-6 depicts an algorithmic approach to hypercalcemia.

Initial laboratory examination includes measurement of electrolytes, BUN, creatinine, phosphorus, chloride, bicarbonate, albumin, and serum total and ionized calcium. A low serum chloride concentration, a high serum bicarbonate concentration, and elevated BUN and creatinine concentrations are characteristic of milk-alkali syndrome. A low serum phosphorus concentration is found in primary hyperparathyroidism and HHM. Calcium should be adjusted for albumin level. If calcium levels are elevated, they should be repeated to confirm hypercalcemia before proceeding to further workup. As a general rule, primary hyperparathyroidism is the etiology in asymptomatic outpatients with a serum calcium concentration ≤11 mg/dL, whereas malignancy is often the cause in symptomatic patients with an abrupt disease onset and serum calcium concentration ≥14 mg/dL. Once hypercalcemia is confirmed, the next step is measuring intact PTH concentration to differentiate PTH-mediated from non–PTH-mediated hypercalcemia:

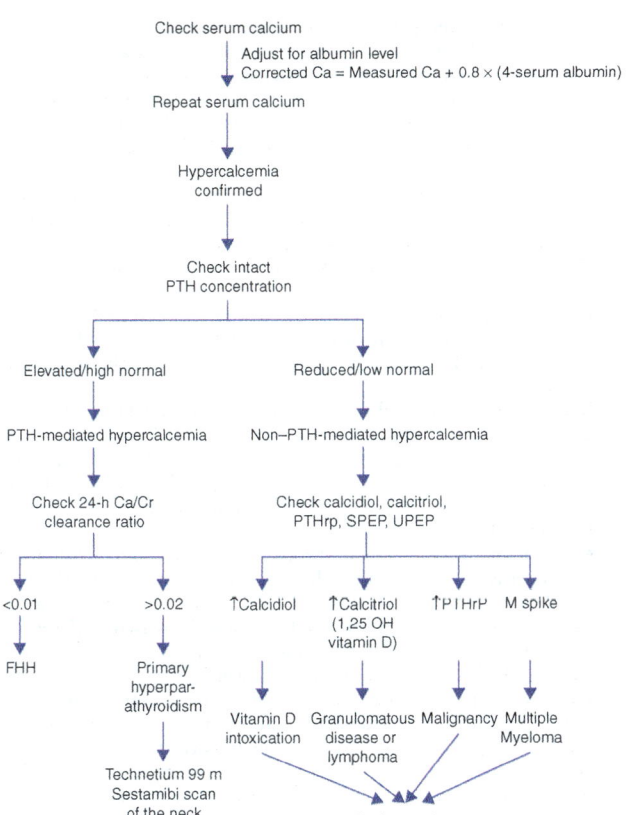

Figure 6-6. Algorithm for workup of hypercalcemia. Ca, calcium; Cr, creatinine; FHH, familial hypocalcuric hypercalcemia; M Spike, monoclonal spike; PTH, parathyroid hormone; PTHrP, parathyroid hormone-related peptide; SPEP, serum protein electrophoresis; UPEP, urine protein electrophoresis.

1. **Elevated or high normal** PTH implies PTH-mediated hypercalcemia. The most common cause of an elevated PTH concentration is primary hyperparathyroidism, although an elevated PTH concentration may also be seen with lithium use and in 15% to 20% of patients with FHH. Occasionally, in primary hyperparathyroidism, PTH concentration will be inappropriately within the normal range compared to the serum calcium concentration. In all other conditions, PTH will be suppressed by hypercalcemia. As mentioned previously, differential diagnosis includes primary and tertiary hyperparathyroidism and FHH. Tertiary hyperparathyroidism is unlikely in the absence of hyperphosphatemia and CKD or ESKD. A 24-hour urine for calcium and creatinine should be checked for calculation of the calcium to creatinine clearance ratio. The calcium/creatinine clearance ratio can be calculated using the formula below:

$$\text{Calcium/Creatinine clearance ratio} = \frac{(24\text{-hour urine Calcium} \times \text{serum Creatinine})}{(\text{serum Calcium} \times 24\text{-hour urine Creatinine})}$$

A positive family history, young age, and reduced urine calcium <100 to 200 mg/dL or 24-hour calcium:creatinine clearance ratio <0.01 can help differentiate primary hyperparathyroidism from FHH. The optimal calcium-to-creatinine clearance ratio for separation of FHH from primary hyperparathyroidism appears to be a value of 0.0115. This yields a sensitivity of 80% and a specificity of 88%. It can be seen that even at this cutoff there is still overlap between FHH and primary hyperparathyroidism, especially in those with primary hyperparathyroidism that are also vitamin D deficient. The presence of a high serum chloride concentration and a low serum phosphorus concentration in a ratio greater than 33:1 is suggestive of primary hyperparathyroidism resulting from the effect of PTH decreasing proximal tubular phosphate reabsorption. If primary hyperparathyroidism is suspected, a technetium 99m sestamibi scan of the neck should be performed to identify parathyroid adenomas that might need to be surgically excised (please refer to the treatment section below).

2. **Reduced or low normal PTH** imply appropriate PTH suppression in the setting of non–PTH-mediated hypercalcemia. Differential diagnosis is wide, as discussed previously. Clinical cues should be used to guide the next steps. In the absence of clinical cues, the following should be checked:
   - Twenty-five (25) and 1,25-hydroxy vitamin D levels
   - Serum PTHrP
   - Serum and urine protein electrophoresis with serum immunofixation

   Increased 25-OH vitamin D is suggestive of vitamin D toxicity and should prompt a reevaluation of the patient's medication list, including over-the-counter supplements and vitamins. Increased $1,25(OH)_2$ vitamin D levels are suggestive of granulomatous diseases or hematologic malignancies. A chest x-ray, serum angiotensin convertase enzyme levels, and serum chiotriosidase activity can help diagnose sarcoidosis. If calcitriol concentration is increased without an apparent cause, occult granulomatous disease can be evaluated with a **hydrocortisone suppression test**. After administration of 40 mg of hydrocortisone every 8 hours for 10 days, the hypercalcemia will resolve if it is the result of granulomatous disease. A monoclonal spike raises suspicion of multiple myeloma and might prompt a bone marrow biopsy. An elevated PTHrP should raise suspicion for malignancy and further radiologic investigation is warranted. A computed tomography scan can help identify primary malignancies and a skeletal survey can help identify osteoclastic lesions secondary to bone resorption and metastases. Finally, a tissue biopsy might be needed to ultimately provide a definitive diagnosis.

D. **Treatment** of hypercalcemia varies depending on the severity of the serum calcium elevation. It is directed at increasing urinary calcium excretion, inhibiting bone resorption, and decreasing intestinal calcium absorption. Table 6-4 highlights the treatment options for hypercalcemia.
   1. **Urinary calcium excretion is increased** by first expanding the ECF volume with isotonic saline and, subsequently, administering loop diuretics (forced diuresis). Calcium reabsorption in the proximal tubule is passive and parallels sodium reabsorption. ECF volume contraction, therefore, increases proximal sodium reabsorption and helps maintain hypercalcemia. Patients with hypercalcemia are often volume-contracted. Hypercalcemia decreases sodium reabsorption in the thick ascending limb of the loop of Henle through activation of the CaSR, and it also antagonizes the effects of antidiuretic hormone. In the setting of a reduced GFR, higher doses of loop diuretics may be required. In the presence of little or no kidney function and severe hypercalcemia, hemodialysis is indicated.

TABLE 6-4 Treatment Options for Hypercalcemia

Treatment	Mechanism of Action	Dose	Adverse Reactions/Comments
Intravenous Normal Saline	Expansion of the ECF → ↑ urinary calcium excretion.	Start with 200–300 mL/h, titrate according to urine output	Nonanion gap metabolic acidosis, volume overload
Loop diuretics	↑ urinary calcium excretion.	Furosemide 20–160 IV mg/d. Preferably used after ECF volume expansion with intravenous normal saline for forced diuresis.	Hypernatremia, hypokalemia, metabolic alkalosis, volume contraction, and ototoxicity at high doses.
Salmon Calcitonin	Inhibits bone resorption. ↑ urinary calcium excretion.	4 IU/kg SC Q12Hs	Local adverse events: Rash, pruritis, allergic reaction. Short-acting but exhibits risk of tachyphylaxis.
Calcimimetics: Cinacalcet, Etalcalcetide	Mimics calcium and thus allosterically activates CaSR → downregulate PTH production	Cinacalcet: Start with 30 mg twice daily. Etelcalcetide: Start with 2.5 mg IV thrice weekly at the end of HD sessions.	GI side effects: Nausea, vomiting, and diarrhea (more with Cinacalcet). Arrhythmias and prolonged QTc interval (more with Etalcalcetide). Etelcalcetide is longer-acting so more beneficial for patients on HD with nonadherence to oral medications.
Bisphosphonates: Pamidronate, Zoledronate	Inhibit bone resorption	Pamidronate: 60–90 mg IV over 2–4 h. Zoledronate: 4 mg over 15 min. Adjust dose to kidney function	Hypocalcemia, hypophosphatemia, fever, acute kidney injury (do not use with CrCl <30/mL/1.73 m^2). Osteonecrosis of the jaw, esophagitis.
Denosumab	Inhibit bone resorption	Starting dose is 60 mg SC.	**Hypocalcemia (severe, must monitor calcium postinfusion)**, Hypophosphatemia
Glucocorticoids	Decrease GI calcium absorption and 1,25-OH vitamin D synthesis	Hydrocortisone 200–300 mg IV daily for 3–5 d	Hypertension, hyperglycemia, peptic ulcers, infection, weight gain, acne, myopathy, avascular necrosis
Hemodialysis	Remove calcium through the dialysis membrane	4-h sessions using low calcium bath	Hypotension, infection, dialysis disequilibrium syndrome, arrhythmias

CaSR, calcium-sensing receptor; CrCl, creatinine clearance; ECF, extracellular fluid; GI, gastrointestinal; HD, hemodialysis; IU, international units; IV, intravenous; PTH, parathyroid hormone; SC, subcutaneously.

2. **An agent that inhibits bone resorption** is often required when hypercalcemia is moderate or severe. In the acute setting, **calcitonin** is often helpful because of its rapid onset of action (2 to 4 hours). Calcitonin inhibits osteoclastic bone reabsorption and increases kidney calcium excretion. It reduces serum calcium concentration, however, by only 1 to 2 mg/dL, and tachyphylaxis often develops with repeated use. For these reasons, calcitonin should not be used as the sole agent to inhibit bone resorption.
   a. **Bisphosphonates** are the agents of choice for the management of hypercalcemia due to bone resorption. These analogs of inorganic pyrophosphate are selectively concentrated in bone, where they interfere with osteoclast attachment and function. Bisphosphonates have a slow onset (2 to 3 days) and long duration of action (several weeks). Caution should be exercised in patients with milk-alkali syndrome. These patients do not have a defect in bone turnover and are susceptible to hypocalcemia with treatment, and post-treatment hypocalcemia may be exacerbated by bisphosphonates.

   Pamidronate is given at a dose of either 60 or 90 mg intravenously over 4 hours. If serum calcium concentration is ≤13.5 mg/dL, 60 mg is given. If serum calcium concentration is greater than 13.5 mg/dL, 90 mg is administered. Serum calcium concentration gradually falls over the ensuing 2 to 4 days. A single dose is usually effective for 1 to 2 weeks. In most patients, serum calcium concentration normalizes after 7 days.

   Zoledronic acid is now the most commonly used bisphosphonate because it can be given intravenously, which avoids esophageal damage from oral doses and can be administered over a short interval (4 mg over 15 minutes). It is administered every 3 to 4 weeks if needed and it may be longer lasting than pamidronate. The dose must be adjusted in patients with kidney dysfunction as follows given the creatinine clearance: greater than 60 mL/min–4 mg; 50 to 60 mL/min–3.5 mg; 40 to 49 mL/min–3.3 mg; 30 to 39 mL/min–3.0 mg; less than 30 mL/min–no data available. The manufacturer recommends that the drug be discontinued if the serum creatinine concentration increases ≥0.5 mg/dL above a normal baseline or greater than 1.0 mg/dL in those with a serum creatinine concentration ≥1.4 mg/dL. Zoledronic acid is superior to Pamidronate, especially in hypercalcemia of malignancy.

   Bisphosphonates are associated with significant toxicity including focal glomerular sclerosis and acute kidney injury. Most of these cases occurred in patients with preexisting CKD or when recommended doses were exceeded. Patients with multiple myeloma are at particular risk because kidney disease is a common complication and management of osteoporosis and/or hypercalcemia may require higher than recommended doses. In addition, when bisphosphonates are used long-term in patients with malignancy, especially multiple myeloma and breast cancer, they are associated with osteonecrosis of the jaw. Most of these patients have had recent tooth extraction or surgical tooth removal. Radiation to the jaw also increases the risk of osteonecrosis.
   b. **Denosumab** inhibits osteoclast-induced bone resorption and can be used in cases of refractory hypercalcemia or in those with contraindications to bisphosphonate therapy. The initial dose is 60 mg with cautious monitoring of serum calcium levels due to the serious risk of hypocalcemia.
   c. **Calcimimetics** such as Cinacalcet mimic calcium and thus stimulate the CaSR to downregulate PTH secretion. Though it has no structural similarity with elemental calcium, it can bind to the receptor and cause allosteric activation. CaSRs are located in the gastrointestinal tract, kidney, bone, and parathyroid glands. Allosteric activation results in a reduction of PTH release, less calcium release from bone, less intestinal calcium absorption,

and an increase in kidney calcium excretion. This results in a lowering of calcium and PTH levels. The lower PTH level's effect on serum phosphorus concentration is dependent on kidney function. In patients on dialysis with no kidney function, decreased PTH levels can reduce phosphorus concentration by limiting bone resorption. In patients with significantly impaired kidney function, such as kidney transplant recipients with persistent tertiary hyperparathyroidism, the initial phosphorus concentration can be low because of persistently elevated PTH levels. Treatment with cinacalcet will reduce PTH levels, reduce kidney phosphate wasting, and increase rather than decrease serum phosphorus levels in these patients. The brain also has CaSRs and a significant dose-limiting side effect is nausea. Cinacalcet is approved for use in the United States for the treatment of secondary and tertiary hyperparathyroidism and parathyroid carcinoma. In Europe, it is also approved for the medical treatment of primary hyperparathyroidism. Etelcalcetide, a longer-acting calcimimetic with an estimated half-life of 4 days, was FDA-approved in 2017. Etelcalcetide carries less risk of gastrointestinal side effects but can significantly prolong QT interval and thus, monitoring with serial ECGs is warranted.

d. **Historical agents:** Gallium nitrate and plicamycin have been used historically for the treatment of malignancy-induced hypercalcemia but have fallen out of favor due to side effect profile, particularly nephrotoxicity with gallium nitrate and hepatotoxicity with plicamycin. These agents were replaced by the newer agents described above.

3. **Measures to decrease intestinal calcium absorption** are often employed in outpatients with mild disease. Corticosteroids may be helpful in vitamin D intoxication, granulomatous disease, and certain neoplasms (lymphoma and multiple myeloma). Alternatives to corticosteroids include ketoconazole and hydroxychloroquine. Oral phosphate can be administered, provided the patient does not have an elevated serum phosphorus concentration or advanced CKD. Oral phosphate, however, often causes diarrhea and only lowers the serum calcium concentration by approximately 1 mg/dL.

4. **Treatment of asymptomatic hyperparathyroidism** is controversial. It is generally accepted that symptomatic hyperparathyroidism should be treated with a parathyroidectomy. Symptoms can include bone pain from excessive bone demineralization, kidney stones from hypercalciuria, or symptoms from hypercalcemia such as fatigue, confusion, depression, nausea, polyuria, and polydipsia. In 1991, a consensus conference made recommendations for the treatment of asymptomatic hyperparathyroidism. Updated recommendations were made in 2002, 2009, and again in 2013. It is recommended that asymptomatic patients with elevated PTH levels undergo parathyroidectomy if they meet one or more of the following criteria:
   - Age <50 years old
   - Calcium >1.0 mg/dL above the upper limit of normal
   - Bone mineral density T score of less than −2.5 at the lumbar spine, hip, femoral neck, or distal radius
   - Radiologic evidence of vertebral fractures or nephrolithiasis
   - Creatinine clearance <60 cc/min
   - 24-hour urine calcium >400 mg/d or high risk on biochemical stone analysis

Surgery has become less extensive because of the ability to preoperatively scan for parathyroid adenomas with a technetium 99 sestamibi scan and parathyroid ultrasound, as well as being able to measure PTH concentration in the operating room. This allows for a minimally invasive approach that does not require general anesthesia. The surgeon can localize the adenoma preoperatively instead of having to explore both sides of the neck and possibly the mediastinum. Intraoperative PTH levels can confirm that the adenoma was successfully resected because the half-life of PTH is only 4 minutes and should drop very quickly after adequate surgical resection. If the PTH level does not fall greater than 50% in 10 minutes, this suggests that a second adenoma may be present and the patient can then be placed under general anesthesia and the neck explored.

Asymptomatic patients who do not undergo surgery because of physician/patient preferences should be monitored yearly with serum calcium and creatinine levels and every 1 to 2 years with a bone mineral density and encouraged to proceed with parathyroidectomy if these values worsen. Medical treatment with cinacalcet is approved in Europe for primary hyperparathyroidism but was not recommended by the consensus conference. Cinacalcet increases bone density, lowers calcium levels, increases phosphorus levels, and reduces PTH levels. Bisphosphonates have also been used for medical management. Bisphosphonates improve bone density and reduce hypercalcemia but do not lower PTH levels. Carcinoma of the parathyroid gland is a rare cause of primary hyperparathyroidism. Surgical resection is the preferred treatment but recurrence is common and may require numerous resections. Cinacalcet is used as a medical treatment for hypercalcemia in recurrent disease.

5. **Treatment of Secondary and Tertiary Hyperparathyroidism in Patients with CKD.** Medical management involves regulating PTH levels in the desired range depending on the CKD stage. In CKD stage 3, the desired PTH range is 35 to 70 pg/mL. In CKD stage 4, the desired range is 70 to 110 pg/mL. In CKD stage 5 and patients on dialysis, the desired range is within two to nine times the upper limit of the assay. In patients not yet on dialysis, if the 25-OH vitamin D_3 level is low, it is replaced with ergocalciferol or cholecalciferol. This will give enough precursor to allow the kidney to convert it to $1,25(OH)_2$ vitamin D_3, which will suppress PTH. If correcting 25-OH vitamin D_3 is not adequate to suppress PTH, then oral calcitriol or paracalcitol is used. Cinacalcet is not used because these patients are often hypocalcemic and a significant side effect of cinacalcet is hypocalcemia.

Patients on hemodialysis are treated with a variety of different $1,25(OH)_2$ vitamin D_3 analogs that can be given intravenously during the hemodialysis treatment. A high PTH level can cause high bone turnover disease with calcification of blood vessels, heart valves, and the lens of the eye, as well as bone fractures, and can progress to tertiary hyperparathyroidism. A low PTH level can result in low bone turnover disease with increased fracture rates, as well as calcification of tissues. Once tertiary hyperparathyroidism develops, the use of vitamin D analogs is limited by hypercalcemia. The elevated calcium and PTH levels can be treated medically with cinacalcet. Cinacalcet allows the use of higher doses of vitamin D analogs by lowering calcium levels. Surgical parathyroidectomy is performed when medical treatment with cinacalcet and vitamin D analogs is no longer effective, particularly for >6 months. Other indications for parathyroidectomy in patients on dialysis include refractory hypercalcemia, hyperphosphatemia, refractory calciphylaxis, or anemia of kidney disease that is nonresponsive to erythropoietin.

SUGGESTED READINGS

Amanzadeh J, Reilly RF Jr. Hypophosphatemia: an evidence-based approach to its clinical consequences and management. *Nat Clin Pract Nephrol.* 2006;2(3):136–148.

Bilezikian JP, Brandi ML, Eastell R, et al. Guidelines for the management of asymptomatic primary hyperparathyroidism: summary statement from the Fourth International Workshop. *J Clin Endocrinol Metab.* 2014;99(10):3561–3569.

Blaine J, Chonchol M, Levi M. Renal control of calcium, phosphate, and magnesium homeostasis. *Clin J Am Soc Nephrol.* 2015;10(7):1257–1272.

Blaine J, Weinman EJ, Cunningham R. The regulation of renal phosphate transport. *Adv Chronic Kidney Dis.* 2011;18(2):77–84.

Clines GA. Mechanisms and treatment of hypercalcemia of malignancy. *Curr Opin Endocrinol Diabetes Obes.* 2011;18(6):339–346.

Eidman KE, Wetmore JB. Treatment of secondary hyperparathyroidism: how do cinacalcet and etelcalcetide differ? *Semin Dial.* 2018;31(5):440–444.

El-Hajj Fuleihan G, Clines GA, Hu MI, et al. Treatment of hypercalcemia of malignancy in adults: an endocrine society clinical practice guideline. *J Clin Endocrinol Metab.* 2023;108(3):507–528.

Goyal A, Anastasopoulou C, Ngu M, Singh S. Hypocalcemia. In: *StatPearls.* 2023.

Grieff M, Bushinsky DA. Diuretics and disorders of calcium homeostasis. *Semin Nephrol.* 2011;31(6):535–541.

Hanna RM, Ahdoot RS, Kalantar-Zadeh K, Ghobry L, Kurtz I. Calcium transport in the kidney and disease processes. *Front Endocrinol (Lausanne).* 2021;12:762130.

Hannan FM, Thakker RV. Investigating hypocalcaemia. *BMJ.* 2013;346:f2213.

Jacobs TP, Bilezikian JP. Clinical review: rare causes of hypercalcemia. *J Clin Endocrinol Metab.* 2005;90(11):6316–6322.

Kelly A, Levine MA. Hypocalcemia in the critically ill patient. *J Intensive Care Med.* 2013;28(3):166–177.

Khan MI, Waguespack SG, Hu MI. Medical management of postsurgical hypoparathyroidism. *Endocr Pract.* 2011;17(Suppl 1):18–25.

Khoury N, Carmichael KA. Evaluation and therapy of hypercalcemia. *Mo Med.* 2011;108(2):99–103.

Kidney Disease: Improving Global Outcomes (KDIGO) CKD-MBD Update Work Group. KDIGO 2017 clinical practice guideline update for the diagnosis, evaluation, prevention, and treatment of chronic kidney disease-mineral and bone disorder (CKD-MBD). *Kidney Int Suppl.* 2017;7(1):1–59.

Komaba H, Kakuta T, Fukagawa M. Diseases of the parathyroid gland in chronic kidney disease. *Clin Exp Nephrol.* 2011;15(6):797–809.

Maier JD, Levine SN. Hypercalcemia in the intensive care unit: a review of pathophysiology, diagnosis, and modern therapy. *J Intensive Care Med.* 2015;30(5):235–252.

Marcocci C, Cetani F. Clinical practice. Primary hyperparathyroidism. *N Engl J Med.* 2011;365(25):2389–2397.

Minisola S, Pepe J, Piemonte S, Cipriani C. The diagnosis and management of hypercalcaemia. *BMJ.* 2015;350:h2723.

Moe SM. Disorders involving calcium, phosphorus, and magnesium. *Prim Care.* 2008;35(2):215–237, v–vi.

Renkema KY, Alexander RT, Bindels RJ, Hoenderop JG. Calcium and phosphate homeostasis: concerted interplay of new regulators. *Ann Med.* 2008;40(2):82–91.

Riccardi D, Brown EM. Physiology and pathophysiology of the calcium-sensing receptor in the kidney. *Am J Physiol Renal Physiol.* 2010;298(3):F485–F499.

Seisa MO, Nayfeh T, Hasan B, et al. A systematic review supporting the Endocrine Society clinical practice guideline on the treatment of hypercalcemia of malignancy in adults. *J Clin Endocrinol Metab.* 2023;108(3):585–591.

Tinawi M. Disorders of calcium metabolism: hypocalcemia and hypercalcemia. *Cureus.* 2021;13(1):e12420.

Turner J, Gittoes N, Selby P, Society for Endocrinology Clinical Committee. SOCIETY FOR ENDOCRINOLOGY EMERGENCY ENDOCRINE GUIDANCE: emergency management of acute hypocalcaemia in adult patients. *Endocr Connect.* 2019;8(6):X1.

Walker MD, Shane E. Hypercalcaemia: a review. *JAMA.* 2022;328(16):1624–1636.

Zivin JR, Gooley T, Zager RA, Ryan MJ. Hypocalcemia: a pervasive metabolic abnormality in the critically ill. *Am J Kidney Dis.* 2001;37(4):689–698.

7
The Patient With Hypophosphatemia or Hyperphosphatemia

Gates Colbert, Edgar V. Lerma

Phosphorus Regulation

Phosphorus is an important element involved in a variety of homeostasis including signal transduction, energy exchange, and cell membrane function. Serum phosphorus circulates in two forms: an organic fraction made up primarily of phospholipids and an inorganic fraction. Of these two forms the inorganic fraction makes up approximately one-third of total plasma phosphorous and is assayed in the clinical laboratory. The vast majority of inorganic phosphorous (75%) is free in solution and exists as either divalent (HPO_4^{2-}) or monovalent ($H_2PO_4^-$) phosphate. Approximately 1% of body weight in a 70-kg person is phosphorus (600 to 700 g). The distribution is primarily in skeletal bone (80%), other organs (19%), and serum making the final 1% that is reported by laboratory testing. A very small fraction of phosphorus is intracellular where it is inorganic and can be transitioned to adenosine triphosphate (ATP) synthesis. Fifteen percent of phosphorous is protein bound, hence why it is easily dialyzable in end-stage kidney disease (ESKD) patients who are receiving hemodialysis.

Phosphorous is abundant in the Western diet with an average intake between 800 and 1,500 mg daily. When measuring phosphorus it should be noted that it has a diurnal variation with low concentrations early in the morning and a rise throughout the day. It remains intact in some patients with hyperparathyroidism but remains unknown for patients with hypophosphatemia of other causes. When measured for health and sickness in the laboratory a normal range is between 2.5 and 4.5 mg/dL (0.8 and 1.5 mM).

Organ Regulation of Phosphorus Balance

The following organs work together to maintain phosphorus balance: intestinal uptake, bones with retention or release, and tight regulation by the kidney. Inorganic phosphate is absorbed along the length of the small intestine via passive and active transport. The colon plays an insignificant role except for cases of hypophosphatemia as unregulated secretion with diarrhea. The small intestine has a high-affinity phosphorus transporter, Npt2b (type II sodium-dependent phosphate transporter) that is found in the brush border. Regulation of active absorption is by dietary inorganic phosphate intake and serum 1,25-dihydroxy-vitamin D_3 concentration. Parathyroid hormone (PTH) has no effect on Npt2b regulation. There is also a crosstalk between small intestine, kidney, and bone which is revealed in Npt2B knockout mice where fibroblast growth factor 23 (FGF-23) decreases and elevation in active vitamin D_3 occurs to maintain serum phosphorus and calcium concentration. Paracellular phosphorus transport in the intestine is not fully understood at this time.

The kidney plays a pivotal role in phosphorus homeostasis. 200 mmol (20 g) of phosphorus is filtered by the glomeruli per day and is freely filtered given its low protein-bound percentage. Around 85% of the phosphorus is reabsorbed primarily in the proximal convoluted tubule (PCT) and proximal straight tubule (PST) via sodium-dependent phosphate transporters (70% Npt2a and 30% Npt2c). See Figure 7-1 on phosphorus absorption in the nephron. The reabsorption saturates and excretion increases in proportion to the filtered load for normal serum phosphorus levels. PTH and FGF-23 lower the transport maximum. PTH induces removal of Npt2a from apical surface of PCT via PTH1 receptors expressed on the apical and basolateral

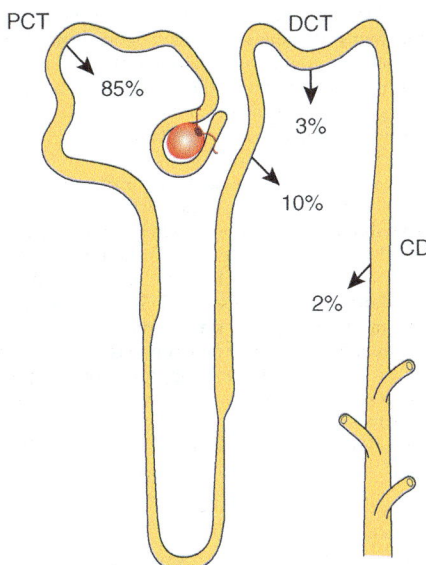

Figure 7-1. Phosphorus absorption in nephron. (Adapted from Carpenter TO. Primary Disorders of Phosphate Metabolism. In: Feingold KR, Anawalt B, Blackman MR, et al., eds. *Endotext* [Internet]. [June 8, 2022]. MDText.com, Inc.; 2000.)

membranes. The PCT does not need FGF-23 or Klotho to have phosphaturic action take place. Phosphatonins, which are circulating phosphaturic peptides, decrease BBM abundance of Npt2a/Npt2c in vivo and suppress 1 alpha-hydroxylase activity in the kidney. FGF-23 is considered a phosphatonin and requires Klotho cofactor to activate its receptor FGF1 in the PCT. FGF-23 is a 351-amino acid protein produced by osteocytes and osteoblasts in response to high phosphorus in the diet, high serum levels of phosphorus, or in the presence of high active vitamin D_3 concentration. Klotho cofactor exists in two forms: secreted and transmembrane. It is highly expressed in distal tubules and in the PCT. How bone cells are able to sense changes in serum phosphorus concentration and alter FGF-23 secretion remains not fully understood.

Role of FGF-23
FGF-23 when injected into experimental animals reduces calcitriol concentration within 3 hours. The mechanism is a result of decreased calcitriol synthesis (decreased expression of 1 alpha-hydroxylase) and increased degradation (increased expression of 24-hydroxylase). The serum phosphorus concentration will then fall within 9 to 13 hours. Elevated FGF-23 levels are also associated with inhibiting PTH secretion from the parathyroid gland. Other factors that can regulate kidney phosphorus regulation include estrogen levels. Estrogen increases serum FGF-23 concentration and decreases Npt2a messenger ribonucleic acid (mRNA) levels.

Hyperphosphatemia
Pathophysiology of Hyperphosphatemia
Hyperphosphatemia commonly results from decreased kidney phosphate excretion, the primary site of physiologic removal. Chronic kidney disease (CKD) is the leading cause of phosphorus retention and is prevalent in more than 90% of cases. A less common cause of retention is inappropriately increased PCT phosphate reabsorption.

Temporary phosphorus loading from exogenous or endogenous sources can also lead to hyperphosphatemia. Signs of aging such as hypogonadism, skin atrophy, osteopenia, vascular calcification, and cognitive impairment that are present in patients with long-standing CKD all may have a link to the toxic effects of high phosphorus levels over time. Table 7-1 lists common etiologies of hyperphosphatemia.

As GFR falls below 60 mL/min/1.73 m^2, phosphate excretion will actually increase in response to higher phosphorus serum levels. Once GFR falls below 30 mL/min/1.73 m^2, phosphate reabsorption is maximally inhibited, and excretion cannot increase to keep serum levels within normal ranges. Dietary intake will exceed excretion and the phosphorus levels will inevitably increase. Approximately 15% of patients with advanced CKD stage G4 between 15 and 30 mL/min/1.73 m^2 and up to 50% of those with CKD stage G5 will have phosphorus serum levels above 4.5 mg/dL. As a mechanism to try and combat rising phosphorus levels in the serum, FGF-23 is released from bones to help with kidney excretion. Unfortunately, CKD state attenuates the response to the phosphaturic effects of FGF-23 secondary to loss of nephron mass. Patients with CKD have high FGF-23 and low calcitriol levels, and this will suppress Klotho expression in the kidney. Thus a vicious cycle ensues with poor Klotho and high FGF-23 levels which cannot work in concert to promote kidney phosphaturic mechanisms. Recent studies have shown that in mice with FGF-23 knockout, hyperphosphatemia, elevated 1,25[OH]$_2$D$_3$ levels, vascular calcification, and early mortality, that reducing serum phosphorus by either ablating the VDR or administering a low phosphorus diet rescues their phenotype.

CKD Risk Factor for Hyperphosphatemia
CKD patients are classically known to have advanced cardiac disease and suffer from high CV mortality. Compared to patients with CKD and serum phosphorus levels less than 6.5 mg/dL, those with equal or greater than 6.5 mg/dL have higher mortality. Many observational studies show a linear relationship between high phosphorus levels and high all-cause and CV mortality. Patients with ESKD have the highest CV mortality, and the highest phosphorus levels, although direct causality remains to be

TABLE 7-1 Etiologies of Hyperphosphatemia

Acute Phosphorus Addition
Endogenous
- Tumor lysis syndrome
- Rhabdomyolysis
- Severe hemolysis

Exogenous
- Sodium phosphate–containing bowel preparations
- High-dose liposomal amphotericin B
- Vitamin D toxicosis
- Improperly purified fresh-frozen plasma

Decreased Kidney Excretion
Decreased glomerular filtration rate
- Acute kidney injury
- Chronic kidney disease

Pseudohyperphosphatemia
- Hyperlipidemia
- Hyperbilirubinemia
- Hemolysis
- Paraproteinemias (multiple myeloma, Waldenstrom's)

proven. However, we do know that elevated phosphorus levels do correlate with vascular calcification severity. Patients with CKD have accelerated atherosclerosis and medial calcification that are known to be risk factors for CV disease. Calcification in large arteries reduces compliance, increases pulse pressure, and subsequently afterload and coronary perfusion. With increased phosphorus levels and its associated CV risk, kidney disease progression is also increased. The REIN (Ramipril Efficacy in Nephropathy) trial showed that each 1 mg/dL rise in serum phosphorus concentration was associated with an 85% excess risk of progression to ESKD.

Uncommon Causes
Other uncommon causes of hyperphosphatemia have been described. Increased kidney PCT reabsorption can occur in hypoparathyroidism as a result of low PTH exposure. Patients with acromegaly have high insulin-like growth factor-1 leading to increased phosphate transport. Bisphosphonates directly increase PCT phosphate reabsorption as well in patients using them for osteoporosis or as a treatment for hypercalcemia. Tumoral calcinosis is an autosomal recessive disease associated with hyperphosphatemia and soft tissue calcium deposition. Exogenous loading of phosphorus can lead to a sudden rise in serum levels. Medications that create phosphorus loading include phosphorus-containing laxatives, enemas, high-dose liposomal amphotericin, and solvent–detergent-treated fresh frozen plasma. Oral sodium phosphate solutions were commonly used as bowel preparation for colonoscopy. A typical oral 90-mL solution contains 43.2 g of monobasic sodium phosphate and 16.2 g of dibasic sodium phosphate. Unfortunately for some patients, a fatal hyperphosphatemia has been reported in several case series of patients undergoing bowel prep with these solutions. Phosphate nephropathy leading to kidney stones or even acute kidney inury (AKI) by tubular injury has been reported from phosphate-based oral bowel preparations. Common releases of phosphorus into the serum are seen in conditions such as tumor lysis syndrome, hemolysis, or rhabdomyolysis. Spurious hyperphosphatemia should be considered in those with hyperlipidemia, hyperbilirubinemia, hemolysis, paraproteinemia, and contaminated blood samples with heparin as these conditions have been reported to interfere with modern assay measurements. Figure 7-2 evaluates hyperphosphatemia based on urinary excretion value.

Exact pathophysiology of elevated phosphorus level exposure and overall morbidity is incompletely understood at this time. One association we do is that patients with CKD and ESKD have decreased elasticity in vascular smooth muscle cells. This may be related to the chronically elevated phosphorus levels and the tendency to be hypocalcemic. Surprisingly, vascular calcification is seen in patients with CKD or ESKD that have normal or near-normal serum phosphorus concentrations, making the direct link of hyperphosphatemia incompletely understood. Phosphate binders, commonly used in advanced CKD and ESKD, remain uncertain in their benefits to reverse or prevent vascular calcification despite their ubiquitous use.

Hyperphosphatemia Treatment
Treatment of hyperphosphatemia depends on the exact cause, as elimination of the primary source is vital to prevent sustained high phosphorus levels. This chapter will focus on treatment of patients with CKD and ESKD, which treatment is most commonly based on decreasing phosphorous absorption in the intestine. Patients with early-stage CKD may be able to control their phosphorus levels by dietary phosphorus restriction. Intestinal absorption is linear over a wide range of intakes between 4 and 30 mg/kg/d. Bioavailability of the phosphorus consumed plays a major role as meat based and additive sources of phosphorus are much more absorbed than plant based. The major dietary sources of phosphorus are found in three food groups: dairy products, meats, and grains. Patients aged 18 to 44 years old consume on average 2.1 fast-food meals per week, accounting for an estimated phosphorus intake of 1,600 mg. Additives are widespread in packaged food to make them more palatable, improve their taste, and prolong shelf life. Inorganic phosphorus salts contained in processed

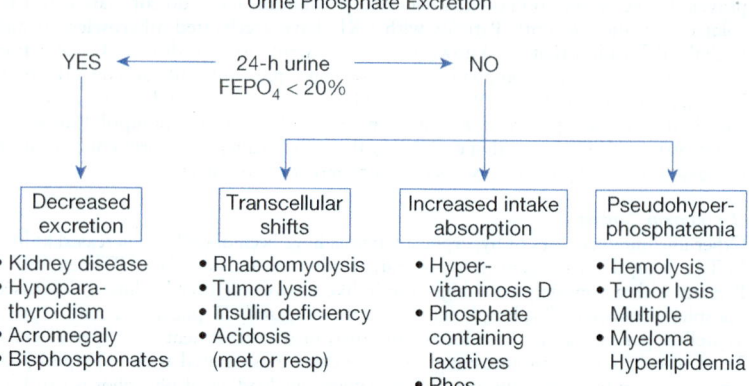

Figure 7-2. Hyperphosphatemia workup approach.

foods are nearly completely absorbed by the intestine. Foods high in these kinds of salts that most Western world patients love to eat include hot dogs, cheese spreads, sodas, and processed deli meats, and these should be counseled for avoidance in those suffering from CKD or hyperphosphatemia. Plant products have much lower bioavailability as they contain phytates, which are not hydrolyzed well for absorption. Thus, vegetarian or plant-based diets should be encouraged for these patients.

Oral Phosphorus Binders

As GFR falls and CKD stages progress, phosphorus excretion decreases which results in the current recommendations to begin phosphorus restrictions and adding a phosphorus intestinal binder. An ideal phosphorus binder should maximize phosphorus binding, have minimal side effects, lower serum phosphorus levels, and be affordable to patients. Unfortunately, as of this publication, none of the currently available binders fulfill these desired criteria. Calcium-containing binders are historically the standard of care but may contribute to a net positive calcium balance and calcium deposition over time with large exposure. Aluminum-containing phosphate binders, now infrequently used in the United States, should only be for short-term use in CKD patients because of aluminum toxicity resulting in dementia and osteomalacia. Sevelamer carbonate has a favorable side-effect profile but is still expensive. Sevelamer hydrochloride was associated with lower serum bicarbonate concentrations and has been changed over to sevelamer carbonate. Lanthanum is a newer binder with excellent intestinal binding capacity but remains at a high cost. Iron-based binders are the newest category of intestinal binding agents. Ferric citrate and sucroferric oxyhydroxide are the two newest phosphate binders that are primarily bound with iron. Ferric citrate has been shown to raise iron levels but both lower phosphorus levels with taken with meals. Sucroferric oxyhydroxide offers lower pill burden and may be more palatable as a chewable or breakable medication. Both agents are still branded drugs and can be expensive depending on insurance coverage.

Mortality benefits have not been associated with using any of the available phosphorus-binding agents. One trial of 2,103 hemodialysis patients compared sevelamer carbonate to other calcium-based binders. In that study, there was no benefit in all-cause or cause-specific mortality between any of the phosphorous binding agents. Additionally, there were limitations of the trial with a high dropout rate. Lanthanum has been shown to be superior in phosphorus-binding compared to sevelamer, but hard outcomes are still lacking. Current standards of ESKD in the United States remain counseling on a low phosphorus diet, including plant-based diets with caution on potassium intake, and use of an oral phosphorus binder that is affordable and results in an improved serum phosphate response.

Hypophosphatemia

Hypophosphatemia Causes

Hypophosphatemia can occur from one or several different mechanisms in the body. A decreased intestinal phosphorous absorption, increased kidney phosphorus excretion, or a redistribution of extracellular fluid phosphorus into the intracellular fluid are all possible mechanisms that should be considered. Classic etiologies of hypophosphatemia are listed in Table 7-2. Phosphorus shift into cells can commonly be seen in a respiratory alkalosis and refeeding syndrome that are readily apparent in critically ill patients who are hospitalized. Severe hypophosphatemia with phosphorus levels less than 0.5 to 1.0 mg/dL is common in alcoholics who have a combination of processes that lead to hypophosphatemia.

With refeeding syndrome, the rapidity of onset of hypophosphatemia depends on the degree of malnourished state of the patient. In those with severe deficiency, patients develop hypophosphatemia within 2 to 5 days from reintroduction of nutrition. The degree of phosphorus depletion is most dramatic in those with liver disease. If given glucose alone, the fall usually does not go below a phosphorus level of 0.5 mg/dL. Carbohydrate repletion and subsequent insulin release enhance intracellular phosphorus, glucose, and potassium uptake. Phosphorus also moves into cells with correction of diabetic ketoacidosis. Phosphorus movement in "hungry bone syndrome" occurs after subtotal parathyroidectomy for hyperparathyroidism seen in patients with advanced

TABLE 7-2 Etiologies of Hypophosphatemia

Increased Kidney Excretion
Primary hyperparathyroidism
Secondary hyperparathyroidism from vitamin D deficiency
X-linked hypophosphatemic rickets
Autosomal dominant hypophosphatemic rickets
Oncogenic osteomalacia
Fanconi syndrome
Decreased Net Gastrointestinal Absorption
Decreased dietary intake
Phosphate-binding agents
Alcohol use disorder
Redistribution of Phosphorus
Shifts into intracellular space
Refeeding syndrome
Respiratory alkalosis
Diabetic ketoacidosis (and its treatments)
Hungry bone syndrome
Sepsis
Pseudohypophosphatemia

CKD. Calcium along with the phosphorus levels decrease rapidly after surgical parathyroid removal, and expectant monitoring of these levels should be performed.

Dietary Issues
Decreased gastrointestinal absorption alone is an uncommon cause of hypophosphatemia as the Western diet phosphorus intake is usually very high and the kidney is very effective at conserving phosphate in response to a low serum state. Poor phosphorus intake is usually combined with intake of an oral phosphate binder or ongoing diarrhea losses causing hypophosphatemia. Incredibly, in Bartter's original description of hypophosphatemia secondary to diet alone, 75 to 100 days of a low phosphorus diet combined with intake of phosphate-binding antacids were needed before a patient would experience symptoms. Other rare gastrointestinal causes such as steatorrhea and malabsorption can result in calcitriol deficiency, secondary hyperparathyroidism, and increased kidney phosphate wasting. The drug sorafenib for the treatment of advanced renal carcinoma is associated with hypophosphatemia.

Increased Phosphate Wasting by Kidney
Increased kidney phosphate excretion is seen in primary hyperparathyroidism, as well as secondary disorders from vitamin D metabolism. We know that PTH can increase kidney phosphate excretion, but this is partially offset by PTH action to increase calcitriol in the kidney which will lead to a secondary increase in gastrointestinal phosphorus absorption. On the contrary, secondary hyperparathyroidism from calcitriol deficiency may be associated with severe hypophosphatemia if the kidney function is normal. There are other rare disease states that lead to isolated kidney phosphate wasting: X-linked hypophosphatemia (XLH); autosomal dominant hypophosphatemic rickets (ADHR); and oncogenic hypophosphatemic osteomalacia. These should be considered for investigation in a patient with phosphorus levels less than 2.5 mg/dL and plasma FGF-23 greater than 30 pg/mL by intact FGF-23 assay. All of these rare disease states have low or normal calcitriol levels.

Medication Causes
Medications should be considered as a culprit of hypophosphatemia. Iron carboxymaltose can induce hypophosphatemia by stimulating FGF-23 release unnecessarily. Sirolimus use may also induce expression of klotho which works in concert with FGF-23. Fanconi syndrome, whether idiopathic or induced by drugs such as cisplatin, can lead to phosphaturia, glucosuria, and aminoaciduria. Inherited conditions associated with Fanconi syndrome include cystinosis, Wilson disease, hereditary fructose intolerance, and Lowe syndrome. Tenofovir is known as a cause of Fanconi syndrome in patients treated for human immunodeficiency virus, although this drug is being used less often due to a variety of secondary effects. The Chinese herb Boui-ougi-tou used for obesity is another agent associated with Fanconi syndrome. Figure 7-3 evaluates hypophosphatemia based on urinary excretion levels.

Signs and Symptoms of Hypophosphatemia
An astute clinician should be on the lookout for signs and symptoms of hypophosphatemia, as it is usually not part of a complete metabolic panel on routine labs. Moderate hypophosphatemia between 1.0 and 2.5 mg/dL does not impair myocardial contractility but is associated with impaired insulin sensitivity. Correction of moderate hypophosphatemia has been associated to improve diaphragmatic function in patients with respiratory failure and those who are failing to be liberated from mechanical ventilation. A cross-sectional study of patients with serum phosphorus less than 2.4 mg/dL was associated with a 20% increase in ventilator wean as compared to those with a normal phosphorus level. Nephrologists and Intensivists must be vigilant in those patients on continuous dialysis for hypophosphatemia as there usually is no phosphorus content in the dialysate fluid and removal of serum phosphorus is continuous as well. Once serum phosphorus levels fall below 1.0 mg/dL morbidity becomes apparent.

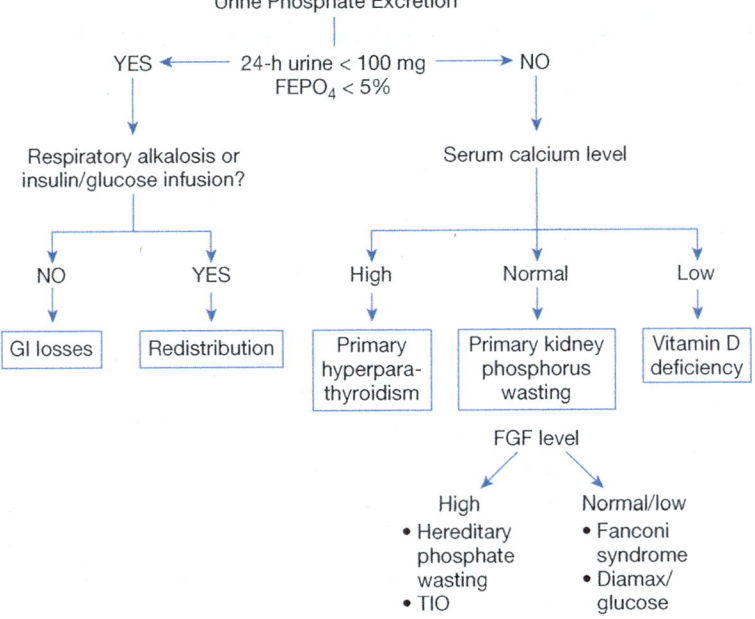

Figure 7-3. Hypophosphatemia workup approach.

This level of phosphorus is seen with reversible myocardial dysfunction and impaired response to cardiac pressors. Prolonged ventilation, longer hospital and ICU stays, and overall increased morbidity are associated with severely low phosphorus levels.

Diagnostic Workup

Workup for hypophosphatemia should be completed to determine the physiologic cause or causes. A 24-hour urinary phosphorus level can be diagnostic, but cumbersome for some patients. FGF-23 levels using an assay are possible but not available in all laboratories. The serum calcium, PTH, and total 24-hydroxy vitamin D levels should concurrently be measured as well. A fractional excretion of phosphorus can be measured using an early first-morning void with the following calculation: $(U_p \times P_{cr})/(U_{cr} \times P_p)$ multiplied by 100. An excretion below 5% indicates that the kidney is responding properly to decreased intestinal absorption or to a phosphorus shift into cells. Excretion above 5% indicates kidney losses that are inappropriate in the setting of hypophosphatemia and thus a kidney cause should be investigated.

Treatment of Hypophosphatemia

Treatment of hypophosphatemia is fairly straightforward. Once a diagnosis is made, the offending drug should be stopped or secondary cause corrected (such as dialysis phosphorus removal). There is currently low evidence that treatment of phosphorus levels above 1.0 mg/dL is necessary with the exception of a mechanically ventilated patient. Severe hypophosphatemia <1 mg/dL or a patient with symptoms should be treated aggressively, however. When treating hypophosphatemia, one should be aware that the serum level may not be reflective of total body phosphorus content, as a cellular shift may have occurred. Most patients can be corrected with up to 1 g of supplemental oral phosphorus per day. Oral repletion can be limited in efficacy in those with

TABLE 7-3	Suggested Replacement Amount for Phosphorus (P) Levels			
Phosphorus Level		Weight-Based Replacement		
mg/dL	mmol/L	40–60 kg	61–80 kg	81–120 kg
1.0	<0.32	30 mmol P	40 mmol P	50 mmol P
1.0–1.7	0.32–0.54	20 mmol P	30 mmol P	40 mmol P
1.7–2.2	0.55–0.70	10 mmol P	15 mmol P	20 mmol P

diarrhea or steatorrhea. Suggested rates of phosphorus replacement per measurement of serum phosphorus are available in Table 7-3.

Intravenous phosphorus repletion is common in hospitalized patients, and may only be reserved for symptomatic patients or those on continuous dialysis. Sodium phosphate should be used except in patients who require concomitant potassium repletion. Oral preparations should be considered once symptoms have resolved and/or serum phosphorus level is above 1.0 mg/dL. Refeeding syndrome should be repleted slowly secondary to cellular shifts. As well recent kidney transplant patients should be corrected slowly as the patient likely has a secondary or tertiary hyperparathyroidism. Phosphate nephropathy should be avoided and considered in those with rising creatinine with supplementation.

SUGGESTED READINGS

Amanzadeh J, Reilly RF Jr. Hypophosphatemia: an evidence-based approach to its clinical consequences and management. *Nat Clin Pract Nephrol*. 2006;2:136–148.

Blaine J, Weinman EJ, Cunningham R. The regulation of renal phosphate transport. *Adv Chronic Kidney Dis*. 2011;18(2):77–84.

Carpenter TO. Primary disorders of phosphate metabolism. [Updated 2022 Jun 8.] In: Feingold KR, Anawalt B, Blackman MR, et al., eds. *Endotext [Internet]*. MDText.com, Inc.; 2000. https://www.ncbi.nlm.nih.gov/books/NBK279172/

Cheng C-Y, Kuro-o M, Razzaque MS. Molecular regulation of phosphate metabolism by fibroblast growth factors-23-klotho system. *Adv Chronic Kidney Dis*. 2011;18:91–97.

Felsenfeld AJ, Levine BS. Approach to treatment of hypophosphatemia. *Am J Kidney Dis*. 2012;60(4):655–661.

Felsenfeld AJ, Levine BS, Rodriguez M. Pathophysiology of calcium, phosphorus, and magnesium dysregulation in chronic kidney disease. *Semin Dial*. 2015;28(6):564–577.

Gore MO, Welch BJ, Geng W, et al. Renal phosphate wasting due to tumor-induced osteomalacia: a frequently delayed diagnosis. *Kidney Int*. 2009;76(3):342–347.

Hutchison AJ, Smith CP, Brenchley PEC. Pharmacology, efficacy and safety of oral phosphate binders. *Nat Rev Nephrol*. 2011;7:578–589.

Martin KJ, González EA. Prevention and control of phosphate retention/hyperphosphatemia in CKD-MBD: what is normal, when to start, and how to treat? *Clin J Am Soc Nephrol*. 2011;6(2):440–446.

Naderi ASA, Reilly RF. Hereditary disorders of renal phosphate wasting. *Nat Rev Nephrol*. 2010;6(11):657–665.

Negri AL, Torres PAU. Iron-based phosphate binders: do they offer advantages over currently available phosphate binders? *Clin Kidney J*. 2015;8(2):161–167.

Reilly RF, Perazella MA. Nephrology in 30 days. Second edition. 2014.

Silver J, Naveh-Many T. FGF-23 and secondary hyperparathyroidism in chronic kidney disease. *Nat Rev Nephrol*. 2013;9(11):641–649.

Vervloet MG, van Ballegooijen AJ. Prevention and treatment of hyperphosphatemia in chronic kidney disease. *Kidney Int*. 2018;93(5):1060–1072.

The Patient With Hypomagnesemia or Hypermagnesemia

Neil Samuel Umles, Joel Topf

Magnesium Homeostasis

Magnesium is a divalent cation. Magnesium plays an important role in neuromuscular function, cardiac excitability, vasomotor tone, mitochondrial function, and energy metabolism. Magnesium is a cofactor for many reactions involved in energy metabolism, hormone release, as well as DNA and protein synthesis. Magnesium is also involved in the regulation of sodium, potassium, and calcium.

The atomic weight of magnesium is 24.3, and it has a valence of 2. See Table 8-1.

Adults have approximately 24 g of magnesium. Of those 24 g, 50% to 60% is found in the bone. The large bone reservoir provides an exchangeable source of magnesium which may release magnesium in response to magnesium deficiency. Of the magnesium not found in bone, almost all of it (99%) is in the intracellular compartment, where it is the second most prevalent cation, leaving only 1% for the extracellular compartment. Serum magnesium exists in one of three states:

1. Ionized (55% to 70%)
2. Protein bound (20% to 30%)
3. Complexed to anions (5% to 15%). Typically citrate, phosphate, or oxalate

It is important to keep in mind that serum magnesium may or may not reflect total body magnesium and that only the ionized fraction is physiologically active.

Intestinal Absorption of Magnesium

Dietary sources of magnesium include nuts, green vegetables, cereal, and milk. Magnesium is poorly absorbed by the intestines. Dietary magnesium ranges from 300 to 400 mg a day with roughly a third (100 to 130 mg) being absorbed. There are two primary routes of magnesium absorption, an active, transcellular, pathway, and a nonsaturable, passive, concentration-dependent, paracellular pathway. The active pathway is mediated by transient receptor potential melastatin (TRPM) type 6 and 7 channels to move magnesium from the gut into the enterocyte. How magnesium leaves the enterocyte is less clear, with evidence for both SLC41A2 and cyclin M family of proteins (CNNM). The passive paracellular route is nonsaturable, meaning higher concentrations of gut magnesium result in more magnesium absorption. However, since magnesium is cathartic, as more magnesium is ingested, colonic transit time decreases, resulting in diarrhea, as well as decreased magnesium absorption.

Renal Handling of Magnesium

The kidney can widely adjust its magnesium handling to maintain homeostasis. With high magnesium loads, fractional excretion of magnesium (FeMg) can reach 80%; while in magnesium-depleted states, it can fall to 0.5% (see Fractional Excretion of Magnesium equation later in the chapter). Both ionized magnesium and complexed magnesium are freely filtered at the glomerulus. The tubules are responsible for reabsorbing the majority of filtered magnesium to maintain homeostasis. Magnesium handling by the kidney is distributed across the proximal convoluted tubule, thick ascending loop of Henle, and the distal convoluted tubule (Fig. 8-1).

The proximal convoluted tubule is responsible for 10% to 20% of total magnesium reabsorption and this is not an important site for regulation of renal magnesium handling.

TABLE 8-1 Magnesium Formulations

Magnesium Salt	Molecular Weight (g/mol)	Elemental Magnesium (mg | mEq | mmol)	Typical Dosing
Magnesium oxide (400 mg tablet)	40	240 | 20 | 10	1 tab tid
Magnesium carbonate (100 mg)	84	29 | 2.4 | 1.2	variable
Magnesium chloride (535 mg tablet)	95	135 | 11 | 5	1 tab tid
Magnesium glycinate (665 mg tablet)	172	93 | 8 | 4	1 tab tid
Magnesium glycerophosphate (425 mg tablet)	194	53 | 4.4 | 2.2	2 tabs tid
Magnesium lactate (84 mg tablet)	202	10 | 0.8 | 0.4	4 tabs tid
Magnesium phosphate (710 mg tablet)	262	65 | 5.4 | 2.7	4 tabs tid
Magnesium aspartate hydrochloride (685 mg tablet)	246	67 | 5.6 | 2.8	2 tabs tid
Magnesium gluconate (500 mg tablet)	417	29 | 2.4 | 1.2	4 tabs tid
Magnesium citrate (625 mg capsule)	214	70 | 5.8 | 2.9	1 tab tid

Most salts come in various doses, to calculate the elemental magnesium divide the total dose by the molecular weight to get mmol, then multiply this by 24 to get the mg of elemental Mg or by 2 to get mEq.

Magnesium is reabsorbed via a paracellular route and passively down its concentration gradient. The tubular magnesium concentration rises as water is reabsorbed along the proximal tubule. But since two-thirds of filtered water is reabsorbed in the proximal tubule and only 20% of filtered magnesium is reabsorbed here, the tubular magnesium concentration rises through the proximal tubule and is then delivered to the loop of Henle.

The bulk of magnesium reabsorption occurs in the thick ascending limb of the loop of Henle. Up to 75% of magnesium reabsorption goes through a paracellular pathway. Magnesium reabsorption is driven by the electrical potential difference generated by the diffusion of potassium out of the cell via the ROMK transporter. This positive charge drives the reabsorption of magnesium and calcium paracellularly by claudins. The claudins are a family of at least 26 proteins that are expressed throughout the nephron. In the TALH specifically, mutations in claudins 16 and 19 lead to decreased Mg and Ca reabsorption and the disease *familial hypomagnesemia with hypercalciuria and nephrocalcinosis* (see Fig. 8-2).

In the distal convoluted tubule, apical TRPM6/7 channel facilitates transcellular magnesium reabsorption from the tubular fluid. This requires intact sodium chloride cotransporter and potassium excretion into the tubular fluid by Kv1.1, allowing magnesium to efflux from the cell on the basolateral membrane are the CNNM2 and SLC41A3 pores. Epithelial growth factor (EGF) increases the deposition of TRPM6/7 channels and inhibiting it with chemotherapy or immunosuppressant drugs can cause hypomagnesemia.

Magnesium, unlike other ions, does not have a well-understood hormonal regulating system. It is primarily regulated by serum magnesium. Three factors are important in regulating renal magnesium handling:

1. Magnesium concentration. TALH magnesium handling is affected by serum magnesium concentration. Increased serum magnesium slows reabsorption, while hypomagnesemia stimulates reabsorption, minimizing renal losses.

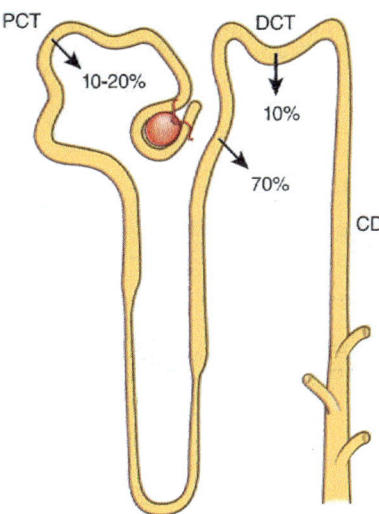

Figure 8-1. Handling of magnesium by the nephron. (Adapted with permission from Blaine J, Chonchol M, Levi M. Renal control of calcium, phosphate, and magnesium homeostasis. *Clin J Am Soc Nephrol.* 2015;10(7):1257–1272. Erratum in: *Clin J Am Soc Nephrol.* 2015; 10(10):1886–1887.)

2. Serum calcium concentration. In the TALH, calcium and magnesium are both reabsorbed by the same paracellular pathway. Hypercalcemia blocks calcium and magnesium reabsorption. When the calcium-sensing receptor (CaSR) is activated on the basolateral membrane, a number of intermediates are tripped before ultimately upregulating the expression of Claudin 14, which acts to block the paracellular reabsorption of calcium and magnesium via Claudin 16/19.
3. While multiple hormones (PTH, calcitonin, glucagon, ADH) alter magnesium handling, it is unclear how important this is, or if it is a significant factor in magnesium homeostasis. Magnesium is generally considered an *orphan ion* without specific hormonal regulation.

Hypomagnesemia

When talking about hypomagnesemia there are two related but distinct entities. *The first is a low blood magnesium level.* As described above, only 1% of total body magnesium is found in the extracellular compartment. So this low magnesium may not reflect total body magnesium stores. *The second entity is a normal serum magnesium with depleted total body magnesium.* The former situation, a low magnesium, is like any other ion, the low levels may cause symptoms, and these symptoms resolve with treatment. The latter case is tricky. In some cases, patients have classic symptoms of low magnesium despite normal magnesium levels and those symptoms improve with magnesium replacement. Good examples are hypocalcemia or hypokalemia resistant to standard replacement that responds only after magnesium supplementation. However, sometimes the improvement in the symptoms may be due to pharmacologic properties of magnesium rather than replacing a magnesium deficit. Magnesium is a natural calcium channel blocker. Is the ability to abrogate torsades de pointes due to correcting an underlying magnesium deficiency or from the pharmacologic and electrophysiologic properties of magnesium? Similar questions arise regarding magnesium's role in preeclampsia and asthma.

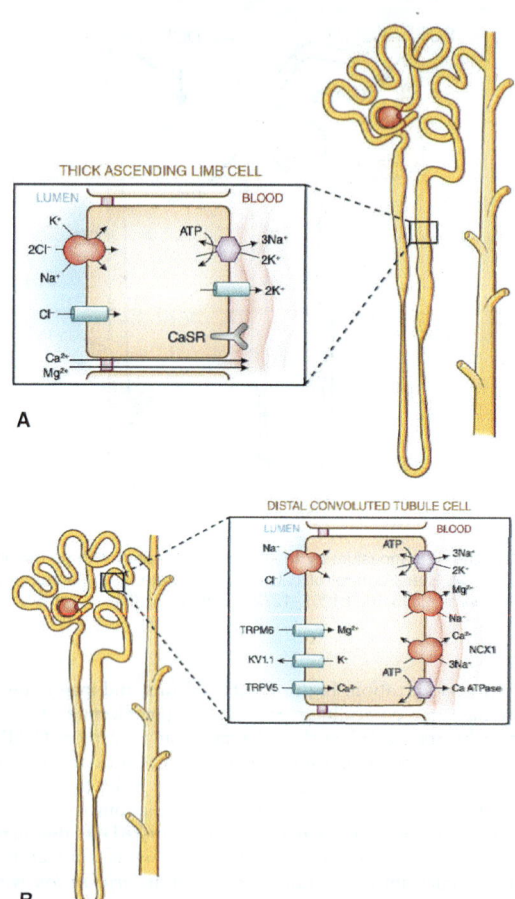

Figure 8-2. A: In the model of magnesium absorption by thick ascending limb of Henle, 40% to 70% of filtered magnesium is absorbed in the thick ascending limb by a paracellular pathway, mostly enhanced by lumen-positive transepithelial voltage. The apical Na-K-2Cl cotransporter mediates apical absorption of Na, K, and Cl. The apical renal outer medullary K channel mediates apical recycling of K back to the tubular lumen and generates lumen-positive voltage. Cl channel Kb mediates Cl exit through the basolateral membrane. Here Na,K-ATPase also mediates Na exit through the basolateral membrane and generates the Na gradient for Na absorption. The tight junction proteins claudin-16 and claudin-19 play a prominent role in magnesium absorption. The calcium-sensing receptor was also recently determined to regulate magnesium transport in this segment: upon stimulation, magnesium transport is decreased. CaSR, calcium-sensing receptor. **B:** In the model of magnesium absorption by distal convoluted tubules, approximately 5% to 10% of magnesium is reabsorbed in the distal convoluted tubule mainly by active transcellular transport mediated by TRPM6. The absorbed magnesium is then extruded via a recently identified magnesium/sodium exchanger across the basolateral membrane. The apical K channel Kv1.1 potentiates TRPM6-mediated magnesium absorption by establishing favorable luminal potential. In addition, the basolateral K channel Kir4.1 and the γ-subunit of Na,K-ATPase also regulate magnesium reabsorption. (Adapted with permission from Blaine J, Chonchol M, Levi M. Renal control of calcium, phosphate, and magnesium homeostasis. *Clin J Am Soc Nephrol.* 2015;10(7):1257–1272. Erratum in: *Clin J Am Soc Nephrol.* 2015;10(10):1886–1887.)

This section will focus on typical magnesium depletion (low serum levels) but will explore some ideas associated with normal magnesemia with total body depletion.

Epidemiology

Hypomagnesemia is a serum magnesium less than 0.62 mmol/L (1.5 mg/dL). Hypomagnesemia is found in approximately 2% of ambulatory, noninstitutionalized Americans and from 10% to 20% of hospitalized patients. However, in some populations it can exceed 60%. Cheungpasitporn et al. looked at patients admitted to the Mayo Clinic with a normal magnesium and found that 13% developed hypomagnesemia during hospitalization and this was associated with increased hospital mortality (OR 1.77).

In addition to hypomagnesemia, there is also an estimated high prevalence of magnesium deficiency with normal serum magnesium. The large pool of both skeletal magnesium and intracellular magnesium, allows these sources to "cover" for magnesium deficiency and maintain a normal serum magnesium level. An estimated 60% of Americans have inadequate nutritional intake of magnesium. Some authors advocate for tests of magnesium retention following diagnostic loading of IV magnesium. The theory is that patients with magnesium deficiency will retain a greater fraction of a slow IV magnesium load, while patients without deficiency will excrete a larger fraction of the load. This, however, will provide the wrong conclusion in patients with acquired (drug-induced, alcohol) or congenital renal magnesium leaks. In a review of 54 randomized controlled trials of magnesium supplementation, only one study used a magnesium loading study to assess magnesium status and the authors concluded that these diagnostics were "more suitable for research units and impractical for most clinical settings."

Clinical Manifestations of Hypomagnesemia

Clinical signs and symptoms of hypomagnesemia are uncommon until serum levels are less than 0.49 mmol/L (1.2 mg/dL). Hypomagnesemia often occurs with other electrolyte abnormalities so determining if the symptoms are due to the low magnesium or concomitant hypokalemia or hypocalcemia can be difficult to determine. Major clinical manifestations include:

- Neuromuscular manifestations including tremors, tetany, convulsions, weakness, confusion, and coma.
- Cardiovascular manifestations, including ECG changes, atrial and ventricular arrhythmias, and hypertension.
- Electrolyte abnormalities, including hypocalcemia, hypokalemia.

Magnesium and Cardiovascular Disease

There have been many associations between lower magnesium levels and various axes of cardiovascular health, but frustratingly few of these have been verified with interventional studies to show improved outcomes with magnesium correction or supplementation. At this time, no major guideline organization recommends magnesium supplementation for asymptomatic hypomagnesemia. A few of the interesting associations will be reviewed here.

HYPERTENSION

Magnesium deficiency is associated with the development of hypertension as well as the worsening of existing hypertension. Data from observational studies have revealed an inverse correlation between Mg serum concentration and hypertension.

Magnesium plays a pivotal role in regulating vascular tone through multiple mechanisms. It promotes the release of nitric oxide (NO) from the coronary endothelium and counteracts the effects of vasoconstrictors. Experimental studies have established a link between dietary magnesium intake or supplementation and improvements in hypertension. Furthermore, magnesium acts as a natural calcium channel blocker and can regulate vascular tone. A meta-analysis looked at 11 randomized controlled trials of magnesium supplementation and its effect on blood pressure. They found in 11 trials of 545 patients, a dose of 365 to 450 mg of magnesium resulted in a statistically significant drop in systolic blood pressure of 0.20 (0.37 to 0.03) mmHg and a diastolic drop of 0.27 (0.52 to 0.03) mmHg when compared to placebo. The longest trial was 6 months, with a mean of only 3.6 months.

MYOCARDIAL INFARCTION

Some early trials of magnesium in patients with acute myocardial infarction showed promise. The LIMITS-2 trial reported a 24% reduction in 28-day mortality and a 25% reduction in left ventricular failure in MI patients treated with intravenous (IV) magnesium sulfate during thrombolysis. However, later two larger, definitive trials, ISIS-4 (ISIS-4) and MAGIC (MAGIC), failed to show any effect. Magnesium is not currently a recommended therapy for myocardial infarction in major clinical practice guidelines.

ARRHYTHMIAS

The role of hypomagnesemia in the development of arrhythmias is not entirely clear, but several mechanisms have been proposed. Magnesium is essential for stabilizing electrolyte concentrations in heart muscle cells and membranes. It also acts as a calcium antagonist, improves oxygen utilization, and reduces the release of adrenaline and noradrenaline. Hypomagnesemia affects the activity of the sodium-potassium pump and potassium channels, depolarizing the cardiac myocyte contributing to arrhythmogenesis. EKG findings associated with hypomagnesemia include flattened T-waves, U-waves, prolonged QT intervals, and widened QRS complexes, all of which can also be seen in hypokalemia.

Torsade de pointes, a polymorphic ventricular tachycardia with prolonged QT intervals, has been observed in cases of hypomagnesemia. The American Heart Association and the American College of Cardiology recommend the use of magnesium and potassium in the management of torsade de pointes.

Electrolyte Abnormalities

Hypokalemia and hypomagnesemia are linked. Hypokalemia can be refractory in the setting of hypomagnesemia due to increased renal potassium losses. Since magnesium is a critical cofactor for reactions involving ATP, low magnesium can slow the Na-K ATPase. Magnesium can also affect the CaSR in the thick ascending limb of the loop of Henle. In the presence of magnesium, the calcium receptor is activated and inhibits the ROMK channel from creating a lumen-positive potential that drives paracellular magnesium reabsorption. Conversely, in magnesium depletion, the lack of activation of the CaSR leads to disinhibition of the ROMK channel, and increased renal potassium wasting.

Hypocalcemia frequently accompanies hypomagnesemia, particularly in cases of moderate to severe magnesium deficiency. Symptomatic hypocalcemia is more common in such patients, and it is important to note that treating hypocalcemia with calcium or vitamin D alone is ineffective; magnesium therapy is essential for resolving hypocalcemia in these cases. Various mechanisms have been proposed, including impaired parathyroid hormone (PTH) secretion, resistance of target organs to PTH, increased PTH metabolism, and decreased levels of 1,25 dihydroxy-vitamin D.

Diabetes Mellitus and Hypomagnesemia

Magnesium plays a significant role in glucose and insulin metabolism, primarily by influencing gluconeogenesis, glucose transporter activity, and directly affecting the insulin receptor. Multiple meta-analyses and prospective studies have established an inverse relationship between magnesium intake and the incidence of type 2 diabetes mellitus. A randomized control trial in individuals newly diagnosed with prediabetes demonstrated that a high magnesium intake reduced the progression to diabetes. Complicating the association of hypomagnesemia and diabetes is that diabetes is often a cause of hypomagnesemia, due to increased renal losses from osmotic diuresis. The American Diabetes Association currently has no recommendations for use of magnesium in the treatment or prevention of diabetes.

Magnesium in Preeclampsia and Eclampsia

Preeclampsia is a pregnancy disorder characterized by hypertension, proteinuria, and pathologic edema. When preeclampsia progresses to seizures, it is termed eclampsia.

TABLE 8-2 Causes of Hypomagnesemia

Renal		Extrarenal		Redistribution
Acquired	**Congenital**	**Acquired**	**Congenital**	
Calcineurin Inhibitors	Familial hypomagnesemia with hypercalciuria and nephrocalcinosis	Nasogastric Suctioning	Congenital achlorhydria	IV glucose
Diuretics				IV hyperalimentation and refeeding syndrome
Cisplatin		Proton-pump inhibitors		
EGFR-monoclonal ABs: cetuximab, panitumumab		Patiromer		
		Lactation		Refeeding syndrome
	Tubulointerstitial renal disease	Profuse sweating, burns, sepsis		
EGFR-related tyrosine kinase inhibitors: afatinib, erlotinib, and gefitinib	Gitelman syndrome	Acute and chronic diarrhea		Hungry bone syndrome
	Bartter syndrome	Malabsorptive syndromes		Pamidronate
		Acute pancreatitis		Massive blood transfusion
Pentamidine		Laxative abuse		
Foscarnet		Malnutrition or inadequate IV alimentation		Pancreatitis and soponification
Alcohol		Small bowel resection		
Aminoglycosides				
Amphotericin B				
Vitamin D intoxication				
Osmotic diuresis				
Postobstructive diuresis				
Post-transplant diuresis				
Diuretic phase of ATN				
Chronic metabolic acidosis				
Hypophosphatemia				
Hypokalemia				

ABs, antibodies; ATN, acute tubular necrosis; EGFR, Epidermal growth factor receptor; IV, intravenous.

Magnesium sulfate is a primary prophylaxis and treatment for preeclampsia and eclampsia. The Magpie trial in 2002 demonstrated a 58% reduction in the risk of eclampsia with magnesium sulfate compared to a placebo. The exact mechanisms of magnesium sulfate's action are not entirely clear but are likely multifactorial. It may act as a vasodilator, protect the blood–brain barrier, limit cerebral edema, and have a central anticonvulsant effect. One proposed mechanism may involve its role as an N-methyl-D-aspartate (NMDA) antagonist, which inhibits seizures, and its potential to promote cerebral vasodilation and lower intracellular calcium, limiting cerebral edema and seizure activity.

Etiologies of Hypomagnesemia

The causes of hypomagnesemia can be broken into three categories (Table 8-2).

1. Decreased intake
2. Redistribution from extracellular to intracellular compartment
3. Increased renal losses

Decreased Intake
Decreased magnesium intake can be seen with anorexia or with magnesium-poor diets. Magnesium content of foods has decreased overtime due to food processing and decreased soil magnesium due to overfarming with inadequate fertilizer. Despite an adequate diet, decreased magnesium absorption can occur with diarrhea, steatorrhea, or malabsorption from the use of a proton pump inhibitor (PPI). Due to the low concentration of magnesium in upper GI secretions, vomiting is an uncommon cause of hypomagnesemia.

PROTON PUMP INHIBITORS
Hypomagnesemia was first observed with PPI in 2006. Evaluation of those cases found that renal magnesium excretion was appropriately reduced, implicating decreased gut absorption of magnesium. PPIs will increase the pH in the intestines by 0.5 which alters TRPM6/7channel affinity for magnesium. Often the hypomagnesemia is compensated by decreased renal excretion of magnesium. But when an insult compromises renal retention of magnesium (diuretics, alcohol), hypomagnesemia can be uncovered. Importantly, H2-antagonists do not cause a similar decline in serum magnesium levels.

Renal Magnesium Wasting
Since a significant portion of magnesium is reabsorbed passively in the proximal tubule, factors that decrease sodium reabsorption in the proximal tubule (IV fluids and volume expansion) will increase renal magnesium loss. Both thiazides and loop diuretics block magnesium reabsorption and can cause hypomagnesemia. Osmotic diuresis also increases renal magnesium losses.

CHEMOTHERAPY
Monoclonal antibody epidermal growth factor receptor (EGFR) inhibitors can cause symptomatic hypomagnesemia from increased renal wasting. These are often used in metastatic colon cancer. They decrease magnesium reabsorption in the distal convoluted tubule by decreasing TRPM6 activity. Since TRPM6 channels are also present in the gut, there may be a component of decreased absorption but FeMg studies are consistent with renal wasting. Cetuximab and panitumumab are most commonly linked to hypomagnesemia. Zalutumumab has a lower rate of hypomagnesemia. Hypomagnesemia is seen in around 30% of cases. EGFR-related tyrosine kinase inhibitors have also been associated with hypomagnesemia, but the rate and severity are less than found with the monoclonal antibodies.

Platinum-based chemotherapeutics can cause protean electrolyte disorders and hypomagnesemia is common. Cisplatin causes more hypomagnesemia than carboplatin. The renal wasting is due to damage to epithelial cells of the thick ascending limb and distal convoluted tubule and can persist for years.

MAGNESIUM IN ASTHMA
IV magnesium sulfate may be a beneficial adjunct therapy for patients with moderate to severe asthma who show limited improvement with beta-agonists. Magnesium appears to enhance the effect of albuterol by inhibiting calcium influx through voltage-dependent calcium channels, leading to smooth muscle relaxation. Magnesium also has an immunoregulatory effect, reducing proinflammatory mediators and promoting the synthesis of bronchodilatory and vasodilatory agents like prostacyclin and NO.

While several systematic reviews and meta-analyses have assessed the role of IV or nebulized magnesium sulfate in acute asthma, results have been mixed. A definitive 1,100-person RCT of IV magnesium, versus nebulized magnesium, versus placebo by Goodacre concluded that there was no role for magnesium in the management of severe acute asthma in adults.

Treatment of Hypomagnesemia
Hypomagnesaemia and chronic magnesium deficiency are distinct conditions with different characteristics and treatment approaches. Magnesium supplementation may

TABLE 8-3	Normal Magnesium Levels	
mmol/L	mEq/L	mg/dL
0.62–0.91	1.2–1.8	1.5–2.2

be beneficial in high-risk individuals or those with specific medical conditions or on magnesium-wasting medications.

The ideal magnesium intake is often suggested to be based on body weight, with recommendations ranging from 4 to 6 mg/kg/d. Magnesium supplements are available in various forms, including magnesium oxide, magnesium chloride, magnesium citrate, magnesium taurate, and magnesium orotate. Organic magnesium salts (citrate, gluconate, orotate, aspartate) may have better bioavailability. Serum magnesium may not always reflect the total body magnesium status, and individuals at risk of deficiency or displaying symptoms of hypomagnesaemia should be considered for treatment regardless of their serum magnesium (see Table 8-3).

In cases of symptomatic hypomagnesemia or when magnesium concentrations are below 0.5 mmol/L, parenteral magnesium supplementation is indicated. In critical situations, such as hemodynamically unstable patients or those with severe arrhythmias, 1 to 2 g (4 to 8 mmol) of magnesium sulfate should be infused over 2 to 15 minutes. This can be repeated if the patient remains in extremis. In noncritical situations, 4 to 8 g (16 to 32 mmol) of IV magnesium sulfate should be infused over 12 to 24 hours. Roughly, half of IV magnesium is rapidly and uselessly excreted in the urine. The slow infusion is an attempt to minimize these renal losses. Magnesium replacement should be approached cautiously in individuals with decreased kidney function and a 50% dose reduction is appropriate in patients with a GFR of less than 30 mL/min (see Fig. 8-3).

In cases of renal magnesium wasting, there are two treatment strategies. The potassium-sparing diuretic, amiloride reduces urine magnesium and improves serum magnesium in treatment-resistant hypomagnesemia. Doses up to 20 mg a day are often employed. Amiloride is not effective at reducing the hypomagnesemia associated with Gitelman syndrome or thiazide use. SGLT2i are also able to ameliorate magnesium wasting. SGLT2i consistently reduced magnesium wasting and increased serum magnesium in large diabetes clinical trials. Additionally, case reports have demonstrated improved serum magnesium and renal magnesium retention in calcineurin- and cisplatin-induced magnesium wasting (see Fig. 8-4).

Hypermagnesemia

Hypermagnesemia is rare, and symptomatic hypomagnesemia rarer still. Hypermagnesemia may be the best-tolerated electrolyte disorder; patients can be largely asymptomatic despite magnesium levels reaching two to three times the upper limit of normal. When seen, hypermagnesemia is usually due to decreased GFR paired with increased absorption, often from increased magnesium loads or GI pathology. Symptoms are largely neuromuscular in nature. Treatment of severe, symptomatic hypermagnesemia usually relies on extracorporeal dialysis.

Epidemiology

The prevalence of hypermagnesemia varies across different populations and clinical settings. Among an ambulatory, urban, Iranian population, the prevalence of hypermagnesemia was 3.0% (hypermagnesemia was defined as a magnesium >1.04 mmol/L). Within hospital settings, the prevalence of hypermagnesemia has been variously reported from 1.8% to 9.3%, and up to 13.5% in the ICU. Much of this variability comes from a lack of consensus on the definition of hypermagnesemia. Patients with kidney disease

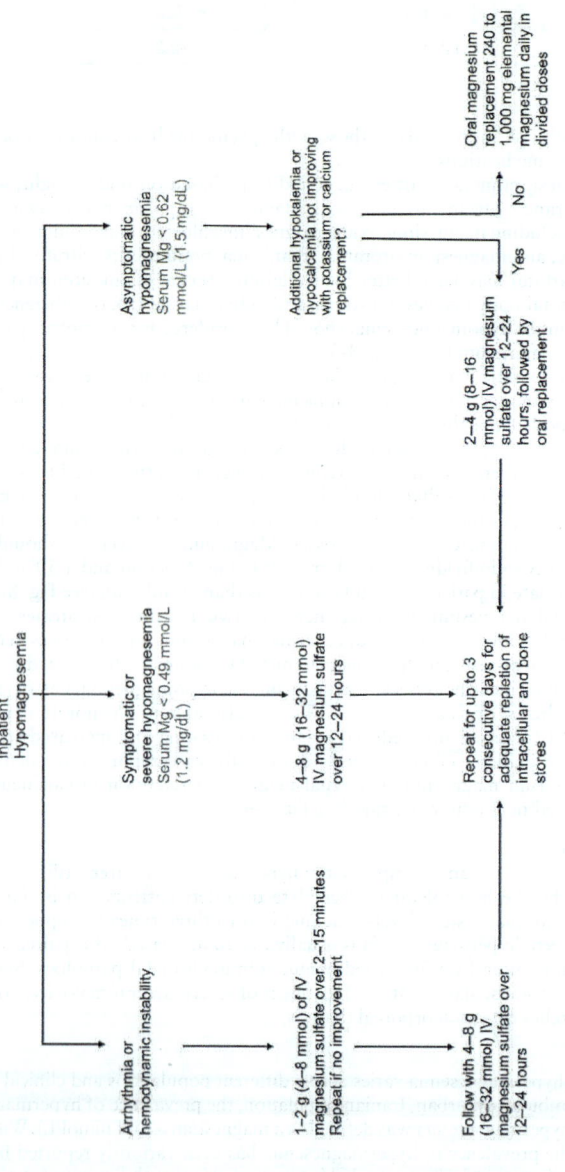

Figure 8-3. Inpatient hypomagnesemia algorithm. There are no clinical practice guidelines to guide the treatment of hypomagnesemia. This algorithm is based on the authors' opinions, expertise, and experience.

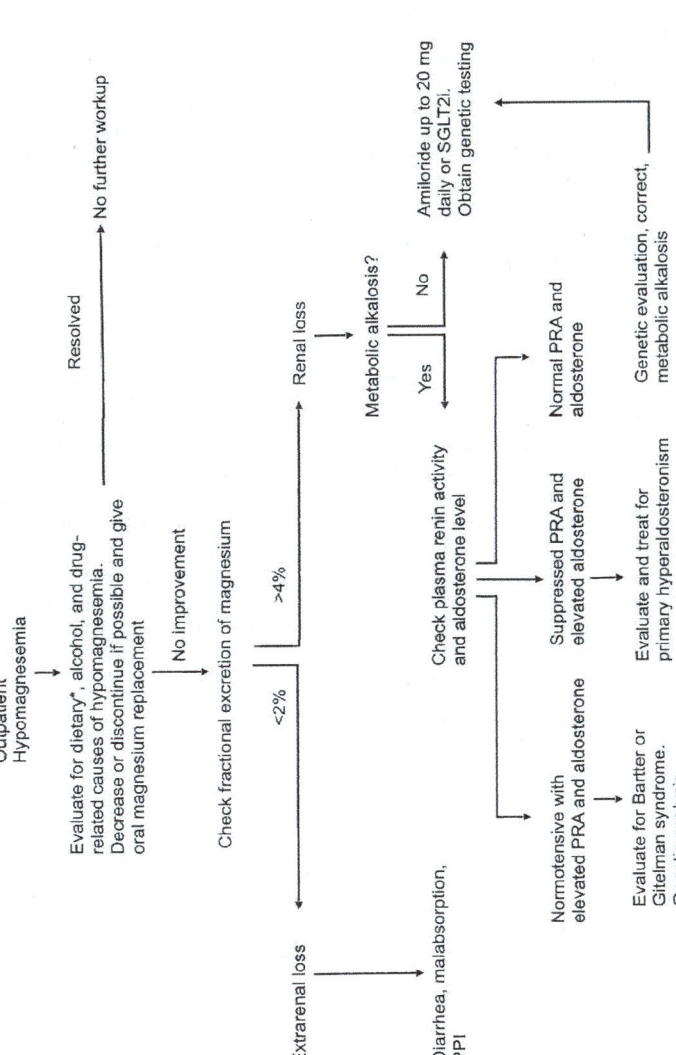

Figure 8-4. Outpatient hypomagnesemia algorithm. There are no clinical practice guidelines to guide the diagnosis of hypomagnesemia. This algorithm is based on the authors' opinions, expertise, and experience.

are at increased risk of developing hypermagnesemia due to reduced renal magnesium clearance. Hypermagnesemia, like most electrolyte disorders, is associated with adverse health outcomes, including increased in-hospital mortality and 1-year mortality rates.

Clinical Manifestations of Hypermagnesemia
The clinical presentation of hypermagnesemia can vary widely, and it is generally well tolerated within a certain range of serum magnesium concentrations (see Fig. 8-5). Concentrations between 1.05 and 2.2 mmol/L (2.55 to 5.35 mg/dL) are usually asymptomatic. As levels increase to 2.2 to 3.5 mmol/L (5.35 to 8.50 mg/dL), patients may experience nausea, weakness, and confusion. Over 3.5 mmol/L (8.5 mg/dL) patients have confusion, somnolence, muscle weakness, ileus, and depressed deep-tendon reflexes. Cardiac effects of hypermagnesemia include hypotension, bradycardia, prolonged PR, QRS, QT intervals, and ultimately asystole.

Etiologies
The causes of hypermagnesemia can be organized by increased intake, decreased excretion, and altered distribution (Table 8-4).

Increased Intake
PARENTERAL MAGNESIUM
Symptomatic hypermagnesemia can result from IV magnesium infusions, often used in the treatment of preterm labor or preeclampsia/eclampsia. These infusions can lead to serum magnesium levels ranging from 4 to 8 mg/dL, though routine laboratory monitoring of magnesium levels is usually not done. In trials of patients with preeclampsia treated with IV magnesium sulfate therapy, magnesium was well-tolerated with only minor side effects reported, including sensations of warmth, flushing, pain, numbness at the infusion site, dry mouth, and malaise. Dialysate mixing errors can result in a high magnesium content and hypermagnesemia, a typical dialysate magnesium concentration is only 0.5 mmol/L.

ORAL MAGNESIUM
Hypermagnesemia can occur even in individuals with normal kidney function, particularly among elderly patients with certain gastrointestinal conditions that enhance magnesium absorption or reduce gut motility, such as inflammatory bowel diseases and constipation. Patients with GI disorders including constipation often take magnesium-containing medications including Epsom salts which are largely magnesium oxide. This can result in a large magnesium load with concurrent prolonged transit time increasing magnesium absorption. Decreased kidney function increases the risk of hypermagnesemia from oral ingestions.

OTHER MAGNESIUM SOURCES
Hypermagnesemia has been reported in cases involving the use of magnesium-containing enemas, and even fatalities have occurred. Additionally, near-drowning incidents in the Dead Sea, known for its extremely high magnesium concentration, can result in hypermagnesemia due to aspiration or ingestion of magnesium-rich seawater.

Decreased Excretion
Magnesium balance is influenced by kidney function. As GFR falls tubular reabsorption of magnesium falls to allow patients to maintain magnesium balance. As this tubular reabsorption falls, there is less room for patients to ramp this up in response to a magnesium load, increasing the risk of hypermagnesemia.

Intracellular Shift
Since magnesium, like potassium, is largely an intracellular cation, cell lysis can cause hypermagnesemia. This cell death is seen with hemolysis, tumor lysis syndrome, and rhabdomyolysis. Metabolic acidosis is also reported to cause hypermagnesemia.

Treatment of Hypermagnesemia
The treatment of hypermagnesemia depends on its severity. Mild cases with normal renal function may not require treatment other than discontinuing the source of

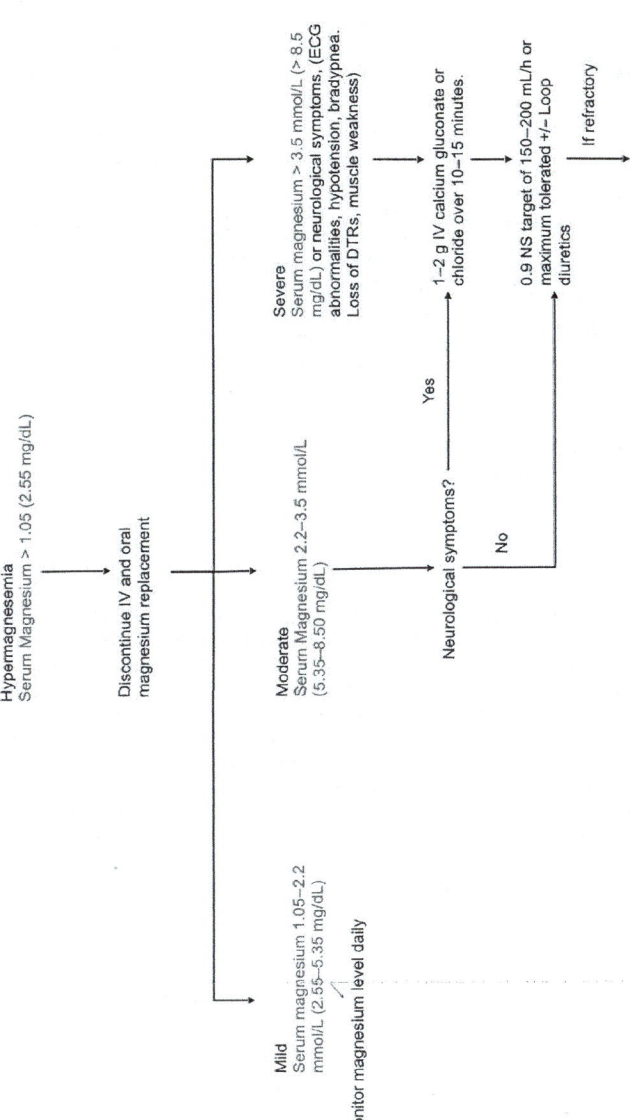

Figure 8-5. Hypermagnesemia algorithm. There are no clinical practice guidelines to guide the treatment of hypermagnesemia. This algorithm is based on the authors' opinions, expertise, and experience.

TABLE 8-4 Causes of Hypermagnesemia

Increased Intake	Decreased Excretion	Altered Distribution
Mg intoxication	Acromegaly	Tumor lysis syndrome
Laxatives	Familial hypocalciuric hypercalcemia	Hemolysis
Antacids		Rhabdomyolysis
Epsom salts	Adrenal insufficiency	Severe burns
Magnesium-containing enemas	Hyperparathyroidism. This decreases renal magnesium clearance, but hypermagnesemia is rare in cases of primary hyperparathyroidism.	Crush injury
Oral magnesium supplementation (mostly in the setting of decreased renal or gastrointestinal excretion)		Metabolic acidosis
Increased absorption		
Inflammatory bowel disease	Kidney failure/decreased GFR (contributor in cases with increased Mg intake)	
Constipation		
Other		
Dead Sea water poisoning		
Magnesium administration for preeclampsia and eclampsia		
Magnesium in dialysate		
Administration error		

GFR, glomerular filtration rate.

magnesium and monitoring. Severe hypermagnesemia with symptoms like neurologic issues, ECG abnormalities, hypotension, and reduced respiratory rate, necessitates immediate intervention. After stopping any exogenous sources of magnesium, the initial treatment is administration of IV calcium gluconate or chloride. Patients should be given 1 to 2 g over 10 to 15 minutes. Additional calcium can be considered if there is no improvement. Then normal saline should be given at the highest tolerated rate (with a target of 150 to 200 mL/h) to increase renal magnesium excretion. Loop diuretics can be added to block magnesium reabsorption in the loop of Henle. Last, dialysis can be used. Hemodialysis, peritoneal dialysis, and continuous dialysis have all been used to successfully lower magnesium in hypermagnesemia, but hemodialysis is the quickest method.

$$\text{Fractional excretion of Mg} = \frac{sCr \times uMg}{(0.7 \times sMg) \times uCr} \times 100$$

The FeMg provides a rapid assessment of the renal response to hypomagnesemia. The 0.7 constant in the denominator represents the fraction of serum magnesium filtered at the glomerulus (nonprotein bound). In the presence of hypomagnesemia, a FeMg less than 2% indicates an appropriate renal response to hypomagnesemia. Levels of 0.5% are more typical and implicate extrarenal magnesium losses or decreased intake. Results over 4% are consistent with renal wasting.

SUGGESTED READINGS

Aal-Hamad AH, Al-Alawi AM, Kashoub MS, Falhammar H. Hypermagnesemia in clinical practice. *Medicina (Mex)*. 2023;59(7):1190.

Ahmed F, Mohammed A. Magnesium: the forgotten electrolyte-a review on hypomagnesemia. *Med Sci (Basel)*. 2019;7(4):56.

Altman D, Carroli G, Duley L. Do women with pre-eclampsia, and their babies, benefit from magnesium sulphate? The magpie trial: a randomised placebo-controlled trial. *Lancet*. 2002; 359(9321):1877–1890.

Antman EM. Magnesium in acute MI. Timing is critical. *Circulation*. 1995;92:2367–2372.

Blaine J, Chonchol M, Levi M. Renal control of calcium, phosphate, and magnesium homeostasis. *Clin J Am Soc Nephrol*. 2015;10(7):1257–1272.

Blanchard A, Vargas-Poussou R, Vallet M, et al. Indomethacin, amiloride, or eplerenone for treating hypokalemia in Gitelman syndrome. *J Am Soc Nephrol*. 2015;26(2):468–475.

Catalano A, Bellone F, Chilà D, et al. Rates of hypomagnesemia and hypermagnesemia in medical settings. *Magnes Res*. 2021;34(1):1–8.

Cheuk DKL, Chau TCH, Lee SL. A meta-analysis on intravenous magnesium sulphate for treating acute asthma. *Arch Dis Child*. 2005;90(1):74–77.

Cheungpasitporn W, Thongprayoon C, Chewcharat A, et al. Hospital-acquired dysmagnesemia and in-hospital mortality. *Med Sci (Basel)*. 2020;8(3):37.

Cheungpasitporn W, Thongprayoon C, Qian Q. Dysmagnesemia in hospitalized patients: prevalence and prognostic importance. *Mayo Clin Proc*. 2015;90(8):1001–1010.

Chrysant SG, Chrysant GS. Association of hypomagnesemia with cardiovascular diseases and hypertension. *Int J Cardiol Hypertens*. 2019;1:100005.

Dibaba DT, Xun P, Song Y, Rosanoff A, Shechter M, He K. The effect of magnesium supplementation on blood pressure in individuals with insulin resistance, prediabetes, or noncommunicable chronic diseases: a meta-analysis of randomized controlled trials. *Am J Clin Nutr*. 2017;106(3):921–929.

Duley L, Metin Gülmezoglu A, Henderson-Smart DJ, Chou D. Magnesium sulphate and other anticonvulsants for women with pre-eclampsia. *Cochrane Database Syst Rev*. 2010;2010(11): CD000025.

Elasy AN, Nafea OE. Critical hypermagnesemia in preeclamptic women under a magnesium sulfate regimen: incidence and associated risk factors. *Biol Trace Elem Res*. 2023;201(8): 3670–3678.

Forbes JM, Cooper ME. Mechanisms of diabetic complications. *Physiol Rev*. 2013;93(1):137–188.

Fulgoni VL III, Keast DR, Bailey RL, Dwyer J. Foods, fortificants, and supplements: where do Americans get their nutrients? *J Nutr*. 2011;141(10):1847–1854.

Goodacre S, Cohen J, Bradburn M, et al. Intravenous or nebulised magnesium sulphate versus standard therapy for severe acute asthma (3Mg trial): a double-blind, randomised controlled trial. *Lancet Respir Med*. 2013;1(4):293–300.

Gröber U, Schmidt J, Kisters K. Magnesium in prevention and therapy. *Nutrients*. 2015;7(9): 8199–8226.

Groenestege WMT, Thébault S, van der Wijst J, et al. Impaired basolateral sorting of pro-EGF causes isolated recessive renal hypomagnesemia. *J Clin Invest*. 2007;117(8):2260–2267.

Guerrero-Romero F, Flores-García A, Saldaña-Guerrero S, Simental-Mendía LE, Rodríguez-Morán M. Obesity and hypomagnesemia. *Eur J Intern Med*. 2016;34:29–33.

Guerrero-Romero F, Simental-Mendía LE, Hernández-Ronquillo G, Rodriguez-Morán M. Oral magnesium supplementation improves glycaemic status in subjects with prediabetes and hypomagnesaemia: a double-blind placebo-controlled randomized trial. *Diabetes Metab*. 2015; 41(3):202–207.

Hansen B-A, Bruserud Ø. Hypomagnesemia in critically ill patients. *J Intensive Care Med*. 2018;6:21.

ISIS-4: A randomised factorial trial assessing early oral captopril, oral mononitrate, and intravenous magnesium sulphate in 58,050 patients with suspected acute myocardial infarction. ISIS-4 (Fourth International Study of Infarct Survival) Collaborative Group. *Lancet North Am Ed*. 1995;345(8951):669–685.

Ismail AAA, Ismail Y, Ismail AA. Chronic magnesium deficiency and human disease; time for reappraisal? *QJM*. 2018;111(11):759–763.

Ismail Y, Ismail AA, Ismail AAA. The underestimated problem of using serum magnesium measurements to exclude magnesium deficiency in adults; a health warning is needed for "normal" results. *Clin Chem Lab Med*. 2010;48(3):323–327.

Jahnen-Dechent W, Ketteler M. Magnesium basics. *Clin Kidney J*. 2012;5(Suppl 1):i3–i14.

Kanbay M, Goldsmith D, Uyar ME, Turgut F, Covic A. Magnesium in chronic kidney disease: challenges and opportunities. *Blood Purif*. 2010;29(3):280–292.

Kim DJ, Xun P, Liu K, et al. Magnesium intake in relation to systemic inflammation, insulin resistance, and the incidence of diabetes. *Diabetes Care*. 2010;33(12):2604–2610.

Kingston ME, Al-Siba'i MB, Skooge WC. Clinical manifestations of hypomagnesemia. *Crit Care Med*. 1986;14(11):950–954.

Larsson SC, Wolk A. Magnesium intake and risk of type 2 diabetes: a meta-analysis. *J Intern Med*. 2007;262(2):208–214.

Magnesium in Coronaries (MAGIC) Trial Investigators. Early administration of intravenous magnesium to high-risk patients with acute myocardial infarction in the Magnesium in Coronaries (MAGIC) Trial: a randomised controlled trial. *Lancet North Am Ed.* 2002;360(9341):1189–1196.

Mori H, Tack J, Suzuki H. Magnesium oxide in constipation. *Nutrients.* 2021;13(2):421.

Morrison AR. Magnesium homeostasis: lessons from human genetics. *Clin J Am Soc Nephrol.* 2023;18:969–978.

Murdoch DL, Forrest G, Davies DL, McInnes GT. A comparison of the potassium and magnesium-sparing properties of amiloride and spironolactone in diuretic-treated normal subjects. *Br J Clin Pharmacol.* 1993;35(4):373–378.

Palmer BF, Clegg DJ. Electrolyte and acid-base disturbances in patients with diabetes mellitus. *N Engl J Med.* 2015;373(6):548–559.

Palmer BF, Clegg DJ. Electrolyte disturbances in patients with chronic alcohol-use disorder. *N Engl J Med.* 2017;377(14):1368–1377.

Pelczyńska M, Moszak M, Bogdański P. The role of magnesium in the pathogenesis of metabolic disorders. *Nutrients.* 2022;14(9):1714.

Perazella MA. Proton pump inhibitors and hypomagnesemia: a rare but serious complication. *Kidney Int.* 2013;83:553–556.

Pham P-CT, Pham P-AT, Pham SV, Pham P-TT, Pham P-MT, Pham P-TT. Hypomagnesemia: a clinical perspective. *Int J Nephrol Renovasc Dis.* 2014;7:219–230.

Piuri G, Zocchi M, Porta MD, et al. Magnesium in obesity, metabolic syndrome, and type 2 diabetes. *Nutrients.* 2021;13(2):320.

Razzaque MS. Magnesium: are we consuming enough? *Nutrients.* 2018;10(12):1863.

Rodríguez-Ramírez M, Simental-Mendía LE, González-Ortiz M, et al. Prevalence of prehypertension in Mexico and its association with hypomagnesemia. *Am J Hypertens.* 2015;28(8):1024–1030.

Rosanoff A. Changing crop magnesium concentrations: impact on human health. *Plant Soil.* 2013;368(1):139–153.

Shah CV, Hammad N, Bhasin-Chhabra B, Rashidi A. SGLT2 inhibitors in management of severe hypomagnesemia in patients without diabetes: a report of 4 cases. *Kidney Medicine.* 2023;5(9):100697.

Silverman RA, Osborn H, Runge J, et al. IV magnesium sulfate in the treatment of acute severe asthma: a multicenter randomized controlled trial. *Chest.* 2002;122(2):489–497.

Syedmoradi L, Ghasemi A, Zahediasl S, Azizi F. Prevalence of hypo- and hypermagnesemia in an Iranian urban population. *Ann Hum Biol.* 2011;38(2):150–155.

Tang H, Zhang X, Zhang J, et al. Elevated serum magnesium associated with sglt2 inhibitor use in type 2 diabetes patients: a meta-analysis of randomized controlled trials. *Diabetologia.* 2016;59(12):2546–2551.

Titan SM, Moysés RMA. Calcium regulation and management of hypo- and hypercalcemia. *Nephrology Self-Assessment Program: NephSAP.* 2020;19(3):195–205.

Topf JM, Murray PT. Hypomagnesemia and hypermagnesemia. *Rev Endocr Metab Disord.* 2003;4(2):195–206.

Whang R, Chrysant S, Dillard B, Smith W, Fryer A. Hypomagnesemia and hypokalemia in 1,000 treated ambulatory hypertensive patients. *J Am Coll Nutr.* 1982;1(4):317–322.

Woods KL, Fletcher S, Roffe C, Haider Y. Intravenous magnesium sulphate in suspected acute myocardial infarction: results of the second Leicester Intravenous Magnesium Intervention Trial (LIMIT-2). *Lancet North Am Ed.* 1992;339(8809):1553–1558.

Workinger JL, Doyle RP, Bortz J. Challenges in the diagnosis of magnesium status. *Nutrients.* 2018;10(9):1202.

Zehender M, Meinertz T, Faber T, Caspary A, Jeron A, Bremm K, Just H. Antiarrhythmic effects of increasing the daily intake of magnesium and potassium in patients with frequent ventricular arrhythmias. Magnesium in Cardiac Arrhythmias (MAGICA) Investigators. *J Am Coll Cardiol.* 1997;29(5):1028–1034.

Zhang X, Del Gobbo LC, Hruby A, et al. The circulating concentration and 24-h urine excretion of magnesium dose- and time-dependently respond to oral magnesium supplementation in a meta-analysis of randomized controlled Trials. *J Nutr.* 2016;146(3):595–602.

Zipes DP, John Camm A, Borggrefe M, et al. ACC/AHA/ESC 2006 guidelines for management of patients with ventricular arrhythmias and the prevention of sudden cardiac death: a report of the American College of Cardiology/American Heart Association Task Force and the European Society of Cardiology Committee for Practice Guidelines (writing committee to develop Guidelines for Management of Patients With Ventricular Arrhythmias and the Prevention of Sudden Cardiac Death): developed in collaboration with the European Heart Rhythm Association and the Heart Rhythm Society. *Circulation.* 2006;114(10):e385–e484...

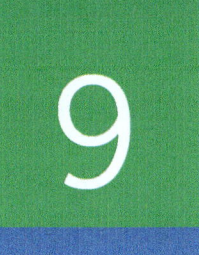

The Patient With Urinary Tract Obstruction (Emphasis on Kidney Stones)

Alexander Hlepas, Anna Zisman

Urinary tract obstruction (UTO) is a blockage of urine flow through the urinary tract and can occur at the level of the kidney, ureter(s), bladder, or urethra. The prevalence of UTO ranges from 5 in 10,000 to 5 in 1,000 depending on the cause. UTO has a bimodal age distribution with the first peak in childhood and the second peak in older adults. In children, the most common causes are anatomic abnormalities including posterior urethral valves and stricture and stenosis at the ureterovesical or ureteropelvic junction. In older adults, causes for external compression and infiltration include benign prostatic hyperplasia (BPH), prostate cancer, retroperitoneal or pelvic tumors (including metastatic cancer), and retroperitoneal fibrosis. Causes of intrinsic blockage include nephrolithiasis, urothelial carcinoma, blood clots, and sloughed papillae. In younger adults the most common cause is kidney stone disease (KSD).

The mechanism of UTO leading to renal dysfunction involves increase in pressure proximal to the obstruction, counteracting the intraglomerular pressure gradient and subsequently lowering the glomerular filtration rate (GFR). Over time secondary vasoconstriction mediated by angiotensin II and thromboxanes will lead to further reduction of GFR. Prolonged UTO eventually causes tubular injury and release of chemotactic substances which contribute to tubular injury and eventually intrinsic fibrosis and atrophy of the obstructed kidney(s).

If obstruction is bilateral and chronic, chronic kidney disease (CKD) may develop. Decreased GFR may rarely occur when obstruction is unilateral because autonomic-mediated vascular or ureteral spasm may affect the functioning kidney. Patients with a single kidney and UTO will present similarly to patients with bilateral obstruction.

When assessing suspected obstruction imaging modalities play a major role (Fig. 9-1). Ultrasound is most commonly utilized for detection and characterization of obstructive uropathy. Hydronephrosis is the typical finding in unilateral upper UTO involving the ureteropelvic junction or ureter. If bladder outlet obstruction is present, a distended urinary bladder may also be detected. Notably, during the first 1 to 3 days (early obstruction) or in an anuric or volume-depleted state, hydronephrosis may be subtle or absent. Doppler ultrasonography can be used to calculate renal arterial resistive indices, augmenting the sensitivity and specificity of ultrasound for diagnosing obstruction. A resistive index of >0.70 is typically considered discriminating for obstruction in setting of hydronephrosis. A more detailed evaluation of hydronephrosis, hydroureter, and/or bladder distension from outlet obstruction can be obtained via computed tomography (CT) scanning. The delayed contrast phase of the scan can demonstrate contrast proceeding from the kidneys to the bladder, localizing the intraureteral and extra-ureteral forms of obstruction, and identifying potential causes (Table 9-1). A MAG-3 (mercaptoacetyltriglycine) nuclear medicine renal scan can assess differential kidney function and, with administration of a loop diuretic, can quantify drainage times for each kidney.

With relief of obstruction, a physiologic diuresis occurs with the excretion of excess total body salt and water, along with a potential additional osmotic diuresis stimulated by the excretion of urea. This process can turn pathologic if tubular injury is present, with both decreased expression of aquaporin channels in the collecting duct and decreased sensitivity to antidiuretic hormone, and abnormalities in

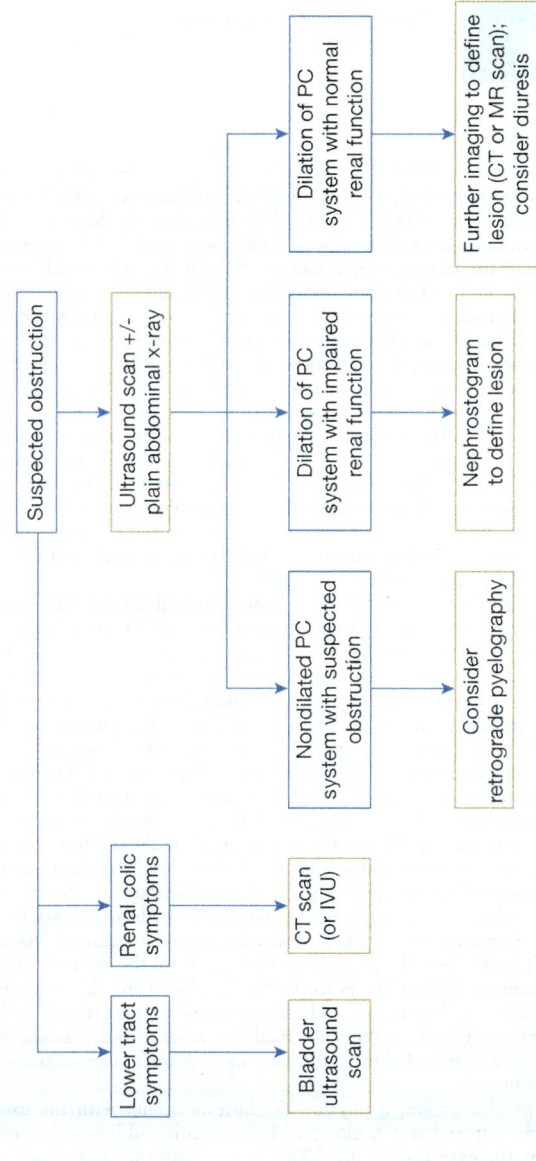

Figure 9-1. Approach to Imaging in Patients With Suspected Urinary Obstruction. The recommended imaging tests for patients with suspected obstruction is related to presenting symptoms. Without localizing symptoms, renal ultrasound is generally preferred while CT scan or bladder scan may be more appropriate in patients with renal colic or lower urinary symptoms, respectively.

TABLE 9-1 Etiologies of UTO

Cause	Kidney	Ureter	Bladder	Urethra
Calculi	+	+		+
Urothelial carcinoma	+	+	+	
Sloughed papilla	+	+		
Extrinsic tumors		+		
Retroperitoneal fibrosis		+		
Infection		+		
Obstructed stent		+		
Blood clot		+	+	
Trauma		+		
Ectopia		+		
Edema/Inflammation			+	
Bladder dysfunction			+	
Posterior urethral valves			+	
Prostatic enlargement				+
Stricture				+

UTO, urinary tract obstruction.

Data from Zeidel ML, O'Neill WC. Clinical manifestations and diagnosis of urinary tract obstruction (UTO) and hydronephrosis. In: *UpToDate*. Curhan GC and Baumgarten DA, eds. Wolters Kluwer. https://www.uptodate.com/contents/clinical-manifestations-and-diagnosis-of-urinary-tract-obstruction-uto-and-hydronephrosis?search=Zeidel%20ML%2C%20O'Neill%20WC.%20Clinical%20manifestations%20and%20diagnosis%20of%20urinary%20tract%20obstruction%20%28UTO%29%20and%20hydro-%20%5BAU3%5D%20nephrosis&source=search_result&selectedTitle=3%7E150&usage_type=default&display_rank=3#topicGraphics. Accessed on May 30, 2024.

the corticomedullary gradient leading to inability to appropriately concentrate the urine. Patients most at risk for pathologic postobstructive diuresis (POD) with relief of obstruction are those with severe urinary retention (postvoid residuals >1,100 mL), high serum creatinine, and elevated blood urea nitrogen (BUN). Management of POD requires close attention to volume status and electrolytes, along with adequate access to oral fluids. Intravenous fluids may be required if volume loss continues, with fluid type dictated by serum and urine electrolyte concentrations. It is important not to replace fluids excessively, however, so as not to perpetuate the supraphysiologic diuresis. Degree of renal recovery after resolution of obstruction is dependent on underlying kidney function, as well as degree and duration of obstruction.

UTO due to KSD presents at more common areas of lodgment including the ureteropelvic junction, the distal ureter (at the level of the iliac vessels), and the ureterovesical junction. Typically, stones greater than 5 mm are more likely to obstruct. Those less than 5 mm are more likely to pass spontaneously.

When the flow of urine is obstructed, kidney stones (KS) are more likely to form. Concurrently, KS themselves can be the causes of UTO. Therefore, it is pertinent to focus on KSD in the context of UTO. KSD has been rapidly increasing in both incidence and prevalence across the world. Reports from multiple countries including

Iceland, New Zealand, Germany, and the United States indicate rising incident rates over the last several decades. The National Health and Nutrition Examination Survey (NHANES), for example, demonstrates a rise in KSD prevalence from 3.2% in 1980 to 10.1% in 2016. Historically, men were threefold more likely than women to suffer from KS, but prevalence rates in women are rapidly increasing, from 2.4% of the female population in 1980 to 9.4% in 2014. KSD appears to be most common in non-Hispanic Whites and Hispanics and less common in non-Hispanic Blacks or non-Hispanic Asians, though this too is quickly changing. Blacks have previously comprised a minority of those affected, with less than 1.7% prevalence noted in the 1988–1994 NHANES dataset. More recently, however, Blacks represent the fastest growing KS demographic, with the population adjusted prevalence rising to 5.8% by 2014. In the United States, there is a higher prevalence among persons with functional disabilities (16%) than among those without disabilities (9%).

Calcium-containing KS make up approximately 90% of all KS; they contain primarily calcium oxalate (CaOx) and are often admixed with contain calcium phosphate (CaP) in the form of apatite or brushite, or occasionally uric acid. The remaining 10% are composed of uric acid (8%), struvite-carbonate, and cystine. KSD is a major cause of morbidity due to associated renal colic, UTO, urinary tract infection (UTI), and renal parenchymal damage, with 0.8% to 3.2% of ESRD attributed to KSD. Struvite stones have been found to account for up to 42.2% of these cases. Although the effect was small, an analysis of NHANES III data revealed an association between history of KS and estimated GFR that was dependent on body mass index (BMI). KS formers with a BMI greater than 27 kg/m^2 had a mean estimated GFR that was 3.4 mL/min/1.73 m^2 lower than similar nonstone formers.

Most cases of nephrolithiasis are currently understood to be dependent on an interplay between environmental factors and genetic susceptibility with a complex and polygenic mode of inheritance. Overall KSD has been reported to occur threefold more frequently in individuals with a positive family history of KS. Genome-wide association studies have implicated a series of genes involved in renal tubular handling of lithogenic substrates, an inhibitor of crystallization in KSD in the general population. However, precise genomic determinants remain ill-defined.

KS can form only when urine is supersaturated with respect to a stone-forming salt. Notably, urine in many healthy subjects is often supersaturated with respect to CaOx or uric acid and crystalluria has been described in as many as 15% to 20% of healthy subjects. However, urine of recurrent KS formers was noted to contain crystals in first morning voided specimens much more frequently than that of KS formers without subsequent recurrence, suggesting that recurrence may depend on the degree and severity of crystalluria.

CaOx can crystallize as either calcium oxalate monohydrate (COM) or calcium oxalate dihydrate (COD). COM is the predominant form found in KS and is more pathogenic and typical of hyperoxaluria. It is thermodynamically more stable and has stronger adhesive capabilities. COD is more physiologic than pathogenic and more associated with hypercalciuria with or without hyperoxaluria. Macromolecular inhibitors block COM growth and favor COD formation. This suggests that a shift toward more COD crystals in urine might protect against KS formation given their reduced capacity to form stable aggregates and adhere to epithelial cells. Another important factor in the pathogenesis of KS formation that is incompletely understood is the interplay of crystallization inhibitors in urine with the procrystallization components. Normal urine contains a variety of inorganic and organic substances that act as crystallization inhibitors and that are not completely accounted for in the supersaturation calculations clinically in use. The most clinically important of these are citrate, magnesium, and pyrophosphate.

Sufficient thermodynamic energy must be generated for a crystal to form in solution. Once a crystal forms, it was once thought that it must either grow to sufficient size to occlude the tubular lumen or anchor itself to the urinary epithelium, which would in turn provide a surface upon which it can grow. The typical transit time of a crystal through the nephron is on the order of 3 minutes, and this is likely too short a period for it to nucleate, grow, and occlude the tubular lumen. More recent work has elucidated a different model. Calcium reabsorption in the thick ascending limb (TAL) occurs via the paracellular pathway and is driven by transepithelial voltage difference between tubule and blood. It has been suggested that reabsorbed calcium is then further transported with the help of descending vasa recta along the thin limbs of the loops of Henle toward the papilla which has been described as "vas washdown." The initial site of crystal formation is found to be in the form of a plaque in the basement membrane of the thin limb of the loop of Henle. Subsequently, either by extension or additional formation, plaque appears in the papillary interstitium, which is known as Randall plaque. The plaque consists of an amalgamation of apatite crystals in an organic matrix that contains osteopontin, inter–α-trypsin inhibitor, heavy chain 3 and other molecules that have yet to be determined. The plaque is then bathed in urine supersaturated with stone-forming constituents upon which CaOx is deposited. In addition to plaque formation tubular plugging of Bellini ducts and inner medullary collecting ducts has been described in various KS types. Tubule plugs give rise to overgrowth that resemble KS in their composition but have not been proven to produce clinical disease.

I. Initial Presentation

KSD can be asymptomatic and may be incidentally found on imaging for other indications. Acute renal colic most commonly presents with severe flank pain, sudden onset, and is often associated with nausea and vomiting. The radiation of the pain may provide some clue as to where in the urinary tract the KS is lodged. KS in the ureteropelvic junction cause flank pain that may radiate to the groin, whereas those lodged in the narrowest portion of the ureter, where it enters the bladder, are associated with signs of bladder irritation (dysuria, frequency, and urgency). A careful abdominal examination and, in women, a pelvic examination are important to rule out other potential causes of abdominal pain.

A. Laboratory evaluation should include a complete blood cell count, serum chemistries, and urinalysis. The white blood cell count may be mildly elevated but is generally less than $15,000/mm^3$. A white blood cell count greater than $15,000/mm^3$ is suggestive of another intraabdominal cause or an associated infection behind an obstructing calculus. An elevation of the serum BUN and creatinine concentrations indicates prerenal azotemia, parenchymal renal disease, or obstruction of a solitary functioning kidney. A urinalysis should be performed routinely in any patient with abdominal pain. Microscopic hematuria is observed in approximately 90% of patients with renal colic.

B. Once the diagnosis is suspected based on the history, physical examination, and preliminary laboratory studies, **establishing a definitive diagnosis** is the focus of the next stage of the evaluation.

1. A **flat radiographic plate of the abdomen** is often obtained and can identify radiopaque KS (CaOx, CaP, struvite-carbonate, and cystine) that are ≥2 mm in size. It will miss radiolucent KS, the most common of which are composed of uric acid, and KS that overlie the bony pelvis. For these reasons, an abdominal flat plate is most valuable in ruling out other intraabdominal processes.

2. An **ultrasonographic examination of the genitourinary tract** often identifies KS in the renal pelvis; however, in acute presentations KS are frequently lodged in the ureter, and the ultrasonographic examination may miss these. However, hydronephrosis can be identified by ultrasound which can help stratify severity of the acute obstruction. Recent trials have shown further utility of fast-track point-of-care ultrasound or ultrasound-first clinical decision support. Time spent in the ED and CT use were significantly reduced and complication rates were similar compared to traditional approaches.

TABLE 9-2 Likelihood of Spontaneous Passage

	Likelihood of Spontaneous Passage (%)
Size	
>6 mm	25
4–6 mm	60
<4 mm	90
Location	
Upper ureter, >6 mm	1
Upper ureter, <4 mm	81
Lower ureter, <4 mm	93

3. **Spiral CT** is the test of choice in the patient with suspected renal colic. The advantages of spiral CT include higher sensitivity, faster scan times, and lack of need for contrast, while also assessing for alternate diagnoses. Digital tomosynthesis has been shown to offer similar detection rates at lower cost and lower radiation exposure.
4. The **intravenous pyelogram** (IVP) was formerly considered the gold standard for the diagnosis of nephrolithiasis. Given advances in CT techniques, this is rarely utilized in the acute setting.

C. **Management.** After the diagnosis is established, subsequent management is determined by (a) the presence or absence of associated infection; (b) whether parenteral narcotics are required for pain control; and (c) the likelihood of spontaneous stone passage. The likelihood of spontaneous passage is determined by stone size and location in the ureter (Table 9-2). Small stones in the distal ureter will likely pass, whereas large stones in the upper ureter will likely require urologic consultation and intervention. Tamsulosin, an α1-receptor antagonist, and calcium channel blockers can be used to aid stone passage (medical expulsive therapy). Obstructing calculi can be managed with observation alone if pain can be controlled with oral analgesics, kidney function is stable, and spontaneous passage is likely. Extracorporeal shock wave lithotripsy or ureteroscopic lithotripsy may need to be employed for KS lodged in the upper ureter. Calculi in the lower ureter can be removed by cystoscopy and ureteroscopy. Hospital admission is necessary if there is evidence of renal parenchymal infection; when nausea, vomiting, or severe pain precludes oral analgesic use; or the stone is unlikely to pass spontaneously.

II. Types of Stones

A. **Calcium-containing stones** make up 90% of all stones and are generally composed of a mixture of CaOx and CaP. In mixed stones, CaOx usually predominates, and pure CaOx stones are more common than pure CaP stones. CaP tends to precipitate in more alkaline urine, as occurs with renal tubular acidosis (RTA), whereas the precipitation of CaOx is less sensitive to pH. The major risk factors for the formation of calcium-containing stones include hypercalciuria, hypocitraturia, hyperuricosuria, hyperoxaluria, low urine volume, and medullary sponge kidney. These risk factors can occur either alone or in combination. Their relative frequency is shown in Table 9-3.

1. **Hypercalciuria** is often defined for research purposes as urinary calcium excretion greater than 250 mg/24 hours in women and greater than 300 mg/24 hours in men. It is critical to note that this is a continuous

TABLE 9-3   Risk Factors for Calcium-Containing Kidney Stones

Risk Factor	Alone (%)	Combined (%)
Hypercalciuria	60	80
Low urine volume	10	50
Hypocitraturia	10	50
Hyperuricosuria	10	40
Hyperoxaluria	2	15

relationship, so the higher the value, the greater the risk of stone formation. Hypercalciuria is present in approximately two-thirds of patients with calcium-containing stones and may result from an increased filtered load, decreased proximal reabsorption, or decreased distal reabsorption. Proximal calcium reabsorption parallels sodium. Any situation that decreases proximal sodium reabsorption such as extracellular fluid (ECF) volume expansion also decreases proximal calcium reabsorption, thus hypercalciuria from any cause will be exacerbated by a high dietary sodium intake. Distal tubular calcium reabsorption is stimulated by parathyroid hormone (PTH), thiazides, and amiloride and inhibited by acidosis and phosphate depletion.

Hypercalciuria may be idiopathic or secondary. Secondary causes are primary hyperparathyroidism, RTA, sarcoidosis, immobilization, Paget disease, hyperthyroidism, milk-alkali syndrome, and vitamin D intoxication. The idiopathic group makes up 90% of all hypercalciuria. This category of patients is characterized by increased $1,25(OH)_2$ vitamin D_3 concentration, suppressed PTH, and reduced bone mineral density and is often familial.

2. **Hypocitraturia** has historically been defined as excretions of less than 320 mg citrate/d, with the understanding that like calcium, this is not a binary variable. Women typically have higher citrate excretions than men. Citrate combines with calcium in the tubular lumen to form a nondissociable but soluble complex. As a result, less free calcium is available to combine with oxalate. Citrate also prevents nucleation and aggregation of CaOx. Chronic metabolic acidosis from any cause enhances proximal tubular citrate reabsorption and decreases urinary citrate excretion; this is the mechanism whereby chronic diarrhea, RTA, and increased dietary protein load result in hypocitraturia. Another important cause of hypocitraturia is hypokalemia, which increases expression of the sodium-citrate cotransporter present in the proximal tubular luminal membrane.

3. **Hyperuricosuria** is defined as uric acid excretion greater than 800 mg/d in men and greater than 750 mg/d in women. Uric acid and monosodium urate decrease CaOx solubility in urine. Addition of increasing concentrations of uric acid and sodium urate to normal human urine can induce CaOx precipitation. This is thought to be through *salting out* which implies reduced solubility (of CaOx) with increasing ionic strength in the urine.

4. **Hyperoxaluria** is defined as urinary oxalate excretion greater than 45 mg/d. The etiologies of hyperoxaluria include enteric hyperoxaluria and a group of rare genetic disorders of primary hyperoxaluria (PH). Enteric hyperoxaluria is a possible complication of inflammatory bowel disease, small bowel resection, jejunoileal bypass, Roux-en-Y gastric bypass or dietary excess (e.g., spinach, Swiss chard, rhubarb, or almonds).

The majority of urinary oxalate is derived from endogenous production in liver (80% to 90%) and the remainder is obtained from dietary oxalate or ascorbic acid metabolism. In enteric hyperoxaluria, intestinal oxalate hyperabsorption occurs through two mechanisms. First, free fatty acids bind calcium and limit the amount of free calcium available to complex oxalate, thereby increasing the oxalate pool available for absorption. Second, bile salts and fatty acids increase colonic oxalate permeability. Additional risk factors for stone formation in these patients include intestinal fluid losses that decrease urine volume; and intestinal bicarbonate and potassium losses that result in hypocitraturia.

Several studies suggest a correlation between decreased activity of the oxalate-degrading bacteria *Oxalobacter formigenes* and the development of recurrent CaOx–containing KS. *O. formigenes* utilizes oxalate as its sole energy source and has the capacity to degrade 0.5 to 1.0 g of oxalate/d. In this process it converts oxalate to CO_2 and formate. It is unclear why intestinal colonization with *O. formigenes* decreases with increasing age and in patients who form CaOx stones. One possibility is that antibiotic therapy, especially recurrent courses of fluoroquinolones, act to eradicate the organism. Studies in colons of colonized rats showed that colonization with *O. formigenes* results in net oxalate secretion across the colonic mucosa and a decrease in urinary oxalate excretion. Control rats showed net oxalate reabsorption. Sel1-like proteins and small peptides have been identified as the major *O. formigenes*-derived secreted factors stimulating oxalate transport by human intestinal epithelial cells. These exciting findings raise the potential for new future therapies in hyperoxaluric CaOx stone formers. To date, however, studies in humans with *O. formigenes* replacement have yielded conflicting results. A more recent mendelian randomization study showed no evidence of a causal association between *O. formigenes* and KS and was suggestive of a more complex association of several genera of gut microbiota and KS.

PH is a group of rare autosomal recessive inborn errors of glyoxylate metabolism characterized by the overproduction of oxalate which deposits as CaOx in the kidney and later on also manifests as systemic oxalosis. PH can be classified into types 1, 2, and 3 with decreasing severity with regard to oxalate excretions and, consequently, KSD. Plasma oxalate and eGFR have been found to inversely correlate in pediatric PH patients with maintained kidney function.

5. **Low Urinary Volume.** This is perhaps the most intuitively obvious of risk factors for all KS types. The lower the volume of solvent, the more likely that a given amount of salt will be supersaturating. This risk factor is particularly prominent in warm climates with low humidity.

6. **Medullary sponge kidney** is a congenital disorder which should be suspected in women, or in men with no other risk factors for calcium-containing stones. It has a prevalence of approximately 1 in 5,000 and affects males and females equally. The anatomic abnormality is an irregular enlargement of medullary and inner papillary collecting ducts. The diagnosis is usually established in the fourth or fifth decade by an IVP that reveals radial, linear striations in papillae or cystic collections of contrast media in ectatic collecting ducts or by a surgeon on direct visualization. Patients present with stones or recurrent UTI, often associated with distal RTA. Malformations of the terminal collecting duct result in urinary stasis that promotes crystal precipitation and attachment to the tubular epithelium.

7. **Obesity** is increasingly being recognized as a risk factor for CaOx and uric acid stone formation. As body size increases, urinary oxalate and uric acid excretion also increase. In a prospective study of three large cohorts with

4,827 incident stones detected, body weight, BMI, waist circumference, and weight gain after age 21 years were all associated with an increased risk of KS formation. This effect was even more pronounced in women than in men. In another study of 4,883 patients with nephrolithiasis who underwent stone evaluation in two different stone clinics, urinary pH was inversely related to BMI. A persistently low urinary pH is the most important risk factor for uric acid nephrolithiasis, which may in part explain the increasing incidence of stone formation observed over the last several decades in the United States. As the BMI of the population increases, it would be expected that the incidence of stone formation will continue to rise well into the future.

B. Uric acid stones represent approximately 5% to 8% of all cases of nephrolithiasis in Western countries. The highest incidence was reported from Israel and the Middle East, where as many as 30% of all KS consist solely of uric acid. This may be the result of the arid climate and reduced urinary volume. Uric acid is the major metabolic end-product of purine metabolism in humans. Unlike most other mammals, humans do not express uricase, which degrades uric acid into the much more soluble allantoin. Uric acid stones are the most common radiolucent stone.

1. **Pathophysiology.** The principal determinant of uric acid crystallization is its relative insolubility at acidic pH. Uric acid is a weak organic acid with two dissociable protons. The first has a pK_a (-log of acid dissociation constant) of 5.3 in the urine, and the second a pK_a of 10. As a result, only the first proton is dissociated in urine. At pH less than 5.5, undissociated acid predominates, and it is more likely to crystallize (solubility 80 mg/L). As pH increases, uric acid dissociates into the more soluble sodium urate (solubility 1 g/L). Because of the great increase in solubility with increasing pH, uric acid stones are the only KS that can potentially be completely dissolved with medical therapy. The main determinants of uric acid crystallization are pH, concentration, and other cations present in urine. A higher sodium concentration and a lower potassium concentration increase uric acid solubility. Sodium-containing alkali may also increase urinary calcium excretion secondary to ECF volume expansion, though this is controversial.

2. **Risk Factors and Presentation.** Patients with uric acid stones exhibit a lower mean urinary pH and ammonium ion excretion rate. As many as 75% demonstrate a mild defect in renal ammoniagenesis in response to an acid load. Urinary buffers other than ammonia are titrated more fully than in unaffected individuals, with a resultant urine pH approximating 4.5. Those with defects in ammoniagenesis, such as the elderly and patients with polycystic kidney disease, are at increased risk for uric acid lithiasis. Patients with type 2 diabetes mellitus are also at increased risk for uric acid stone formation, as they have a lower urine pH compared with healthy individuals. In one study, 33% of unselected uric acid stone formers had type 2 diabetes mellitus and 23% had impaired glucose tolerance. The low urine pH in patients with insulin resistance is due to impairment in urinary ammonium excretion. Insulin stimulates ammonia synthesis, as well as the activity of the Na^+/H^+ exchanger in the proximal tubule. Low insulin bioactivity leads to defective ammonia synthesis or transport into the lumen. In addition, insulin deficiency causes an increase in plasma free fatty acid concentration. Ammoniagenesis uses glutamine as substrate; the presence of an alternative nonnitrogen metabolic substrate such as free fatty acids or ketoanions inhibits ammoniagenesis. Uric acid stone formers also have a blunted urinary response to acute acid load due to low NH_3 availability. Patients with type 2 diabetes mellitus also tend to have higher BMI and increasing weight is associated with lower urinary pH. In addition, type 2 diabetic patients also consume more dietary acid and this may contribute

to their lower urinary pH. However, neither the increased acid consumption nor body weight alone completely explains the low urinary pH.

The second most important risk factor is decreased urine volume. Hyperuricosuria is the least important risk factor and is seen in less than 25% of patients with recurrent uric acid stones.

C. **Struvite-carbonate stones** are also known as *infection stones* and are composed of a mixture of magnesium ammonium phosphate (struvite: $MgNH_4PO_4 \cdot 6H_2O$) and carbonate apatite [$Ca_{10}(PO_4)_6CO_3$]. Struvite-carbonate stones likely make up about 5% of KS and are a frequent cause of staghorn calculi, although cystine, CaOx, CaP, and uric acid stones may occasionally form staghorns. Struvite-carbonate becomes supersaturating in urine only in one circumstance: infection by urea-splitting organisms that express urease. The most common urease-producing bacteria include *Proteus*, *Morganella*, *Providencia*, *Pseudomonas*, and *Klebsiella*. Of note, *Escherichia coli* and *Citrobacter* do not produce urease.
   1. **Pathophysiology.** For struvite-carbonate stones to form, urine must be alkaline, with a pH greater than 7.0 and supersaturated with ammonium hydroxide. Bacterial urease hydrolyzes urea to ammonia and carbon dioxide. The ammonia then hydrolyzes spontaneously to form ammonium hydroxide; the carbon dioxide hydrates to form carbonic acid and, subsequently, bicarbonate. At high pH, bicarbonate loses its proton to become carbonate. UTI with a urease-producing organism is the only situation in which urinary pH, ammonium, and carbonate are elevated simultaneously. The bacteria produce supersaturation in their own immediate environment. Crystals form around bacterial clusters, and bacteria permeate every crevice of a struvite-carbonate stone. The stone itself is an infected foreign body and treatment with antibiotics alone is almost never sufficient to eliminate the infection: source control is required by removal of the stone.
   2. **Risk Factors and Presentation.** Patients with recurrent UTI, indwelling bladder catheters, spinal cord injury, other forms of neurogenic bladder, or ileal diversions of the ureter are most prone to form struvite-carbonate stones. Struvite stones may present in a variety of ways, including fever, hematuria, flank pain, recurrent UTI, and septicemia. They can grow to a very large size and fill the renal pelvis as a staghorn calculus. The carbonate apatite component makes them radiopaque. Rarely, if ever, do they pass spontaneously, and 25% are discovered incidentally. If untreated, they may result in loss of the affected kidney with potential complications of xanthogranulomatous pyelonephritis or with diffuse obstruction of the renal papillae.

D. **Cystine Stones.** Cystinuria is the result of an autosomal recessive defect in proximal tubular and jejunal reabsorption of the dibasic amino acids cysteine, ornithine, lysine, and arginine. Excessive amounts of these amino acids are excreted in urine, but clinical disease is due solely to the poor urinary cystine solubility. Cystine is a dimer of cysteine. Cystine stones make up less than 1% of all calculi in adults but may constitute as many as 5% to 8% of KS in children. The prevalence of cystinuria is approximately 1 per 15,000 individuals in the United States. Pure cystine stones form only in homozygotes. A healthy adult excretes less than 20 mg of cystine per gram of creatinine in 24 hours. Excretion of greater than 250 mg/g of creatinine is almost always indicative of homozygous cystinuria. Cystine stones are radiopaque due to the sulfhydryl moiety of cysteine.
   1. **Pathophysiology.** Cystine solubility is approximately 250 mg/L at a urinary pH of 7.0, and this rises with increasing pH. The pK_a of cysteine is 6.5; therefore, a gradual increase in solubility occurs as urinary pH rises from 6.5 to 7.5. Supersaturation occurs at cystine concentrations greater than

250 mg/L. If the cystine concentration can be maintained below 200 mg/L continuously, cystine stones should not form. In patients with severe cystinuria (>1,000 mg/d) as much as 4 L of urine is required at normal urinary pH to keep cystine concentration within the soluble range and additional treatment is usually required.

2. **Signs and Symptoms.** Cystine stones begin to form in the first to fourth decades. Presentations can vary from a single stone to bilateral obstructive staghorn calculi with associated renal failure. Characteristic hexagonal crystals may be identified, particularly in first morning urine, which is usually acidic. Heterozygotes can form stones either with no cystine or with cystine as only a minor component, given that cystine can act as a nidus for crystallization of both CaOx and CaP.

E. Drug-Related Stones. A variety of drugs can precipitate in urine, including sulfonamides, triamterene, acyclovir, and the antiretroviral agent indinavir. Microscopic hematuria occurs in up to 20% of patients on indinavir. Nephrolithiasis develops in 3%, and 5% experience either dysuria or flank pain that resolves when the drug is discontinued. Reports show that patients with flank pain may have abnormal CT scans with a decrease in contrast excretion in the medullary rays.

Topiramate and other inhibitors of carbonic anhydrases such as zonisamide and acetazolamide are often used in the treatment of migraines and seizure disorders and are associated with an increased risk of KS formation. These carbonic anhydrase inhibitors are associated with metabolic acidosis, hypercalciuria, and increased urinary pH, factors which result in urinary CaP supersaturation that can subsequently lead to CaP stone formation.

III. Evaluation of the Patient

A. Calcium-Containing Stones. The first question to be addressed in the patient with calcium-containing stones is whether the stone disease is simple or complicated. Simple disease is defined as a single stone in the absence of an associated systemic disorder. Complicated calcium-containing stone disease is present if the patient has multiple stones, evidence of new stone formation, enlargement of old stones, or passage of gravel. This distinction is made based on the initial evaluation. A history should be obtained, looking for a family history of stone disease, skeletal disease, inflammatory bowel disease, and UTI. Environmental risk factors are evaluated, such as fluid intake, urine volume, immobilization, diet, medications, and ingestion of supplements including vitamins and protein powders. Initial laboratory evaluation includes blood chemistries, urinalysis, and a renal ultrasound and flat radiographic plate of the abdomen to assess stone burden. Stone analysis should always be carried out if the patient has saved the stone. Stone analysis is inexpensive. It is also the only way to establish the diagnosis of a specific disorder and often helps to direct therapy. In addition, it was shown that in 15% of cases, analyses of 24-hour urine would not have predicted the chemical composition of the stone.

In the patient with complicated disease, two to three measurements of serum calcium concentration should be performed. If any serum calcium level is above 10 mg/dL, PTH concentration should be evaluated. Blood chemistries are examined. First morning void urine should be examined for cystine crystals. Upper urinary tract imaging with US or CT is required if not already performed. At least two 24-hour urine collections should be obtained on the patient's usual diet for calcium, citrate, uric acid, oxalate, sodium, phosphate, volume, pH, and creatinine. Further therapeutic intervention depends on the results of these collections. Normal values for 24-hour urine collection are shown in Table 9-4. If a therapeutic intervention is undertaken, a 24-hour urine collection should be repeated in 6 to 8 weeks to verify its expected effect and then repeated yearly.

TABLE 9-4 Normal Values for 24-Hour Urine Collection

Substance	Male (mg/24 h)	Female (mg/24 h)
Calcium	<300	<250
Uric acid	<800	<750
Citrate	>320	>320
Oxalate	<45	<45

B. Uric Acid Stones. The etiologies of **uric acid stones** can be subdivided into three pathophysiologic groups based on risk factors. Low urine volume contributes to uric acid stones in gastrointestinal disorders such as Crohn disease, ulcerative colitis, diarrhea, ileostomies, and dehydration. Acidic urinary pH plays an important role in primary gout and gastrointestinal disorders. Hyperuricosuria is divided into those with hyperuricemia (primary gout, enzyme disorders, myeloproliferative diseases, hemolytic anemia, and drugs) and those without hyperuricemia (dietary excess). Hyperuricosuria is not typically a significant contributor to uric acid stone disease which is predominantly driven by pH.

Primary gout is an inherited disorder most likely transmitted in an autosomal dominant manner with variable penetrance. It is associated with hyperuricemia, hyperuricosuria, and persistently acid urine. In affected patients, 10% to 20% have uric acid stones, and in 40% KS precede the first articular gout attack.

Uric acid stones are typically round and smooth and are more likely to pass spontaneously than calcium-containing stones, which are often jagged. A definitive diagnosis is established through stone analysis. The diagnosis is suggested by the presence of a radiolucent stone, or by the presence of uric acid crystals in unusually acidic urine. Xanthine, hypoxanthine, and 2,8-dihydroxyadenine stones are also radiolucent and should be suspected if a radiolucent stone fails to dissolve with alkali therapy.

C. Struvite-Carbonate Stones. Seventy-five percent of all staghorn calculi are composed of struvite-carbonate. Struvite-carbonate stones are large and less radiopaque than calcium-containing stones. As with any KS, the definitive diagnosis is only established on chemical analysis, but a diagnosis of struvite-carbonate stones should be strongly suspected in any patient with an infected alkaline urine. In the presence of an infected acidic urine and a staghorn calculus, one should consider the possibility that the two are unrelated and that the calculus may be either calcium containing or uric acid. Stone analysis and culture should be carried out in all patients undergoing surgical intervention. *Proteus mirabilis* accounts for more than one-half of all urease-producing infections. Stone culture, when possible, is important, because urine culture is not always completely representative of the organisms present in the stone. If no organisms are cultured, then the possibility of infection with *Ureaplasma urealyticum*, which is often difficult to culture, should be considered.

D. Cystine Stones. The presence of characteristic hexagonal crystals in first morning void urine is diagnostic of cystinuria, although this is a very infrequent finding. The simplest and most rapid screening test for cystinuria is the sodium-nitroprusside test, which has a lower limit of detection of 75 mg cystine/g of creatinine. The nitroprusside complex binds to sulfide groups and may yield a false-positive result in patients taking sulfur-containing drugs. Phosphotungstic acid has also been used as an alternative screening test. Patients with a positive screening test result should undergo 24-hour urine cystine quantitation. Cystine stones are usually less radiodense on radiography than calcium-containing or struvite-carbonate stones, but they are not amenable to extracorporeal shock wave lithotripsy (ESWL).

IV. Prevention and Treatment

A. Calcium Oxalate Stones. Approach to prevention of calcium-containing stones is determined by whether the patient has simple or complicated disease. The American College of Physicians advises that the patient with a single, isolated stone and no associated systemic disease be managed with nonspecific forms of therapy alone, including increased fluid intake. This approach is appropriate in patients at low risk of recurrence. One may consider, however, performing more extensive evaluation with 24-hour urine collections in patients at high risk for recurrence (those with family history, those with a systemic disorder) or in those who may experience substantial morbidity with a recurrence (patients who have undergone transplantation or patients with a solitary kidney).

The patient with complicated disease is managed with both nonspecific and specific treatment. Specific therapy varies depending on assessment of risk factors derived from analysis of 24-hour urines.

Although conventional upper limits of daily calciuria (95th percentiles) are defined as 250 mg/d for women and 300 mg/d for men, stone formers in the 70th percentiles (170 mg/d for women and 210 mg/d for men) or lower may benefit from even lower calcium excretion rates. Data linking calcium excretion to stone risk are supportive of the idea that quantity of calciuria is a graded risk factor for development of calcium-containing KS.

1. **Nonspecific therapeutic options** include manipulation of fluid intake and diet. Increasing fluid intake is the cheapest way to reduce urinary supersaturation with CaOx and CaP. In a prospective randomized trial of 199 first-time stone formers followed up for a 5-year period, the risk of recurrent stone formation was reduced from 27% to 12% by raising urinary volume to more than 2 L/d with water ingestion. The average increase in urine volume in patients advised to increase fluid intake is approximately 300 mL/d, so often insufficient as a standalone treatment.

   Lower dietary sodium will lead to lower urinary sodium and increased passive calcium reabsorption in the proximal tubule which decreases calciuria and portends decreased risk for stone formation. A secondary analysis of the large prospective WHI OS (Women's Health Initiative Observational Study) study on women with no history of nephrolithiasis showed higher sodium intake increasing the risk for nephrolithiasis from 11% to 61% after multivariate adjustment.

   Historically, calciuria was thought to be reduced by dietary calcium restriction. Three large prospective cohort studies, however, in both men and women suggest that a low-calcium diet increases the risk of forming calcium-containing stones. The postulated mechanism is that ingested calcium aids in complexing dietary oxalate, and a reduction in dietary calcium results in a reciprocal increase in intestinal oxalate absorption. As a result, urinary supersaturation of CaOx increases and stones form. The WHI OS study showed a 5% decrease in incident KSD with higher dietary calcium intake. By contrast, calcium supplements have shown to slightly increase the propensity to form stones in women. Calcium supplements may be ingested without meals implying with no or less oxalate. This is opposed to dietary calcium which will be ingested with dietary oxalate. There appears to be a reciprocal relationship of calcium and oxalate balance in the gut which affects absorption and the resultant degree of hyperoxaluria and potentially also calciuria. Overall, the lithoprotective effect of dietary calcium intake via oxalate binding is of greater clinical significance than the potential increase in urinary calcium. In addition, patients with idiopathic hypercalciuria often have reduced bone mass and are in negative calcium balance and may depend on adequate calcium intake for bone health. While generally best avoided, if calcium supplements are required due to inability to obtain dietary calcium, they should be ingested at mealtime. A prospective, randomized controlled trial compared patients on a low-calcium diet to those on a normal calcium, low-sodium, low-protein diet. The relative risk for KS formation was reduced by 51% in those on the normal calcium diet. As predicted, urinary oxalate increased in the low-calcium group, compatible with the reciprocal relationship hypothesis.

High nondairy animal protein intake constitutes a high acid load due to the content of sulfur-containing amino acids, which decreases urine pH and citrate and increases urinary calcium excretion, perhaps through bone resorption and/or reduced renal calcium reabsorption.[1] Another study examined the effects of a low-carbohydrate, high-protein diet on risk factors for calcium-containing stone disease. Net acid excretion increased by 56 mEq/d, urinary citrate decreased from an average of 763 to 449 mg/d, urinary pH fell from 6.09 to 5.67, and urinary calcium increased from 160 to 248 mg/d. Notably, there was not an associated increase in fractional absorption of intestinal calcium, suggesting negative systemic calcium balance.

High fructose has also been found to likely be a contributing factor for the development of KSD in part via effects on urate metabolism, urinary pH, and via effects on oxalate.

2. **Specific forms of treatment** are directed by results of the 24-hour urine studies. Therapy is focused on agents shown to reduce the relative risk of stone formation in randomized placebo-controlled clinical trials with more than 1 year of follow-up (results shown in Table 9-5). This is important because of the "stone clinic effect." After patients present for evaluation of nephrolithiasis, the subsequent period is often associated with a reduced risk of new stone formation (the "stone clinic effect"). This is the result of at least two factors: (a) regression to the mean and (b) increased adherence to nonspecific forms of treatment. Trials with less than 12 to 24 months of follow-up should be viewed with skepticism if no effect is detected. At the start of treatment, patients at high risk for recurrence may have stones too small to be detected radiographically that grow and subsequently are identified as new stones. Because calcium-containing stones are often difficult to prevent from increasing in size once a nidus is established, this could minimize the treatment effect in high-risk patients. Agents that were shown to be effective in randomized placebo-controlled trials with a long duration of follow-up include thiazide diuretics, allopurinol, potassium citrate, and potassium-magnesium citrate. More recently sodium-glucose cotransporter-2 (SGLT-2) inhibitors have shown to be associated with a 40% reduced risk in urinary tract stone events in a post hoc analysis of 20 phase I–IV randomized controlled trials including EMPA-REG OUTCOME. SGLT-2 inhibitors may have lithoprotective effects due to increasing urinary flow rate via osmotic diuresis and decreased uric acid levels, decreased urine pH, and increase in urinary citrate excretion.

   a. **Urinary volume** should be increased to at least 2 L/d. This is best accomplished by drinking water, which is the only liquid shown to reduce stone formation rate in randomized controlled clinical trials. Epidemiologic data note benefit of total urine volume regardless of fluid type,

TABLE 9-5 Randomized Trials in Calcium-Containing Nephrolithiasis

Author	Treatment	Dose	Condition	No. of Patients; Length of Follow-Up	Risk Reduction
Borghi	Water	>2 L UO daily	First stone	199; 5 yrs	55%
Laerum	Hydrochlorothiazide	25 mg b.i.d.	Noncategorized, recurrent	50; 3 yrs	54%
Ettinger	Chlorthalidone	25–50 mg	Noncategorized, recurrent	54; 3 yrs	48%
Borghi	Indapamide	2.5 mg	Hypercalciuria, recurrent	75; 3 yrs	79%
Ettinger	Allopurinol	100 mg t.i.d.	Hyperuricosuria, recurrent	60; 3 yrs	45%
Barcelo	Potassium citrate	30–60 mEq	Hypocitraturia, recurrent	57; 3 yrs	65%
Ettinger	Potassium-magnesium citrate	42/21/63 mEq	Noncategorized, recurrent	64; 3 yrs	81%
Ettinger	Potassium phosphate	1.4 g	Noncategorized, recurrent	71; 3 yrs	None
Ettinger	Magnesium hydroxide	650–1,300 mg	Noncategorized, recurrent	52; 3 yrs	None
Dhayat	Hydrochlorothiazide	12.5–50 mg daily	Noncategorized, recurrent	416; 2.9 yrs	None

L, liter; UO, urine output; b.i.d., twice daily; t.i.d., three times daily.

though sweetened beverages are best avoided. A recent study suggests that even in patients with a substantial genetic susceptibility for developing nephrolithiasis, coffee, milk, and perhaps tea might also be protective against stone formation.

b. **Hypercalciuria** is managed initially with low salt diet and thiazide diuretics. Thiazides act directly to increase distal calcium reabsorption and indirectly to increase calcium reabsorption in the proximal tubule by inducing a state of mild volume contraction. Volume contraction must be maintained, and hypokalemia avoided for thiazide diuretics to remain maximally effective. Thiazides generally reduce urinary calcium by up to 50%. The doses used in studies that show an effect are high (25 mg of hydrochlorothiazide [HCTZ] twice a day, 25 to 50 mg of chlorthalidone once a day, or 2.5 mg of indapamide per day). If they are ineffective, noncompliance with the low-sodium diet should be considered. This can be monitored with a 24-hour urine for sodium. Amiloride acts independently of thiazides at a more distal site and can be added if required and is also beneficial for potential hypokalemia. Four randomized controlled trials in recurrent CaOx stone formers demonstrated a reduction in new stone formation risk with thiazide diuretics. Although all patients in these trials were CaOx stone formers, the minority were hypercalciuric. This suggests that thiazides may have additional effects beyond reducing urinary calcium or that the reduction of urinary calcium, even in the absence of hypercalciuria, may reduce the risk of recurrent KS formation. Some have argued that the effect of thiazide diuretics may diminish with time, but this does not appear to be the case. In the recent NOSTONE trial comparing HCTZ with placebo the incidence of symptomatic stone events did not appear significantly different. However, the study had several limitations. HCTZ was not dosed according to urinary calcium levels and was only dosed daily limiting its effect due to its short half-life. In addition, sodium intake was not controlled and was, in fact, quite high, which is known to be the most common reason for thiazide therapy being ineffective. Finally, passage of existing stones was deemed to be a new stone event. Despite these concerns, the study still showed a significant reduction of radiologic stone recurrence from 49% to 32% with higher doses of HCTZ.

In patients who cannot tolerate thiazide diuretics, other potential therapies include sodium cellulose phosphate and orthophosphate. These are often poorly tolerated. Slow-release neutral phosphate appears to be better tolerated and may become the second-line agent of choice. Randomized controlled trials of potassium acid phosphate and magnesium hydroxide showed no benefit when compared with placebo.

c. **Hypocitraturia** is managed with potassium citrate or potassium-magnesium citrate. Each of these agents reduced the relative risk of stone formation in randomized controlled trials. Potassium-magnesium citrate may be especially beneficial in patients receiving thiazide diuretics because potassium and magnesium losses induced by the diuretic are repleted. Patients with struvite-carbonate stones should not be given citrate, because it may increase deposition of magnesium ammonium phosphate and carbonate apatite. Citrate may also increase intestinal aluminum absorption in patients with CKD. Citrate preparations can be difficult for patients to tolerate secondary to nausea or diarrhea. Slow-release preparations such as Urocit-K are well tolerated but may still be unaffordable to socio-economically disadvantaged patient populations. Typically, 60 mEq of citrate should be administered daily in divided doses with meals and carefully titrated to urine citrate values. Caution is required not to over-alkalinize, as this can increase the risk of CaP crystallization.

d. **Hyperoxaluria** is managed with a normal calcium, low-oxalate diet. Enteric hyperoxaluria should be initially treated with a low-fat, low-oxalate diet. If this is unsuccessful, calcium carbonate, cholestyramine, or both can be added. Enteral administration of oxalate-degrading bacterium *O. formigenes* with current formulations has not been found effective in reducing urinary oxalate excretion. For PH1 patients the RNA interference agent Lumasiran is available and has proven to be effective in reducing urinary oxalate excretion. For PH3 Nedosiran is being studied and has shown promising results.

This approach, directed at both specific and nonspecific risk factor reduction, has been shown to decrease frequency of recurrent stone formation and reduce the number of cystoscopies, surgeries, and hospitalizations.

B. **Calcium phosphate stones** remain a controversial area with respect to therapy. All randomized controlled trials to date have enrolled patients with either pure CaOx stones or those containing CaOx and a small percentage of CaP (<20%). Thus, there is little evidence to guide therapy. Stones that are predominantly CaP (≥60% CaP salt; usually either brushite or apatite) may be increasing in frequency over the last several decades. Lowering urinary calcium and increasing fluid ingestion seem prudent and are likely beneficial. However, use of potassium citrate which can raise urinary pH may be harmful, given that rises in urinary pH are associated with increases in CaP supersaturation. Whether the deleterious effects of rising urinary pH on supersaturation would win out over the benefits of increased urinary citrate concentration on reducing CaP supersaturation, as well as crystal aggregation and agglomeration, is difficult to predict. In this situation, it may be prudent to employ citric acid, which can raise urinary citrate concentration without increasing urinary pH (citric acid is acid–base neutral while metabolism of potassium citrate generates three bicarbonates) but larger prospective studies are needed.

C. Uric Acid Stones. Therapy for uric acid stones is directed at the three major risk factors (decreased urine pH, decreased urine volume, and hyperuricosuria). First, urine volume should be increased to 2 to 3 L/d. Second, urine should be alkalinized to a pH of 6.5 using potassium alkali. The starting dose is 20 to 30 mEq twice daily to be titrated upward according to urinary pH. More than 80 to 100 mEq is rarely required. Sodium alkali therapy is second line, because it may result in hypercalciuria, but should be pursued if potassium alkali is contraindicated, as in hyperkalemia. In one study of 12 patients, alkali therapy resulted in a dissolution of stones within a period of 3 weeks to 5 months. Increases in urinary pH above 6.5 should be avoided because of the increased risk of CaP stone formation at high urinary pH.

If hyperuricosuria is present, dietary purine consumption should be reduced. Allopurinol has not been studied in patients with uric acid stones and is rarely required if urine volume and alkalization are achieved. If allopurinol is administered for massive uric acid overproduction, adequate hydration must be maintained to avoid the precipitation of xanthine crystals.

D. Struvite-Carbonate Stones. Complete surgical elimination of the stone burden is the goal of therapy, coupled with appropriate antibiotic therapy. The combination of percutaneous nephrolithotomy and ureteroscopy with laser lithotripsy maybe required depending on stone size. If a struvite-carbonate stone is not removed in its entirety, the patient will likely continue to have recurrent UTI, and the stone will regrow. Stone growth in most patients with residual fragments progresses despite antibiotic treatment. It can be slowed by reducing the bacterial population, but cure with antibiotics alone is unlikely. Urease inhibitors, such as acetohydroxamic acid, reduce urinary saturation of struvite-carbonate and prevent stone growth. These agents, however, are associated with a variety of severe complications including hemolytic anemia, thrombophlebitis, and nonspecific neurologic symptoms (e.g., disorientation, tremor, and headache) and are best avoided if possible. Acetohydroxamic acid is also renally excreted and should not be used in those with a creatinine clearance less than 40 mL/min.

E. Cystine Stones. Lifestyle modification is first-line treatment, which includes hydration, urinary alkalinization, and a low-sodium, moderate animal protein diet. The required fluid intake is based on the patient's urinary cystine excretion, with a target urine cystine concentration of <250 mg/L and a pH of 7.0. Urinary alkalinization is crucial as the dissociation constant of cystine is 6.5. As a result, a pH of 7.5 is required for 90% of cystine to exist in the ionized form. At this pH, CaP stone formation risk is increased, and frequent follow-up urine collections are required to assure that supersaturations for all stone types remain in a safe range. Potassium citrate is the agent of choice and is preferable to sodium-containing alkali because ECF volume expansion increases cystine excretion. Methionine is a substrate for cystine production and fish, red meat, poultry, and dairy products are rich sources of methionine so a diet low in animal protein (target 0.8 g/kg) is prudent. If these measures are ineffective, then either D-penicillamine or tiopronin can be tried. These compounds are thiols that bind preferentially to cysteine, forming compounds that are more soluble than cysteine–cysteine dimers (cystine). Tiopronin causes fewer complications than D-penicillamine and is preferred. D-Penicillamine also binds pyridoxine, and therefore pyridoxine (50 mg/d) should be administered to prevent deficiency. Zinc supplements can usually prevent the anosmia and loss of taste that often occurs with D-penicillamine. More recently SLGT-2 inhibitors, tolvaptan, alpha-lipoic acid, and cystine mimetic agents are being studies for therapeutic effects in cystinuria. Captopril although initially reported to be of benefit has more recently fallen out of favor.

V. Special Patient Populations
  A. **Pregnancy.** Higher risk for a symptomatic KS event in pregnancy has recently been reported. The risk was found increased 2-fold higher during the second semester and 2.7-fold higher during the third trimester and returned to baseline at 0 to 3 months after delivery. KS in pregnancy have also been associated with increased adverse birth outcomes. Potential reasons for the higher risk maybe due to hypercalciuria from supplemental calcium in the prenatal vitamins and in antacids, high 1,25 vitamin D levels from the placenta, increased filtered load due to increased GFR, and perhaps also due to urinary stasis from increased progesterone levels and diminished fluid intake during late pregnancy as a result of decreasing bladder capacity from the gravid uterus. To limit radiation exposure, ultrasound in the preferred initial imaging modality prior to low-dose CT which can be used in the second and third trimesters.
  B. **Transplant.** KSD after kidney transplantation has been reported in 1.8% of patients including both de-novo and donor stones. KS after kidney transplant are often asymptomatic due to the lack of innervation of the graft ureter and are particularly dangerous given the potential for asymptomatic obstruction. Stones may be secondary to infection, local stasis due to anatomy of the transplant ureter, hyperoxaluria from prior oxalate retention, hyperphosphaturia and hypercalciuria from tertiary hyperparathyroidism, and hypocitraturia from calcineurin inhibitors such as cyclosporin or tacrolimus. To date, renal graft stones have not been found to have a long-term impact on graft function or graft survival. Longer dialysis vintage appears to increase the risk for a KS event. A limited retrospective study on living donor gifted lithiasis found no episodes of nephrolithiasis requiring any form of intervention during the 3.5-year follow-up of the recipients. Criteria for accepting living donor transplant w/ KSD differ between centers and no guidelines have been published. Overall data on allograft lithiasis remain sparse.

SUGGESTED READINGS

Alexander RT, Fuster DG, Dimke H. Mechanisms underlying calcium nephrolithiasis. *Annu Rev Physiol.* 2022;84:559–583.

Arvans D, Chang C, Alshaikh A, et al. Sel1-like proteins and peptides are the major *Oxalobacter formigenes*-derived factors stimulating oxalate transport by human intestinal epithelial cells. *Am J Physiol Cell Physiol.* 2023;325(1):C344–C361.

Balasubramanian P, Wanner C, Ferreira JP, et al. Empagliflozin and decreased risk of nephrolithiasis: a potential new role for SGLT2 inhibition? *J Clin Endocrinol Metab.* 2022;107(7):e3003–e3007.

Chewcharat A, Curhan G. Trends in the prevalence of kidney stones in the United States from 2007 to 2016. *Urolithiasis.* 2021;49(1):27–39.

Coe FL, Worcester EM, Evan AP. Idiopathic hypercalciuria and formation of calcium renal stones. *Nat Rev Nephrol.* 2016;12(9):519–533.

Dai JC, Pearle MS. Diet and stone disease in 2022. *J Clin Med*. 2022;11(16):4740.

Dhayat NA, Bonny O, Roth B, et al. Hydrochlorothiazide and prevention of kidney-stone recurrence. *N Engl J Med*. 2023;388(9):781–791.

Doizi S, Poindexter JR, Pearle MS, et al. Impact of potassium citrate vs citric acid on urinary stone risk in calcium phosphate stone formers. *J Urol*. 2018;200(6):1278–1284.

Elia M, Monga M, De S. Increased nephrolithiasis prevalence in people with disabilities: a National Health and Nutrition Survey Analysis. *Urology*. 2022;163:185–189.

Ettinger B, Tang A, Citron JT, Livermore B, Williams T. Randomized trial of allopurinol in the prevention of calcium oxalate calculi. *N Engl J Med*. 1986;315(22):1386–1389.

Ferraro PM, Taylor EN, Asplin JR, Curhan GC. Associations between net gastrointestinal alkali absorption, 24-hr urine lithogenic factors, and kidney stones. *Clin J Am Soc Neph*. 2023;18(8):1068–1074.

Ganesan C, Holmes M, Liu S, et al. Kidney stone events after kidney transplant in the United States. *Clin J Am Soc Nephrol*. 2023;18(6):777–784.

Gottlieb M, Long B, Koyfman A. The evaluation and management of urolithiasis in the ED: a review of the literature. *Am J Emerg Med*. 2018;36(4):699–706.

Guerra A, Ticinesi A, Allegri F, Pinelli S, Aloe R, Meschi T. Idiopathic calcium nephrolithiasis with pure calcium oxalate composition: clinical correlates of the calcium oxalate dihydrate/monohydrate (COD/COM) stone ratio. *Urolithiasis*. 2020;48(3):271–279.

Pak CYC, Odvina CV, Pearle MS, et al. Effect of dietary modification on urinary stone risk factors. *Kidney Int*. 2005;68(5):2264–2273.

Reddy ST, Wang CY, Sakhaee K, Brinkley L, Pak CYC. Effect of low-carbohydrate high-protein diets on acid-base balance, stone-forming propensity, and calcium metabolism. *Am J Kidney Dis*. 2002;40(2):265–274.

Rimer JD, Sakhaee K, Maalouf NM. Citrate therapy for calcium phosphate stones. *Curr Opin Nephrol Hypertens*. 2019;28(2):130–139.

Singh P, Harris PC, Sas DJ, Lieske JC. The genetics of kidney stone disease and nephrocalcinosis. *Nat Rev Nephrol*. 2022;18(4):224–240.

Thongprayoon C, Vaughan LE, Chewcharat A, et al. Risk of symptomatic kidney stones during and after pregnancy. *Am J Kidney Dis*. 2021;78(3):409–417.

Tran TV, Maalouf NM. Uric acid stone disease: lessons from recent human physiologic studies. *Curr Opin Nephrol Hypertens*. 2020;29(4):407–413.

Wang RC, Fahimi J, Dillon D, et al. Effect of an ultrasound-first clinical decision tool in emergency department patients with suspected nephrolithiasis: a randomized trial. *Am J Emerg Med*. 2022;60:164–170.

10 The Patient With Urinary Tract Infection

Abdul-Rehman Syed, Jessica Kendrick

Urinary tract infections (UTIs) are some of the most common infections experienced by humans, exceeded in frequency among ambulatory patients only by respiratory and gastrointestinal infections. Over 8 million episodes of acute cystitis occur annually in the United States. Bacterial infections of the urinary tract are the most common cause of both community-acquired and nosocomial infections for patients admitted to hospitals in the United States.

The prognosis and management of UTIs depend on the site of infection and any predisposing factors.

I. Definitions

Some definitions are necessary because infection of the urinary tract may result from microbial invasion of any of the tissues extending from the urethral orifice to the renal cortex. Although the infection and resultant symptoms may be localized at one site, the presence of bacteria in the urine (bacteriuria) places the entire urinary system at risk for invasion by bacteria.

A. Significant bacteriuria is defined as the presence of 100,000 or more colony-forming units (CFUs) of bacteria per milliliter of urine, although smaller colony counts can be of diagnostic importance, particularly in young women, where 1,000 bacteria per CFU may be associated with cystitis or acute urethral syndrome.

B. Anatomic Location. The first useful distinction is between upper (kidney) and lower (bladder, prostate, and urethra) UTIs. Infections confined to the bladder (cystitis), the urethra (urethritis), and the prostate (prostatitis) commonly cause dysuria, frequency, and urgency. Pyelonephritis is the nonspecific inflammation of the renal parenchyma; acute bacterial pyelonephritis is a clinical syndrome characterized by chills and fever, flank pain, and constitutional symptoms caused by the bacterial invasion of the kidney. Chronic pyelonephritis has a histopathology that is similar to tubulointerstitial nephritis, a renal disease caused by a variety of disorders such as chronic obstructive uropathy, vesical ureteral reflux (reflux nephropathy), renal medullary disease, drugs and toxins, and possibly chronic or recurring renal bacteriuria.

C. Recurrence of UTI is the result of either relapse or reinfection; making this distinction is clinically important. Recurrent UTI is defined as two uncomplicated infections within 6 months or three infections within a year and are often considered reinfections. Most recurring episodes of cystourethritis are due to reinfection. While the pathogenesis of recurrent UTIs is classically attributed to different pathogens, recent studies indicate that over 50% of recurrent infections occur with genetically identical pathogens and are usually drug susceptible. Relapse is a return of infection due to the same microorganism, is often drug resistant, and may require further urologic evaluation, longer treatment courses, and potential surgical intervention. Most relapses occur after treatment of acute pyelonephritis or prostatitis. Finally, asymptomatic bacteriuria is an important clue to the presence of parenchymal infection somewhere in the urinary tract; however, the importance of the infection and the need for treatment depend on the age, sex, and underlying condition of the patient.

D. Complicated and Uncomplicated UTIs. For the clinician, another important distinction is made between uncomplicated and complicated infections. An uncomplicated infection is an episode of cystourethritis following bacterial colonization of the urethral and bladder mucosae in the absence of upper tract disease. This type of infection is considered *uncomplicated* because sequelae are rare and exclusively due to the morbidity associated with reinfections in a subset of women. Complicated UTIs increase the risk of potentially life-threatening infectious sequelae such as bacteremia and sepsis or treatment failure. Complicated UTIs may occur with pregnancy, diabetes, immunosuppression, structural abnormalities of the urinary tract, symptoms lasting for more than 2 weeks, and previous pyelonephritis. Young women constitute a subset of patients with pyelonephritis (acute uncomplicated pyelonephritis) who often respond well to therapy and may also have a low incidence of sequelae. In contrast, complicated infections include those involving parenchyma (pyelonephritis or prostatitis) and frequently occur in the setting of obstructive uropathy or after instrumentation. Episodes may be refractory to therapy, often resulting in relapses, and occasionally leading to significant sequelae such as sepsis, metastatic abscesses, and, rarely, acute renal failure.

E. Several authors have proposed a **clinical classification** for the practicing clinician.
1. Asymptomatic Bacteriuria
2. Acute Uncomplicated Cystitis in Women
3. Recurrent Infections in Women
4. Acute Uncomplicated Pyelonephritis in Women
5. Complicated UTIs in Both sexes
6. Catheter-Associated UTIs

II. Risk Factors and Pathogenesis

Early recognition and possible prevention depend on an understanding of the pathogenesis and epidemiology of UTIs. Figure 10-1 shows the major risk periods of life for symptomatic UTIs; the increasing prevalence of asymptomatic bacteriuria that accompanies aging is apparent. Much has been learned about the risk factors for UTIs. Several host factors contribute to the promotion of bacterial colonization in the urinary tract. These include: (a) obstruction to urine flow, such as congenital anomalies, renal calculi, or ureteral occlusions; (b) vesicoureteral reflux; (c) instrumentation of the urinary tract, such as urinary catheterization, urethral dilation, or cystoscopy; and (d) the presence of residual urine in the bladder, associated with conditions like neurogenic bladder, urethral strictures, or prostatic hypertrophy. Associations have been established between UTI and age; pregnancy; sexual intercourse; use of diaphragms, condoms, and spermicides, particularly Nonoxynol-9; delayed postcoital micturition; menopause; and a history of recent UTI. Factors that do not seem to increase the risk include diet, use of tampons, clothing, and personal hygiene, including directions for cleansing after defecation and bathing practices. Studies on pathogenesis have elucidated specific interactions between the host and microbes that are causally related to bacteriuria. Bacteria in the enteric flora periodically gain access to the genitourinary tract. How such bacteria actually migrate from the gastrointestinal tract to the periurethra is not known; the close proximity of the anus in women is a likely factor. The subsequent bacterial colonization of uroepithelial cells is the biologic phenomenon that sets the stage for persistent bacteriuria. The colonization of the periurethra often precedes the onset of bladder bacteriuria. P-fimbriated strains of *Escherichia coli* adhere to uroepithelial cells, in which glycolipids function as receptors in women who secrete blood group antigens. *E. coli* that encode for the type 1 pilus, which contains the adhesin FimH, recognizes multiple cell types associated with cystitis, sepsis, and meningitis. Immunocompromised patients may become infected with less virulent *E. coli* strains. Opposing colonization are

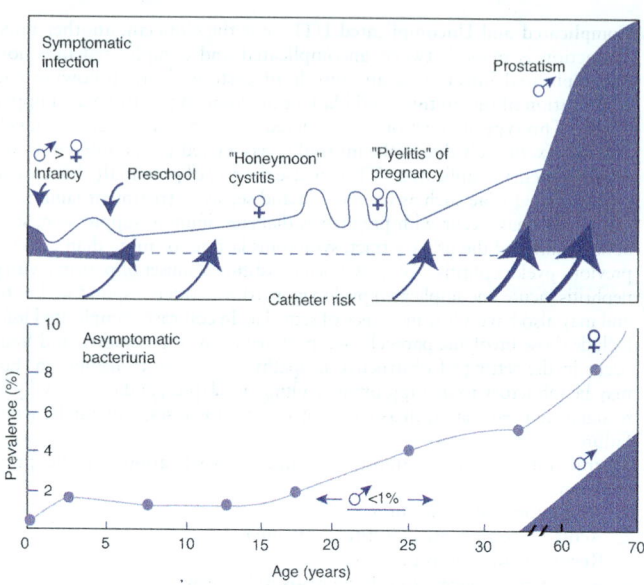

Figure 10-1. Frequency distribution of symptomatic urinary tract infections and prevalence of asymptomatic bacteriuria by age and sex (male, shaded area; female, line). (From Kunin CM. *Urinary Tract Infections: Detection, Prevention, and Management*. 5th ed. Williams & Wilkins; 1997.)

several host factors, most notably acid pH, normal vaginal flora, and type-specific cervicovaginal antibodies.

After periurethral colonization, uropathogens gain access to the bladder through the urethra, to the kidneys through the ureters, and to the prostate through the ejaculatory ducts. The urethra and ureterovesical junction are mechanical barriers that prevent ascension. Besides instrumentation and mechanical obstruction, however, factors promoting ascent of bacteria are not as well understood. In the bladder, organisms multiply, colonize the bladder mucosa, and invade the mucosal surface. Although urine adequately supports the growth of most uropathogens, the bladder has several mechanisms that prevent bacteriuria: (a) a mucopolysaccharide (urine slime) layer covers the bladder epithelium and prevents colonization; (b) Tamm–Horsfall protein, which is a component of uromucoid, adheres to P fimbriae and prevents colonization; and (c) urine flow and bladder contraction serve to prevent stasis and colonization. Bladder bacteriuria sets the stage for subsequent migration to the kidneys, where organisms such as P-fimbriated *E. coli* adhere to renal tubular cells. In fact, outside the setting of obstructive nephropathy, this strain of *E. coli* is the most common cause of pyelonephritis. With obstruction, however, bacterial adherence is ostensibly unimportant. Other host factors that prevent a renal infection are high urine osmolality, high ammonium concentration, phagocytes, and increased urine flow rate.

In the presence of a urethral catheter, defense mechanisms against bacterial–epithelial cell interactions are impaired both by disruption of the protective glycosaminoglycan layer of the bladder and by the formation of biofilm on the catheter. Microorganisms in the biofilm are protected from antibiotics, host defenses, and mechanical flushing. Effective therapy ultimately requires removal of the catheter.

Pathogens colonizing indwelling urinary catheters often have reduced virulence, for example, *E. coli* strains lacking P fimbriation, which accounts for the low incidence of febrile UTIs and bacteremia.

Chronic urinary catheters are associated with lower tract obstruction due to catheter blockage with encrustation and urinary tract stones and may be complicated by scrotal abscesses, epididymitis, and prostatitis. The incidence of bladder cancer may be increased with prolonged catheter use that exceeds 10 years as in patients with spinal cord injuries.

III. Clinical Setting

A. Asymptomatic bacteriuria is especially common in women, as evidenced by a minimum prevalence of 2% to 4% in young and 10% in elderly women and a three to four times higher prevalence of asymptomatic bacteriuria in diabetic women compared with their nondiabetic counterparts. The higher incidence of asymptomatic bacteriuria in diabetic women is attributed to lower urinary cytokine and leukocyte concentrations and enhanced adherence to uroepithelial cells of *E. coli* that express type 1 fimbriae.

The cumulative prevalence of asymptomatic bacteriuria in women increases by approximately 1% per decade throughout life. Of note, this phenomenon has been observed in different ethnic groups and geographic locations. In contrast to women, the occurrence of asymptomatic bacteriuria in men is rare until after the age of 60 years, at which time the prevalence increases per decade and often approaches the rate in elderly women. For example, in noncatheterized, institutionalized elderly men, the prevalence of bacteriuria exceeds 20%. Prostatic hypertrophy and increased likelihood of instrumentation are thought to account for the bacteriuria of older men. Moreover, differences between men and women in the rates of bacteriuria have been attributed to the shorter female urethra and its proximity to the vaginal and rectal mucosae and the abundant microbial flora of these areas. Screening for and treatment of asymptomatic bacteriuria is not warranted unless the patient is at high risk for serious complications (e.g., pregnant women and patients undergoing urologic surgery).

Patients in long-term care facilities have an increased risk of asymptomatic bacteriuria as do patients with spinal cord injuries owing to intermittent catheters, sphincterotomies, or condom catheters. Bacteriuria related to indwelling catheters increases at a rate of 3% to 10% per day and is predominantly asymptomatic. In the absence of UTI symptoms, a positive urine culture for 10^5 CFU/mL of bacteria is consistent with asymptomatic catheter-associated bacteriuria. Asymptomatic catheter-associated candiduria is defined as 10^3 per mL of yeast. The incidence of significant morbidity with asymptomatic bacteriuria and candiduria is low, and antimicrobial therapy is not recommended while the catheter is present.

B. Symptomatic UTIs occur in all age groups. Among newborns and infants, boys are affected more often than girls. When the urinary tract is the source of neonatal sepsis, serious underlying congenital anomalies are frequently present. During childhood, persistent bacteriuria, with or without repeated symptomatic episodes, occurs in a small group (less than 2%) of school-aged girls. Such girls, and also school-aged boys with bacteriuria, should have a urologic evaluation to detect correctable structural abnormalities when UTIs are documented. Sexually active women have a markedly increased risk of episodes of cystitis. *E. coli* is the predominant organism in 75% to 90% of cases, whereas *Staphylococcus saprophyticus* is found in 5% to 15%, primarily in young women. The remainder of cases are due to *enterococci* and aerobic gram-negative rods, such as *Klebsiella* species and *Proteus mirabilis*.

In the absence of prostatitis, bacteriuria and symptomatic UTIs are unusual in men. In fact, asymptomatic prostatitis is very common in men presenting with febrile UTIs. More recently, uropathogenic strains of *E. coli* have been recognized as causes of cystitis in young men at risk because of homosexuality and anal intercourse, lack of circumcision, or having a partner with vaginal colonization with such P-fimbriated *E. coli*. At any age, both sexes may develop symptomatic infections in the presence of risk factors that alter urinary flow. *Mycoplasma hominis* has been well recognized as a sexually transmitted infection and cause of bacterial vaginosis in females and nongonococcal urethritis in males. *Ureaplasma urealyticum* is a cause of nongonococcal urethritis and chronic prostatitis and can be isolated from expressed prostatic secretions and urine voided after prostatic massage.

IV. Clinical Features

A. Acute Urethral Syndrome. The cardinal symptoms of frequency and dysuria occur in more than 90% of ambulatory patients with acute genitourinary tract infections. One-third to one-half of all patients with frequency and dysuria, however, do not have significant bacteriuria, although most have pyuria. These patients have acute urethral syndrome, which can mimic both bladder and renal infections. Vaginitis, urethritis, and prostatitis are common causes of acute urethral syndrome. Although certain signs and symptoms help to differentiate these clinical entities, a classic UTI can be definitively diagnosed only by quantitative cultures of urine.

1. **Vaginitis.** Approximately 20% of women in the United States have an episode of dysuria each year, and one-half of these seek medical care. The presence of an abnormal vaginal discharge (leukorrhea) and irritation make vaginitis the likely cause of dysuria, unless a concomitant UTI can be confirmed by culture. *Candida albicans*, the most common specific cause of vaginitis, can be demonstrated readily by culture or by finding yeast cells in a Gram-stained smear of vaginal secretions or in a saline preparation with potassium hydroxide added. Trichomoniasis can be documented with a saline preparation that shows the motile protozoa of *Trichomonas vaginalis*. Nonspecific vaginitis most often is associated with *Gardnerella vaginalis*. A clue to this diagnosis is the presence of many small gram-negative bacilli that adhere to vaginal epithelial cells.

2. **Urethritis.** Acute urinary frequency, dysuria, and pyuria in the absence of vaginal symptoms favor a diagnosis of urethritis or UTI rather than vaginitis. *Chlamydia trachomatis* is a common cause of the acute urethral syndrome in women, as well as nonspecific urethritis in men. *Neisseria gonorrhoeae* is also a widespread cause of urethritis and dysuria. The diagnosis and treatment of gonorrhea are now well standardized. Low colony count (100 to 1,000 CFU) infections with coliforms are now a recognized cause of urethritis in symptomatic young women with pyuria. Herpes simplex virus, usually type 2, is another sexually transmitted agent that can cause severe dysuria through ulcerations in close proximity to the urethral orifice. The diagnosis of herpes progenitalis can be confirmed by real-time HSV PCR assays, by isolating the virus in tissue culture, by direct fluorescent antibody test, or finding giant multinucleated transformed cells in epidermal scrapings stained with Wright stain.

3. **Prostatitis.** Prostatitis is a common affliction in men that causes dysuria and urinary frequency in middle-aged and younger men more frequently than UTIs do. In addition, more than 90% of men with febrile UTIs have asymptomatic prostatitis manifested by elevated prostate-specific antigens (PSAs) and prostate volume. The PSA may remain elevated for up to 12 months. Prostate syndromes have classically been divided into four clinical entities: (a) acute bacterial prostatitis, (b) chronic bacterial prostatitis, (c) nonbacterial prostatitis, and (d) prostatodynia.

a. **Acute bacterial prostatitis** is easily distinguished from the other prostatitis syndromes by its acute characteristics. The patient often appears acutely ill, with the sudden onset of chills and fever, urinary frequency and urgency, dysuria, perineal and low back pain, and constitutional symptoms. Rectal examination should not be performed because of the risk of precipitating sepsis, but it may disclose an exquisitely tender, hot, and swollen prostate gland. Microscopic examination of the urine usually displays numerous white blood cells. Urine culture is usually positive for enteric gram-negative bacteria (especially *E. coli*); gram-positive bacteria (staphylococci and enterococci) are less frequently isolated.
b. **Chronic Bacterial Prostatitis.** A hallmark of chronic prostatitis is relapsing UTIs. Urinary frequency, dysuria, nocturia, and low back and perineal pain are the usual symptoms, although patients may have a minimum of symptoms between UTIs. The patient is often afebrile, does not appear acutely ill, and may have an unremarkable prostate examination. A proposed mechanism to explain the migration of bacteria into the prostate is by reflux of urine and bacteria into the prostatic ducts from the urethra. This syndrome is distinguished from other forms of chronic prostatitis by displaying an initial negative midstream urine examination and culture; after prostate massage, however, the urine displays a positive microscopic examination for white blood cells, and a uropathogen can be cultured (see Section V). Nonbacterial prostatitis is the most common form of chronic prostatitis. It mimics chronic bacterial prostatitis clinically and displays inflammatory cells on postprostate massage specimens. However, bacteriologic cultures of urine and prostatic secretions are sterile. The etiology is unknown, but some evidence exists for an infectious etiology involving organisms that are difficult to culture.
c. **Prostatodynia** has also been referred to as *chronic noninflammatory prostatitis*. Clinically, it presents with symptoms similar to other forms of chronic prostatitis. It is distinguished by the absence of inflammatory cells or uropathogens from all specimens.

B. **UTIs.** Despite the mimicking syndromes, a presumptive diagnosis of infections of the urinary tract can be established economically by analyzing urine in patients with characteristic, albeit nonspecific, signs and symptoms. Acute uncomplicated UTIs occur mainly in women of childbearing age. The presenting features are only suggestive of the site of infection. Patients with bacterial cystourethritis, as distinct from urethritis caused by a sexually transmitted disease (STD) pathogen, will have had prior episodes, will have experienced symptoms for less than 1 week, and will experience suprapubic pain.

V. Laboratory Diagnosis
The diagnostic approach to UTIs is shown in Figure 10-2.
A. **Urine Specimens for Culture**
1. **Indications.** The diagnosis of UTI, from simple cystitis to complicated pyelonephritis with sepsis, can be established with absolute certainty only by quantitative cultures of urine. The major indications for urine cultures are as follows:
   a. **Patients with Symptoms or Signs of UTIs**
   b. **Follow-Up of Recently Treated UTI**
   c. **Removal of Indwelling Urinary Catheter**
   d. **Screening for Asymptomatic Bacteriuria during Pregnancy**
   e. **Patients with Obstructive Uropathy and Stasis Before Instrumentation**
2. When universally applied, the first two indications may not be the most cost-effective approach to diagnosing UTIs in nonpregnant, young adult women. These individuals present with dysuria, urgency, and pyuria due to

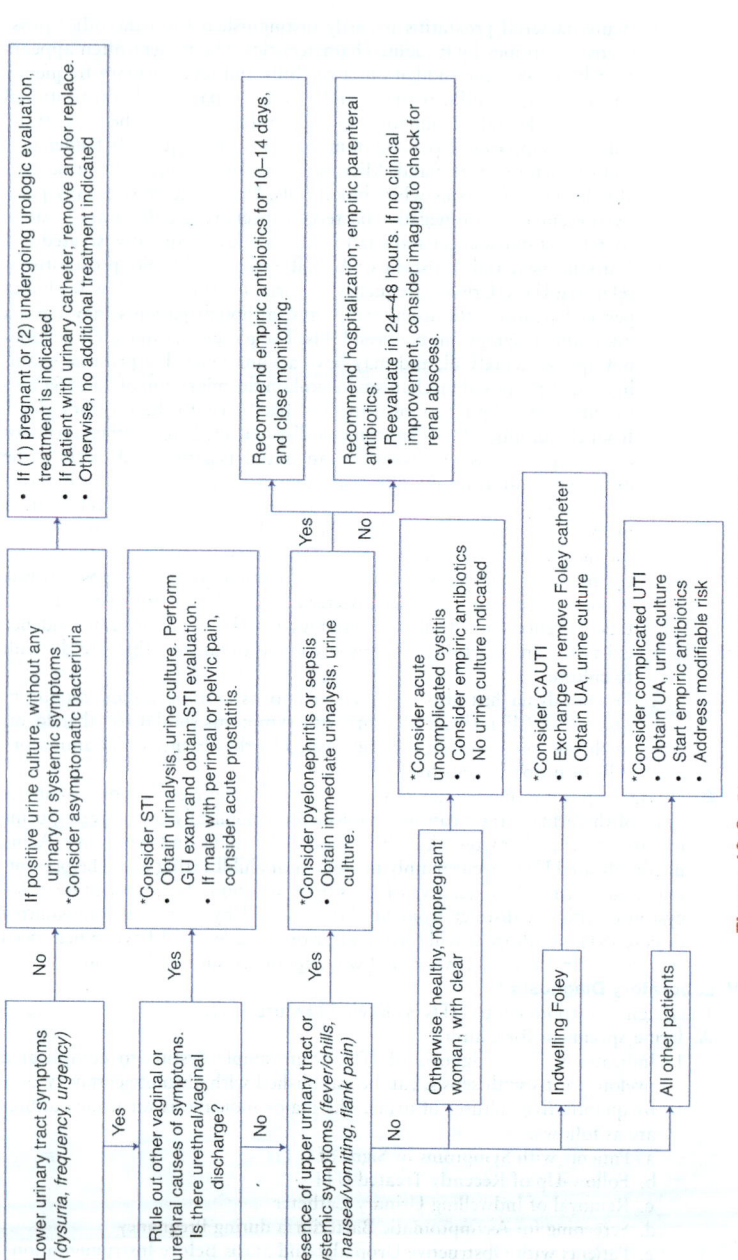

Figure 10-2. Diagnostic approach to urinary tract infections.

an uncomplicated episode of cystourethritis, with organisms usually susceptible to a variety of antimicrobial agents, or due to an STD pathogen such as *gonococcus* or *chlamydia*. Moreover, because the beneficial outcome of therapy is to minimize morbidity rather than prevent life-threatening complications, laboratory costs and use of resources can be minimized if pretreatment cultures are not ordered in this clinical setting. Therefore, women with symptoms consistent with simple uncomplicated lower tract disease and a positive urine dipstick can be treated without obtaining a urine culture. In addition, if symptoms completely resolve, post-treatment cultures are also unnecessary for patients with uncomplicated infections.
3. **Methods.** Urine specimens must be cultured promptly within 2 hours or be preserved by refrigeration or a suitable chemical additive (e.g., boric acid sodium formate preservative). Acceptable methods of collection are the following:
   a. **Midstream urine voided into a sterile container after careful washing (water or saline) of external genitalia (any soap must be rinsed away)**
   b. **Urine obtained by single catheterization or suprapubic needle aspiration of the bladder**
   c. **Sterile needle aspiration of urine from the tube of a closed catheter drainage system (do not disconnect tubing to get specimen)**
4. Not acceptable, because of constant contamination and the impossibility of quantitative counts, are tips from indwelling urinary catheters and urine obtained randomly, without adequate patient preparation. The clean-voided, midstream technique of collection is preferred whenever possible to avoid the risk of introducing infection at the time of catheterization, a hazard in elderly patients confined to bed, in men with condom catheters, and in diabetic patients with dysfunctional bladders. Because contamination is exceedingly rare in circumcised men, a clean-catch, midstream specimen is unnecessary in such patients. Occasionally, suprapubic aspiration of the bladder is necessary to verify infection. This technique has been most helpful in obtaining specimens from possibly septic infants and from adults in whom repeated clean-voided specimens have yielded equivocal colony counts on culture.
5. **The usual microbial pathogens** isolated from patients with UTIs are listed in Table 10-1. Results of cultures highly depend, however, on the clinical setting in which bacteriuria occurs. For example, *E. coli* is found in the urine of 80% to 90% of patients with acute uncomplicated cystitis and acute uncomplicated pyelonephritis. *S. saprophyticus* is another common cause of UTI, but rarely causes acute pyelonephritis. Many patients with staghorn calculi of the kidneys harbor urea-splitting *Proteus* organisms in their urine. *Klebsiella, Pseudomonas aeruginosa*, and *Enterobacter* infections are commonly acquired in the hospital. The presence of *Staphylococcus aureus* in the urine most often is a clue to concomitant staphylococcal bacteremia, unless an underlying risk factor exists. Microorganisms in young men are similar to the organisms that cause uncomplicated infections in women. Enterococci and coagulase-negative staphylococci are more common in elderly men, most likely representing recent instrumentation or catheterization. *C. albicans* is rarely encountered, except in patients with indwelling catheters, nosocomial UTIs, or relapsing infections after multiple courses of antibiotic therapy. Most urinary catheter-related infections originate from the patient's colonic flora with long-term catheterization exceeding 28 days. Multidrug-resistant organisms such as *Providencia stuartii, Pseudomonas spp., Proteus spp., Morganella spp.*, and *Acinetobacter spp.* are found more frequently owing to antibiotic exposure. In addition, polymicrobial bacteriuria is found in up to 95% of urine cultures from patients with long-term catheter use. Although the likely microorganism and

TABLE 10-1 Microbial Pathogens of Kidney and Bladder

Organism	Uncomplicated Cystitis: Young Women[a] (%)	Pyelonephritis: Outpatient, Women[b] (%)	UTI: Men[c] (%)	Bacteremic UTIs[d] (%)	Nosocomial UTIs[e] (%)
Gram-Negative Bacteria					
Escherichia coli	79	86	41	54	29
Klebsiella pneumoniae	3	4	3	9	8
Proteus	2	3	6	8	4
Enterobacter	0	0	1	2	4
Pseudomonas aeruginosa	0	0	NS	3	9
Gram-Positive Bacteria					
Staphylococcus saprophyticus	11	3	NS	0	0
Staphylococcus aureus	0	1	1	13	0
Staphylococcus nonaureus	0	0	5	1	5
Enterococci	2	0	5	6	13
Other Bacteria	0	4	19	4	15
Mixed Infections	3	3	18	2	NS
Yeast	0	0	0	3	13

NS, not stated; UTI, urinary tract infection.

[a]Data from 607 episodes of cystitis; from Stamm WE. Urinary tract infections. In: Root RK, ed. *Clinical Infectious Diseases: A Practical Approach*. 1st ed. Oxford University Press; 1999.

[b]Eighty-four episodes from Stamm 1992 and 54 nonhospitalized women; from Pinson AG, Philbrock JT, Lindbeck GH, Schorling JB, eds. Management of acute pyelonephritis in women: a cohort study. *Am J Emerg Med*. 1994;12: 271–278.

[c]Data from 223 outpatient males with symptoms; from Pead L, Maskell R. Urinary tract infections in adult men. *J Infect*. 1981;3:71–78.

[d]185 cases (excluding five cases of *Candida albicans*); from Ackermann RJ, Monroe PW. Bacteremic urinary tract infections in older people. *J Am Geriatr Soc*. 1996;44:927–933.

[e]90% catheter-associated infections, 1991 experience at the University of Iowa (900-bed hospital); from Bronsema DA, Adams JR, Pallares R, Wenzel RP. Secular trends in rates and etiology of nosocomial urinary tract infections at a university hospital. *J Urol*. 1993;150:414–416.

usual susceptibility patterns are sufficient to guide the initial empiric therapy of uncomplicated cystitis, adequate treatment of acute bacterial pyelonephritis and complicated UTIs necessitates precise therapy based on isolation of the causative bacterium and standardized antimicrobial susceptibility testing using the disk-diffusion or the broth-dilution or agar-dilution methods.

B. Interpretation of Urine Cultures. Organisms residing in the distal urethra and on pubic hairs contaminate voided, clean-catch specimens. This bacterial contamination must be distinguished from "true infection" or "significant bacteriuria" in urine cultures. Quantitative bacteriology makes this distinction. Because quantitation of bacteriuria is so important clinically, methods for culture of urine must enable the CFU number of a potential pathogen per milliliter of urine to be assessed. The standard procedure involves the use of calibrated bacteriologic loops that deliver a known volume of urine to the surface of agar plates. Proper plating techniques achieve isolated colonies that can be enumerated accurately. A satisfactory alternative for the diagnosis of uncomplicated UTIs is the dip slide method, which is particularly well suited to quantitative urine cultures in smaller clinics. Rapid methods based on filtration and colorimetry, bioluminescence, growth kinetics, and biochemical reactions are used increasingly to screen urine specimens for the presence of bacteria. The sensitivities of these rapid assays are in the range of 10^4 to 10^5 CFU/mL. The simplest screen is the paper-strip test for detection of leukocyte esterase and nitrite in first-morning urine specimens. However, these methods are not a substitute for standard cultures in symptomatic patients with complicated UTIs.

1. **Colony Counts.** Figure 10-3 shows a basic guide to the interpretation of quantitative cultures of urine. Colony counts greater than 10^5 CFU/mL in properly collected and transported specimens usually indicate infection. Colony counts of 10^3 or fewer CFU/mL from untreated patients are uncommon with true UTIs, except in symptomatic young women with pyuria and urethritis, in whom colony counts of *E. coli* as low as 10^3 may be interpretable if the urine was obtained by single catheterization. Intermediate counts, especially with mixed flora, usually imply poor collection or delayed transport and culture. Brisk diuresis may transiently reduce an otherwise high colony count.

2. **Suprapubic Needle Aspiration.** Any growth from urine obtained by suprapubic needle aspiration may be important; recent guidelines suggest a threshold of 1000 CFU/mL. Use of a 0.01 mL quantitative loop for culturing aspirated urine permits the detection of as few as 100 CFU/mL. Two or more colonies (≤200 CFU/mL) of the same microorganism ensure the purity of growth from such specimens and permit standardized antimicrobial susceptibility testing. Similar criteria should be used for patients who are receiving antimicrobials at the time of culture. Except in unusual circumstances, the isolation of diphtheroids, α-hemolytic streptococci, and lactobacilli indicates contamination of the urine specimen with vaginal or periurethral flora.

3. **Prostatic Secretions.** In men, the distinction between a urinary source and a prostatic focus of infection must be made. The procedure for obtaining voided urine and expressed prostatic secretions in partitioned segments that enable proper interpretation is diagrammed in Figure 10-4. Leukocytes (greater than 10 to 15 white blood cells per high-power field) and lipid-laden macrophages are seldom observed in the expressed prostatic secretion of healthy men. These agents signify prostatic inflammation. Therefore, a prostatic focus of infection should be considered when a significant step-up of pyuria or colony counts occurs in the prostate specimens. A UTI of prostatic origin is indicated by colony counts of 10^5 or more CFU/mL of the same microorganism in all four specimens. Both urologists and primary care physicians underuse this procedure. In one study, a two-step procedure involving microscopic examination and culture of pre- and postprostate massage urine specimens compared favorably to this four-step procedure. This simplified approach was able to arrive at a similar diagnosis in 91% of patients. Further trials are needed to evaluate this approach, which may improve physician use.

C. **Microscopic Examination of Urine.** Procedures for the microscopic examination of urine are poorly standardized; nonetheless, visualization of bacteria,

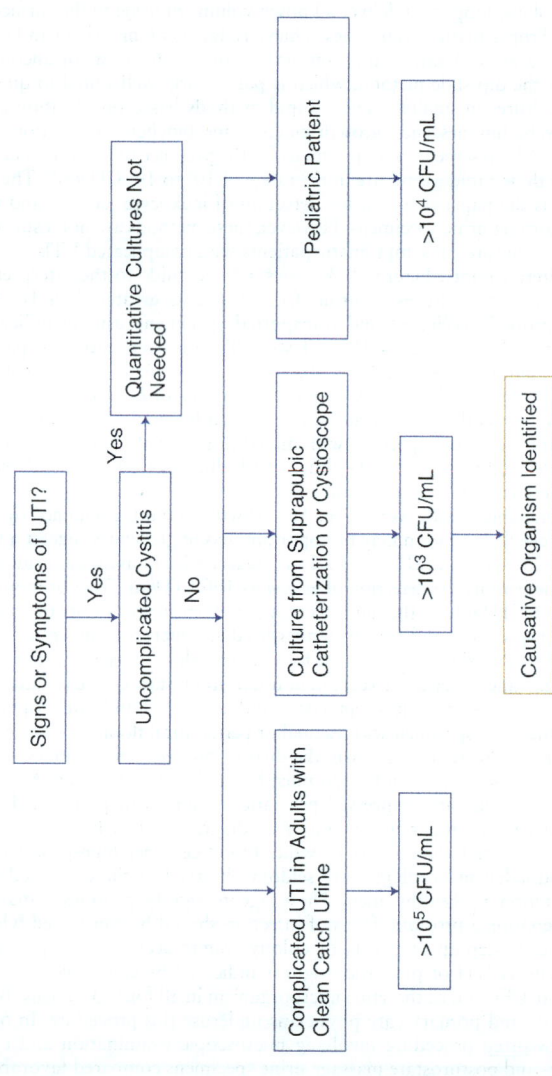

Figure 10-3. Use of quantitative urine cultures. CFU, colony forming units.

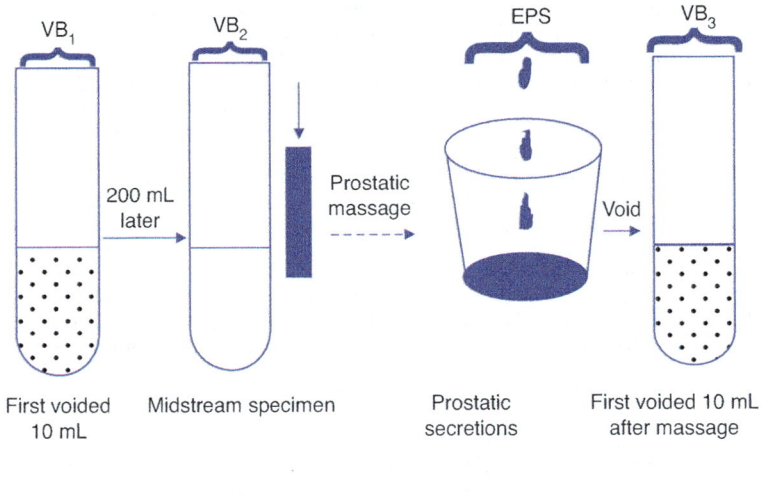

Figure 10-4. Localization of infection with segmented cultures of the lower urinary tract in men. VB_1 is the first 10 mL of voided urine, and VB_2 is the midstream specimen of urine obtained before prostatic massage. Subsequently, the expressed prostatic secretions (EPS) are collected before the final voided urine specimen (VB_3). When the bacterial colony counts in the urethral culture exceed by 10-fold or more those of the midstream and prostatic cultures, the urethra is the source of the infection. The diagnosis is bacterial prostatitis if the quantitative counts of the prostatic specimens exceed those of the urethral and midstream samples. (From Meares EM, Stamey TA. Bacteriologic localization patterns in bacterial prostatitis and urethritis. *Invest Urol.* 1968;5:492. Reprinted with permission.)

leukocytes, and epithelial cells in urine can provide some useful information and enable the clinician to make a presumptive diagnosis of UTI. The advantages of microscopic analysis are immediate availability and low cost. The disadvantages, depending on the method, are lack of sensitivity, specificity, or both. Only properly collected and processed specimens for quantitative urine cultures can provide definitive diagnosis. The microscopic examination can be done on either unspun urine or the centrifuged sediment. A critical comparison of these two techniques is not available. The presence of squamous epithelial cells and mixed bacterial flora indicates contamination and the need for a repeat specimen.

1. **Unspun Urine.** When fresh, unspun urine from patients with significant bacteriuria (greater than 10^5 CFU/mL) is examined microscopically ($\times 1,000$), 90% of specimens show one or more bacteria, and 75% of specimens show one or more white blood cells per oil-immersion field. The best assessment of pyuria is the finding of approximately 10 white blood cells per mm^3 of unspun urine examined in a counting chamber.
2. **Centrifuged Sediment.** After 10 mL of urine is centrifuged in a standard 15-mL conical tube for 5 minutes at 2,500 revolutions/min in a clinical centrifuge, three or four drops of the sediment are examined under a coverslip at high power ($\times 400$) in diminished light. Patients with significant bacteriuria usually show bacilli in the urinary sediment, whereas only approximately 10% of patients with fewer than 105 CFU/mL show bacteria. Approximately 60% to 85% of patients with significant bacteriuria

have 10 or more white blood cells per high-power field in the sediment of midstream voided urine; however, approximately 25% of patients with negative urine cultures also have pyuria (10 or more white blood cells per high-power field), and only approximately 40% of patients with pyuria have 105 or more bacteria per mL of urine by quantitative culture. The principal pitfall is false-positive pyuria owing to leukocytes from a contaminating vaginal discharge.
3. **Gram Stain.** A simple Gram-stained smear of unspun urine or spun sediment can enhance the specificity of the test, because morphology and stain characteristics aid in identifying the likely pathogen and in targeting empiric therapy.
4. **Pyuria.** Although the presence of pyuria in a midstream specimen has low predictive value for significant bacteriuria, pyuria is a sensitive indicator of inflammation. Therefore, pyuria may be more accurate than bacteriuria in distinguishing a "true infection" from contamination: 95% of patients with pyuria have a genitourinary tract infection; however, pyuria cannot distinguish a bacterial UTI from acute urethral syndrome. In addition to a UTI, any of the causes of acute urethral syndrome (see Section IV.A) can result in pyuria. For example, tuberculosis is a cause of pyuria with negative routine urine cultures, although mycobacterial cultures are positive in 90% of instances. Analgesic nephropathy, interstitial nephritis, perinephric abscess, renal cortical abscess, disseminated fungal infection, and appendicitis may also result in pyuria.

D. Biochemical Tests for Bacteriuria. Two metabolic capabilities shared by most bacterial pathogens of the urinary tract are use of glucose and reduction of nitrate to nitrite; these are properties of all Enterobacteriaceae. Because small amounts of glucose and nitrate are normally present in urine, the presence of significant numbers of bacteria in urine results in the absence of glucose and presence of nitrite. Dipstick devices are commercially available for both types of testing. Studies with nitrite-indicator strips show that 85% of women and children with culture-confirmed significant bacteriuria show positive results if three consecutive morning urine specimens are tested. A morning urine specimen is preferred for the nitrite test because most bacteria take 4 to 6 hours to convert nitrate to nitrite. A negative nitrite test may be observed in patients taking diuretics or with organisms that do not produce nitrate reductase (*Staphylococcus* species, *Enterococcus* species, and *P. aeruginosa*). The sensitivity of the glucose-use test is approximately 90% to 95% in patients without diabetes mellitus. Both biochemical tests have fewer than 5% false-positive results. Therefore, these biochemical tests can be used by patients or parents, after proper instruction, to determine when quantitative cultures are needed in the management of recurrent episodes of UTI. Spectrum bias in the use of dipsticks must be avoided. Dipsticks should only be used for patients with symptoms suggestive of UTI (i.e., high pretest probability of UTI) and not for asymptomatic screening, as in pregnancy.

E. Localization of the Site of Infection. The site of infection within the urinary tract has great therapeutic and prognostic importance. Upper UTI (pyelonephritis) indicates a much greater likelihood of underlying uropathy (e.g., congenital anomalies, renal stones, ureteral occlusion, vesicoureteral reflux, neurogenic bladder, or prostatic hypertrophy) or previous instrumentation (see Section III.B). Relapses with the same, often multiple, antibiotic-resistant bacteria are common with pyelonephritis or chronic bacterial prostatitis. Treatment is long (minimum 10 to 14 days) and may be arduous. On the other hand, cystitis rarely is complicated, and treatment can be short (single dose or 3 days) and usually is easy. No ready way exists to distinguish between upper and lower UTIs by simple laboratory tests. The difficulty in making this distinction reliably on clinical grounds alone has been discussed (see Section IV.B).

Older, indirect methods (e.g., serum antibodies, urine concentration test, and urinary β-glucuronidase activity) are neither sensitive nor specific. Direct methods for localization (e.g., ureteral catheterization, renal biopsy, and the bladder washout technique) are hazardous, expensive, or both. Eradication of bacteriuria with single-dose or short-course (3-day) antibiotic therapy in symptomatic patients with uncomplicated disease is a practical method for presumptive localization of infection to the bladder or urethra.

F. Radiography and Other Diagnostic Procedures: Indications. The principal role of radiographic and urologic studies for patients with UTIs is to detect vesicoureteral reflux, renal calculi, and potentially correctable lesions that obstruct urine flow and cause stasis. Uncomplicated reinfections (cystitis and urethritis) in women who respond to short-course antimicrobial therapy are not an indication for radiographic and cystoscopic investigation of the urinary tract. Radiologic and urologic evaluation should be considered in all children with a first episode of UTIs (except for school-aged girls). Special emphasis should be on the early detection of urologic abnormalities in all young children and boys with a first infection, as well as any child with pyelonephritis or a complicated course. A review of studies evaluating diagnostic imaging in children with UTIs expressed the need for better outcome-based research in this area. Radiologic and urologic evaluation should be considered in adults with UTIs. In the past, all UTIs in males were considered complicated. The conventional recommendation that all males presenting with initial UTIs undergo urologic evaluation to identify predisposing anatomic or functional abnormalities is still followed. However, several studies have indicated that only approximately 20% of men have previously unidentified abnormalities. Some sexually active males are at a higher risk for cystitis (homosexual males, males with a partner who harbors a uropathogen, and uncircumcised males). The value of urologic evaluation in this high-risk group, with a single episode of cystitis and an uncomplicated course, is not known. In general, urologic evaluations are recommended in the following situations: (a) males with first episode, (b) all patients with a complicated infection or bacteremia, (c) suspected obstruction or renal stones, (d) hematuria following infection, (e) failure to respond to appropriate antibiotic therapy, and (f) patients with recurrent infections.

Some experts recommend the evaluation of all patients with pyelonephritis. The radiologic evaluation of a subgroup of patients with pyelonephritis (young and otherwise healthy women who respond well to therapy) may have a low diagnostic yield. In one study, only 1 of 25 young women with uncomplicated pyelonephritis had a surgically correctable etiology, and 2 of 25 had focal abnormalities that resolved on a follow-up ultrasonography. This has led others to recommend a diagnostic evaluation in young women with uncomplicated pyelonephritis after the second recurrence, or at any time, if a complicating course is present. The ease of obtaining a noninvasive test (ultrasonography) has increased radiologic evaluations for most patients admitted with pyelonephritis.

Ultrasonography with a plain film of the abdomen has replaced intravenous pyelogram (IVP) as the initial radiologic study for most adults. For a detailed evaluation of the ureterovesical junction, bladder, and urethra, a voiding cystourethrogram and measurement of the residual urine after voiding may be necessary. If vesicoureteral reflux is present after acute infection has been treated, a urologist should be consulted. Cystoscopy may be warranted. Contrast-enhanced computed tomography (CT) of the kidneys is the most effective imaging modality in adult patients with pyelonephritis. CT has high sensitivity in detecting renal abnormalities and perirenal fluid collections. Noncontrast spiral CT is the most sensitive test to detect renal calculi as many are not seen on plain radiograph of the abdomen or ultrasound. Radionuclide imaging procedures are not used in the evaluation of adult patients with UTI, but they are useful in children with pyelonephritis. Ordinarily, radiographic studies should not be performed within 6 weeks of acute infections.

Gram-negative bacilli have the ability to impede ureteral peristalsis, and transient abnormalities of the IVP are common with acute pyelonephritis. These include hydroureter, vesicoureteral reflux, diminished pyelogram, loss of renal outline, and renal enlargement. Acute pyelonephritis with an obstructed ureter is a surgical emergency, and a perinephric abscess also requires surgical drainage. These complications, however, are best detected initially by ultrasonography and by CT, respectively. To avoid radiocontrast-induced acute renal failure, excretory urography and other radiocontrast studies should be avoided whenever possible in patients with a serum creatinine above 1.5 mg/dL, diabetes mellitus, dehydration, or advanced age.

VI. Treatment of UTI

A. Principles of Underlying Therapy and Follow-Up. To successfully treat a UTI, the clinician must have knowledge of microbial susceptibility and mechanisms of resistance, pharmacokinetics, and pharmacodynamics, and status of host defenses. First, most uropathogens are susceptible to a wide range of antibiotics; however, resistant gram-negative bacteria frequently are seen with indwelling catheters, in immunocompromised patients, and in patients with relapsing bacteriuria. Second, most antibiotics are filtered by the kidney and therefore achieve a urinary concentration that is many times higher than the minimum inhibitory concentration. Third, although most antibiotics achieve adequate concentration in renal tissue, only tetracyclines, trimethoprim-sulfamethoxazole, and fluoroquinolones achieve any reasonable concentration in the prostate. Finally, patients with systemic or local abnormalities in host defenses usually develop a renal infection that is refractory to therapy. In this case, antibiotics that achieve adequate serum concentrations and are bactericidal are preferable to bacterial static agents. The basic caveats for the effective management of UTIs are outlined here.

1. **Asymptomatic patients** should have colony counts ≥100,000/mL on at least two occasions before treatment is considered.
2. Unless symptoms are present, **no attempt should be made to eradicate bacteriuria** until catheters, stones, or obstructions are removed.
3. Selected patients with chronic bacteriuria may benefit from suppressive therapy.
4. A patient who develops **bacteriuria as a result of catheterization** should have treatment to re-establish a sterile urine after the removal of catheter.
5. **Antimicrobial agents used for treatment** should be the safest and least expensive agents to which the causative microorganisms are susceptible.
6. **Efficacy of treatment** should be evaluated by urine culture 1 week after completion of therapy, except in nonpregnant adult women who respond to therapy for uncomplicated cystitis and uncomplicated pyelonephritis.

B. Antimicrobial Agents

1. **β-Lactams.** Because of increasing antimicrobial resistance observed in *E. coli*, amoxicillin and ampicillin should **not** be used for empiric therapy, unless *enterococcus* or Group B *streptococcus* is determined to be the sole cause of infection. Amoxicillin is effective for uncomplicated cystitis, but short-course therapy (single-dose and 3-day regimens) has generally been less effective than trimethoprim-sulfamethoxazole or fluoroquinolones given for a similar duration. Cefixime and cefpodoxime are oral third-generation cephalosporins with enhanced activity against enteric gram-negative bacteria, longer serum half-life, and less frequent dosing than first-generation cephalosporins. Parenteral β-lactams are generally reserved for more complicated infections. Ceftriaxone is a third-generation cephalosporin with good activity against most community-acquired gram-negative

enteric bacteria (except *P. aeruginosa*). Ceftazidime and cefepime are examples of cephalosporins with good activity against many gram-negative bacteria, including *P. aeruginosa*.

2. **Nitrofurantoin** is active against many uropathogens, including *E. coli*, *S. saprophyticus*, and *Enterococcus faecalis*. Some gram-negative bacteria are resistant to nitrofurantoin (*Klebsiella*, *Enterobacter*, and *Pseudomonas* species), making it a less-than-ideal agent for the empiric therapy of complicated UTIs. No clinically significant increase in resistance has been observed. However, this drug is significantly less active than fluoroquinolones and trimethoprim-sulfamethoxazole against non-*Escherichia coli* aerobic gram-negative rods and is inactive against *Proteus* and *Pseudomonas* species. The major role of nitrofurantoin in therapy includes the treatment of uncomplicated cystitis and as an alternative agent for cystitis caused by *E. faecalis*. Two preparations are available in the United States: (1) a combination nitrofurantoin monohydrate–macrocrystals slow-release capsule and (2) a preparation that is made solely of nitrofurantoin macrocrystals. The usual adult dose for the monohydrate/macrocrystals preparation is 100 mg twice daily for 7 days. The dose for the macrocrystalline preparation is 50 to 100 mg every 6 hours for 7 days. Although a 3-day regimen is successful in many patients with uncomplicated cystitis, one clinical trial found nitrofurantoin to be less effective than a 3-day regimen of trimethoprim-sulfamethoxazole. Patients with renal insufficiency (creatinine clearance less than 60 mL/min) should not receive this agent. Nitrofurantoin has been used in pregnancy (U.S. Food and Drug Administration [FDA] category B), although it is contraindicated in nursing mothers, pregnant women near term, and newborns (in whom it is associated with hemolytic anemia). Suppressive therapy has been successful in some patients, although concern for less common reactions (e.g., peripheral neuropathy, pneumonitis, and hepatitis) may limit long-term use.

3. **Trimethoprim-sulfamethoxazole and Trimethoprim.** Trimethoprim-sulfamethoxazole has a wide spectrum of activity against many uropathogens. However, lack of clinical activity against *enterococci* and *P. aeruginosa*, as well as increased resistance by some enteric gram-negative bacteria (*Klebsiella* species, *Enterobacter* species), makes trimethoprim-sulfamethoxazole a less than ideal agent for the treatment of complicated UTIs. In addition, resistance patterns tabulated by microbiology laboratories show trimethoprim-sulfamethoxazole resistance variability depending on locale; an 18% incidence of resistance is present in the southeastern and western United States for women with acute cystitis who have had a UTI in the last 6 months. Therefore, some authorities recommend the use of trimethoprim-sulfamethoxazole only if (a) the local resistance pattern is less than 20%, (b) no sulfa allergy exists, and (c) no recent antibiotic use is present. Of interest, despite a 30% resistance prevalence in some locales, at least half of the women treated with trimethoprim-sulfamethoxazole have 80% to 85% clinical and microbiologic cures.

Trimethoprim-sulfamethoxazole is well tolerated in most patients. Adverse effects due to sulfonamides are well described and include gastrointestinal symptoms, transient elevation in the serum creatinine, and hematologic and dermatologic reactions. Sulfonamides displace warfarin and hypoglycemic agents from albumin, thereby potentiating these drug effects. Trimethoprim-sulfamethoxazole is highly effective for the prophylaxis and therapy for uncomplicated cystitis and for therapy of uncomplicated pyelonephritis. A randomized trial with four different 3-day drug regimens in women with uncomplicated acute cystitis found that a 3-day regimen of trimethoprim-sulfamethoxazole was the most cost effective. Trimethoprim-sulfamethoxazole should be used with caution in patients with kidney disease (creatinine clearance <30 mL/min) due to the risk of worsening renal failure and hyperkalemia. Complicated UTIs, especially catheter-associated infections and nosocomial UTIs, should have in vitro susceptibility testing performed. Trimethoprim-sulfamethoxazole has been used in pregnancy, but it is not FDA-approved for pregnant women. Other agents such as amoxicillin, nitrofurantoin, and cephalosporins are preferred.

Trimethoprim alone is preferred over trimethoprim-sulfamethoxazole by some experts for the prophylaxis and treatment of uncomplicated cystitis because its efficacy is similar and the side effects are fewer (because of the absence of sulfamethoxazole). This agent should not be used alone for the therapy of complicated UTIs.

Trimethoprim monotherapy also achieves good prostate concentrations and is an alternative to fluoroquinolones depending on the susceptibility pattern of the bacteria.

4. **Fosfomycin.** A novel class of antibiotics that has broad spectrum of activity against both gram-positive and negative organisms, including MDR isolates. Should only be used for uncomplicated cystitis in patients who have risk factors for MDR gram-negative infections. These risk factors include a history of any of the following within the past 3 months: inpatient stay at any health care stay facility, prior MDR gram-negative urinary isolate, recent use of antibiotics, or travel to regions with high rates of MDR. Given as a 3-g powder mixed in water as a single dose. Appears to have inferior efficacy compared with other standard short-course regimens, so not used as commonly.
5. Multiple **fluoroquinolones** are now available for clinical use (Tables 10-2 and 10-3). These agents achieve very high concentrations in the urine and renal tissue, easily exceeding the minimal inhibitory concentration of most uropathogens. Fluoroquinolones should not be used as first-line agents for the therapy of uncomplicated cystitis because of concern for the development of resistance and because of the cost. However, their antimicrobial spectrum and generally low side-effect profile make them excellent choices for empiric therapy of complicated UTIs. Among current agents within this antimicrobial class, no particular drug has demonstrated superior clinical efficacy for the therapy of patients with UTIs. An exception is moxifloxacin, which does not achieve adequate urinary concentrations and should be avoided in the treatment of UTIs. Fluoroquinolones should not be used for enterococcal UTIs (only 60% to 70% susceptible) during pregnancy or in children (until further information is available). Aluminum- and magnesium-containing antacids and iron-, calcium-, and zinc-containing preparations should not be administered with oral fluoroquinolones due to a significant decrease in absorption. In general, these agents are well tolerated by most patients. The most common adverse effects are gastrointestinal and on the central nervous system, but these infrequently lead to drug discontinuation. Photosensitivity may limit the use of some of these agents (e.g., lomefloxacin, sparfloxacin). Many of these agents are available for both parenteral and oral administration. Conversion from parenteral to oral therapy (step-down therapy) should be considered for patients who are clinically stable and tolerating oral medications. The excellent bioavailability of these drugs, good clinical success with oral therapy, and the high cost of parenteral therapy due to intravenous catheter–related complications and cost of intravenous preparations are all good reasons for considering oral therapy.
6. Macrolides—Erythromycin, clarithromycin, and azithromycin may be considered for the treatment of *Mycoplasma* sp and *U. urealyticum*.
7. Tetracyclines—May be used for *Chlamydia* sp and *Mycoplasma* sp.

TABLE 10-2 Oral Antimicrobial Agents Commonly Used for the Treatment of Urinary Tract Infections

	Adult Dose	Comment
Miscellaneous Agents		
Trimethoprim	100 mg every 12 h 100 mg daily (for prophylaxis)	Prophylaxis, uncomplicated cystitis
Trimethoprim-sulfamethoxazole	160 mg/800 mg every 12 h	Uncomplicated cystitis; cost effective
Nitrofurantoin	50–100 mg every 6 h	Prophylaxis, uncomplicated cystitis
Tetracycline	250–500 mg every 6 h	Prophylaxis
β-Lactams[a]		
Amoxicillin	250–500 mg every 8 h	During pregnancy, enterococcal infections
Cephalexin or cephradine	250 mg every 6 h	During pregnancy, uncomplicated cystitis
Cefixime	200 mg every 12 h/400 mg every 24 h	Step-down therapy[a]
Cefpodoxime	100–200 mg every 12 h	Step-down therapy[a]
Fluoroquinolones		
Norfloxacin	400 mg every 12 h	Low-serum drug levels
Ciprofloxacin	250–500 mg every 12 h	First "systemic" fluoroquinolone
Lomefloxacin	400 mg every 24 h	Skin photosensitivity reactions
Enoxacin	400 mg every 12 h	P-450 drug interactions[b]
Ofloxacin	200–400 mg every 12 h	Generally replaced by levofloxacin
Levofloxacin	250–500 mg every 24 h	L-isomer of ofloxacin

Comments for miscellaneous agents and β-lactams relate to role in therapy. The role of fluoroquinolones has been for treatment of complicated urinary tract infections and as an alternative agent for uncomplicated cystitis. Because these agents have not been rigorously compared, comments are related to general spectrum of activity, side-effect profile, and drug interactions.

[a]Short-course therapy for uncomplicated cystitis has generally been less effective than the use of trimethoprim-sulfamethoxazole or fluoroquinolones for a similar duration. The general role of extended-spectrum oral cephalosporins (cefixime, cefpodoxime) has been for the treatment of complicated urinary tract infections (alternative agent) and for intravenous to oral step-down therapy.

[b]Enoxacin is a potent inhibitor of P-450 hepatic isoenzymes. (Inhibition of hepatic isoenzymes causes an elevation of serum levels of theophylline and caffeine.)

C. Treatment of Asymptomatic Bacteriuria

1. **Pregnancy** increases the risk of UTI complications. The rate of premature children born to women who have bacteriuria during pregnancy is increased, and 20% to 40% of these patients develop pyelonephritis. Successful therapy in these patients with bacteriuria decreases the risk of symptomatic infection by 80% to 90%. Therefore, all women should be screened twice during gestation for asymptomatic bacteriuria. Pregnant women with a history of recurrent UTI should have monthly urine cultures

TABLE 10-3 Intravenous Antimicrobial Agents Commonly Used for the Treatment of Urinary Tract Infections (UTIs)

	Adult Dose	Comment
β-Lactams		
Ampicillin	1–2 g every 4 h	*Enterococcus faecalis*; usually combined with gentamicin
Ceftriaxone	1 g every 12–24 h	Pyelonephritis
Ceftazidime	1–2 g every 8–12 h	Complicated UTI, including *P. aeruginosa*
Cefepime	1–2 g every 12 h	Complicated UTI, including *P. aeruginosa*
Aztreonam	1 g every 8–12 h	Penicillin-allergic patient
Fluoroquinolones[a]		
Ciprofloxacin	200–400 mg every 12 h	—
Ofloxacin	200–400 mg every 12 h	Generally changed to levofloxacin
Levofloxacin	500 mg every 24 h	—
Miscellaneous Agents		
Trimethoprim-sulfamethoxazole	160 mg/800 mg every 12 h	Prophylaxis, uncomplicated cystitis
Vancomycin	1 g every 12 h	Methicillin-resistant *S. aureus*; serious enterococcal infection in the penicillin-allergic patient
Gentamicin	4–7 mg/kg every 24 h	Serious gram-negative infection
	1.5–2.0 mg/kg every 8 h	Older dosing schedule; for enterococcus combined with ampicillin

[a]Because oral fluoroquinolones have excellent bioavailability and cost approximately 20% as much as parenteral fluoroquinolones, conversion from intravenous to oral therapy should be done when the patient is clinically stable.

and should undergo imaging of the urinary tract before conception or early in pregnancy to evaluate for structural disease. All patients with bacteriuria should be treated, with follow-up cultures to identify relapses. Long-term prophylaxis offers no advantage over close surveillance. In selecting therapy, the risk to the fetus should be considered. Amoxicillin, amoxicillin-clavulanate, nitrofurantoin, or cephalexin for 3 to 7 days usually suffices, because almost all these infections are caused by susceptible *E. coli*. Tetracyclines (FDA category D), trimethoprim (FDA category C), and fluoroquinolones (FDA category C) should be avoided.

2. **Children.** Asymptomatic bacteriuria in preschool- and school-aged girls may signify underlying vesicoureteral reflux. Moreover, vesicoureteral reflux, when combined with recurring bacteriuria, can result in progressive renal scarring. Therefore, in this at-risk population, asymptomatic bacteriuria should routinely be detected and treated, with follow-up urologic evaluations after 6 weeks.
3. **General Population.** Asymptomatic bacteriuria in men and nonpregnant women, a common condition in the elderly, does not appear to cause renal damage in the absence of obstructive uropathy or vesical ureteral reflux.

Prospective randomized studies of therapy for asymptomatic bacteriuria in the elderly have been recently reviewed. Of the five clinical trials reviewed, three studies had very small sample sizes, and one nonblinded study displayed a nonstatistical significant decrease in symptomatic infections. The largest randomized trial failed to demonstrate any significant difference in mortality between treated and untreated patients. Therefore, repeated attempts to clear the bacteriuria with antimicrobial agents seem unwarranted; they may only select for more resistant microorganisms and create a need for more toxic and costly antibiotics should the patient subsequently develop symptoms. Treatment of asymptomatic catheter-associated UTIs should be avoided due to the risk of developing a reservoir of resistant organisms. Patients with diabetes also have a high incidence of asymptomatic bacteriuria. The bacteriuria does not need to be treated as it is not associated with adverse renal outcomes, and studies have found treatment does not reduce symptomatic infection.

4. **Miscellaneous.** Instrumentation of the genitourinary tract should be avoided in patients with asymptomatic bacteriuria or, if necessary, done under the cover of prophylactic antimicrobial therapy. Treatment of asymptomatic catheter-associated bacteriuria is recommended only for (a) patients undergoing urologic surgery or implantation of a prosthesis, (b) part of a treatment plan to control a virulent organism predominant in a treatment unit, (c) patients at risk for serious infectious complications, such as immunosuppressed individuals, and (d) treatment of pathogens associated with a high risk of bacteremia, such as *Serratia marcescens*.

D. **Treatment of Uncomplicated Cystitis.** Acute cystitis and low colony count coliform urethritis are almost exclusively diseases of women, mostly sexually active women between the ages of 15 and 45 years. Although reinfection is common, complications are rare.

1. **Short-Course Therapy.** Appreciable evidence exists that infections truly confined to the bladder or urethra respond as well to single-dose or short-course (3-day) therapy as to conventional therapy for 10 to 14 days. Indeed, response to single-dose or short-course therapy implies a lower UTI. Reviews of short-course therapy have concluded that 3-day regimens are more effective than single-dose therapy. One randomized trial evaluated four different 3-day drug regimens in women with uncomplicated acute cystitis. A 3-day regimen of trimethoprim-sulfamethoxazole was more effective than a 3-day regimen of nitrofurantoin. Cure rates for cefadroxil (66%) and amoxicillin (67%) were not statistically different from the cure rate for trimethoprim-sulfamethoxazole (82%). The 3-day regimen of trimethoprim-sulfamethoxazole was the most cost-effective regimen. Infectious Diseases Society of America (IDSA) guidelines recommend the use of oral 3-day regimens including trimethoprim-sulfamethoxazole or a fluoroquinolone. This variety of treatments is an important breakthrough in the management of uncomplicated cystitis and coliform urethritis, because all patients were treated formerly with the standard 10 to 14 days of therapy. Diabetic women with uncomplicated infections (i.e., with normal urinary tracts) may also be treated with a 3-day course of antibiotic therapy. Post-treatment urine cultures are not required unless symptoms persist. Formal urologic imaging, such as ultrasonography, IVP, and CT, is not needed in most cases because correctable abnormalities are rarely found.

2. **Seven-Day Regimen.** A longer course of therapy for cystitis should be considered in patients with complicating factors that lead to a lower success rate and a higher risk of relapse. These complicating factors include a history of prolonged symptoms (more than 7 days), recent UTI, diabetic

patients with abnormal urinary tracts, age older than 65 years, and use of a diaphragm. Importantly, the elderly frequently have concurrent renal bacteriuria; therefore, short-course therapy should not be used.

3. **Symptomatic pyuria without bacteriuria** in an otherwise healthy young person suggests chlamydial or gonococcal urethritis. The importance of documenting these infections as well as screening for other STDs (e.g., human immunodeficiency virus infection, syphilis), and the necessity of counseling about STD risk reduction cannot be understated. Recent guidelines suggest that either a single dose of azithromycin or a 7-day course of doxycycline is effective for chlamydial urethritis. Therapy for gonococcal urethritis includes a single dose of ceftriaxone or cefixime, or a fluoroquinolone combined with therapy for chlamydial infection.

E. **Management of Recurrent Cystitis (Reinfections).** Ten percent to 20% of women develop recurrent UTIs within several months. Some infections are related to inadequate antimicrobial therapy. It is common, however, for women whose periurethral and vaginal epithelial cells avidly support attachment of coliform bacteria to have recurrent episodes of cystitis in the absence of recognized structural abnormalities of the urinary tract. A recent prospective study of UTIs in young women identified recent use of a diaphragm and spermicide such as Nonoxynol-9, recent sexual intercourse, and a history of recurrent infection as risk factors for infection.

1. **Antimicrobial Strategies.** Strategies for managing the disease of women with frequent episodes of cystitis include (a) postcoital prophylaxis, (b) continuous low-dose prophylaxis, (c) patient self-administered therapy, and (d) consideration of contraception or barrier methods against STDs without the use of vaginal spermicides. Postcoital prophylaxis is most helpful for patients who associate recurrent UTIs with sexual intercourse. In these women, a single dose of an antimicrobial after sexual intercourse or thrice weekly at bedtime has been shown to significantly reduce the frequency of episodes of cystitis from an average of 3 per patient-year to 0.1 per patient-year. Women with frequent recurrent infections (more than three UTIs per year) are offered these prophylactic regimens. Women with fewer than three UTIs per year can be offered self-administered treatment. Multiple antimicrobial agents have demonstrated efficacy in prophylaxis and self-administered therapy. Some of these regimens include nitrofurantoin, 100 mg; trimethoprim, 100 mg; trimethoprim-sulfamethoxazole, 40 mg/200 mg; and cephalexin, 250 mg. Fluoroquinolones and cephalosporins are also effective but are more expensive. Although antimicrobial prophylaxis is effective and usually safely tolerated for months to years, single-dose therapy for acute cystitis makes prophylaxis more expensive and possibly more hazardous for most patients because of alterations in fecal and vaginal bacterial flora. Indeed, self-administration of a single-dose regimen at the onset of symptoms has proved to be as cost effective as prophylaxis.

2. **Nonantimicrobial Prophylaxis Issues.** Encouraging women to practice regular and complete emptying of the bladder may help prevent recurrent cystitis. Postcoital emptying of the bladder has also been widely recommended, although one prospective study failed to demonstrate any relationship with recurrent infections. Moreover, several theoretic preventive measures relate to the use of an alternative contraceptive method: to use a properly fitted diaphragm, to void frequently when wearing a diaphragm, and to limit diaphragm use to the recommended 6 to 8 hours after intercourse. Women should also increase fluid intake to increase the frequency of micturition. In postmenopausal women, intravaginal administration of estriol can reduce recurrent UTIs by modifying the milieu for vaginal flora.

Cranberry juice (300 mL/d) was effective in decreasing asymptomatic bacteriuria with pyuria in postmenopausal women. The small difference in symptomatic UTIs was not statistically significant.

3. **Emerging Therapies.** Many recurrent UTIs arise from the ability of bacteria to attach and invade the bladder mucosa. Pillicides are small synthetic molecules that interfere with pilus assembly, thereby blocking bacterial adhesion and subsequent reservoir formation. Pillicides have potential as a therapy for recurrent UTIs but their efficacy in animal models has not yet been reported. Mannoside, a soluble receptor analogue, is also an antiadhesive that binds to FimH. FimH allows bacteria to bind to and invade host bladder cells and mannoside prevents FimH from interacting with host receptors. Mannosides have shown great promise as a therapy, both prophylactically and for established infections. In a murine UTI model, mannoside prevented bacterial invasion into bladder tissue. These agents also act synergistically with antibiotics to reduce bacteria titers within the urinary tract of infected mice. Vaccination approaches have also been explored but to date, none have been shown to protect against cystitis.

F. Treatment of Acute Bacterial Pyelonephritis. The occurrence of flank pain, costovertebral angle tenderness, chills, fever, and nausea and vomiting with or without dysuria suggests acute bacterial pyelonephritis. In this clinical setting, blood cultures and quantitative cultures of urine should be obtained. Whether ambulatory patients should be admitted to the hospital for treatment depends in part on a subjective assessment of toxicity, likely compliance with therapy, and the home situation. When the assessment is doubtful, the patient should be treated in the hospital, at least until a clear response to therapy has occurred. This policy also applies to patients with known underlying uropathies because complications are more common in these patients.

1. **Outpatient Therapy.** Recommendations for therapy of uncomplicated pyelonephritis are outlined in Table 10-4. Fluoroquinolone or trimethoprim-sulfamethoxazole is the drug of choice for initial therapy of pyelonephritis in outpatients. Local susceptibility patterns will influence the choice for initial therapy. After culture results and susceptibility tests are available, a full 10- to 14-day course of antimicrobial therapy may be completed with the least expensive drug to which the patient's microorganism is susceptible.

2. **Inpatient Therapy.** Patients who require admission to the hospital should be treated initially with a third-generation cephalosporin or a fluoroquinolone (intramuscular or intravenous), or gentamicin or tobramycin (1.5 to 2.0 mg/kg every 8 hours or 4.0 to 7.0 mg/kg every 24 hours, with appropriate alteration of the dose interval if the serum creatinine exceeds 1 mg/dL) if the urine shows gram-negative bacilli on microscopic examination. If gram-positive cocci are seen in the urine, intravenous ampicillin (1 g every 4 hours) should be given in addition to the aminoglycoside, to cover the possibility of enterococcal infection while the results of urine and blood cultures and antimicrobial susceptibility tests are pending. If no complications ensue and the patient becomes afebrile, the remaining days of a 10- to 14-day course can be completed with oral therapy. However, persistent fever, persistent bacteriuria in 48 to 72 hours, or continual signs of toxicity beyond 3 days of therapy suggest the need for an evaluation to exclude obstruction, metastatic focus, or the formation of a perinephric abscess. The urinary tract is a common source of sepsis and bacteremic shock in patients with underlying uropathies. As with other patients in septic shock, intravenous fluids must be given to maintain adequate arterial perfusion, which usually results in a urinary output in excess of 50 mL/hour. Failure to respond to seemingly appropriate therapy suggests the possibility of undrained pus. Examination by ultrasonography or CT

TABLE 10-4 Recommendations for Therapy for UTIs

Infection	Group	Medication	Duration
Uncomplicated cystitis	Young women	Trimethoprim-sulfamethoxazole, trimethoprim, fluoroquinolone[a]	3 d
Cystitis	Women with risk factors including recent UTI, symptoms >7 d, diaphragm use, age older than 65 yrs, diabetic patients with abnormal GU structures	Trimethoprim-sulfamethoxazole, trimethoprim, fluoroquinolone, nitrofurantoin, cephalosporins	7 d
	Pregnant women	Amoxicillin, cephalosporins[b], nitrofurantoin, sulfonamides, trimethoprim-sulfamethoxazole[c]	7 d
Acute uncomplicated pyelonephritis	Women (outpatient)	Fluoroquinolone, trimethoprim-sulfamethoxazole, oral cephalosporin[d]	10–14 d
	Women (inpatient)	Fluoroquinolone[e], ceftriaxone, ampicillin plus gentamicin[f], trimethoprim-sulfamethoxazole	14 d
Complicated infection	Outpatient	Fluoroquinolone	10–14 d
	Inpatient	Fluoroquinolone[e], cephalosporins[g], ampicillin plus gentamicin[f]	14 d

GU, genitourinary; UTI, urinary tract infection.

[a]Oral fluoroquinolones are listed in Table 10-2; they offer no significant advantage over trimethoprim-sulfamethoxazole in women with uncomplicated cystitis.

[b]Oral cephalosporins: cephradine, cephalexin.

[c]Trimethoprim-sulfamethoxazole has been used in pregnancy, but it has not been approved by the U.S. Food and Drug Administration for pregnant patients.

[d]Oral cephalosporins with an extended spectrum: cefpodoxime, loracarbef.

[e]Fluoroquinolones available for intravenous administration are listed in Table 10-3.

[f]Increasing ampicillin resistance among many enteric bacteria, including *Escherichia coli*, limits ampicillin as a single agent for complicated UTIs. If enterococcus is not likely, then a fluoroquinolone or a parenteral third- or fourth-generation cephalosporin is recommended.

[g]Some examples of parenteral cephalosporins are listed in Table 10-3.

Adapted from Falagas ME. Practice guidelines: urinary tract infections. *Infect Dis Clin Pract.* 1995;4:241–257; Kunin CM. *Detection, Prevention, and Management of Urinary Tract Infections.* 5th ed. Lea & Febiger; 1997; Stamm WE. Urinary tract infections. In: Root RK, ed. *Clinical Infectious Diseases: A Practical Approach.* 1st ed. Oxford University Press; 1999.

may disclose an obstructed ureter or perinephric abscess, both of which require surgical drainage.

G. **Management of Recurrent Renal Infections (Relapses).** Chronic bacterial pyelonephritis is one of the most refractory problems in clinical medicine; relapse rates are as high as 90%. The entity is a heterogeneous one with multiple underlying factors.

1. **Risk Factors.** To improve the success rate, it is of utmost importance that any correctable lesion be repaired, that obstructions to urine flow be relieved,

and that foreign bodies (e.g., indwelling urinary catheters or renal staghorn calculi) be removed if possible. If the risk factors cannot be corrected, long-term eradication of bacteriuria is almost impossible. Attempting eradication in such instances leads only to the emergence of more resistant strains of bacteria or fungi; consequently, the physician must be resigned to treating symptomatic episodes of infection and suppressing bacteriuria in selected patients.

2. **Acute Symptomatic Infection.** The treatment of acute symptoms and signs of UTI in a patient with chronic renal bacteriuria is the same as for patients with acute bacterial pyelonephritis. Urine cultures to detect a possible change in antimicrobial susceptibility of the infecting microorganism are important. Toxic patients should also have blood cultures.

3. **Prolonged Treatment.** Some patients with relapsing bacteriuria after 2 weeks of therapy respond to 6 weeks of antimicrobial therapy. This is especially true of patients with no underlying structural abnormalities. Men may require 6 to 12 weeks of antibiotic therapy for febrile UTIs because more than 90% have associated asymptomatic prostatitis. Patients who fail the longer therapy, who have repeated episodes of symptomatic infection, or who have progressive renal disease despite corrective measures are candidates for suppressive chemotherapy.

4. **Suppressive Therapy.** To reduce the colony counts in their urine, patients selected for suppressive therapy should have 2 to 3 days of specific high-dose antimicrobial therapy, to which their infecting bacteria are susceptible. The preferred agent for long-term suppression is methenamine mandelate, 1 g four times daily in adults. To be most effective, the pH of the urine should be maintained below 5.5; this can be accomplished with ascorbic acid, 500 mg two to four times daily. Alternatively, the dosage of methenamine mandelate alone can be increased to 8 g or even 12 g/d. The dosage should be adjusted to the minimum amount required to keep the urine free of bacteria. To avoid metabolic acidosis, the dosage of methenamine mandelate must be reduced in patients with renal insufficiency, in whom 2 g/d may suffice. In these patients, methenamine mandelate should not be used at all unless the creatinine clearance exceeds 10 mL/min. Alternative therapy is trimethoprim-sulfamethoxazole (160 mg/800 mg tablets twice daily) or nitrofurantoin (50 to 100 mg once or twice daily).

5. **Prognosis.** Although a common cause of appreciable morbidity, UTIs do not play a major role in the pathogenesis of end-stage renal disease. Patients who come to renal dialysis or transplantation because of chronic bacterial pyelonephritis almost always have an underlying structural defect. Most often, the lesion is chronic atrophic pyelonephritis associated with vesicoureteral reflux that started in infancy. The role of surgical correction of vesicoureteral reflux is not clear despite years of debate; what is certain, however, is the importance of meticulous control of infection in children to prevent progressive renal scarring and renal failure by early adulthood.

H. Treatment of Prostatitis

1. **Acute bacterial prostatitis** is commonly accompanied by acute cystitis, which enables the recovery of its causative pathogen by culture of voided urine. Massage of an acutely inflamed prostate gland often results in bacteremia; therefore, this procedure should be avoided unless the patient is already receiving effective antibiotic therapy. Antimicrobial selection depends on the susceptibility pattern of the causative bacteria and the ability of the drug to achieve concentrations in the prostate that exceed the minimum inhibitory concentrations of the bacteria. The drug of choice most commonly is either the combination of trimethoprim-sulfamethoxazole (cotrimoxazole) or a fluoroquinolone; treatment, however, must be

based ultimately on an accurate microbiologic diagnosis. β-Lactam antibiotics should be avoided because of the low concentrations achieved in prostatic tissue and lower cure rates. Treatment should be given for 30 days to prevent chronic bacterial prostatitis. After acute symptoms subside, a suitable oral antibiotic can be given in full dose for at least 30 days. Urethral catheterization should be avoided. If acute urinary retention develops, drainage should be by suprapubic needle aspiration or, if prolonged bladder drainage is required, by a suprapubic cystostomy tube, placed while the patient is under local anesthesia.

2. **Chronic Bacterial Prostatitis.** The hallmark of chronic bacterial prostatitis is relapsing UTI. It is most refractory to treatment. Although erythromycin with alkalinization of the urine has been effective against susceptible gram-positive pathogens, most instances of chronic bacterial prostatitis are caused by gram-negative enteric bacilli. Cotrimoxazole or a fluoroquinolone is the drug of choice. Approximately 75% of patients improve, and 33% are cured with 12 weeks of cotrimoxazole therapy (160 mg/800 mg twice daily). For patients who cannot tolerate cotrimoxazole or a fluoroquinolone, nitrofurantoin, 50 or 100 mg once or twice daily, can be used for long-term (6 to 12 months) suppressive therapy.

3. The therapy for **nonbacterial chronic prostatitis** is difficult because an exact etiology has not been identified. Owing to a concern for *C. trachomatis*, *U. urealyticum*, and other fastidious and difficult-to-culture organisms, many experts recommend a 6-week trial of a tetracycline or erythromycin. Symptomatic therapy with nonsteroidal anti-inflammatory drugs and α-receptor blockers has also been used.

I. **Recommendations for the Care of Urinary Catheters.** Urinary catheters are valuable devices for enabling drainage of the bladder and while they may be associated with asymptomatic bacteriuria, their use is also associated with an appreciable risk of infection in the urinary tract, specifically pyelonephritis. In addition, bacteremia and sepsis are recognized complications.

On August 1, 2007, the Centers for Medicare and Medicaid Services issued a decision to implement a modification to the Inpatient Prospective Payment System whereby additional payment for the complication or comorbidity of a catheter-related UTI will not be reimbursed. Therefore, it is imperative that guidelines for the prevention and expeditious treatment of catheter-related UTIs be enforced. In addition, documentation of an existing UTI at the time of admission is recommended.

For a single (in-and-out) catheterization, the risk is small (12%), although this prevalence is much higher in diabetic and elderly women. Intermittent catheterization is a safe alternative for patients in four situations: (a) children with neurogenic bladders (such as spina bifida), (b) uncontrolled reflex detrusor contraction resulting in incontinence in women, (c) chronic urinary retention due to ineffective or absent detrusor contraction, and (d) bladder outlet obstruction in men who are not surgical candidates.

In the absence of outlet obstruction, condom catheters are an alternative method of urinary drainage that has a lower incidence of bacteriuria.

Explicit recommendations for the prevention of catheter-associated UTIs, formulated by the Centers for Disease Control and Prevention, are as follows:

1. **Indwelling Urinary Catheters Should Be Used Only When Absolutely Necessary.** They should never be used solely for nurse or physician convenience and be removed as soon as possible. Duration of catheter use is the most important risk factor for the development of bacteriuria.

2. **Catheters Should Be Inserted Only by Adequately Trained Personnel.** If practical, a team of individuals should be given responsibility for catheter insertion and maintenance.

3. **Urinary Catheters Should Be Aseptically Inserted Using Proper Sterile Technique and the Following Sterile Equipment:** gloves, a fenestrated drape, sterile sponges and an iodophor solution for periurethral cleansing, a lubricant jelly, and an appropriately sized urinary catheter. After insertion, catheters should be properly secured to prevent movement and urethral traction.
4. Once- or twice-daily **perineal care for catheterized patients** should include cleansing of the meatal-catheter junction with an antiseptic soap; subsequently, an antimicrobial ointment may be applied.
5. **A Sterile Closed Drainage System Should Always Be Used.** The urinary catheter and the proximal portion of the drainage tube should not be disconnected (thereby opening the closed system) unless it is required for irrigation of an obstructed catheter. Sterile technique must be observed whenever the collecting system is opened and catheter irrigation is done. A large-volume sterile syringe and sterile irrigant fluid should be used and then discarded. If frequent irrigations are necessary to ensure catheter patency, a triple-lumen catheter that permits continuous irrigation within a closed system is preferable.
6. **Small volumes of urine for culture can** be aspirated from the distal end of the catheter with a sterile syringe and 21-gauge needle. The catheter must first be prepared with tincture of iodine or alcohol. Urine for chemical analyses can be obtained from the drainage bag in a sterile manner.
7. **Nonobstructed Gravity Flow Must Be Maintained at All Times.** This requires emptying the collecting bag regularly, replacing poorly functioning or obstructed catheters, and ensuring that collection bags always remain below the level of the bladder.
8. **All closed collecting systems contaminated by inappropriate technique, accidental disconnection, leaks, or other means should be immediately replaced.**
9. **Routine catheter change is not necessary** for patients with urinary catheterization of fewer than 2 weeks' duration, except when obstruction, contamination, or other malfunction occurs. In patients with chronic indwelling catheters, replacement is necessary when concretions can be palpated in the catheter or when malfunction or obstruction occurs.
10. **Catheterized patients should be separated from each other whenever possible** and should not share the same room or adjacent beds if other arrangements are available. Separation of patients with bacteriuria and those without it is particularly important.

These guidelines should be adhered to meticulously, and the use of indwelling urinary catheters should be kept to a responsible minimum.

J. **Catheter-Associated Infections.** Catheter-associated bacteriuria should only be treated in the symptomatic patient. When the decision to treat a patient with a catheter-associated infection is made, removal of the catheter is an important aspect of therapy. If an infected catheter remains in place, relapsing infection is very common. The interaction between the organisms and catheter (foreign body) causes the organism to form a biofilm or area in which antibiotics are unable to completely eradicate these organisms. Recommendations for empiric therapy are similar to recommendations for complicated UTIs (see Table 10-4). The choice of empiric therapy is based on an initial Gram stain of the urine, local susceptibility patterns, host factors, and the patient's recent antibiotic use. The final choice of an antibiotic and duration of therapy should be based on the identification and susceptibility of the etiologic agent and the host's response to therapy. Patients who respond rapidly to therapy may be treated for 7 days, although making firm conclusions about duration of therapy is very difficult.

Patients with candiduria may fall into several different clinical categories. Otherwise healthy patients with asymptomatic candiduria often require only a urinary catheter change and may not require antifungal therapy. On the other end of the spectrum is the immunocompromised host, in whom candiduria may represent disseminated infection. The patient with disseminated candidiasis requires systemic therapy with either fluconazole or amphotericin B or a liposomal preparation of amphotericin. General recommendations for treating patients with candiduria and without evidence of disseminated infection include the removal of the urinary catheter and discontinuation of antibiotics. Antifungal options include fluconazole (200 mg the first day, then 100 mg for 4 days), continuous bladder irrigation with amphotericin B (50 mg/1,000 mL of sterile water through a three-way catheter for 5 days), or low-dose intravenous therapy with amphotericin (0.3 mg/kg in a single dose). Occasionally, longer systemic therapy with oral 5-fluorocytosine, intravenous amphotericin B, or both is required.

SUGGESTED READINGS

Ang BSP, Telenti A, King B, Steckelberg JM, Wilson WR. Candidemia from a urinary source: microbiological aspects and clinical significance. *Clin Infect Dis.* 1993;17(4):662–666.

Barber AE, Norton JP, Spivak AM, Mulvey MA. Urinary tract infections: current and emerging management strategies. *Clin Infect Dis.* 2013;57(5):719–724.

Domingue GJ, Hellstrom WJG. Prostatitis. *Clin Microbiol Rev.* 1998;11:604–613.

Edelstein H, McCabe RE. Perinephric abscess: modern diagnosis and treatment in 47 cases. *Medicine (Baltimore).* 1988;67(2):118–131.

Fihn SD. Acute uncomplicated urinary tract infection in women. *N Engl J Med.* 2003;349:259–266.

Fisher JF, Newman CL, Sobel JD. Yeast in the urine: solutions for a budding problem. *Clin Infect Dis.* 1995;20:183–189.

Fowler JE Jr, Pulaski ET. Excretory urography, cystography, and cystoscopy in the evaluation of women with urinary-tract infection. *N Engl J Med.* 1981;304:462–465.

Gupta K, Hooton TM, Naber KG, et al; Infectious Diseases Society of America; European Society for Microbiology and Infectious Diseases. International clinical practice guidelines for the treatment of acute uncomplicated cystits and pyelonephritis in women: A 2010 update by the Infections Diseases Society of America and the European Society for Microbiology and Infectious Diseases. *Clin Inf Dis.* 2011;52(5):e103–e120.

Gupta K, Hooton TM, Roberts PL, Stamm WE. Patient-initiated treatment of uncomplicated recurrent urinary tract infections in young women. *Ann Intern Med.* 2001;135(1):9–16.

Harding GK, Zhanel GG, Nicolle LE, Cheang M; Manitoba Diabetes Urinary Tract Infection Study Group. Antimicrobial treatment in diabetic women with asymptomatic bacteriuria. *N Engl J Med.* 2002;347(20):1576–1583.

Hooton TM, Fihn SD, Johnson C, Roberts PL, Stamm WE. Association between bacterial vaginosis and acute cystitis in women using diaphragms. *Arch Intern Med.* 1989;149(9):1932–1936.

Hooton TM, Scholes D, Hughes JP, et al. A prospective study of risk factors for symptomatic urinary tract infection in young women. *N Engl J Med.* 1996;335(7):468–474.

Hooton TM, Winter C, Tiu F, Stamm WE. Randomized comparative trial and cost analysis of 3-day antimicrobial regimens for treatment of acute cystitis in women. *JAMA.* 1995;273(1):41–45.

Kincaid-Smith P, Becker G. Reflux nephropathy and chronic atrophic pyelonephritis: a review. *J Infect Dis.* 1978;138:774–780.

Krieger JN. Complications and treatment of urinary tract infections during pregnancy. *Urol Clin North Am.* 1986;13:685–693.

Kunin CM. *Detection, Prevention, and Management of Urinary Tract Infections.* 5th ed. Lea & Febiger; 1997.

Kunin CM, Chin QF, Chambers S. Indwelling urinary catheters in the elderly: relation of "catheter life" to formation of encrustations in patients with and without blocked catheters. *Am J Med.* 1987;82:405–411.

Lachs MS, Nachamkin I, Edelstein PH, Goldman J, Feinstein AR, Schwartz JS. Spectrum bias in the evaluation of diagnostic tests: lessons from the rapid dipstick test for urinary tract infection. *Ann Intern Med.* 1992;117(2):135–140.

Langner JL, Chiang KF, Stafford RS. Current prescribing practices and guideline concordance for the treatment of uncomplicated urinary tract infections in women. *Am J Obstet Gynecol.* 2021;225(3):272.e1–272.e11.

Lipsky BA, Baker CA. Fluoroquinolone toxicity profiles: a review focusing on new agents. *Clin Infect Dis.* 1999;28:352–364.

Miller JM, Binnicker MJ, Campbell S, et al. Guide to utilization of the microbiology laboratory for diagnosis of infectious diseases: 2024 Update by the Infectious Diseases Society of America (IDSA) and the American Society for Microbiology (ASM). *Clin Infect Dis.* 2024:1–123.

Neuhauser MM, Weinstein RA, Rydman R, Danziger LH, Karam G, Quinn JP. Antibiotic resistance among gram-negative bacilli in US intensive care units: implications for fluoroquinolone use. *JAMA.* 2003;289:885–888.

Nickel JC. The Pre and Post Massage Test (PPMT): a simple screen for prostatitis. *Tech Urol.* 1997;3:38–43.

Nicolle LE, Bjornson J, Harding GK, MacDonell JA. Bacteriuria in elderly institutionalized men. *N Engl J Med.* 1983;309(23):1420–1425.

Nicolle LE, Bradley S, Colgan R, Rice JC, Schaeffer A, Hooton TM; Infectious Diseases Society of America; American Society of Nephrology; American Geriatric Society. Infectious Diseases Society of America guidelines for the diagnosis and treatment of asymptomatic bacteriuria in adults. *Clin Infect Dis.* 2005;40:643–654.

Nicolle LE, Gupta K, Bradley SF, et al. Clinical practice guideline for the management of asymptomatic bacteriuria: 2019 update by the Infection Diseases Society of America. *Clin Infect Dis.* 2019;68(10):e83–e110.

Nicolle LE, Harding GK, Preiksaitis J, Ronald AR. The association of urinary tract infection with sexual intercourse. *J Infect Dis.* 1982;146(5):579–583.

Nicolle LE. Asymptomatic bacteriuria in the elderly. *Infect Dis Clin North Am.* 1997;11:647–662.

Silverman DE, Stamey TA. Management of infection stones: the Stanford experience. *Medicine (Baltimore).* 1983;62:44–51.

Stamm WE. Guidelines for prevention of catheter-associated urinary tract infections. *Ann Intern Med.* 1975;82:386–390.

Stamm WE, Counts GW, Wagner KF, et al. Antimicrobial prophylaxis of recurrent urinary tract infections: a double-blind, placebo-controlled trial. *Ann Intern Med.* 1980;92(6):770–775.

Stapleton A, Latham R, Johnson C, Stamm WE. Postcoital antimicrobial prophylaxis for recurrent urinary tract infection: a randomized, double-blind, placebo-controlled trial. *JAMA.* 1990;264(6):703–706.

Stapleton A, Stamm WE. Prevention of urinary tract infection. *Infect Dis Clin North Am.* 1997;11:719–733.

Strom BL, Collins M, West SL, Kreisberg J, Weller S. Sexual activity, contraceptive use and other risk factors for symptomatic and asymptomatic bacteriuria: a case-control study. *Ann Intern Med.* 1987;107(6):816–823.

Talan DA, Klimberg IW, Nicolle LE, Song J, Kowalsky SF, Church DA. Once daily, extended release ciprofloxacin for complicated urinary tract infections and acute uncomplicated pyelonephritis. *J Urol.* 2004;171(2):734–739.

Tenke P, Kovacs B, Bjerklund Johansen TE, Matsumoto T, Tambyah PA, Naber KG. European and Asian guidelines on management and prevention of catheter-associated urinary tract infections. *Int J Antimicrob Agents.* 2008;31(Suppl 1):68–78.

Ulleryd P. Febrile urinary tract infection in men. *Int J Antimicrob Agents.* 2003;22:S89–S93.

Velasco M, Horcajada JP, Mensa J, et al. Decreased invasive capacity of quinolone-resistant Escherichia coli in patients with urinary tract infections. *Clin Infect Dis.* 2001;33(10):1682–1686.

Velasco M, Martinez JA, Moreno-Martinez A, et al. Blood cultures for women with uncomplicated acute pyelonephritis: are they necessary? *Clin Infect Dis.* 2003;37(8):1127–1130.

Wald HL, Kramer AM. Nonpayment for harms resulting from medical care: catheter-associated urinary tract infections. *J Am Med Assoc.* 2007;298(23):2782–2784.

Warren JW. Catheter-associated urinary tract infections. *Infect Dis Clin North Am.* 1997;11(3):609–622.

Warren JW, Abrutyn E, Hebel JR, Johnson JR, Schaeffer AJ, Stamm WE. Guidelines for antimicrobial treatment of uncomplicated acute bacterial cystitis and acute pyelonephritis in women. *Clin Infect Dis.* 1999;29(4):745–758.

Zhanel GG, Hisanaga TL, Laing NM, et al. Antibiotic resistance in Escherichia coli outpatient urinary isolates: final results from the North American Urinary Tract Infection Collaborative Alliance (NAUTICA). *Int J Antimicrob Agents.* 2006;27(6):468–475.

The Patient With Glomerular Disease or Vasculitis

Russell S. Whelan, Joshua Thurman

I. Overview

Glomerular diseases are defined by their clinical presentations and the histologic findings seen on biopsy. Glomerular diseases can also be categorized as primary processes in which the disease is confined to the kidney, or as secondary processes in which a systemic disease impacts the kidney. Many glomerular diseases are autoimmune in nature, in which case injury to the kidney is caused by the deposition of immune complexes, complement activation, or production of cytokines. The small vessels of the kidney and the glomerular capillaries are also frequently the target of small vessel vasculitides. Clinically, the presence of a glomerular disease should be considered when proteinuria or hematuria is present.

When hematuria and/or proteinuria has been identified and glomerular disease is determined to be the most likely etiology, further clinical information and serologic testing can assist in the classification of the underlying disease. Patients frequently present with clinical and laboratory evidence of either the "nephritic syndrome" or the "nephrotic syndrome," and recognition of these syndromes can guide further serologic testing. However, the definitive diagnosis of the underlying disease often requires a kidney biopsy. The primary glomerular diseases are listed in Table 11-1, with the prominent histologic findings on biopsy that define the disorder.

II. Clinical Patterns of Glomerular Disease

A. The Nephritic Syndrome. Patients with nephritic syndrome typically present with microscopic or gross hematuria, dysmorphic red blood cells and/or red blood cell casts, and proteinuria. The proteinuria can range from 200 mg/d to heavy proteinuria (greater than 10 g/d). Clinically, it is accompanied by hypertension and edema. Reduced kidney function is common and typically progressive. The term *rapidly progressive glomerulonephritis* (RPGN) refers to diseases with a nephritic syndrome that leads to a rapid deterioration in kidney function, defined as a doubling of serum creatinine or a 50% decrease in glomerular filtration rate (GFR) over 3 months or less (Table 11-2).

B. The Nephrotic Syndrome. Patients with nephrotic syndrome present with proteinuria (often defined as greater than 3.5 g of proteinuria per day in adults and greater than 40 mg/kg in pediatric patients), hypoalbuminemia (serum albumin less than 3.0 mg/dL), and edema. Dysmorphic red blood cells and casts are typically absent, but there are exceptions. Focal segmental glomerulosclerosis (FSGS), for example, usually presents with the nephrotic syndrome, but patients can also have low-grade hematuria. Complications of the nephrotic syndrome include hyperlipidemia, thrombosis, and infection. The diseases that cause the nephrotic syndrome can lead to chronic, progressive kidney failure, but typically are more slowly progressive than diseases presenting as the nephritic syndrome.

III. Clinical Assessment of Glomerular Disease

A. The Nephritic Syndrome. In cases in which the nephritic syndrome is the predominant clinical presentation, a search for systemic diseases is warranted (Table 11-3). The history and physical examination should particularly focus

TABLE 11-1 Primary Glomerular Diseases, Defined by Histology

Nephritic	Histologic Findings	Nephrotic	Histologic Findings
Kidney-limited vasculitis/microscopic polyangiitis	Necrotizing capillary lesions, crescents; negative IF, EM	Minimal change disease	Normal light microscopy, effaced foot processes on EM
Anti-GBM	Linear IgG staining along glomerular basement membrane	Membranous nephropathy	Thickened GBM on light microscopy, granular IgG and C3 on IF; subepithelial "spikes" on EM
IgA nephropathy	IgA in mesangium on IF	Focal segmental glomerulosclerosis	Sclerosis in portions of glomeruli
Immune-complex membranoproliferative glomerulonephritis	Thickened mesangial matrix, splitting ("double contour") of the glomerular basement membrane, Granular deposits of IgG and C3 by IF	Immunotactoid and fibrillary glomerulonephritis	Microtubular and fibrillary deposits on EM, respectively. Positive staining for monoclonal IgG (usually λ). Staining for DNAJB9 is a specific finding in fibrillary glomerulonephritis
C3 glomerulopathy	Glomerular C3 deposits two orders of magnitude brighter than immunoglobulin deposits on IF	Amyloidosis	Fibrillary deposits on EM. Positive staining for monoclonal IgG (κ or λ). Positive Congo red staining

EM, electron microscopy; GBM, glomerular basement membrane; IF, immunofluorescence; Ig, immunoglobulin; DNAJB9, DnaJ homolog subfamily B member 9.

TABLE 11-2	Histologic Classification of Crescentic (or Rapidly Progressive) Glomerulonephritis		
Linear Immunofluorescence	**Granular Immunofluorescence**	**Absent (Pauci-immune) Immunofluorescence**
Goodpasture disease Anti-GBM disease	Lupus nephritis IgA nephropathy/IgA vasculitis Cryoglobulinemia	ANCA-associated vasculitis (GPA, eosinophilic GPA, microscopic polyangiitis)

ANCA, antineutrophil cytoplasmic antibody; GBM, glomerular basement membrane; GPA, granulomatosis with polyangiitis; Ig, immunoglobulin.

on the assessment of rashes, lung disease, neurologic abnormalities, evidence of viral or bacterial infections, and musculoskeletal and hematologic abnormalities. Laboratory assessment should be tailored to the clinical findings in the history and physical examination. A complete blood count (CBC), electrolyte panel, 24-hour urine collection for protein and creatinine clearance or a spot urine to protein measurement, and liver function tests should be obtained. Serum complement (C3 and C4) levels are helpful in the diagnosis (Table 11-4). Further laboratory assessment may be performed based on these findings, and may include an antistreptolysin titer, antinuclear antibody (ANA), anti–double-stranded DNA (anti-dsDNA), antineutrophil cytoplasmic antibody (ANCA), cryoglobulins or rheumatoid factors, anti-GBM antibody, serum protein electrophoresis (SPEP) and immunofixation, and urine protein electrophoresis (UPEP) (see Table 11-3). These early assessments may provide a presumptive diagnosis and should lead the clinician to an appropriate therapeutic intervention while awaiting kidney biopsy results, but are usually not an adequate substitute for direct evaluation of kidney tissue by biopsy. Proper management of the glomerular diseases requires a tissue diagnosis to confirm the clinical findings and provide information regarding the acuity and chronicity of the disease process.

B. The Nephrotic Syndrome. Secondary causes of nephrotic syndrome should be considered in patients with significant proteinuria (Table 11-5). History and physical examination should evaluate for evidence of viral and bacterial infections, malignancies (particularly lung, breast, and lymphomas), and chronic diseases (such as diabetes). Medications should be reviewed for their potential to cause glomerular proteinuria. Laboratory assessment initially includes CBC, electrolyte panel, 24-hour urine collection for protein and creatinine clearance, liver function tests, and a cholesterol panel. Serologic assessment may include antiphospholipid A2 receptor (PLA2R) antibodies, hepatitis and human immunodeficiency virus (HIV) serologies, ANA, rapid plasma reagin, SPEP, and UPEP (see Table 11-5). It is also important to note that all glomerular diseases can eventually result in glomerulosclerosis, which is probably irreversible.

C. Clinicopathologic Correlation. Kidney biopsy is often necessary to confirm the underlying etiology of disease and to determine the extent of irreversible kidney damage. Contraindications for biopsy include small kidneys (which may have had an irreversible loss of function, pyelonephritis or a perinephric abscess), a solitary kidney or horseshoe kidney, uncontrolled hypertension (>140 mmHg), a bleeding disorder (including aspirin or anticoagulants), hydronephrosis, a renal mass, and a large cyst or multiple cysts. Uremia may

TABLE 11-3 Systemic Diseases That Cause Glomerular Injury and a Nephritic Clinical Presentation

Disease	Specific Examples	Laboratory Findings
Infections	Hepatitis C (Hepatitis B less commonly)	Low C3, hepatitis C Ab, hepatitis C viral PCR, cryoglobulins, or rheumatoid factors
	Poststreptococcal GN	Low C3, antistreptolysin Ab
	Bacterial endocarditis	Low C3, positive blood cultures
	Methicillin-resistant *Staphylococcus aureus* infection	Low C3, positive blood cultures
Autoimmune diseases	Lupus nephritis	Low C3, ANA, anti-dsDNA Ab
	Goodpasture syndrome	Anti-GBM Ab
Vasculitides	Granulomatosis with polyangiitis	c-ANCA
	Microscopic polyangiitis	p-ANCA
	Eosinophilic granulomatosis with polyangiitis	p-ANCA
	IgA vasculitis	IgA in skin biopsy
	Polyarteritis nodosa	ANCA in 20% (c- or p-ANCA)
	Mixed cryoglobulinemia	Rheumatoid factor, low C4
Thrombotic microangiopathy	Scleroderma renal crisis	Anti–Scl-70
	Thrombotic thrombocytopenic purpura	Low platelets, hemolysis, low ADAMTS13 activity
	Hemolytic uremic syndrome	Low platelets, hemolysis. *Shigatoxin HUS:* evidence of Shiga producing *E. Coli* (toxin or PCR studies), Atypical: low C3 or other evidence of complement activation, biopsy results
	Malignant hypertension	

Ab, antibody; ANA, antinuclear antibody; ANCA, antineutrophil cytoplasmic antibody; anti-dsDNA, anti–double-stranded DNA; GN, glomerulonephritis; Ig, immunoglobulin; PCR, polymerase chain reaction.

also increase a patient's bleeding diathesis. Finally, the patient must be able to cooperate with the procedure, and the body habitus can affect the ability to obtain a suitable sample.

The pathologic diagnosis of glomerular diseases incorporates the histologic pattern defined by light microscopy, immunofluorescence staining for immunoglobulins (Igs; IgG, IgM, and IgA; Fig. 11-1) and complement proteins (C3 and sometimes C1q), and examination of the glomerular ultrastructure by electron microscopy. The primary glomerular diseases are listed in Table 11-1, with the prominent histologic findings on biopsy that define the disorder. Several patterns of glomerular injury are also depicted in Figure 11-2. The clinician must also consider if there is a systemic process that is causing the kidney

TABLE 11-4 Clinical Approach to Glomerulonephritis Based Upon Serum Complement

Low Serum Complement Level		Normal Serum Complement Level	
Systemic diseases	Primary kidney diseases	Systemic diseases	Primary kidney diseases
SLE Subacute bacterial endocarditis "Shunt" nephritis Cryoglobulinemia Atypical hemolytic uremic syndrome	Poststreptococcal glomerulonephritis Membranoproliferative glomerulonephritis C3 glomerulopathy	Polyarteritis nodosa Hypersensitivity vasculitis Granulomatosis with polyangiitis IgA vasculitis Goodpasture syndrome Visceral abscess	IgA nephropathy Idiopathic rapidly progressive glomerulonephritis (antiglomerular basement membrane disease, pauci-immune glomerulonephritis, immune complex disease)

Ig, immunoglobulin; SLE, systemic lupus erythematosus.

Adapted from Madaio MP, Harrington JT. Current concepts. The diagnosis of acute glomerulonephritis. *N Engl J Med.* 1983;309:1299, with permission.

TABLE 11-5 Systemic Diseases That Cause Glomerular Injury and a Nephrotic Clinical Presentation

Disease State	Common Etiologies	Laboratory Findings
Infections	Hepatitis B (hepatitis C less common) HIV Syphilis	Hepatitis B sAg, hepatitis B eAg HIV Ab RPR
Chronic diseases	Diabetes Amyloidosis Sickle cell disease Obesity	Elevated HgbA$_{1c}$, blood glucose UPEP/IEP (when associated with light chains) Hemoglobin electrophoresis
Malignancies	Multiple myeloma Adenocarcinoma (lung, breast, colon most common) Lymphoma	SPEP, UPEP Abnormal cancer screening studies (usually clinically evident tumor burden)
Rheumatologic	Systemic lupus erythematosus Rheumatoid arthritis Mixed connective tissue disease	ANA, anti-dsDNA Ab Rheumatoid factor Anti-RNP (ribonuclear protein) Ab
Medications	NSAIDs Lithium Penicillamine Ampicillin	—

Ab, antibody; ANA, antinuclear antibody; anti-dsDNA Ab, anti–double-stranded DNA antibody; HIV, human immunodeficiency virus; IEP, immunoelectrophoresis; NSAID, nonsteroidal anti-inflammatory drug; RPR, rapid plasma reagin; SPEP, serum protein electrophoresis; UPEP, urine protein electrophoresis.

injury. Primary glomerular diseases often cannot be distinguished histologically from the injury pattern seen in systemic diseases, so this distinction is made clinically.

The nephritic syndrome is usually caused by glomerular inflammation and manifests with an "active" urine sediment (e.g., cells and/or cellular casts; Fig. 11-3). Immune complexes that deposit in the mesangium or in the subendothelial space (immune-complex membranoproliferative glomerulonephritis [IC-MPGN], IgA nephropathy, and many forms of lupus nephritis) generate inflammatory mediators that have access to the circulation and can cause an influx of inflammatory cells. Glomerular endothelial injury is also caused by autoantibodies to the glomerular basement membrane (anti-GBM), and with necrotizing injury of the glomerular capillaries as occurs in the ANCA-associated vasculitis (AAV). C3 glomerulopathy (C3G) is a disease in which the complement system is activated within the glomerulus in the relative absence of immunoglobulin or immune complexes. C3G typically presents as a nephritic syndrome.

Diseases that present with the nephrotic syndrome disrupt the size and charge-selective barriers that ordinarily prevent the ultrafiltration of

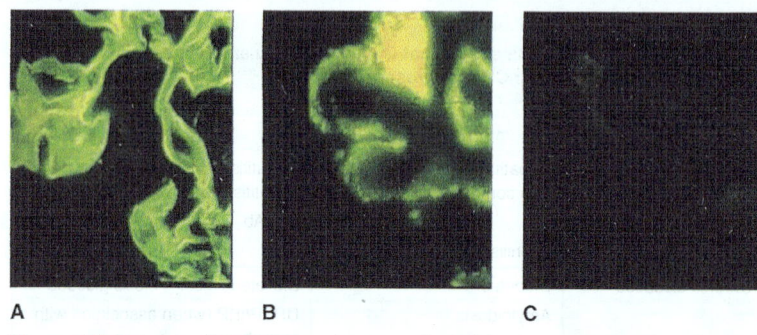

A   **B**   **C**

Figure 11-1. Immunofluorescence microscopy for IgG in glomerulonephritis. Immunofluorescence microscopy patterns of glomerular staining for immunoglobulin G (IgG) that are indicative of antiglomerular basement membrane (GBM) (**A**), immune complex (**B**), and pauci-immune (**C**) glomerulonephritis. Note the linear staining of anti-GBM disease compared with the granular staining of immune complex disease and the scanty background staining of pauci-immune disease (fluorescein isothiocyanate anti-IgG). (Reproduced with permission from Nachman P, Lerma E, Michelle R. *Handbook of Glomerulonephritis*. Lippincott Wolters Kluwer; 2023.)

macromolecules across the glomerular capillary wall. In general, these diseases affect podocytes without causing overt glomerular inflammation.

IV. Therapy for Glomerular Disease

The management of systemic diseases that cause secondary glomerular injury is rapidly changing (e.g., the success of new antiviral therapies for HIV and hepatitis B and C). Therefore, the reader is encouraged to refer to recent disease-specific reviews of the literature for current management strategies for these systemic diseases. An overview of the general approach to treatment of glomerular disease is shown in Figure 11-4.

A. General Management of Proteinuric Glomerular Disease. Untreated nephrotic syndrome is associated with significant morbidity due to chronic kidney disease (CKD) progression, accelerated atherosclerosis and coronary heart disease, dyslipidemia, thromboembolic events, and infections. Treatment often requires both general management and disease-specific treatment to achieve remission and lessen morbidity. The general treatment strategies that should be considered in the patient with nephrotic syndrome include management of proteinuria, hypertension, edema, hyperlipidemia, and hypercoagulability.

1. **Proteinuria.** In nephrotic syndrome, treatment to reduce the degree of proteinuria to the nonnephrotic range will often result in an elevation or normalization of serum proteins (such as albumin) and slow CKD progression. A reduction in proteinuria is associated with a reduction in the symptoms of nephrotic syndrome, thus improving patients' quality of life. The cornerstone of management of proteinuria is the inhibition of the renin–angiotensin system using either angiotensin-converting enzyme (ACE) inhibitors or angiotensin receptor blockers (ARBs). ACE inhibitors and ARBs are particularly effective at reducing proteinuria when compared with other antihypertensive agents. Treatment with an ACE inhibitor or an ARB has been shown to reduce proteinuria by up to 30% to 50% in a dose-dependent manner. The reduction in proteinuria is more pronounced if the patient complies with dietary salt restriction. Likewise, studies have demonstrated that the antiproteinuric efficacy of ACE inhibitors and ARBs can be reversed in the setting of a high-salt diet.

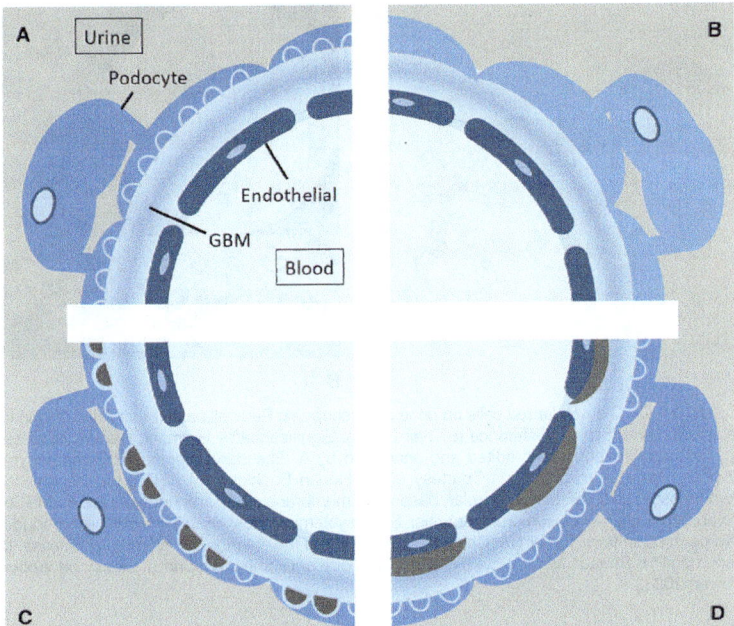

Figure 11-2. Patterns of injury in the glomerular capillary. **A:** Represents the glomerular capillary. Endothelial cells line the capillary wall and face the blood. Underneath the endothelial cells, the glomerular basement membrane (GBM) constitutes the central portion of the capillary wall. Podocytes form the outer layer of the capillary wall and face the urine. The podocytes contact the GBM through interdigitating "foot processes" that support the capillary wall. Slit diaphragms link adjacent foot processes and serve as a filtration barrier to plasma proteins. **B:** The foot processes are effaced in most types of nephrotic syndrome. In minimal change disease, there is effacement of the foot processes, but immune deposits are not seen. **C:** Subepithelial immune deposits are associated with podocyte injury and proteinuria. These deposits are typical of membranous nephropathy. **D:** Subendothelial immune deposits are seen in several forms of glomerulonephritis. The deposits are associated with capillary wall injury, and inflammatory mediators can enter the bloodstream and attract immune cells to the kidney.

The benefit of ACE inhibitors in diabetic kidney disease is well established. ACE inhibitor and ARB therapy have been shown to slow the development of overt diabetic nephropathy and reduce the incidence of end-stage kidney disease (ESKD) and overall mortality in patients with type 1 or type 2 diabetes. Studies have demonstrated that the renoprotective benefits of ACE inhibitor or ARB therapy extend to CKD patients with nondiabetic proteinuria as well. Therapy with ACE inhibitors or ARBs in this patient population reduces progression to ESKD. The benefits of ACE inhibitors and ARBs are likely mediated through a reduction in glomerular pressure due to efferent arteriolar vasodilation, thereby resulting in a reduced amount of protein filtration. This is likely accompanied by a reduction in podocyte damage. Filtered proteins may also be directly toxic to the tubulointerstitium. In addition, ACE inhibitors and ARBs may have direct antifibrotic effects.

Sodium-glucose cotransporter-2 (SGLT2) inhibitors were first studied as antihyperglycemic agents in patients with diabetes. Studies have shown that they reduce proteinuria and slow CKD progression in patients with

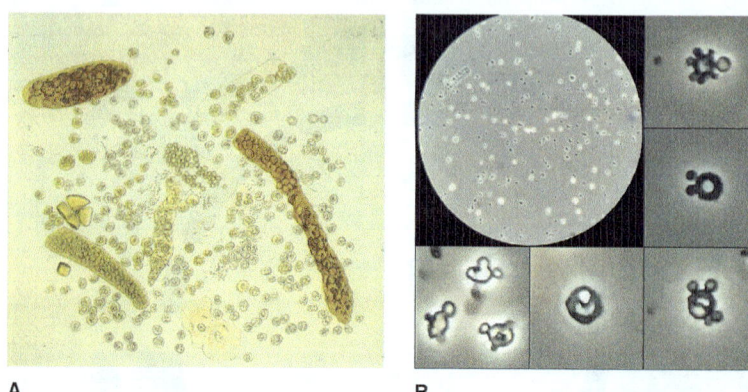

Figure 11-3. Glomerular red cells on urine microscopy. **A:** Red cell cast. (From Atlas of Urinary Sediments: With Special Reference to Their Clinical Significance/by Hermann Rieder; translated by Frederick Craven Moore; edited and annotated by A. Sheridan Delépine.) **B:** Acanthocytes by phase-contrast microscopy. (Courtesy of Dr. Florian Buchkremer.) FSGS, focal segmental glomerulosclerosis; GBM, glomerular basement membrane; IgA, immunoglobulin A; MPGN, membranoproliferative glomerulonephritis; SLE, systemic lupus erythematosus. (Reproduced with permission from Turner NA, Chapter 3: Approach to the diagnosis of glomerular disease. In: Nachman PH, Rheault MN, Lerma EV, eds. *Handbook of Glomerulonephritis*. Lippincott Wolters Kluwer; 2023.)

diabetic kidney disease. The mechanisms by which this class of drugs protects the kidney are incompletely understood, but they extend beyond the drugs' effects on blood glucose levels. Small studies and subgroup analyses have shown that SGLT2 inhibitors are protective in FSGS and IgA nephropathy. It is possible, therefore, that this class of medications will be beneficial in all patients with proteinuric kidney disease, although specific studies in the various types of glomerular disease are still ongoing.

2. **Hypertension.** The recommended goal blood pressure in patients with proteinuric nondiabetic CKD is less than 130/80 mmHg. For reasons described above, the first-line antihypertensive therapy should be with an ACE inhibitor or ARB. Treatment to achieve goal blood pressure should include lifestyle modification (salt restriction, weight normalization, regular exercise, and smoking cessation). In addition, in a large study in which proteinuric nondiabetic CKD patients had their blood pressure lowered below 130/80 mmHg, there was a significantly lower rate of (1) kidney failure (defined as dialysis or kidney transplantation) and (2) the combined endpoint of kidney failure or all-cause mortality at long-term follow-up, with these protective effects seen for both patients excreting more than 3 g of proteinuria per day and those excreting 1 to 3 g/d.

3. **Edema.** Edema associated with nephrotic syndrome should be treated with dietary sodium restriction (1.5 to 2 g of sodium/24 hours) and diuretics. Thiazides are a reasonable treatment choice for patients with mild edema. However, most patients, particularly those with impaired kidney function, will require a loop diuretic such as furosemide for adequate sodium balance. Nephrotic patients are often diuretic-resistant even if the patient's GFR is normal. Oftentimes combining a loop diuretic with a thiazide diuretic or with metolazone is required to overcome diuretic resistance. The use of intravenous albumin infusions with diuretics to treat diuretic resistance has not been shown to be effective. Occasionally, mechanical ultrafiltration is required for resistant edema with severely impaired kidney function.

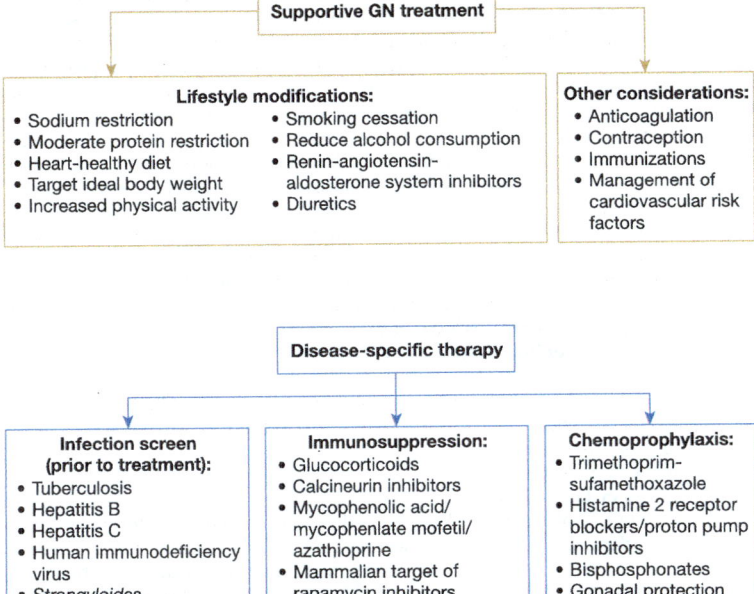

Figure 11-4. Summary of supportive management of patients with glomerular disease. (Reproduced with permission from Kidney Disease: Improving Global Outcomes (KDIGO) Glomerular Diseases Work Group. KDIGO. 2021 Clinical Practice Guideline for the Management of Glomerular Diseases. Supplement to Kidney International. 2021;100:4S.)

4. **Hyperlipidemia.** Treatment of hyperlipidemia in nephrotic syndrome should follow the guidelines for those patients at high risk for the development of cardiovascular disease. For the treatment of hyperlipidemia, statins (3-hydroxy-3-methylglutaryl-coenzyme A [HMG-CoA] reductase inhibitors) or agents such as gemfibrozil are well tolerated and effective in correcting the lipid profile. Some studies have shown that treatment with statins slows the decline in GFR, but they have not been proven to reduce cardiovascular events in patients with nephrotic syndrome. In patients undergoing treatment for nephrotic syndrome, there is an increased risk of myositis and rhabdomyolysis when statins are combined with calcineurin inhibitors.

5. **Hypercoagulability.** Patients with nephrotic syndrome have an increased incidence of arterial and venous thrombosis, and the risk is particularly high in patients with membranous nephropathy. The development of a thrombophilic state in nephrotic syndrome is not entirely understood; however, some of the predisposition is attributed to loss of antithrombotic factors such as antithrombin III and plasminogen. In addition, some studies have demonstrated increased platelet activation and high fibrinogen levels. The risk of thromboembolism increases as serum albumin values fall below 2.5 g/dL (25 g/L). Full-dose anticoagulation with low–molecular-weight heparin or warfarin is

required in patients with a diagnosed arterial or venous thrombosis or pulmonary embolism. Prophylactic anticoagulation is reasonable in patients with a serum albumin concentration of less than 2.0 g/dL, particularly those with membranous nephropathy. Treatment should continue as long as proteinuria remains in the nephrotic range. Anticoagulation is also indicated in patients with concomitant risks of thromboembolism, such as pregnancy.
   6. **Infection.** Infection was the major cause of morbidity and mortality in children with nephrotic syndrome prior to the antibiotic era. The increased risk of infection with nephrotic syndrome may be due to urinary losses of immunoglobulin and other immune system mediators. Studies show that patients with GN and nephrotic syndrome are at increased risk of invasive pneumococcal infection. These patients should receive pneumococcal vaccination as well as annual influenza vaccination. Vaccination with live vaccines is contraindicated for patients receiving treatment with immunosuppressive or cytotoxic agents.

V. Treatment of Specific Glomerular Diseases

The specific management of glomerular diseases requires the information obtained by kidney biopsy but is also influenced by the patient's clinical presentation. For example, more aggressive treatment may be undertaken in patients with a faster rate of progression or a greater degree of proteinuria.

A. Nephritic Syndrome
   1. **Kidney Limited Disease**
      a. **IgA Nephropathy.** IgA nephropathy is the most common form of primary glomerular disease in the world. The term IgA vasculitis is now used for patients with extra-kidney involvement (typically arthralgias, abdominal pain and palpable, purpuric rash). IgA nephropathy is particularly prevalent in Asia and Australia (perhaps due to sampling bias resulting from the screening of school-aged children and a more frequent rate of biopsy in these regions), and it is rare in African Americans. Although generally considered to be a slowly progressive kidney disease, ESKD occurs in 20% to 40% of patients within 20 years. A minority of patients may experience RPGN with crescent formation on biopsy, and approximately 10% of patients present with the nephrotic syndrome.
         i. **Diagnosis.** Patients with IgA nephropathy usually present with hematuria and subnephrotic proteinuria, which may be an incidental finding on urinalysis. Some patients develop gross hematuria, which classically develops in the setting of an upper respiratory tract infection ("synpharyngitic"). The definitive diagnosis of IgA nephropathy requires a kidney biopsy, which reveals immunodominant deposits of IgA. IgA deposits are typically seen in the mesangium. By light microscopy, mesangial expansion and mesangial proliferation are usually seen. IgA is also present in the capillary loops of some patients, a finding that is associated with endocapillary proliferation. In autopsy series, some patients without clinical disease also have glomerular IgA deposits.
         ii. **Pathophysiology.** IgA nephropathy has been linked with the aberrant glycosylation of IgA1 molecules. Affected patients develop IgG and IgA autoantibodies that recognize the abnormally glycosylated IgA1 and form immune complexes that deposit in the mesangium. Genome-wide association studies have linked some major histocompatibility complex loci with IgA nephropathy, further supporting an immunologic basis of the disease. Polymorphisms in complement system genes are also associated with disease risk.
         iii. **Treatment.** ACE inhibitors have been shown to slow the progression of IgA nephropathy, and all patients should be treated with either

ACE inhibitors or ARBs. Sparsentan is an angiotensin II receptor antagonist and endothelin-1 receptor blocker. It has been conditionally approved for treatment of IgA nephropathy. SGLT2 inhibitors also reduce proteinuria and slow progression of disease and may be a useful adjunctive therapy.

Several clinical trials have demonstrated that glucocorticoids are effective at slowing the progression of IgA nephropathy, and patients with proteinuria greater than 1 g/d may benefit. Budesonide is a delayed-release formulation glucocorticoid that may effectively target B-cells in the ileum. Studies have shown that budesonide reduces proteinuria in IgA nephropathy, and it has been approved by the Food and Drug Administration (FDA). Proteinuria is a surrogate endpoint, although a review of IgA nephropathy studies demonstrated that an early reduction in proteinuria predicts a lower likelihood of kidney disease progression. Recent studies have also shown that mycophenolate mofetil is effective in patients with patients whose proteinuria is greater than 1.0 g/d. Rituximab, on the other hand, does not appear to be effective. Some studies support the use of fish oil in slowing the progression of kidney insufficiency, although not all studies showed a benefit.

For crescentic disease or rapidly progressive disease, short-term, high-dose prednisone may be of benefit. Cytotoxic agents, such as cyclophosphamide, are sometimes employed.

b. **C3 Glomerulopathy and Immune-Complex Membranoproliferative GN.** Historically, patients were diagnosed with MPGN based on the histologic pattern of glomerular injury seen by light microscopy. More recently it has been observed that some of these patients have immunodominant glomerular C3 deposits, and these patients are now classified as having C3G. Patients who also have immunoglobulin deposits and an MPGN pattern of injury are classified as having IC-MPGN. IC-MPGN is associated with a variety of systemic conditions, including autoimmune diseases (e.g., systemic lupus erythematosus) and infection-associated glomerular disease (e.g., hepatitis C). Patients with an identified autoimmune or infectious cause of their disease are categorized according to the primary disease.

   i. **Diagnosis.** The clinical presentations of idiopathic C3G and IC-MPGN are variable. Patients can present with mild nephritic findings, a rapid decline in kidney function, or with the nephrotic syndrome. On biopsy, the glomeruli usually demonstrate mesangial expansion and hypercellularity; endocapillary proliferation, duplication, or splitting of the GBM (referred to as "double contours" or "tram tracks"); and lobulation of the glomerular tuft. The diagnosis of C3G is based on detection of C3 deposits which are at least two orders of magnitude brighter than that of immunoglobulin by immunofluorescence. Not all patients with C3G have an MPGN pattern of injury, so the diagnosis is primarily based on the immunofluorescence findings. C3G can be further subdivided into two subsets based on ultrastructural examination of the glomeruli by electron microscopy. C3G patients with electron-dense deposits within the GBM and are classified as having "dense deposit disease (DDD)," and patients without these deposits are classified as C3 glomerulonephritis (C3GN).

   ii. **Pathophysiology.** In IC-MPGN, the deposition of the immune complexes activates the classical pathway of complement, causing glomerular inflammation and injury. C3G, on the other hand, is caused by uncontrolled activation of the alternative pathway of complement. Many patients have "nephritic factors," autoantibodies that impair the body's endogenous regulators of the complement system. Other patients have mutations in complement genes, impairing the body's ability to control complement activation. It is not clear, however, whether IC-MPGN and C3G are completely distinct diseases. In some patients with C3G, disease starts as a postinfectious process but persists as C3G. It is possible that these patients are unable to restore control of complement activity in the glomerulus.

   iii. **Treatment.** In any case of IC-MPGN, secondary causes must be fully evaluated, because diseases such as chronic bacterial infection, hepatitis C infection, and cryoglobulinemia, as well as leukemias and lymphomas, all have therapies that may lead to remission of the kidney disease. In patients with C3G, particularly those older than 50, tests should be performed to look for an underlying monoclonal gammopathy. The blood pressure should be controlled in all patients, and treatment should include an ACE inhibitor. Unfortunately, there is not currently any established specific treatment for IC-MPGN or C3G. A randomized controlled trial demonstrated a benefit to treating children and teenagers with alternate-day corticosteroids, although this study included patients with all forms of MPGN. In C3G, retrospective studies have shown that treatment with mycophenolate mofetil is associated with better outcomes.

B. **Nephritic Syndrome with Systemic Manifestations**
   1. **Anti-GBM Disease and Goodpasture Syndrome.** Anti-GBM disease is a severe and rapidly progressive form of GN caused by antibodies to targets expressed within the GBM. The same epitopes are expressed within the basement membranes of other tissues, and patients can present with isolated kidney dysfunction (anti-GBM disease) or with kidney disease in conjunction with pulmonary involvement (Goodpasture syndrome).
      a. **Diagnosis.** Anti-GBM disease causes a nephritic pattern of injury, and the loss of kidney function can be rapid. Patients with Goodpasture syndrome can have pulmonary hemorrhage at the time of presentation, and this diagnosis should be considered in all patients who present with a pulmonary-renal syndrome. The anti-GBM antibodies can be detected in patient serum using an enzyme-linked immunosorbent assay (ELISA) test. Kidney biopsy typically reveals fibrinoid necrosis and crescents. Immunofluorescence microscopy is central to the diagnosis of the disease and is characterized by linear deposition of immunoglobulin (usually IgG) along the glomerular capillaries.
      b. **Pathophysiology.** Strong evidence indicates that anti-GBM antibodies cause glomerular inflammation and are pathogenic. Passive transfer of the antibodies into rodents causes glomerular disease. The disease-inducing antibodies bind to specific epitopes in type IV collagen.
      c. **Treatment.** Treatment for anti-GBM disease and Goodpasture syndrome includes high-dose steroids, cyclophosphamide, and plasmapheresis to remove the anti-GBM antibody. Patients who present with oliguria have poor kidney outcomes, but occasionally may avoid chronic dialysis with aggressive and early therapy.
   2. **Pauci-immune Renal Vasculitis.** Small vessel vasculitis frequently involves the kidneys. Several diseases can cause immune complex–mediated vasculitis (e.g., cryoglobulinemia, lupus, and anti-GBM disease). Patients with small vessel vasculitis of the kidneys who do not have evidence of immune complex deposition in vessels are considered to have *pauci-immune* vasculitis. Approximately 90% of patients with pauci-immune small

vessel vasculitis have detectable ANCA. ANCAs recognize several different antigens, including myeloperoxidase (MPO) and proteinase-3 (PR-3). Antibody to MPO results in perinuclear staining of neutrophils (p-ANCA) by immunofluorescence, whereas antibody to PR-3 results in cytoplasmic staining of neutrophils (c-ANCA). ANCA-associated small vessel vasculitis of the kidney typically presents as one of three different syndromes: granulomatosis with polyangiitis (GPA), microscopic polyangiitis (MPA), and eosinophilic granulomatosis with polyangiitis (EGPA).

   a. **Diagnosis.** All forms of pauci-immune small vessel vasculitis can affect multiple organ systems, including the skin, lungs, and gastrointestinal system. EGPA is associated with asthma and eosinophilia. The clinical presentation of small vessel pauci-immune vasculitis is variable, but patients generally present with a nephritic pattern of kidney disease. This kidney disease can progress rapidly, making it very important to diagnose the disease promptly. Because the lungs are frequently involved in all forms of ANCA-associated vasculitis, patients can present with alveolar capillaritis and pulmonary hemorrhage ("pulmonary-renal syndrome"). GPA is most commonly associated with anti–PR-3 (c-ANCA). MPA and EGPA are more commonly associated with anti-MPO (p-ANCA). However, there is an overlap in the clinical presentation and ANCA specificity among all three diseases. Histologically, the glomeruli in patients with kidney involvement in all forms of pauci-immune small vessel vasculitis typically demonstrate fibrinoid necrosis and crescents. GPA is associated with granulomas on tissue biopsy, whereas granulomas are not seen in patients with MPA and EGPA. Immune complexes must be sparse or absent in order to make the diagnosis of pauci-immune vasculitis.
   b. **Pathophysiology.** There is evidence that ANCA is pathogenic in small vessel vasculitis. Experiments in rodents have demonstrated that injection of the antibodies can cause glomerular disease. The ANCA titer does not always correlate with disease severity, however, and ANCA is not detected in some patients. Experiments have also shown that complement activation contributes to disease pathogenesis.
   Treatment. Whether systemic or kidney-limited, patients with pauci-immune small vessel vasculitis are treated with immunosuppressive drugs. The most commonly used protocols include high-dose steroids in combination with rituximab and/or cyclophosphamide (either oral or intravenous). Approximately 80% of patients respond to therapy, although patients with a serum creatinine greater than 6 mg/dL at presentation are less likely to respond than patients with a lower serum creatinine. Several studies and systematic reviews have examined the benefits of plasma exchange. The results of these studies have been mixed, but some experts still advocate its use in patients with severe disease or pulmonary hemorrhage. Avacopan, a C5a receptor antagonist, has been approved for use in combination cyclophosphamide or rituximab.

3. **Lupus Nephritis.** More than half of the patients with lupus develop clinically evident kidney involvement. Kidney disease is an important cause of morbidity in these patients, and mortality is higher in patients with lupus who have kidney involvement than in those who do not.

   a. **Diagnosis.** The manifestations of lupus nephritis are variable among patients, and in individual patients, the nature of the disease can change over time and in response to therapy. Kidney involvement is usually discovered by the detection of proteinuria and hematuria, but patients can present with either nephritic or nephrotic patterns of injury. Because the

histologic pattern of injury in lupus nephritis is variable, different classifications have been developed to better predict the prognosis. In patients with lupus nephritis, immune complexes may be seen within the mesangium, the subendothelial space, and the subepithelial space. The location of the immune deposits often correlates with the clinical presentation. Subepithelial deposits, for example, cause injury that is clinically and histologically similar to MN. Patients with this pattern of injury often present with the nephrotic syndrome. Mesangial and subendothelial deposits, on the other hand, can cause glomerular inflammation and a nephritic syndrome. Immunofluorescence typically, but not always, demonstrates positive staining for C3, C1q, IgG, IgM, and IgA, within the same kidney (a "Full house" pattern). These deposits are granular, and are distinguishable from the linear pattern seen in anti-GBM disease.
  b. **Pathophysiology.** Lupus is caused by the loss of tolerance to self-antigens and the generation of autoantibodies. Most of the autoantibodies react with antigens present in the cell nucleus, such as DNA, RNA, and histone. Preformed immune complexes may deposit in the kidney, or the antibodies and antigen may deposit separately. There is also evidence that some autoantibodies cross-react with proteins expressed within the kidney. Antibodies that deposit within the kidney or that bind to glomerular structures can cause injury to nearby cells through activation of the complement system or via signaling through Fc receptors.
  c. **Treatment.** In general, therapy for lupus nephritis includes high-dose corticosteroids in combination with either mycophenolate mofetil or cyclophosphamide, particularly for the treatment of diffuse proliferative lupus nephritis. Patients with severe disease are usually treated with high doses of these drugs for an induction period, typically about 6 months. In patients who respond well, the dose of immunosuppression can be reduced, but patients are usually continued on some form of maintenance regimen for another 18 months or longer. Several additional drugs have been approved by the FDA for treatment of lupus nephritis, including belimumab and voclosporin. It is not yet known how these drugs can best be integrated into the treatment protocols for the disease.
4. **Cryoglobulinemia (Cryoglobulinemia).** Cryoglobulins are antibodies that precipitate in the cold. In vivo, they can form immune complexes that precipitate in small vessels, causing vasculitis. Cryoglobulins are most frequently associated with hepatitis C infection, although they are also seen in other conditions.
   a. **Diagnosis.** Cryoglobulinemia can affect numerous different tissues throughout the body. Most patients with symptomatic disease develop palpable purpura, arthralgias, and generalized weakness. In the kidney, cryoglobulinemia causes an immune complex GN. Patients typically have proteinuria, hematuria, and slowly progressive disease. Some patients have nephrotic range proteinuria, however, and patients can have a rapid loss of kidney function. Labs that support the diagnosis of cryoglobulinemia include a low C4 level and the cryoglobulins often have rheumatoid factor activity. On kidney biopsy, affected patients usually have a membranoproliferative pattern of injury and subendothelial immune deposits. Microtubular structures are seen on electron microscopy, and the deposits can form a characteristic "fingerprint" appearance.
   b. **Pathophysiology.** Three categories of cryoglobulins have been identified. They can be composed of monoclonal antibodies (type I); a monoclonal IgM that binds to polyclonal IgG (type II, "mixed"); and polyclonal IgM that binds to polyclonal IgG (type III; "mixed"). Cryoglobulinemia is associated with lymphoproliferative disorders, autoimmune disease

(particularly Sjögren syndrome), and infections (particularly hepatitis C). Cooling of blood in the extremities may favor precipitation of cryoglobulins in blood vessels. In organs such as the kidneys, immune complexes formed by IgM with rheumatoid activity may favor precipitation.

   c. **Treatment.** Antiviral therapies have significantly reduced the incidence of hepatitis C–associated cryoglobulinemia and are associated with clinical improvement for those with active disease. B-cell–depleting therapies, such as rituximab, are beneficial in patients with an underlying B-cell lymphoproliferative disease and in those with rapidly progressive or resistant disease. Plasmapheresis removes the cryoglobulins and can be beneficial in patients with rapidly progressive disease.

5. **Infection-related GN.** Various forms of infection-related GN can develop in patients with bacterial, viral, fungal, and helminthic infections. Some pathogens are associated with specific patterns of kidney disease, and there is a range of clinical presentations among different organisms. Chronic hepatitis B is associated with MN and nephrotic syndrome, for example, and HIV infection is associated with FSGS. The most common form of infection-related GN is poststreptococcal GN, although the incidence of this disease is declining due to improved recognition and treatment of these infections. Bacterial endocarditis and infected atrioventricular shunts are also associated with the development of immune complex GN, and the incidence of *Staphylococcus aureus*–related GN is growing due to an increase in the prevalence of resistant organisms.

   a. **Diagnosis.** Most patients with bacterial infection–related GN present with a nephritic pattern of injury. Streptococcal infections have often resolved by the time that GN develops ("poststreptococcal"). Patients with endocarditis or infected shunts (historically ventriculoatrial [VA] shunts, but less common now with the predominance of ventriculoperitoneal [VP] shunts) may have fevers and arthralgias. Levels of C3 in plasma are often low (see Table 11-4). Light microscopy in patients with postinfectious disease typically reveals proliferative glomerular changes and is often described as "exudative" (abundant neutrophils). By immunofluorescence microscopy, large granular deposits of IgG, IgM, and C3 are seen in the mesangium and capillary loops of patients with poststreptococcal disease, and electron-dense deposits are seen in the subendothelial, mesangial, and subepithelial spaces by electron microscopy. Large subepithelial deposits ("humps") are characteristic of poststreptococcal GN.

   b. **Pathophysiology.** Immune complexes formed by antibodies bound to bacterial antigens may deposit in the kidneys, triggering local inflammation. Although C3 is consistently seen within the glomeruli of patients with poststreptococcal GN, C4 is often absent. One possible explanation is that bacterial antigens may directly activate the alternative pathway of complement.

   c. **Treatment.** In general, eradication of the underlying infection is the best treatment for infection-related GN. Although steroids have been used in patients with rapidly progressive poststreptococcal GN, there is no evidence that it improves outcomes.

C. Nephrotic Syndrome
1. **Renal Limited Disease**
   a. **Primary MN.** Approximately 30% to 40% of cases of idiopathic nephrotic syndrome in adults are due to MN.
      i. **Diagnosis.** MN typically presents in the fourth or fifth decade with a 2:1 male predominance. MN is often slowly progressive; however, some patients have spontaneous remission of disease. The hallmark

of MN is the thickened glomerular capillary basement membrane visible on light microscopy. Silver stain of the tissue reveals a characteristic "spike-and-dome" feature of the capillary basement membrane. Electron microscopy demonstrates subepithelial deposits within the capillary basement membrane. Immunofluorescence microscopy demonstrates IgG and C3 along the glomerular capillary walls. The M-type phospholipase A2 receptor (PLA2R) is the target antigen in 70% to 80% of cases of primary MN. Immunostaining reveals PLA2R in the glomeruli of patients with anti-PLA2R MN. Detection of anti-PLA2R antibody in the serum by ELISA is also diagnostic of MN. Recent studies have identified several additional antigens in subsets of patients with MN. Approximately 5% of patients have antibodies against thrombospondin type-1 domain-containing 7A (THSD7A). Some patients with autoimmune disease have exostosin 1/exostosin 2 within the glomerular deposits. Neural epidermal growth factor-like 1 (NELL1) is another possible antigen and may be associated with cancer-associated disease. Currently, PLA2R is the only target antigen that can be identified with clinically available tests.

ii. **Pathophysiology.** Antibodies to PLA2R, when present, are believed to be pathogenic in MN. Some patients have autoantibodies reactive with other podocyte antigens. Once the autoantibodies bind within the glomerulus they activate complement and cause podocyte injury.

iii. **Treatment.** All patients with MN should be treated with ACE inhibitor or ARB therapy. Treatment with immunosuppressive agents is indicated for those patients at high risk for progressive loss of kidney function. Risk factors include heavy proteinuria (greater than 8 g/d), hypertension, diminished GFR (creatinine greater than 1.2 mg/dL for women, greater than 1.4 mg/dL for men), male gender, and greater than 20% tubulointerstitial fibrosis in kidney biopsy, and high anti-PLA2R titers.

Immunosuppressive therapy is indicated for patients with persistent nephrotic range proteinuria after antiproteinuric therapy with an ACE inhibitor or ARB over an observation period of 6 months, development of severe symptoms due to the nephrotic syndrome, or progressive kidney impairment. Provided there is no absolute contraindication to immunosuppressive therapy (active untreated infection, malignancy, preexisting leukopenia, or an inability to comply with treatment), initial therapy consists of glucocorticoids in combination with rituximab or cyclophosphamide. Calcineurin inhibitors (tacrolimus or cyclosporine) are also capable of inducing remission, although patients frequently relapse after discontinuation of treatment. Mycophenolate mofetil may also be effective in the management of low- to moderate-risk patients as shown in short-term studies.

b. **Primary FSGS.** Approximately 20% of cases of idiopathic nephrotic syndrome in adults are due to FSGS.

   i. **Diagnosis.** Patients with FSGS present with features of the nephrotic syndrome and often have hypertension. Light microscopy in FSGS demonstrates focal areas of segmental glomerular sclerosis and electron microscopy demonstrates foot process effacement.

   ii. **Pathophysiology.** Segmental areas of sclerosis occur as a result of damaged podocytes or as a repair process after segmental glomerular inflammation. It has long been suspected that primary FSGS can be caused by circulating factors, underscored by rapid recurrence of nephrotic-range proteinuria shortly after FSGS patients receive a kidney transplant, although the identity of these "permeability factors" has remained elusive.

   iii. **Treatment.** The natural history of primary FSGS is variable, but spontaneous remission in primary FSGS associated with nephrotic syndrome is low (<10%). The strongest predictor of progression to ESKD is resistance to corticosteroids. In patients who do not achieve remission of disease, the 5-year kidney survival is poor (on average 65%) and the 10-year kidney survival is 30%. Even in patients who achieve remission, relapse rates can be as high as 40%. Treatment for the initial presentation of primary FSGS with nephrotic syndrome consists of prednisone at a daily single dose of 1 mg/kg (maximum 80 mg) or alternate-day dose of 2 mg/kg (maximum 120 mg). High dose of corticosteroids should be continued for 12 to 16 weeks before tapering. Calcineurin inhibitors (cyclosporine, tacrolimus) can be considered as first-line therapy for patients with contraindications or intolerance to high-dose corticosteroids (e.g., uncontrolled diabetes, psychiatric conditions, and severe osteoporosis). However, while calcineurin inhibitors have been successful at inducing remission they are associated with a high relapse rate and difficulty discontinuing the medication.

  c. **Minimal Change Disease.** Approximately 10% to 15% of cases of idiopathic nephrotic syndrome in adults and 85% in children are due to MCD.
     i. **Diagnosis.** Patients with MCD may have a sudden onset of edema and signs of the nephrotic syndrome. On kidney biopsy glomeruli appear normal by light microscopy and immunofluorescence is typically negative. However, histologic variants with immunofluorescence demonstrating IgM deposits within the mesangium may be seen, which may portend a poorer prognosis. Electron microscopy shows the characteristic effacement of the podocyte foot processes but no electron-dense deposits.
     ii. **Pathophysiology.** The etiology of MCD is not well understood. Some studies suggest that T-cell dysfunction, autoantibodies to podocyte proteins, or podocyte-related factors are involved.
     iii. **Treatment.** For a first episode, treatment consists of high-dose prednisone (1 mg/kg daily [maximum 80 mg] or alternate-day single-dose 2 mg/kg [maximum 120 mg]), for a minimum of 4 weeks and up to 16 weeks. After achieving complete remission, prednisone can be slowly tapered over a total period of up to 6 months. Whereas greater than 90% of children with MCD will achieve complete remission of proteinuria within 2 months of starting steroid therapy, rates of remission drop to approximately 50% to 75% in adults. Extending the duration of high-dose prednisone to 5 to 6 months increases the rate of complete remission to 80%. After remission, prednisone should be slowly tapered over approximately 4 months. A number of studies have shown that B cell depleting therapies may reduce the risk of disease flares and can reduce the need for glucocorticoids. In adults, relapses are common, with relapse rates as high as 60% to 70%. For relapsed disease, the corticosteroid regimen is to be repeated as if it is the first episode. In cases where steroids cannot be tapered (steroid dependence or frequently relapsing), second-line agents (rituximab, cyclophosphamide, cyclosporine, tacrolimus, or mycophenolate mofetil) may be effective as steroid-sparing agents.

D. **Nephrotic Syndrome Due to Systemic Illness**
  1. **Secondary MN.** Approximately 20% of MN cases are secondary in etiology. MN can be caused by secondary factors such as malignancy (colon,

lung, or prostate cancer), autoimmune disease (systemic lupus erythematosus), infectious disease (hepatitis B virus, hepatitis C virus), drugs (nonsteroidal anti-inflammatory drugs [NSAIDs], gold, penicillamine), and others. Factors on biopsy that favor a secondary form of MN include subendothelial and/or mesangial deposits, a "full house" of immunoglobulins and complement (suggestive of lupus nephropathy), tubuloreticular inclusions in endothelial cells, and mesangial or endocapillary proliferation. Secondary MN due to malignancy is more prominent in patients greater than 65 years old. In cases of malignancy-related MN, a clinical remission of cancer is associated with a reduction in proteinuria.
2. **Secondary FSGS.** Secondary causes of FSGS include viral nephropathies (HIV-associated nephropathy and parvovirus B19), drug-induced nephropathy (pamidronate, interferon alpha, heroin), and adaptive hemodynamic changes (congenital or acquired solitary kidney, reflux nephropathy, obesity). Secondary causes of FSGS typically have patchy foot process effacement instead of global effacement on biopsy. Patients with secondary FSGS are not treated with immunosuppressive therapy. Instead, treatment should be focused on treatment of the underlying disorder.
3. **Secondary MCD.** Systemic conditions associated with secondary MCD include Hodgkin disease, and medications such as lithium and NSAIDs.
4. **Diabetic Nephropathy.** Diabetes is the leading cause of ESKD in dialysis patients in the United States. The earliest clinical manifestation of diabetic nephropathy is microalbuminuria. Risk factors for progression of diabetic nephropathy to ESKD include nephrotic range proteinuria and kidney dysfunction at diagnosis.
    a. **Diagnosis.** Diabetic nephropathy is characterized by persistent proteinuria. It is recommended that diabetic patients are screened regularly with a urine albumin/creatinine ratio. Diabetes affects the microvascular circulation, and it has been shown that the presence of diabetic retinopathy correlates well with overt diabetic nephropathy. Diagnosis can typically be made on clinical history. If a kidney biopsy is performed, it classically shows mesangial and matrix expansion, GBM thickening, and nodular glomerulosclerosis with the characteristic nodular Kimmelstiel–Wilson lesions.
    b. **Pathophysiology.** The kidney disease associated with diabetes progresses over the span of years. Glomerular hyperfiltration develops in most patients with an initial increase in GFR. Parenchymal hypertrophy develops, which can be seen as large kidneys on ultrasound imaging. Glomerular hypertension occurs with subsequent development of clinical abnormalities such as microalbuminuria, glomerular lesions, macroalbuminuria, and a progressive loss of GFR.
    c. **Treatment.** Hypertension is a modifiable risk factor of the GFR decline in diabetic nephropathy. The antihypertensive agent of choice in diabetes is an ACE inhibitor or ARB. Treatment with ACE inhibitors or ARB has been shown to reduce the rate of decline in GFR in patients with hypertension and diabetes. SGLT2 inhibitors also reduce proteinuria and have been shown to reduce kidney and cardiovascular disease progression in patients with type II diabetes. Finerenone, a nonsteroidal mineralocorticoid receptor antagonist, slows the decline of eGFR in patients with proteinuric diabetic kidney disease.
5. **Monoclonal Immunoglobulin Deposition and Amyloidosis.** Monoclonal gammopathies are disorders in which B-cells or plasma cells produce immunoglobulin or immunoglobulin fragments that cause injury of the kidney. Although B-cell malignancies and multiple myeloma can cause the same pattern of kidney disorders, deposition of the immunoglobulin in the kidney

may be the only pathologic manifestation of the abnormal immunoglobulin production ("monoclonal gammopathy of renal significance," or MGRS). This group of diseases includes AL amyloidosis, immunotactoid GN, fibrillary GN, and proliferative GN with monoclonal immunoglobulin deposits (PGNMID). Monoclonal gammopathies are also associated with the development of C3G, but immunoglobulin is not deposited in the glomeruli of these patients.

  a. **Diagnosis.** SPEP with immunofixation and UPEP can help identify monoclonal gammopathies. Immunostaining of kidney biopsies detects deposits of intact immunoglobulin, light chains, and/or heavy chains. Isotype staining of the tissue for λ and κ light chains reveals whether the deposits are monoclonal. In amyloidosis and fibrillary GN, the deposited immunoglobulin is organized into fibrils. In immunotactoid GN, in contrast, the deposited immunoglobulin is organized into microtubules. In PGNMID, light chain deposition disease, and heavy chain deposition disease, the deposited Ig or Ig fragments are not organized. Congo red staining of biopsy tissue from patients with amyloid deposits demonstrates green birefringence under polarized light. Kidneys with fibrillary GN stain positively for DnaJ homolog subfamily B member 9 (DNAJB9).
  b. **Treatment.** Treatment of MGRS is aimed at reducing the concentration of the pathologic immunoglobulin or immunoglobulin fragment. This typically involves the use of chemotherapy to reduce the pathologic B-cell or plasma cell clone.

VI. The Thrombotic Microangiopathies

Systemic disorders that can cause kidney injury include thrombotic thrombocytopenic purpura (TTP), hemolytic uremic syndrome (HUS), scleroderma, malignant hypertension, and antiphospholipid antibody syndrome (APS) (Fig. 11-5). These diseases are characterized by direct injury to small vessels, and can present with hematuria, hypertension, and proteinuria (although usually less than 1 to 1.5 g/d). Common histologic findings on kidney biopsy in HUS, TTP, and APS include glomerular capillary thrombi and afferent arterioles with fibrinoid necrosis from endothelial injury. These diseases can also cause an MPGN pattern of injury by light microscopy, but immunofluorescence is typically negative except for fibrinogen. Electron microscopy is also usually unremarkable, with no deposits noted. In addition, malignant hypertension and scleroderma can cause subintimal proliferation within blood vessels, leading to an "onion skin" appearance of arterioles. Microthrombi may be present as well.

The specific management of the thrombotic microangiopathies differs significantly from other disorders that lead to a nephritic clinical presentation; highlighting the need for an appropriate work-up and appropriate index of suspicion when evaluating nephritic disease. For treatment of malignant hypertension and scleroderma renal crisis, proactive blood pressure control is paramount, given the severe activation of the renin–angiotensin–aldosterone pathway. ACE inhibitor therapy is the first-line therapy in the setting of scleroderma, because data demonstrates improved patient survival and kidney outcomes using this form of therapy.

  A. **Hemolytic Uremic Syndrome.** In HUS, the clinical picture is predominantly one of acute kidney failure, thrombocytopenia, and hemolysis resulting from Shiga toxin (usually from *Escherichia coli* 0157:H7 gastrointestinal infection). Therapy is primarily supportive and 85% of cases of diarrhea-associated HUS will completely recover, although 5% die within the acute phase and >5% may have persistent kidney and systemic complications. Patients who develop HUS in the absence of a Shiga toxin-producing infection are regarded as having atypical HUS, a disease that is usually caused by dysregulated activation of the alternative pathway of complement. These patients have a worse prognosis

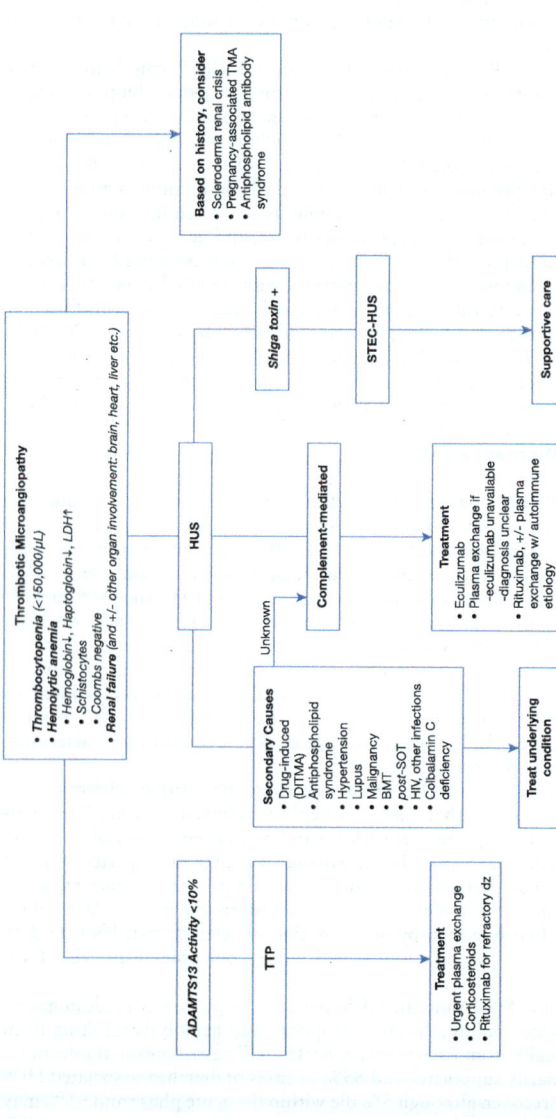

Figure 11-5. Approach to patients with thrombocytopenia and hemolytic anemia. Thrombotic microangiopathy is a clinical diagnosis based on the detection of thrombocytopenia and hemolytic anemia. Associated small-vessel thromboses of affected tissues can also lead to organ ischemia, and commonly injured tissues include the kidney and central nervous system. ADAMTS13 activity and detection of Shiga toxin should be performed in all patients suspected of having thrombotic microangiopathy. Depending on the clinical history and exam findings, specific tests should be performed for other causes of thrombotic microangiopathy. All patients with suspicion of having thrombocytopenic thrombotic purpura should be treated with plasma exchange while awaiting the results of ADAMTS13 activity. Patients suspected of having complement-mediated hemolytic uremic syndrome should be treated with targeted anticomplement therapy, with eculizumab being the prototypical drug. ADAMTS13, a disintegrin and metalloproteinase with a thrombospondin type 1 motif, member 13; BMT, bone marrow transplant; DITMA, drug-induced TMA; HUS, hemolytic uremic syndrome; LDH, lactate dehydrogenase; STEC-HUS, Shiga toxin–producing *Escherichia coli*–associated HUS; SOT, solid-organ transplant; TMA, thrombotic microangiopathy; TTP, thrombotic thrombocytopenic purpura.

than those with diarrhea-associated HUS. Eculizumab (a therapeutic complement inhibitor) is considered the standard of care treatment of atypical HUS.
B. Thrombotic Thrombocytopenic Purpura. The "classic pentad" of signs of TTP includes (1) thrombocytopenia, (2) hemolytic anemia, (3) kidney failure, (4) fever, and (5) neurologic abnormalities. Most patients do not present with all five of these symptoms, however, and these findings can wax and wane. Secondary forms of TTP exist, and include pregnancy-, malignancy-, and HIV-associated causes. Primary TTP is triggered by endothelial injury in patients who have persistence of abnormally large von Willebrand factor (vWF) multimers, which are normally cleaved as part of homeostatic coagulation control. This combination of vascular injury and propensity for clotting leads to platelet aggregation and thrombi formation. This failure to cleave large vWF multimers is usually caused by a functional deficiency of the metalloproteinase ADAMTS13, which is most commonly caused by inhibitory autoantibodies, but rarely genetic defects in function ADAMTS13 expression can also result in TTP. ADAMTS13 activity can be tested clinically. A very low ADAMTS13 level supports the diagnosis of TTP, but given the associated high morbidity and mortality, the decision to treat TTP is usually made on clinical grounds while awaiting ADAMTS13 results. The "PLASMIC score" algorithm utilizes lab data and historical factors and can estimate the likelihood of disease while awaiting results of ADAMTS13 testing. Plasma exchange or infusion is the most effective therapeutic intervention for TTP. It is felt that plasma exchange may remove autoantibody when it is present and replace ADAMTS13 when there is a deficiency of this protein. Plasma exchange should be continued until the platelet count has normalized and the serum lactate dehydrogenase enzyme level returns to normal range. Additional therapies that are used in some patients, include high-dose prednisone, rituximab, vincristine, and other chemotherapeutic agents. Caplacizumab is a monoclonal antibody to vWF. It has been approved by the FDA and is used as part of the initial treatment of TTP by some clinicians.

SUGGESTED READINGS

Heerspink HJL, Stefansson BV, Correa-Rotter R, et al. Dapagliflozin in patients with chronic kidney disease. *N Engl J Med*. 2020;383(15):1436–1446.

Kopp JB, Anders HJ, Susztak K, et al. Podocytopathies. *Nat Rev Dis Primers*. 2020;6(1):68.

Lv J, Wong MG, Hladunewich MA, et al. Effect of oral methylprednisolone on decline in kidney function or kidney failure in patients with IgA nephropathy: the TESTING randomized clinical trial. *JAMA*. 2022;327(19):1888–1898.

Mejia-Vilet JM, Malvar A, Arazi A, Rovin BH. The lupus nephritis management renaissance. *Kidney Int*. 2022;101(2):242–255.

Noris M, Remuzzi G. Atypical hemolytic-uremic syndrome. *N Engl J Med*. 2009;361:1676–1687.

Ronco P, Beck L, Debiec H, et al. Membranous nephropathy. *Nat Rev Dis Primers*. 2021;7(1):69.

Waldman M, Crew RJ, Valeri A, et al. Adult minimal-change disease: clinical characteristics, treatment, and outcomes. *Clin J Am Soc Nephrol*. 2007;2:445–453.

Wong E, Marchbank K, Lomax-Browne H, et al. C3 glomerulopathy and related disorders in children. *Clin J Am Soc Nephrol*. 2021;16(11):1639–1651.

Wyatt RJ, Julian BA. IgA nephropathy. *N Engl J Med*. 2013;368:2402–2414.

12. The Patient with Acute Kidney Injury

Sarah Faubel, Charles Edelstein

I. Definition and Recognition of Acute Kidney Injury (AKI)

AKI, formerly known as acute renal failure, is a sudden decrease in kidney function characterized by a reduction in the glomerular filtration rate (GFR). AKI may occur in patients with previously normal kidney function or patients with chronic kidney disease (CKD); in either case, the clinical approach to find and treat the cause remains similar.

The Kidney Disease/Improving Global Outcomes (KDIGO) Clinical Practice Guidelines for AKI provide the simplest definition of AKI (Table 12-1): (1) Increase in SCr from baseline by ≥0.3 mg/dL within 48 hours; OR (2) increase in SCr to ≥1.5 times baseline, which is known or presumed to have occurred within the prior 7 days; OR (3) urine volume <0.5 mL/kg/h for 6 hours after exclusion of causes of decreased urine output like obstruction. This standardized definition is now the most commonly accepted definition for both clinical care and clinical trials of AKI.

Staging criteria for AKI have been established by the Acute Kidney Injury Network (AKIN) and the Risk, Injury, Failure, Loss, End-stage kidney disease (RIFLE) criteria (Table 12-2). The AKIN and RIFLE criteria convey the concept that AKI is not only significant when it requires kidney replacement therapy (KRT), but that it is a spectrum ranging from early disease to long-term failure. Based on the AKIN and RIFLE criteria, the definition of stage 1 AKI is as follows: (1) an increase in serum creatinine from baseline by ≥0.3 mg/dL within 48 hours, or (2) an increase in serum creatinine ≥1.5 times baseline which is known or presumed to have occurred within the prior 7 days, or (3) urine volume <0.5 mL/kg/h for 6 hours. For example, an increase in serum creatinine from 2.0 to 2.3 mg/dL within 48 hours is diagnostic of stage 1 AKI; similarly, an increase from 1.0 to 1.3 within 48 hours is diagnostic of stage 1 AKI. The AKIN and RIFLE criteria have been validated in multiple studies. Furthermore, an increase in serum creatinine by 0.3 mg/dL is associated with an independent increased risk of mortality.

After the onset of AKI, patients with normal baseline kidney function may recover kidney function back to normal or may progress to CKD. To capture a potentially nebulous time period between the onset of AKI and the development of CKD (which requires 3 months to be diagnosed), the term acute kidney disease (AKD) has been proposed. AKD was first introduced in the KDIGO 2012 guidelines and the definition was recently updated in 2021. AKD is defined as the following: AKI or GFR <60 mL/min/1.73 m^2 or decrease in GFR by ≥35%, or increase in serum creatinine by >50% for less than or equal to 3 months; and/or presence of a marker of kidney damage such as albuminuria, hematuria, or pyuria.

A. Serum Creatinine as a Marker of AKI and GFR. Normal serum creatinine is 0.6 to 1.2 mg/dL and is the most commonly used parameter to assess kidney function. Unfortunately, the correlation between serum creatinine concentration and GFR may be confounded by several factors.

1. **Creatinine Excretion Is Dependent on Factors Independent of Kidney Function.** Certain medications such as trimethoprim or cimetidine interfere with

TABLE 12-1 KDIGO Definition of AKI

Increase in SCr by ≥0.3 mg/dL within 48 h;
Or
Increase in SCr to ≥1.5 times baseline, which is known or presumed to have occurred within the prior 7 d;
Or
Urine volume <0.5 mL/kg/h for 6 h

AKI, acute kidney injury; SCr, serum creatinine.

TABLE 12-2 AKIN and RIFLE Criteria for Diagnosis and Classification of AKI

AKIN Criteria			RIFLE Criteria		
Stage	SCr	Urine Output	Class	SCr	GFR
1	Increase of ≥0.3 mg/dL or increased ≥1.5- to 2-fold from baseline	<0.5 mL/kg/h for >6 h	Risk	Increased × 1.5	Decreased >25%
2	Increased >2- to 3-fold from baseline	<0.5 mL/kg/h for >12 h	Injury	Increased × 2	Decreased >50%
3	Increased >3-fold from baseline, or baseline ≥4.0 mg/dL with an acute rise of ≥0.5 mg/dL or on KRT	<0.5 mL/kg/h for >24 h or anuria for 12 h	Failure	Increased × 3 or baseline >4 mg/dL with an acute rise >0.5 mg/dL	Decreased >75%
			Loss		Persistent AKI = complete loss of kidney function >4 wk
			ESRD		ESRD >3 mo
Time	<48 h		1–7 d Sustained >24 h		

AKI, acute kidney injury; AKIN, Acute Kidney Injury Network; ESRD, end-stage renal disease; GFR, glomerular filtration rate; RIFLE, Risk, Injury, Failure, Loss, End-stage kidney disease; KRT, kidney replacement therapy; SCr, serum creatinine.

TABLE 12-3	Medications and Other Conditions That Affect Serum Creatinine without Actually Affecting Renal Function
Mechanism and Medication	

Increased serum creatinine by the inhibition of creatinine secretion
  Trimethoprim
  Cimetidine	

Increased serum creatinine due to interference with creatinine measurement
  Ascorbic acid
  Cephalosporins
  Flucytosine
  Plasma ketosis	

Falsely low serum creatinine due to interference with creatinine measurement Very high serum bilirubin levels (usually 5.85 mg/dL)	
Enhanced creatinine production Cooked meat (creatine is converted to creatinine by cooking)	

proximal tubular creatinine secretion and may cause a rise in serum creatinine without a fall in GFR (Table 12-3). Once filtered, creatinine cannot be reabsorbed.

2. **Serum Creatinine is Dependent on Factors Independent of Kidney Function.** For example, creatinine production is dependent on muscle mass. Muscle mass declines with age and illness. Therefore, a serum creatinine of 1.2 mg/dL in an elderly, 40-kg patient with cancer and wasted muscles may represent a severely impaired GFR, whereas a serum creatinine of 1.2 mg/dL in a 100-kg weightlifter with large muscle mass may represent a normal GFR. Serum creatinine is also dependent on other factors such as nutritional status, infection, volume of distribution, age, gender, race, body habitus, presence of amputations, malnutrition, and diet.

3. **Creatinine Production and Excretion Must Be in a Steady State Before Creatinine Levels Accurately Reflect the Decline in Kidney Function.** The most commonly used formulae to estimate GFR in CKD patients, in a steady state, are the Chronic Kidney Disease Epidemiology Collaboration (CKD-EPI) equations using either serum creatinine or serum cystatin C. The CKD-EPI creatinine-cystatin C equation (which employs both markers) is thought to be the most accurate marker of GFR in CKD patients but has not been validated in AKI. Other formulae such as Cockcroft–Gault, modification of diet in renal disease (MDRD), and the modified MDRD have fallen out of favor having been shown to be less reliable than the CKD-EPI formula. The CKD-EPI and other formulae are often applied to estimate eGFR in patients with AKI. This may be necessary, for example, for medication dosing (which commonly uses the Cockcroft–Gault formula since many of the early drug dosing studies used this formula). It is important to note, however, that estimation of eGFR in patients with AKI needs to be done with caution, mindful that formulae are inaccurate if a steady state has not yet been reached. For example, after an acute insult, it takes several days for creatinine excretion and production to reach a steady state, and kidney function will be worse than what the formulae suggest.

For example, if a 60-kg, 30-year-old woman with a serum creatinine of 1.0 mg/dL suddenly loses all kidney function, her serum creatinine may only rise to 1.8 mg/dL after 1 day. By CKD-EPI, her GFR is 37 mL/min; by Cockcroft–Gault it is 43 mL/min, but it is actually 0 mL/min. (The CKD-EPI and other formulae to estimate eGFR are available through numerous free online calculators.)

B. Creatinine clearance (CrCl) may be measured in the acute setting to give an estimate of kidney function; more reliable results will be obtained when creatinine production and excretion are in a steady state. Steady state may be suggested when the creatinine reaches its peak and then stabilizes (e.g., if creatinine [mg/dL] is 1.0 at baseline, 2.0 on day 2, 4.0 on day 3, and 4.0 on the subsequent days, one may reasonably conclude that a steady state has been achieved at a creatinine of 4.0). Normal ranges for CrCl are 120 ± 25 mL/min for men and 95 ± 20 mL/min for women. The formula for CrCl performed on a 24-hour urine collection is as follows:

$$\text{CrCl} = [\text{urine creatinine (mg/dL)} \times \text{urine volume (mL/24 hours)}] / [\text{serum Cr (mg/dL)} \times 1{,}440 \text{ minutes}]$$

When the reduction in kidney function is severe, both CrCl and urea clearance may be determined on the same 24-hour urine collection; the average of CrCl and urea clearance may be a more accurate assessment of kidney function than CrCl alone (due to the increase in creatinine secretion that may occur with kidney dysfunction which will increase the amount of creatinine in the urine not related to GFR).

C. Blood urea nitrogen (BUN) as a Marker of AKI and GFR. Normal BUN is 8 to 18 mg/dL. An increase in BUN typically accompanies a rise in serum creatinine in the setting of AKI. Urea is filtered, but not secreted. Increased reabsorption of urea by the proximal tubule and arginine vasopressin (AVP)–sensitive urea transporters in the collecting duct occurs in states of volume depletion. In this setting, BUN can rise without a rise in creatinine, resulting in a BUN to serum creatinine ratio that is greater than 20. BUN levels are affected by multiple factors not related to GFR. Because BUN production is related to protein metabolism, an increase in BUN without a decline in GFR may occur with hypercatabolic states, protein loading, upper gastrointestinal (GI) bleeding, and high-dose steroid administration. Conversely, a low BUN may be present in the setting of reduced GFR in patients who are on a low-protein diet, are severely malnourished, or have severe liver disease.

D. Cystatin C as a Marker of AKI and GFR. Cystatin C is a protein produced by all nucleated cells. It is freely filtered by the glomerulus, completely reabsorbed by the proximal tubules, and is not secreted by the renal tubules. Therefore, some of the limitations of serum creatinine, for example, effect of muscle mass, are not a problem with cystatin C. In AKI, changes in cystatin C are generally observed to occur sooner after changes in kidney function than serum creatinine. In the recovery phase of AKI, the serum cystatin C decreases faster than serum creatinine. In studies, serum cystatin C correlated better with GFR than did serum creatinine and was diagnostically superior to creatinine, especially in patients with liver cirrhosis. Cystatin C is best measured by an immunonephelometric assay. Cystatin C is particularly useful in patients with reduced muscle mass due to frailty, amputations, immobilization (e.g., spinal cord injury), or prolonged critical illness where serum creatinine is a less reliable marker of kidney function. Cystatin C should be measured in patients in whom serum creatinine is judged to be a poor marker of kidney function.

E. Biomarkers of AKI. There has been an ongoing investigation into the identification of biomarkers of AKI that might detect kidney injury earlier and with more sensitivity and specificity than the traditional markers of kidney function (e.g., creatinine, BUN, and cystatin C) described above. Nephrocheck® is an assay that measures cell cycle arrest markers metalloproteinase-2 (TIMP-2) and insulin-like growth factor–binding protein 7 (IGFBP7) in the urine. Measurement of urinary TIMP-2/IGFBP7 is an FDA-approved test for the early detection, before serum creatinine, of patients at high risk for AKI after cardiac surgery and in the ICU with sepsis or shock. Nephrocheck® can discriminate the septic shock patients with an AKIN stage 1 or 2 AKI who will not progress to the AKIN stage 3 level. Urinary interleukin-18 (IL-18), neutrophil gelatinase–associated lipocalin (NGAL), kidney injury molecule-1 (Kim-1), and tubular enzymes have been found to increase 1 to 2 days before serum creatinine in patients with ischemic AKI. Higher levels of IL-18, NGAL, KIM-1, and liver fatty acid binding protein (L-FABP) also predict worsening AKI and death. Urine NGAL is available in some health care systems.

F. Distinguishing AKI from CKD. CKD is defined by the presence of kidney damage or reduced GFR for 3 or more months. Distinguishing AKI from CKD may be challenging. Laboratory findings such as hyperphosphatemia, hypoalbuminemia, and hyperkalemia are unreliable factors to distinguish AKI from CKD and may be present in either case. Symptoms such as nausea, vomiting, and malaise may also occur in AKI or CKD. Potential methods to distinguish between the two include the following:

1. **Old Records.** The most reliable way to distinguish AKI from CKD is an evaluation of old records. Assessment of serum creatinine in a stable outpatient setting is the most reliable method to determine baseline creatinine and the presence of CKD. Multiple creatinine levels should be reviewed as patients may have had episodes of AKI which do not represent their true baseline.

2. **Kidney Ultrasonography.** As summarized in Table 12-4, ultrasound may be a useful technique to distinguish AKI from CKD. Increased echogenicity (i.e., the kidney appears brighter than the normal liver) does not distinguish between AKI and CKD and may be present or absent in either. That said, increased echogenicity is abnormal, and suggests that some level of kidney pathology is present. Useful ultrasound features to identify CKD include decreased kidney length (<9 cm) or cortical thinning (<1 cm), and are not features of AKI. It is important to note that since AKI is common in patients with CKD, the presence of small kidneys or a thin cortex does not necessarily exclude the possibility that AKI is also present. For reference, "normal" kidney size is dependent on age. For example, at age 55, normal kidney length is approximately 11 cm; at age 75, normal kidney length is approximately 10 cm (although it is currently unknown whether the decrease in kidney length that is observed in aging is "normal" or represents undetected CKD). Normal cortex length is generally considered to be 1 cm or greater.

TABLE 12-4 Use of Ultrasonography to Distinguish Acute from Chronic Kidney Diseases

Ultrasound Finding	Acute	Chronic
Increased echogenicity	Yes	Yes
Cortical thinning <1 cm	No	Yes
Decrease in renal size <9 cm in length	No	Yes

3. **Anemia.** Normochromic normocytic anemia is common in patients with CKD and a GFR of less than 30 mL/min; in patients with a GFR of 30 to 44 mL/min, only approximately 20% of patients have anemia. Therefore, with a GFR of 30 mL/min or below, the absence of anemia suggests that the decline in kidney function may be acute. In some etiologies of CKD (e.g., autosomal dominant polycystic kidney disease), however, anemia may be absent. In some etiologies of AKI, anemia may be present, for example, hemolytic uremic syndrome (HUS) or thrombotic thrombocytopenic purpura (TTP). Thus, the presence or absence of anemia must be interpreted in context with other clinical indicators when considering the diagnosis of AKI versus CKD.

G. **Urine Output in AKI.** AKI is typically described as either oliguric or nonoliguric. **Oliguria** is defined as a urine output of less than 400 mL/d; in general, 400 mL is the minimum amount of urine that a person in a normal metabolic state must excrete to get rid of the daily solute production. For example, a person with a daily solute production of 500 mOsm who concentrates urine to a maximum of 1,200 mOsm/L would need to pass approximately 400 mL of urine per day to excrete the daily solute production (i.e., 500 mOsm/1,200 mOsm/L = 417 mL of urine per day).

Anuria is defined as a lack of urine (or a minimal amount, i.e., <50 mL/d) obtained from the bladder. It is most often caused by complete bilateral urinary tract obstruction, urinary tract obstruction in a solitary kidney, and shock. Less common causes are HUS, rapidly progressive glomerulonephritis (RPGN), particularly antiglomerular basement membrane (GBM) antibody disease, and bilateral renal arterial or venous occlusion.

II. Classifications of AKI: Definitions and Causes

AKI is classified as either intrinsic renal or postrenal. Prerenal disease (alternatively known as prerenal azotemia or prerenal AKI) may also cause a decline in GFR that is reflected by increased serum creatinine and BUN.

A. **Prerenal Disease** (Fig. 12-1). Prerenal disease is a fall in the GFR due to reduced renal perfusion in which no or minimal injury to the kidney has occurred. Urine sediment is typically bland and hyaline casts may be present. Essential to this diagnosis is that kidney function returns to normal within 24 to 72 hours of correction of the hypoperfused state. Some studies have demonstrated that certain biomarkers of AKI are increased in clinically defined prerenal disease, suggesting that term prerenal AKI could also be used. That said, the use of biomarkers to distinguish prerenal disease from intrinsic kidney injury disease is controversial, with disagreement regarding the appropriate use, interpretation, and levels of clinically relevant biomarkers increase. Prerenal disease occurs in the following situations:

1. **Total Intravascular Volume Depletion.** This condition can occur in a number of settings where intravascular volume is reduced and may be secondary to
   a. Hemorrhage
   b. Renal fluid loss
      - Excessive diuresis (e.g., diuretics)
      - Osmotic diuresis (e.g., glucosuria, mannitol administration)
      - Primary adrenal insufficiency (i.e., hypoaldosteronism)
      - Salt-wasting nephritis
      - Diabetes insipidus
   c. GI fluid loss
      - Vomiting
      - Diarrhea
      - Nasogastric tube drainage

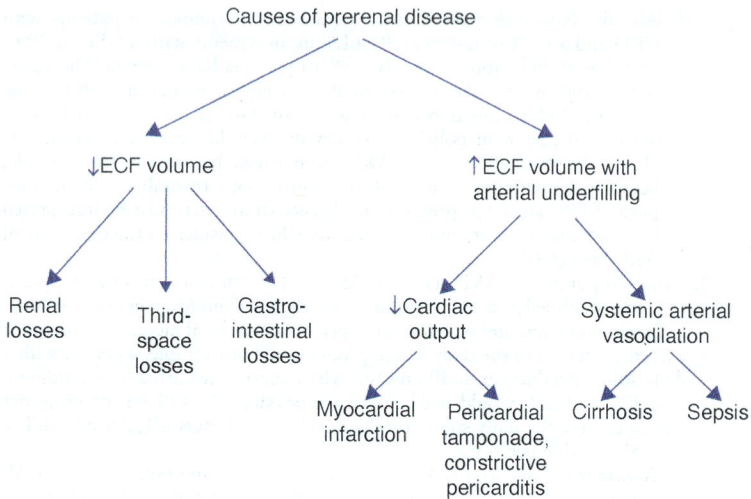

Figure 12-1. Causes of prerenal disease. Prerenal disease may be secondary to true intravascular volume depletion or arterial underfilling from a decrease in cardiac output or arterial vasodilatation. The extracellular fluid (ECF) volume comprises the intravascular and the interstitial body water compartments.

    d. Skin fluid loss
- Burns
- Excessive sweating
- Hyperthermia

    e. Third-space fluid loss
- Peritonitis
- Pancreatitis
- Systemic inflammatory response syndrome
- Profound hypoalbuminemia

2. **Effective Volume Depletion from Arterial Underfilling.** Arterial underfilling is a state in which intravascular volume is actually normal (or even increased) but circulatory factors are inadequate to maintain kidney perfusion pressure. Underfilling may be due to either a decrease in cardiac output or arterial vasodilatation and may occur in a number of clinical settings:

    a. Reduced cardiac output
- Acute decompensated heart failure (ADHF) (previously referred to as congestive heart failure)
- Cardiogenic shock
- Pericardial effusion with tamponade
- Massive pulmonary embolism

    b. Peripheral vasodilatation
- Sepsis
- Antihypertensive medications
- Anaphylaxis
- Anesthesia
- Cirrhosis and other liver diseases

3. **Intrarenal Hemodynamic Changes**
   a. Glomerular afferent arteriole vasoconstriction (preglomerular effect)
      - Nonsteroidal anti-inflammatory drugs (NSAIDs) (prostaglandin inhibition)
      - Cyclooxygenase 2 (Cox-2) inhibitors (prostaglandin inhibition)
      - Cyclosporine
      - Tacrolimus
      - Radiocontrast dye
      - Hypercalcemia
   b. Glomerular efferent arteriole vasodilatation (postglomerular effect)
      - Angiotensin-converting enzyme inhibitors (ACEIs)
      - Angiotensin II receptor blockers (ARBs)

B. Postrenal AKI. Postrenal AKI is caused by the acute obstruction of the flow of urine. Urinary obstruction of both ureters, the bladder, or the urethra may cause postrenal AKI. Patients most at risk for postrenal AKI are elderly men, in whom prostatic hypertrophy or prostatic cancer may lead to complete or partial obstruction of urine flow. In women, complete urinary tract obstruction is relatively uncommon in the absence of pelvic surgery, pelvic malignancy, or previous pelvic irradiation. The causes of postrenal AKI include the following:

1. **Bilateral Ureteral Obstruction or Unilateral Obstruction in a Solitary Kidney (Upper Urinary Tract Obstruction)**
   a. Intraureteral
      - Stones
      - Blood clots
      - Pyogenic debris or sloughed papillae
      - Edema following retrograde pyelography
      - Transitional cell carcinoma
   b. Extraureteral
      - Pelvic or abdominal malignancy
      - Retroperitoneal fibrosis
      - Accidental ureteral ligation or trauma during pelvic surgery
   c. Bladder neck/urethral obstruction (lower urinary tract obstruction)
      - Prostatic hypertrophy
      - Prostatic and bladder carcinoma
      - Autonomic neuropathy or anticholinergic agents causing urinary retention
      - Urethral stricture
      - Bladder stones
      - Fungal infection (e.g., fungus balls)
      - Blood clots

C. Intrarenal or Intrinsic AKI. In contrast to prerenal disease and postrenal AKI, the disorders listed here represent problems that originate within the kidney itself. These problems may be vascular, glomerular, interstitial, or tubular. The diseases may be primary renal or part of a systemic disease. The course of AKI in these situations cannot be changed by manipulating factors outside the kidney (e.g., performing volume repletion, improving cardiac function, correcting hypotension, or removing obstruction).

1. **Vascular.** Vascular disorders causing AKI are classified based on the size of the vessels involved.
   a. Large- and medium-sized vessels
      - Renal artery thrombosis or embolism
      - Operative arterial cross-clamping
      - Bilateral renal vein thrombosis
      - Polyarteritis nodosa

b. Small vessels
- Atheroembolic disease
- TTP-HUS
- Scleroderma renal crisis
- Malignant hypertension
- Hemolysis, Elevated Liver enzymes, and Low Platelets (HELLP) syndrome
- Postpartum AKI

2. **Glomerular.** Glomerular diseases are typically categorized based on urine findings as either nephrotic or nephritic.
   a. **Nephrotic** glomerular disorders are characterized by large proteinuria (greater than 3 g in 24 hours) and minimal hematuria. Nephrotic glomerular disorders are uncommonly associated with AKI, but may occur in minimal-change disease or focal segmental glomerulosclerosis (FSGS), particularly collapsing FSGS.
   b. **Nephritic** glomerular disorders (glomerulonephritis) are characterized by hematuria and proteinuria (typically 1 to 2 g in 24 hours). Patients with known glomerulonephritis may develop AKI; alternatively, glomerulonephritis may present as AKI. Rapidly progressing Glomerulonephritis (RPGN), also called *crescentic nephritis*, should be suspected in a patient with rising creatinine, hematuria, and proteinuria. RPGN is defined clinically as a doubling of serum creatinine in a 3-month period in a patient with glomerulonephritis. RPGN is caused by injury to the glomerular capillary wall, which results in subsequent inflammation, fibrosis, and crescent formation. Urgency is required to make the diagnosis of RPGN, because crescent formation can rapidly destroy the glomeruli; response to therapy is directly correlated with the percentage of glomeruli having crescents. If RPGN is suspected, a biopsy should be performed as soon as possible as waiting even a few days can result in irreversible loss of kidney function. Because the diagnosis is typically made by kidney biopsy, the causes of glomerulonephritis and RPGN are classified according to immunofluorescence staining on kidney biopsy.
      i. **Diseases with Linear (anti-GBM) Immune Complex Deposition**
         - Goodpasture syndrome (renal and pulmonary complications are present)
         - Renal-limited Goodpasture syndrome
      ii. **Diseases with Granular Immune Complex Deposition**
         - Acute postinfectious glomerulonephritis
         - Lupus nephritis
         - Infective endocarditis
         - Immunoglobulin (Ig) A glomerulonephritis
         - Henoch–Schönlein purpura
         - Membranoproliferative glomerulonephritis
         - Cryoglobulinemia
      iii. **Diseases with No Immune Deposits (Pauci-immune)**
         - Granulomatosis with polyangiitis (GPA) (formerly known as Wegener granulomatosis)
         - Microscopic polyangiitis (MPA)
         - Churg–Strauss syndrome (CSS)
         - Idiopathic crescentic glomerulonephritis

3. **Interstitium.** AKI from an interstitial cause is known as *acute interstitial nephritis* (*AIN*). The primary histologic lesion of AIN is marked edema of the interstitial space with a focal or diffuse infiltration of the kidney interstitium with inflammatory cells (lymphocytes and/or eosinophils). AIN (also called *acute tubulointerstitial nephritis*) is most commonly due

to drug hypersensitivity, but may also be a consequence of infections or systemic disease (e.g., systemic lupus erythematosus).
   a. **Drug-Induced AIN.** More than 100 drugs have been implicated in drug-induced AIN. Some of the drugs most commonly associated with AIN are as follows:
      - **Antibiotics** (e.g., methicillin, cephalosporins, rifampicin, sulfonamides, erythromycin, and ciprofloxacin)
      - **Diuretics** (e.g., furosemide, thiazides, chlorthalidone)
      - **Anticonvulsant drugs** (e.g., phenytoin, carbamazepine)
      - **Allopurinol**
   b. **Infection-Associated AIN**
      - **Bacterial** (e.g., *Staphylococcus*, *Streptococcus*)
      - **Viral** (e.g., cytomegalovirus, Epstein–Barr virus)
      - **Tuberculosis**
4. **Tubular.** Acute tubular injury (ATI) (formerly known as acute tubular necrosis [ATN]) is characterized by an abrupt decrease in GFR due to proximal tubular dysfunction most commonly caused by ischemic AKI or nephrotoxic AKI. ATI has long been referred to as ATN, yet—in many cases—true necrosis of tubular cells is not present on histologic examination. Most of the kidney biopsies are, however, late and therefore could miss early tubular necrosis. The tubules may demonstrate morphologic changes of sublethal injury (e.g., swelling, vacuolization, loss of brush border, apical blebbing, and loss of basolateral infoldings). Loss of viable and nonviable tubular epithelial cells into the urine also occurs. The continued presence of renal blood flow and reversibility of tubular dysfunction is compatible with the recovery of kidney function that is seen in some patients with ischemic or nephrotoxic AKI.

   Ischemic AKI is a consequence of reduced blood flow to the kidneys, which results from a decreased total blood volume or arterial underfilling with a redistribution of blood away from the kidney. Ischemic AKI is seen most commonly after septic or hemorrhagic shock. **Nephrotoxic AKI** is most commonly caused by aminoglycoside antibiotics and radiocontrast dye. In most cases, the insults are multifactorial.

   Causes of ischemic or nephrotoxic AKI include the following:
   a. **Kidney Ischemia**
      - Shock
      - Hemorrhage
      - Trauma
      - Sepsis
      - Pancreatitis
      - Hypotension from any cause
   b. **Nephrotoxic Drugs**
      - Aminoglycoside antibiotics
      - Amphotericin B
      - Pentamidine
      - Foscarnet
      - Acyclovir
      - Indinavir
      - Antineoplastic agents (e.g., cisplatin)
      - Radiocontrast dye
      - Organic solvents (e.g., carbon tetrachloride)
      - Ethylene glycol (antifreeze)
   c. **Endogenous Toxins**
      - Myoglobin (e.g., rhabdomyolysis)
      - Hemoglobin (e.g., incompatible blood transfusion, acute falciparum malaria)
      - Uric acid (e.g., acute uric acid nephropathy)

5. **Sepsis.** Sepsis is the most common cause of AKI in the intensive care unit (ICU). The pathophysiology of AKI in sepsis is complex, and many aspects of the cause of kidney function decline in sepsis remain controversial. Although previously thought to be similar to ischemic AKI, it is now understood that septic AKI is a separate entity from ischemic AKI—although ischemic AKI may ultimately occur in severe sepsis or shock from reduced renal blood flow. Kidney function decline in sepsis is likely due to a combination of vascular factors (affecting autoregulation and resulting in decreased GFR) as well as intrinsic tubular damage.

III. Epidemiology of AKI (Table 12-5)
A. **Community-Acquired AKI.** The most common causes of community-acquired AKI include prerenal (70%) and postrenal (17%). The overall mortality of patients presenting with community-acquired AKI is 15%.

TABLE 12-5 Characteristics of AKI in Regard to the Location of Its Development

History/Symptoms	Predisposing Factor(s)	Type of AKI
Community-Acquired AKI		
Acute systemic illness (e.g., viral influenza, gastroenteritis)	Volume depletion	Prerenal disease or ATI
Streptococcal pharyngitis or pyoderma (vesicular skin lesions, typically located on the extremities, which become pustular and then crust)	Immune complex deposition in the glomeruli	Acute poststreptococcal glomerulonephritis
Trauma, crush injury, prolonged immobilization, "found down"	Extensive muscle damage and tissue breakdown	Rhabdomyolysis
Urinary tract symptoms such as difficulty voiding, incontinence, dribbling	Obstruction to urine flow or neurogenic bladder	Postrenal
Fever and/or rash in a patient recently prescribed a new medication	NSAIDs, antibiotics, and diuretics are frequently prescribed on an outpatient basis	Allergic interstitial nephritis
Accidental or intentional overdose of a nephrotoxin (altered mental status may be a frequent accompaniment)	Heavy metal compounds, solvents, ethylene glycol, salicylates, and acetaminophen	Nephrotoxic AKI
AKI Occurring Inside the Hospital		
Excessive fluid loss from aggressive diuresis, nasogastric suction, surgical drains, diarrhea, etc.	Volume depletion	Prerenal disease or ischemic AKI
Surgery with or without concomitant volume depletion	Anesthesia causes renal vasoconstriction, which reduces renal blood flow	Prerenal disease or ischemic AKI
Radiologic (contrast CT) or other procedures (e.g., coronary angiography)	Intravenous contrast dye	Nephrotoxic AKI
Sepsis	Infection, volume depletion, hypotension, nephrotoxic antibiotics (e.g., aminoglycosides)	Ischemic or nephrotoxic AKI

AKI, acute kidney injury; ATI, acute tubular injury; CT, computed tomography; NSAID, nonsteroidal anti-inflammatory drug.

B. **Hospital-Acquired AKI.** The development of AKI in hospitalized patients is common and carries with it a significant independent risk of mortality. Up to 20% of hospitalized patients may develop AKI. The most common causes of AKI in hospitalized patients include ischemia, sepsis, medications, and radiocontrast dye. Prerenal disease and ATI (including sepsis) account for the majority of cases of hospital-acquired AKI. In the ICU, AKI is typically multifactorial and may be part of multiple organ dysfunction syndrome.

C. **Prevention of AKI.** Numerous factors predispose hospitalized patients to the development of AKI: sepsis, volume depletion, drugs that affect renal blood flow (e.g., NSAIDs and COX-2 inhibitors), and the use of nephrotoxic medications and contrast dye. Although data are limited on treatments to prevent AKI, it is prudent to carefully follow volume status and maintain adequate hydration; discontinue (when possible) medications that are potentially nephrotoxic; choose alternate nonradiocontrast imaging techniques (e.g., magnetic resonance imaging without gadolinium); and use nonnephrotoxic antibiotics. It is important to carefully weigh the benefits of contrast procedures—including CT scans that require contrast as well as cardiac catheterization against the potential harm of contrast-associated AKI (CA AKI). It is often appropriate to accept the risk of CA AKI in patients who need contrasted CT studies or cardiac catheterization for appropriate evaluation and management.

D. **Morbidity and Mortality Associated with AKI.** It was previously thought that AKI is a completely reversible disorder. Recent data suggest that of patients who develop AKI in the ICU and require dialysis, 10% to 30% may require maintenance dialysis after discharge from the hospital. Severe AKI has been associated with an increase in cardiovascular events, heart failure, and numerous other long-term consequences after discharge. Another previously held belief is that patients die with AKI, not from AKI. Numerous well-controlled studies have found that after adjusting for comorbidities, the development of AKI in hospitalized patients is an independent and significant predictor of in-hospital mortality, regardless of whether the AKI is mild or requires KRT. Clinical and animal data suggest that AKI is a multisystem disease that affects the lung, brain, liver, metabolic function, and immune function. These multisystem effects likely contribute to the increased mortality observed in patients with AKI. AKI requiring KRT has one of the highest mortality rates of any hospitalized condition, for example, AKI requiring KRT in the ICU has a mortality of 45% to 55%.

IV. Evaluation of the Patient with AKI

A stepwise evaluation approach to the patient with AKI is recommended. A comprehensive **history** and thorough **physical examination** suggest the diagnosis in most patients.

Whether the patient is seen for the first time in the office, emergency room, hospital, or ICU, careful tabulation and recording of data are the first steps in determining the diagnosis. Vital signs, daily weights, records of intake and output, past and current laboratory data, and the fluid and medication list should be recorded on a flow sheet and included in the patient's chart. When the patient has been hospitalized for several days or weeks with a complicated course before developing AKI, a carefully prepared flow sheet may often be the only way to comprehend the problem and guide the selection of proper therapy.

Urinalysis by dipstick and the evaluation of **urine sediment** by microscopy should always be performed in patients with AKI. **Urine chemistries** that may be helpful in the diagnosis of AKI include sodium, creatinine, urea, osmolality, and proteinuria.

Clinical features of the common causes of AKI are described in the following sections.

A. **Prerenal Disease.** This may occur in patients who are clinically hypovolemic (total intravascular volume depletion) or hypervolemic (arterial underfilling).
  1. **History.** The following history is suggestive of prerenal disease from true volume depletion or hypovolemia: thirst, decreased fluid intake, fever, nausea, vomiting, diarrhea, burns, peritonitis, and pancreatitis. Prerenal disease from arterial underfilling occurs most commonly in patients with ADHF or liver disease. Features of the history that are suggestive of ADHF include recent myocardial infarction, orthopnea, paroxysmal nocturnal dyspnea, or dyspnea on exertion. Features suggesting liver disease and cirrhosis include a history of alcohol abuse or hepatitis. A complete documentation of medications (prescribed and over-the-counter) is important in the evaluation of prerenal disease. Medications that affect intrarenal hemodynamics include cyclosporine, tacrolimus, NSAIDs, Cox-2 inhibitors, ACEIs, and ARBs.
  2. **Physical Examination.** Assessment of volume status and the adequacy of the extracellular fluid (ECF) volume are critical to the diagnosis of prerenal disease.
     a. **Physical findings that suggest a reduction in intravascular volume** include the following:
        - Absence of axillary sweat
        - A recent reduction in body weight
        - Orthostatic hypotension. Defined as a fall in systolic blood pressure of more than 20 mmHg or a rise in pulse rate of more than 10 beats/min after standing
        - Tachycardia
        - Dry mucous membranes
        - "Tenting" of upper thorax skin when pinched between the fingers
        - Jugular venous pressure not visible when supine
        - Point of care ultrasound (POCUS). POCUS is an emerging technique that may be a useful adjunct to physical examination to identify patients who may be responsive to a fluid challenge. The diameter and collapsibility of the inferior vena cava are features that are typically assessed. The procedure requires specific training.
     b. **Physical examination findings generally found in arterial underfilling states with an excess of ECF** (which is generally characterized by peripheral edema) include the following:
        - Elevated jugular venous pressure
        - Ascites
        - Lower extremity pitting edema
        - Anasarca

        ADHF in particular may be identified by
        - Pulmonary crackles
        - S3 gallop

        Liver failure may be identified by
        - Jaundice
        - Decreased liver size
        - Palmar erythema
        - Spider angiomas
  3. **Urinary Findings.** Regardless of the cause of prerenal disease (hypovolemic, arterial underfilling, or medication induced), the urine dipstick, sediment, and chemistries will be the same (see Table 12-6 for a comparison of urinary findings in various types of AKI).
     a. The urine **dipstick** should be normal with negative protein, heme, leukocyte esterase, and nitrate. The specific gravity is increased (<1.020).
     b. The **urine sediment** may be bland and hyaline casts may be present.

TABLE 12-6 Urinary Findings in Various Causes of AKI

	Prerenal Disease[a]	Postrenal[b]	Small Vessel Vascular	Nephrotic Glomerular	Nephritic Glomerular	AIN	ATI[c]
Dipstick							
Leukocyte esterase	(−)	(−)	(−)	(−)	(−)	(+)	(−)
Heme	(−)	(−)	(+)	(−) or trace	(+)	(+)	(−)
Protein	(−)	(−)	(+)	(+)	(+)	(+)	(−) or trace
Specific gravity	>1.020	1.010	Variable	Variable	Variable	1.010	1.010
Microscopy							
RBCs	(−)	(−)	(+)	(−) or few	(+)	(+)	(−)
WBCs	(−)	(−)	(−)	(−)	(−)	(+)	(−)
RBC casts	(−)	(−)	(+)	(−)	(+)	(−)	(−)
WBC casts	(−)	(−)	(−)	(−)	(−)	(+)	(−)
Granular casts	(−)	(−)	(−)	(−)	(−)	(−)	(+)
Renal tubular epithelial cells	(−)	(−)	(−)	(−)	(−)	(−)	(+)
Tests							
Osmolality (mOsm/L)	>500	≤350	Variable	Variable	Variable	≤350	≤350
Protein (g/d)	(−)	(−)	1–2	>3	1–2	1–2	≤1

[a] Although classically associated with a bland urinary sediment, a few granular casts may occasionally be present.
[b] If a superimposed infection is present due to urine stasis, the leukocyte esterase, heme, protein, RBCs, and WBCs may be positive.
[c] If ATI is secondary to rhabdomyolysis, heme will be positive on dipstick and RBCs will be absent on microscopy.

AKI, acute kidney injury; AIN, acute interstitial nephritis; ATI, acute tubular injury; RBCs, red blood cells; WBCs, white blood cells.

TABLE 12-7 Urinary Diagnostic Indices

Index	Prerenal Disease	ATI
Urine sodium (UNa), mEq/L	<20	>40
Urine osmolality, mOsm/kg H$_2$O	>500	<350
UCr to PCr	>40	<20
BUN/serum creatinine	>20	≤10
Fractional excretion of sodium (FENa): FENa = [(UNa/PNa)/(UCr/PCr)] × 100	<1	>1
Fractional excretion of urea (FEUN): FEUN = [(UUN/BUN)/(UCr/PCr)] × 100	<35	>50

Please note that many causes of ATI may have urine indices that are consistent with prerenal disease. However, in the absence of diuretics (or other causes of diuresis), it is unusual for the urine indices associated with ATI to be present in prerenal disease. Thus, urine indices consistent with ATI are unusual in prerenal disease.

ATI, acute tubular injury; BUN, blood urea nitrogen (mg/dL); PCr, plasma creatinine (mg/dL); PNa, plasma sodium (mEq/L); UCr, urine creatinine; UUN, urine urea nitrogen (mg/dL).

c. **Urine Chemistry and Indices.** Frequently it is difficult to distinguish between prerenal disease and ATI. Laboratory tests and indices characteristic of prerenal disease versus other causes of AKI are summarized in Table 12-7. The pathophysiologic basis of these tests is discussed below. Please note that many causes of ATI may have urine indices that are consistent with prerenal disease. However, in the absence of diuretics (or other causes of diuresis), it is unusual for the urine indices associated with ATI to be present in prerenal disease. Thus, urine indices consistent with ATI are unusual in prerenal disease.
4. **Specific Disorders of Prerenal Disease**
   a. **Hepatorenal syndrome (HRS)** occurs in patients with severe liver failure. It is characterized by peripheral vasodilatation (low systemic vascular resistance) accompanied by intense renal vasoconstriction that causes a fall in GFR. Two forms of HRS are recognized. **Type 1 HRS, also known as HRS-AKI** is the more severe form and is characterized by an abrupt decline of kidney function, defined as a doubling of serum creatinine to greater than 2.5 mg/dL within 2 weeks. Without liver transplantation, the mortality of this condition is very high. Type 2 HRS is characterized by slowly progressing kidney insufficiency (serum creatinine greater than 1.5 mg/dL) in a patient with refractory ascites; it has a much better prognosis. Patients with type 2 HRS may convert to type 1 in the setting of certain insults such as the development of infections (e.g., spontaneous bacterial peritonitis) or the use of NSAIDs. The only permanent cure for HRS is liver transplantation unless there is substantial recovery of liver function.

   Diagnostic Criteria for HRS-AKI:
   - Diagnosis of acute or chronic liver disease with portal hypertension
   - Diagnosis of AKI defined by increase in SCr of ≥0.3 mg/dL within a 48-hour period, or a ≥50% increase from the lowest SCr value observed over the prior 3 months

- No response at 48 hours of plasma volume expansion using albumin 1 g/kg of body weight and withdrawal of diuretics
- Absence of other predominant explanations of kidney injury such as shock, nephrotoxin exposure
- No macroscopic signs of structural kidney injury defined as follows:
  - Absence of proteinuria (<500 mg/d)
  - Absence of microhematuria (<50 RBCs per high-power field)

It should be noted that establishing the diagnosis of HRS-AKI is challenging, and some level of urgency to make the diagnosis is important since early initiation of vasopressor treatment (e.g., terlipressin, discussed below) may be beneficial.

b. **Acute decompensated heart failure (ADHF).** ADHF may occur in patients due to either new HF or exacerbation of chronic HF. Numerous cardiac conditions may lead to ADHF which is characterized by insufficient cardiac function. The reduced system perfusion may lead to reduced kidney perfusion and prerenal disease. Pulmonary and peripheral edema are characteristic.

c. **Vasomotor Prerenal Disease Due to NSAIDs.** A history of NSAID use in all patients with prerenal disease or AKI should be assessed. Under euvolemic conditions with normal kidney, liver, and cardiac function, the administration of NSAIDs does not cause an increase in serum creatinine. In the presence of clinical conditions with increased renal vasoconstrictor activity (e.g., ADHF, cirrhosis, nephrotic syndrome, hypertension, sepsis, volume depletion, anesthesia), NSAIDs can cause prerenal disease. Patients with CKD (e.g., diabetic nephropathy) are also at risk for acute vasomotor decline in kidney function with NSAIDs. Typical clinical features include the presence of risk factors, decreased urinary output, usually bland urine sediment, low (less than 1%) fractional excretion of sodium (FENa), and prompt improvement in kidney function after discontinuation of NSAIDs. NSAIDs may cause AIN and contribute to ischemic AKI.

d. **Cyclosporine and tacrolimus** are calcineurin inhibitors that may cause a dose-dependent, hemodynamically mediated prerenal disease in patients who have undergone solid-organ and bone marrow transplantation. A large increase in renal vascular resistance occurs. The loss of kidney function is generally reversible when the dosage of the drug is reduced. The urine sediment is bland. Animal and human data suggest that concurrent administration of calcium channel blockers may protect against calcineurin inhibitor toxicity.

e. **ACEIs and ARBs** are widely used for the treatment of hypertension, heart failure, and diabetic nephropathy. Prerenal disease may occur in conditions where angiotensin plays a crucial protective role in maintaining GFR by constricting the glomerular efferent arteriole, such as volume depletion, bilateral renal artery stenosis, autosomal dominant polycystic kidney disease, cardiac failure, cirrhosis, and diabetic nephropathy. Diuretic-induced sodium depletion and underlying CKD are other major predisposing factors. The decline in kidney function is usually asymptomatic, nonoliguric, and associated with hyperkalemia; kidney function returns to baseline in most cases after discontinuation of the ACEI or ARB. Prerenal disease from ACEI or ARB can usually be managed in the outpatient setting by discontinuation of the ACEI or ARB and discontinuation of diuretics if present. An increase in BUN and serum creatinine in a patient on an ACEI or ARB should raise the possibility of renal artery stenosis.

B. Postrenal AKI

1. **History.** Symptoms that suggest urinary tract obstruction are anuria or intermittent anuria and polyuria, prostatic symptoms (urinary frequency and urgency, dysuria, straining upon urination), pelvic malignancy or previous radiotherapy, and recurrent kidney stones. Patients may complain of pain over a distended bladder; severe pain (renal colic) may be present if obstruction is due to kidney calculi. Patients with diabetes mellitus, sickle cell anemia, analgesic nephropathy, and benign prostatic hypertrophy are predisposed to papillary necrosis that causes obstruction.

2. **Physical Examination.** The physical examination is important in diagnosing postrenal AKI, especially in the unconscious patient or in the confused patient in whom otherwise unexplained agitation may be the only clue to acute urinary retention. Careful abdominal examination may uncover a distended, tender bladder or bilaterally hydronephrotic kidneys. A digital examination of the prostate should be performed routinely in any male patient with AKI. Although it is tempting to place a Foley catheter immediately to assess urine volume and relieve obstruction, we recommend obtaining an ultrasound first, if it is possible to be done in a timely fashion (within an hour or two) and if complications such as infection and sepsis are absent. As discussed below, ultrasound is the modality of choice to evaluate for obstruction; however, if the obstruction is relieved by catheterization, then the diagnostic utility of ultrasound is lost. Furthermore, catheter placement may significantly alter the diagnostic utility of urinalysis (i.e., red blood cells [RBCs] may be present from catheter placement rather than signifying glomerular diseases). If urine output does not occur, catheter placement is a reasonable and important procedure. The patient should be asked to attempt to void, and urine output after catheterization should be recorded. The normal postvoid residual volume should be less than 50 mL.

3. **Urine Findings.** The typical urinalysis and sediment finding in postrenal AKI compared with other causes of AKI is presented in Table 12-6.
   a. **Urinalysis.** The urine dipstick should be normal with negative protein, heme, leukocyte esterase, and nitrite. The specific gravity is typically isosmotic (1.010). Heme test for RBCs may be positive if obstruction is due to kidney calculi. A secondary infection may be present due to urine stasis; in this setting, the dipstick may be positive for leukocyte esterase, nitrite, heme, and trace protein.
   b. **Urine sediment** is typically bland without cells or casts. As noted, hematuria may be present if obstruction is due to kidney calculi. Prostatitis and some cases of benign prostatic hypertrophy may also be associated with hematuria. In the setting of a secondary urinary tract infection, the sediment may contain white blood cells (WBCs), RBCs, and/or bacteria.

4. **Radiologic Tests.** Kidney ultrasonography is sufficient to diagnose urinary obstruction in most patients.
   a. **Kidney ultrasonography** is the radiologic test of choice to evaluate for obstruction which is characterized by dilatation of the urinary tract (hydronephrosis). The absence of hydronephrosis virtually excludes important urinary tract obstruction; hydronephrosis may be absent, however, in the following settings: early obstruction (before the urinary tract has been able to dilate) and obstruction due to the encasement of the urinary system by retroperitoneal fibrosis or tumor.

   Hydronephrosis that is not functionally significant may occur in pregnancy and in people with anatomic variants of the collecting system. If the functional importance of hydronephrosis is in doubt, a furosemide isotope renogram can evaluate the functional significance of the obstruction.

b. **Isotope renography** is performed by the intravenous injection of a radionucleotide and furosemide. Furosemide increases urinary flow and normally causes a rapid washout of the radionucleotide. Persistence of the isotope in the kidney parenchyma suggests obstruction. Poor kidney function limits the usefulness of this test because the diuretic response may be blunted, thereby making interpretation of the test difficult.
c. **Noncontrast computed tomography** (CT) of the kidneys, ureters, and abdomen is often done following kidney ultrasonography to identify the cause and location of urinary obstruction.
d. **Cystoscopy and Retrograde Pyelography.** In instances of AKI with a high clinical suspicion of urinary tract obstruction (e.g., calculi, pyogenic debris, blood clots, bladder cancer), cystoscopy and retrograde or anterograde pyelography should be performed, even if ultrasonographic findings are negative for obstruction.

C. Intrinsic Kidney Disease—Large Vessel Disease
1. **History.** Renal artery thrombosis or embolism, or bilateral renal vein thrombosis may present with flank pain. Predisposing disorders such as membranous nephropathy or antiphospholipid antibody syndrome may be present.
2. **Urine Findings**
   a. **Urinalysis.** The urine dipstick is positive for heme.
   b. **Urine Sediment.** RBCs.
3. **Laboratory Findings and Radiology.** An elevated serum lactic dehydrogenase (LDH) may be present. Doppler ultrasonography may be used to assess renal blood flow and to evaluate for renal vein thrombosis. CT or MR angiography is useful for detecting clots in the renal vein or inferior vena cava. Angiography may be required in emergent cases (e.g., acute anuria due to acute renal embolization).

D. Intrinsic Kidney Disease—Small Vessel Disease. Intrinsic kidney disease due to small vessel disease is caused by either atheroembolic disease or thrombotic microangiopathy. The clinical and laboratory features of these disorders are as follows:
1. **Atheroembolic disease** is caused by the detachment of atheromatous plaques from the intimal surface of large vessels. These plaques travel distally and occlude small arteries or large arterioles of the kidney. Showers of cholesterol crystals or microemboli from the surface of ulcerated plaques may also occur, traveling distally to occlude small arterioles throughout the body (e.g., kidney, gut, or skin). The presentation and clinical findings of atheroembolic disease like peripheral necrotic areas, blue toe syndrome, and livedo reticularis can be confused with those of polyarteritis nodosa, allergic vasculitis, subacute bacterial endocarditis, or left atrial myxoma. The usual course is progressive kidney insufficiency. However, milder forms of kidney injury with some recovery of function have been described. No treatment is known. Prevention of the disease involves avoiding unnecessary invasive procedures (e.g., renal arteriogram in patients with clinical evidence of widespread atherosclerosis).
   a. **History.** A history of AKI occurring after cardiovascular surgery, angiography, or administration of intravenous thrombolytics or heparin should raise a suspicion of atheroembolic disease as the cause of AKI, particularly in a patient with known atherosclerosis. Occasionally, the disease occurs spontaneously.
   b. **Physical Examination.** Skin manifestations of cholesterol emboli include discrete peripheral necrotic areas, blue toe syndrome, and livedo reticularis. Small cholesterol emboli to the gut and pancreas may cause abdominal pain. Focal neurological defects. Retinal cholesterol crystal emboli (Hollenhorst plaques) seen on fundoscopy.

c. **Laboratory investigation** may reveal an increased erythrocyte sedimentation rate, eosinophilia, and hypocomplementemia (C3 is reduced whereas C4 remains normal). Biopsy of the skin, muscle, or kidney reveals intravascular cholesterol crystals.
d. **Urinary Evaluation**
   i. **Urinalysis.** Dipstick is frequently negative although heme or protein or both may be positive. Specific gravity is variable.
   ii. **Urine Sediment.** Sediment is often bland, although RBCs, granular casts, RBC casts, or all may be present.
   iii. **Urine Tests.** Proteinuria is typically less than 1 g in 24 hours.
2. **Thrombotic microangiopathies** (TMA) are characterized by microangiopathic hemolytic anemia, thrombocytopenia, and variable kidney and neurologic manifestations. These disorders begin with endothelial injury followed by secondary platelet thrombi formation in renal arterioles; renal cortical necrosis may result from the arterial lesions. The primary site of injury is the glomerulus or the vascular supply of the glomerulus; the proximal tubule and interstitium are relatively uninvolved. The primary TMAs are (1) TTP (deficiency of ADAMTS13), (2) complement-mediated TMA (antibodies to complement factor H or I), (3) Shiga toxin–mediated hemolytic uremic syndrome (ST-HUS), and (4) drug-induced TMA (quinine, cyclosporine, cancer therapies). ADAMTS13 is a von Willebrand factor (VWF)-cleaving protease that cleaves ultralarge molecules of VWF made by endothelial cells preventing ultralarge multimers from accumulating in blood vessels.
   a. **History and Physical Examination.** HUS-TTP should be suspected in patients with anemia, AKI, and thrombocytopenia. Malignant hypertension causing thrombotic microangiopathy is characterized by high blood pressure associated with papilledema and/or retinal hemorrhages; other organ involvement may manifest as chest pain, shortness of breath from pulmonary edema, and confusion from brain involvement. Scleroderma renal crisis should be considered in patients with scleroderma and an abrupt rise in serum creatinine associated with hypertension.
   b. **Laboratory Findings.** Peripheral blood smear demonstrates increased RBC fragmentation (schistocytes) and thrombocytopenia. Indices of hemolysis (e.g., LDH) are elevated. Severe decrease of ADAMTS13 activity to <10% or a detectable ADAMTS13 inhibitor (autoantibody) in cases of TTP.
   c. **Urine Findings**
      i. **On Dipstick.** Variable specific gravity; heme positive, protein positive, or both.
      ii. **Urine sediment** is characterized by granular casts, RBC casts, or both.

E. Intrinsic Kidney Disease—Glomerular Disease from a Nephrotic Cause. Nephrotic glomerular disorders are characterized by a urine protein excretion of greater than 3 g in 24 hours. Nephrotic glomerular disorders are uncommonly associated with AKI, but they may occur in patients with minimal-change disease (especially in the elderly) and FSGS (especially from collapsing FSGS). This generally occurs when the serum albumin concentration is less than 2.0 g/dL.
1. **History and Physical Examination.** Clinical symptoms and signs characteristic of a nephrotic disorder include pitting peripheral edema, hypertension, periorbital edema, and anasarca.
2. **Laboratory Findings.** Typically hypoalbuminemia and hypercholesterolemia are present.

3. **Urine Findings.** In cases of minimal-change–induced AKI, urine dipstick and sediment may also include features of ATI.
   a. **Dipstick** is strongly positive for protein. Heme is negative or trace.
   b. **Urine sediment** is typically bland, possibly with few RBCs. Oval fat bodies reflecting lipiduria may be present.
   c. **Urine tests** show proteinuria greater than 3 g in 24 hours.
F. **Intrinsic Kidney Disease—Glomerular Disease from a Nephritic Cause.** Nephritic glomerular disorders (glomerulonephritis) frequently cause AKI. Nephritic glomerular disorders are characterized by hematuria and proteinuria (typically 1 to 2 g in 24 hours). RPGN should be suspected in a patient with an increase in serum creatinine associated with hematuria and proteinuria.
   1. **History and Physical Examination.** Clinical symptoms and signs that suggest that the glomerulonephritis is part of a systemic disease include palpable purpura, skin rash, arthralgias, arthritis, fever, cardiac murmurs, sinusitis, hemoptysis, abdominal pain, and acute neuropathy. Hemoptysis is an ominous symptom in a patient with AKI and may indicate a life-threatening vasculitis, such as Goodpasture syndrome or GPA (formerly known as Wegener granulomatosis).
   2. **Urine Findings.** Glomerulonephritis is characterized by hematuria and proteinuria. The identification of RBC casts confirms the presence of glomerular disease.
   3. **Laboratory Findings.** ANCAs are helpful in determining the cause of glomerulonephritis. ANCA staining by immunofluorescence is either cytoplasmic (c-ANCA) or perinuclear (p-ANCA). Although c-ANCA and p-ANCA are sensitive screening tests, numerous conditions other than vasculitis and glomerulonephritis may result in c-ANCA or p-ANCA positivity. Therefore, all positive results must be confirmed with enzyme-linked immunosorbent assay (ELISA) tests for the more specific antigen targets proteinase 3 (PR3) and myeloperoxidase (MPO). The PR3-ANCA antibody is typically responsible for c-ANCA staining and the MPO-ANCA antibody for the p-ANCA staining.

      Of patients with active GPA (formerly known as Wegener granulomatosis), up to 90% are ANCA positive (the majority are PR3-ANCA positive). Of patients with MPA, 70% are ANCA positive (the majority are MPO-ANCA positive). Of patients with CSS, 50% are ANCA positive (PR3- and MPO-ANCA detected with about equal frequency). More than 90% of patients with kidney-limited, idiopathic pauci-immune vasculitis are ANCA positive (the majority are MPO-ANCA positive).
   4. **Anti-GBM antibodies** are useful for the diagnosis of Goodpasture disease, although false-negative results may occur.
   5. Evaluation of **serum complement** (C3 and C4) may be helpful in the evaluation of patients with AKI and glomerulonephritis. Hypocomplementemia is common in postinfectious glomerulonephritis, lupus nephritis, membranoproliferative glomerulonephritis, and mixed cryoglobulinemia. Another cause of AKI associated with hypocomplementemia includes atheroembolic kidney disease. It is important to recognize that other nonrenal conditions may lower serum complement levels (e.g., sepsis, acute pancreatitis, and advanced liver disease).
G. **Intrinsic Kidney Disease—AIN.** Intrinsic kidney disease due to AIN may be secondary to medications, infections, or a systemic illness such as lupus. On kidney biopsy, it is characterized by interstitial inflammation. Urine sediment generally has WBCs, RBCs. Nonnephrotic range proteinuria is characteristic. WBCs casts may be present. Drug-induced AIN is caused by a wide variety of medications and generally develops within 1 to 4 weeks of initiation, although onset may vary. Over 100 different medications have been associated with

AIN, and are typically grouped into categories; as examples, categories include antibiotics (e.g., cephalosporins, sulfonamides), proton pump inhibitors (e.g., omeprazole), diuretics (e.g., furosemide), and cancer therapeutics (e.g., immune checkpoint inhibitors). NSAID-induced AIN is a distinct category of AIN which is characterized by nephrotic range proteinuria after prolonged NSAID use (i.e., 6 months).

1. **History.** In NSAID-induced AIN, symptoms and findings do not occur until several months after initiation of drug therapy (average 6 months). AIN from other medications typically occurs within a few weeks of drug therapy. Patients may complain of fever, rash, or flank pain.
2. **Physical Examination.** Physical findings with acute drug-induced interstitial nephritis may be lacking, although fever and a maculopapular or petechial skin eruption may occur with any of the agents, particularly the penicillin derivatives and allopurinol.
3. **Laboratory Findings.** Eosinophilia may be present.
4. **Urine Findings.** RBCs and WBCs are characteristic findings; WBC casts may be present. The urine is typically isotonic, and 20% of cases are oliguric. In NSAID-induced AIN, nephrotic-range proteinuria is present in 80% of cases (greater than 3 g in 24 hours).

   The presence of urinary eosinophils is neither sensitive nor specific for the diagnosis of AIN. Indeed, urinary eosinophils are present in many other kidney diseases such as ATI and glomerulonephritis, and may commonly be absent in patients with AIN.

H. **Intrinsic Kidney Disease—Acute tubular injury (ATI), also known as acute tubular necrosis (ATN).** ATI typically occurs in hospitalized patients as a consequence of ischemia or nephrotoxins. The various causes of ATI may also be referred to as ischemic AKI, sepsis-induced AKI, or nephrotoxin-induced AKI.

1. **History.** The evaluation of a patient with suspected ischemic or nephrotoxic AKI must focus on identifying a predisposing cause. The chart should be reviewed for a history of sepsis, hypotensive episodes, fluid losses, aminoglycoside use, NSAID administration, or radiologic procedures associated with contrast administration.
2. **Physical Examination.** Signs of sepsis or ongoing infection should be evaluated. Volume status should be determined (see Section IV.A.2.a).
3. **Laboratory Findings and Urinalysis.** Distinguishing ischemic or nephrotoxic AKI from prerenal disease is often very difficult; this is an important clinical problem because a decline in GFR in hospitalized patients is most commonly due to either ATI or prerenal disease. Because the causative factors for prerenal disease and ATI overlap, distinguishing between the two may become possible only by the outcome of therapy (e.g., if volume repletion improves kidney function, then prerenal disease was present).

   In general, a urine sediment with muddy brown granular casts is characteristic of ischemic or nephrotoxic ATI. However, this finding may be lacking, and other clinical clues will be necessary to make the diagnosis. To distinguish between the two, numerous diagnostic indices and formulae have been developed based on their pathophysiologic differences.

   Prerenal disease is a hemodynamic condition in which tubular function is normal, whereas ATI is characterized by tubular dysfunction. This distinction is the basis for the following tests (Table 12-7):
   - Urine specific gravity
   - Urine osmolality
   - Urine creatinine/plasma creatinine
   - Urine sodium concentration
   - FENa
   - BUN to plasma creatinine ratio

Prerenal disease is characterized by the increased reabsorption of water and sodium by the nephron. The increased reabsorption of water increases urine-specific gravity and osmolality. Tubular reabsorption of urea increases, thereby increasing the BUN-to-plasma creatinine ratio; creatinine, however, is not reabsorbed, and its concentration increases in the urine and increases the urine-to-plasma creatinine ratio. Sodium reabsorption increases, resulting in a low urine sodium concentration and low FENa. In ATI, these processes typically cannot occur. Therefore, urine specific gravity and osmolality are isotonic (similar to plasma), the urine creatinine to plasma creatinine ratio does not increase above a 20:1 ratio, the serum BUN to creatinine ratio does not increase, and urine sodium and FENa are higher than in prerenal disease. FENa is not always increased in ATI; the causes of ATI that are associated with a low urine sodium concentration and low FENa include radiocontrast nephropathy and rhabdomyolysis.

The use of loop diuretics in AKI is a confounding factor in the use of FENa to distinguish prerenal disease and ATI. Distal-acting diuretics (e.g., furosemide) increase urinary sodium excretion and increase FENa even if the patient is prerenal. A study evaluated the use of the fractional excretion of urea nitrogen (FEUN) to distinguish prerenal disease in the setting of diuretic use from ATI (both of which are typically associated with a FENa of greater than 2%). The basis of this test is that urea absorption increases in the proximal tubule in prerenal disease and would not be affected by the use of diuretics, which act on the distal tubule. In prerenal disease, the FEUN is less than 35% and in ATI it is greater than 50%. Keep in mind that FEUN cannot be used in the setting of osmotic diuretic use (e.g., mannitol) because these agents affect proximal tubular reabsorption.

A recent systematic review and meta-analysis evaluated the ability of the FENa to distinguish prerenal disease from intrinsic AKI and found that performance was excellent in the presence of oliguria without either CKD or diuretic use since both situations can be associated with high FENa despite a prerenal cause of AKI. Thus, urine indices need to be interpreted in context.

A urine sodium of less than 1% is typically used to categorize patients as having prerenal disease. Recent studies suggest that very low urine sodium of less than 0.5% is highly predictive of HRS-AKI in patients who are suspected of this disorder.

4. **Specific Causes of Nephrotoxic AKI**
   a. **Aminoglycoside Nephrotoxicity.** AKI occurs in up to 20% of patients on aminoglycosides, even with careful dosing and therapeutic plasma levels. The incidence of nephrotoxicity correlates better with total cumulative dose than with plasma levels. Predisposing factors are old age, preexisting kidney disease, volume depletion, and combination with other agents (e.g., diuretics, cephalosporins, vancomycin). Nephrotoxicity is usually clinically apparent after 5 to 10 days of therapy; early findings are isosthenuria caused by nephrogenic diabetes insipidus, and magnesium and potassium wasting. An increase in serum creatinine and BUN may not develop for the first time until after the drug has been discontinued; conversely, recovery of kidney function after discontinuation of the nephrotoxic aminoglycoside is often delayed and may require weeks or months to be complete. AKI from aminoglycosides is typically nonoliguric. It is suggested that, in patients with normal kidney function in steady state, aminoglycosides are administered as a single-dose daily rather than multiple-dose daily treatment regimens. It is also suggested that aminoglycoside drug levels are monitored when treatment with single daily dosing is used for more than 48 hours.

b. **Vancomycin with and without Concomitant Piperacillin-Tazobactam.** Vancomycin may cause AKI, especially with increased doses, and this risk is increased with the coadministration of piperacillin-tazobactam. Vancomycin alone is associated with ATI which is typically recognized 5 to 7 days after the first dose. When vancomycin and piperacillin-tazobactam are used together, the onset of AKI recognition is sooner. The mechanisms underlying pathophysiology of AKI associated with this combination of medications are not yet clearly elucidated; ATI with or without AIN is the most common manifestation.
c. **Contrast-Associated AKI** (formerly known as **Contrast-Induced Nephropathy**). Radiocontrast agents cause AKI through a direct nephrotoxic effect and by causing kidney vasoconstriction. Risk factors include old age, high-contrast dose, preexisting kidney disease (especially diabetes mellitus), CKD stage 4 or 5, volume depletion, and recent exposure to other agents, such as NSAIDs. AKI typically develops 1 to 2 days after exposure and is typically nonoliguric and associated with a high urine specific gravity, bland urine sediment, and low FENa. Serum creatinine typically peaks at 3 to 4 days and returns to baseline after about a week.
   i. **Prevention.** Either iso-osmolar or low-osmolar contrast media, rather than high-osmolar iodinated contrast media is recommended in patients at increased risk for contrast-induced AKI. Drugs that affect kidney hemodynamics (e.g., NSAIDs) and diuretics should be discontinued before the procedure if possible.

   Although numerous agents have been studied to prevent contrast nephropathy, the only therapies that have been shown to be beneficial are intravenous hydration with either isotonic saline or isotonic sodium bicarbonate before and after the contrast load.

   The Prevention of Serious Adverse Events Following Angiography (PRESERVE) trial is the largest clinical trial comparing different prevention strategies for iodinated contrast-induced AKI in high-risk patients. The PRESERVE trial showed that oral acetylcysteine and intravenous sodium bicarbonate are not superior to i.v. hydration with isotonic saline. The PRESERVE trial concludes that simple i.v. hydration with sodium chloride is a sufficient preventative measure to prevent contrast-induced AKI in high-risk patients. Prophylactic hemofiltration or hemodialysis (HD) is probably harmful and is not a recommended measure to prevent contrast-induced AKI.

   The clinical significance of contrast-induced AKI should not be underestimated. It has been demonstrated that the development of AKI after contrast administration is associated with an adjusted odds ratio of death of 5.5 versus patients who do not develop AKI.

   Other agents tested and demonstrated to be ineffective in the prevention of contrast-induced AKI include furosemide, mannitol, theophylline, dopamine, fenoldopam, and atrial natriuretic peptide.
d. **Rhabdomyolysis** is caused by muscle injury (traumatic or atraumatic) that leads to the systemic release of muscle contents including myoglobin. Myoglobin is a heme pigment that is directly nephrotoxic; the intratubular precipitation of myoglobin causes obstruction and also contributes to the development of AKI. Rhabdomyolysis should be considered in patients with trauma, muscle pain, and dark brown urine. However, rhabdomyolysis is frequently atraumatic, and up to 50% of patients have no muscular complaints. In Table 12-8, predisposing factors for rhabdomyolysis are listed.

   The characteristic **urine finding** is a heme-positive urine with absence of RBCs. Pigmented granular casts are typically present on

TABLE 12-8 Causes of Rhabdomyolysis

Direct muscle damage (e.g., crush injuries, polymyositis, prolonged immobilization associated with unconsciousness)
Muscle ischemia (e.g., arterial occlusion or embolism)
Excess energy consumption (e.g., seizures, hyperthermia, delirium tremens)
Decreased energy production (e.g., severe hypophosphatemia, hypokalemia, myxedema, genetic defect)
Drugs and toxins (e.g., alcohol, heroin, cocaine, amphetamines, poisonous insect, and snake bites)
Severe infections (e.g., tetanus, Legionnaire disease, influenza)

urine sediment. Laboratory clues to the diagnosis include a rapid rise of serum creatinine, massively increased creatine phosphokinase, hyperphosphatemia, hyperuricemia, hypocalcemia, increased anion gap, and disproportionate hyperkalemia. Serum calcium is reduced due to the sequestration of calcium into injured muscle; this calcium is released from the tissue during the recovery phase and may cause hypercalcemia. Therefore, replacement of serum calcium should be avoided unless symptoms of hypocalcemia are present.

The only proven **therapy** in the treatment of rhabdomyolysis is early and vigorous infusion of intravenous isotonic saline. In crush injury, it is recommended that intravenous saline be administered even before extrication. Mannitol and other diuretics, and urinary alkalinization with bicarbonate, were previously thought to have theoretical benefits in the treatment of rhabdomyolysis. Since their efficacy has not been demonstrated treatment with these agents is not recommended.

e. **Acute Uric Acid Nephropathy.** Uric acid causes AKI due to the intratubular deposition of uric acid crystals. A very high serum uric acid concentration is present (e.g., ≥15 mg/dL). The condition typically occurs during induction chemotherapy for malignancies with high cell turnover (e.g., leukemias and lymphoproliferative malignancies). Acute uric acid nephropathy and AKI occur in tumor lysis syndrome but may occur spontaneously in patients with high tumor burden. Clinical features of acute uric acid nephropathy are hyperuricemia, hyperkalemia, hyperphosphatemia, and a urine urate to creatinine ratio higher than 1. Preventive measures include allopurinol administration (300 to 600 mg/d) and vigorous hydration and forced diuresis with mannitol. Rasburicase, a recombinant urate oxidase, can lower uric acid levels rapidly allowing earlier initiation of chemotherapy, and may reduce the risk of acute uric acid nephropathy. Patients at high risk for tumor lysis syndrome, for example, Burkitt lymphoma, should receive rasburicase 0.2 mg/kg daily for 5 to 7 days.

V. AKI in Special Clinical Circumstances

A. **Crystal-Associated AKI.** A number of important causes of AKI may be due to the formation of urinary crystals. In Table 12-9, the causes of AKI associated with crystal formation are listed.

B. **Abdominal Compartment Syndrome (ACS).** ACS is an important cause of AKI to be aware of since rapid diagnosis and treatment are necessary to reverse

TABLE 12-9 Urinary Crystals Associated with AKI

Type of AKI	Crystal	Shape/Appearance
AKI from ethylene glycol	Calcium oxalate monohydrate or Calcium oxalate dihydrate	Needle shaped Envelope shaped
AKI from uric acid nephropathy	Uric acid	Diamond shaped, yellow or brown
AKI from sulfadiazine (intratubular obstruction)	Sulfadiazine	Needle shaped or shocks of wheat
AKI from acyclovir (intratubular obstruction)	Acyclovir	Needle shaped, birefringent
AKI from indinavir, atazanavir (intratubular obstruction)	Indinavir sulfate or atazanavir	Needle shaped, occasionally forming rosettes
AKI from methotrexate	Methotrexate	Compact or needle-shaped golden crystals arranged in annular structures
AKI from ciprofloxacin	Ciprofloxacin	Varying shapes, lamellar structure, strongly birefringent under polarizing light

AKI, acute kidney injury.

ongoing kidney damage. ACS is diagnosed when the intra-abdominal pressure is 20 mmHg or greater and leads to organ dysfunction, including AKI. It may occur in a variety of settings associated with increased abdominal pressure such as trauma, postsurgery, and ascites. Presentation is typically a tense abdomen and reduced urine output. The diagnosis is confirmed with measurement of intra-abdominal pressure which may be accomplished by assessing bladder pressure using a Foley catheter. Abdominal decompression is the mainstay of treatment with a variety of approaches depending on the clinical scenario; surgical decompression is typically indicated.

C. Acute Phosphate Nephropathy. Acute phosphate nephropathy is an uncommon cause of AKI that is associated with the use of oral sodium phosphate (OSP) (used as a bowel purgative) resulting in hyperphosphatemia, hypocalcemia, and the development of acute nephrocalcinosis, AKI, and CKD. OSPs are contraindicated in patients with kidney disease since the risk of complications is greater in this population.

D. AKI in Hematopoietic Cell Transplant (HCT) Patients. AKI is common after HCT. AKI rates are higher in patients who receive allogeneic as opposed to autologous transplantation and myeloablative as opposed to nonmyeloablative transplants. The incidence of AKI is high in HCT because of the life-threatening nature of the underlying diseases and the toxicity of the cancer drugs, immunosuppressive regimens, and antibiotics. Patients who have undergone autologous HCT do not receive immunosuppressive drugs and have less AKI than allogeneic HCT.

Factors that predispose to ATI are vomiting and diarrhea due to radio/chemotherapy or acute graft-versus-host disease; nephrotoxic drugs such as aminoglycosides and amphotericin B; and hemorrhagic and septic shock.

Hepatic sinusoidal obstruction syndrome also known as hepatic veno-occlusive disease, which is more common in allogeneic than in autologous bone marrow transplants, is a syndrome that may resemble HRS. A sodium retention state occurs and leads to weight gain, edema, and a low FENa of less than 1%, despite the use of diuretics. Progressive hyperbilirubinemia and nonoliguric AKI occur.

The most common time for development of AKI is 7 to 21 days after the transplant. The renal syndromes unique to HCT recipients are classified according to the time of presentation:

- **Immediate (first few days)**
  Tumor lysis syndrome
  Stored marrow toxicity
- **Early (7 to 21 days)**
  Hepatic veno-occlusive disease
  Sepsis-induced, ischemic, or nephrotoxic AKI
  Cyclosporin or FK506 toxicity
- **Cytokine release storm. HLA-haploidentical. AKI due to hemodynamic insults. Late (6 weeks to 1 year)**
  Bone marrow transplant–associated HUS
  Chronic cyclosporine nephrotoxicity
  Nephrotic syndrome (membranous glomerulonephritis related to graft-vs.-host disease)

E. AKI in the Setting of Liver Disease. In addition to HRS, AKI in patients with liver disease may also occur in other clinical settings. Jaundice and AKI may be due to HUS, leptospirosis, mismatched blood transfusion, acute hemorrhage, or falciparum malaria. Simultaneous AKI and acute liver failure suggest acetaminophen overdose, bacteremia, or carbon tetrachloride exposure. Glomerulonephritis and liver cirrhosis are associated with cryoglobulinemia, IgA nephropathy, membranous glomerulonephritis (associated with hepatitis B), and membranoproliferative glomerulonephritis (associated with hepatitis C).

F. AKI due to COVID-19. The approach to the diagnosis and management of AKI in COVID-19 patients is the same as other causes of AKI. However, there are some issues in the management of AKI that are specific to COVID-19 patients: (1) Circuit thrombosis during KRT is common and it is recommended that COVID-19 patients should receive anticoagulation during dialysis; (2) conservative use of IV fluids in patients with COVID-19 pneumonia. Incidence of AKI increases with the severity of disease. Rates of AKI have declined over the duration of the pandemic. COVID-19 can cause ATI or glomerular disease. Tubular injury is the predominant pathological finding in kidney biopsy. Renal Tropism of SARS-CoV-2 may contribute to the tubular injury. In 30-day survivors of COVID-19, there is a risk of developing CKD in nonhospitalized and hospitalized patients and patients admitted to the ICU.

G. Indications for Kidney Biopsy in AKI. Kidney biopsy may be useful in certain settings to establish the diagnosis of AKI and are listed below. Perirenal hematomas are commonly noted (>50% of the time), yet clinically significant bleeding is uncommon and PRBC transfusions are needed in approximately 1% of biopsies. Major complications requiring intervention or nephrectomy are rare (<1% and <0.1%, respectively). Some potential settings to consider kidney biopsy are the following:

1. **AKI of Unknown Etiology.** In patients with an unclear cause of AKI, kidney biopsy may be useful. In particular, a biopsy may be helpful if the possible causes of AKI have divergent treatment strategies. A classic example of this scenario is a patient with AKI who is receiving a nephrotoxic antibiotic with an infection and thus ATI, AIN, and an infection-associated GN

are all possibilities; while treatment of AIN rests on steroid administration and removal of the offending medication, infection-associated GN requires antibiotic treatment.
2. **Suspicion of glomerulonephritis** or systemic disease (e.g., vasculitis) as the cause of AKI. A kidney biopsy in such circumstances may provide the basis and justification for aggressive and life-saving therapy (e.g., high-dose steroids, cytotoxic agents, plasmapheresis).
3. **Suspicion of AIN.** Early initiation of steroids, in addition to discontinuation of offending medications, may facilitate kidney recovery in patients with AIN. Although not always possible, it is generally advisable to perform a kidney biopsy to confirm the diagnosis if steroids are being considered for suspicion of AIN.
4. AKI in patients with known lupus nephritis.

VI. Management
A. Prerenal AKI
1. **True Volume Depletion or Hypovolemia.** Therapy in this setting is directed toward correcting volume deficits. If volume depletion is due to hemorrhage, then the administration of packed RBCs is indicated; otherwise, the administration of an isotonic crystalloid fluid such as 0.9% saline (also known as normal saline) or lactated Ringer's is appropriate. When 1 L of isotonic crystalloid is given, approximately 250 mL remains in the plasma compartment, whereas 750 mL enters the interstitial compartment. The Saline versus Albumin Fluid Evaluation (SAFE) study, a randomized controlled trial comparing 4% human albumin in 0.9% saline with isotonic saline in ICU patients, demonstrated that albumin is no more effective than isotonic saline for fluid resuscitation.

The most appropriate choice of isotonic crystalloid (normal saline versus lactated Ringer's) for volume resuscitation remains uncertain. Normal saline is composed of 154 mEq/L of sodium and 154 mEq/L chloride. Since normal plasma sodium is approximately 140 mEq/L and normal chloride concentration is approximately 110 mEq/L, it has been argued that normal saline is not normal. Studies clearly demonstrate that normal saline administration increases the risk of hyperchloremic metabolic acidosis; other complications—including AKI—may also occur. Lactated Ringer's is composed of 130 mEq/L of sodium, 109 mEq/L of chloride, 28 mEq/L of lactate, 4 mEq/L of potassium, and 3 mEq of calcium. Clearly, lactated Ringer's should be avoided in patients with hyperkalemia and those who cannot metabolize lactate.

The amount of intravenous fluid (IVF) and the rapidity of administration depend on the clinical situation. In a young, stable patient, IVF should be given in one-time boluses (e.g., 500 to 1,000 mL over 1 hour). Smaller boluses (e.g., 250 mL over 1 hour) may be prudent in elderly patients in whom cardiac status is unknown. After a bolus, the patient should be evaluated clinically for signs of hypovolemia or volume overload. Bedside evaluation includes monitoring of orthostatic changes in blood pressure and pulse and jugular venous pulsation (JVP). JVP is a gross indicator of pressure in the central venous area of the right heart. In a euvolemic patient, JVPs are visible when the patient is supine but disappear when the patient assumes the sitting position. JVPs are not visible in the volume-depleted patient; therefore, their reappearance following fluid administration suggests that the central venous pressure has returned to normal. The presence of basilar crackles or a third heart sound implies too vigorous fluid replacement, with resultant cardiopulmonary congestion. Intravenous boluses of fluid should continue until euvolemia is achieved. Electrolyte deficits (e.g., potassium) should be monitored and replaced if necessary. In addition to

clinical evaluation of fluid status, ultrasound of the IVC may help in the evaluation of volume status.
   2. **Arterial Underfilling with an ECF Excess.** Prerenal disease in this setting is usually a secondary problem overshadowed by primary cardiac or liver disease. The management goal, therefore, is to treat the underlying cause; if the primary disease cannot be treated, then conservative management of symptoms is desirable.
      a. **Heart Failure.** Numerous medications may be employed to improve cardiac output in patients with cardiac disease including diuretics, beta blockers, ACEIs, ARBs, nitrates, and hydralazine. Improved cardiac output may improve renal blood flow and improve kidney function. However, with advanced heart failure that is refractory or only partially responsive to these agents, the physician may be forced to accept mild to moderate prerenal disease as a trade-off. Such disease rarely leads to symptomatic uremia.

      In hospitalized patients with ADHF who are diuretic resistant, fluid may be removed with continuous venovenous hemofiltration (CVVH), slow continuous ultrafiltration (SCUF), or intermittent ultrafiltration, without dialysis. Diuretic resistance has been defined as (1) persistent hypervolemia despite maximum doses of intravenous loop diuretics or combination diuretics, (2) FENa <0.2%, and (3) failure to excrete at least 90 mmol of sodium within 72 hours of maximum diuretic doses. Patients should not be called diuretic resistant in the presence of excess fluid intake.
      b. **Liver Disease.** (i) Ordinarily, the management goal is to reduce symptoms and treat ascites and edema with a sodium-restricted diet (1 to 2 g of salt per day), an aldosterone antagonist (e.g., spironolactone 200 to 400 mg/d), and a loop diuretic (e.g., furosemide) while the usually mild prerenal state may persist. Diuretic-resistant patients can be treated with intermittent large-volume paracentesis, transjugular intrahepatic portosystemic stent shunt (TIPS), or liver transplantation. (ii) Treatment of hospitalized patients with type I HRS may include vasopressin analogs with albumin, or TIPS (see Chapter 2) in an attempt to decrease splanchnic vasodilatation and improve renal blood flow. The vasopressin analogue, terlipressin is now FDA approved for the treatment of HRS-AKI. The recommended Dosage Regimen for terlipressin is shown in Table 12-10. Terlipressin can cause acute pulmonary edema, especially in patients that have received large doses of intravenous albumin. Terlipressin should not be used in patients with hypoxia (e.g., SpO_2 <90%) until oxygenation levels improve and should be discontinued if SpO_2 decreases below 90%. To date, liver transplant is the only definitive cure for HRS.
B. Postrenal Failure. Foley catheter drainage is usually successful for acute obstruction secondary to prostatic hypertrophy. The decision regarding further therapy must be made in consultation with a urologist. Medical therapy with finasteride or an α-blocker, or surgical removal of prostatic tissue may be recommended.

With ureteral obstruction, cystoscopy and the placement of ureteral drainage nephrostomy tubes or stents may allow passage of obstructing stones, sludge, or pus, but if this fails, surgical intervention is required. With ureteral obstruction due to more chronic conditions like tumor infiltration, prograde stents, and nephrostomies are often placed by interventional radiology.

C. Primary Kidney Disease: Vasculitis and Glomerulonephritis. When AKI develops in the course of a systemic or vascular disorder, it is usually a grave sign. A comprehensive discussion of the treatment of these systemic and vascular

TABLE 12-10	Dosage Regimen for Terlipressin

Days 1–3 administer 0.85 mg intravenously every 6 h.
Day 4: Assess serum creatinine (SCr) versus baseline.
If SCr has decreased by at least 30% from baseline, continue 0.85 mg intravenously every 6 h.
If SCr has decreased by less than 30% from baseline, dose may be increased to 1.7 mg intravenously every 6 h.
If SCr is at or above baseline value, discontinue.
Continue terlipressin until 24 h after two consecutive SCr ≤1.5 mg/dL values at least 2 h apart or a maximum of 14 days.

disorders is beyond the scope of this chapter. Obtaining an urgent kidney biopsy early after presentation is essential to make the diagnosis and to guide appropriate therapy. Therapeutic options include immunosuppressive therapy with steroids and/or cyclophosphamide. A subset of patients may benefit from plasmapheresis (e.g., Goodpasture syndrome).

D. Acute Interstitial Nephritis (AIN). When a therapeutic agent is identified as a potential cause of AIN, removal of the agent is the obvious first step in therapy. A confirmatory kidney biopsy within days, especially if the patient requires KRT, should be strongly considered. This is because early treatment with steroids within 1 week of recognition has been shown in a retrospective analysis to be beneficial in terms of improvement of kidney function and reduction in kidney fibrosis versus late (after 2 weeks) initiation of steroids. Although a prospective randomized trial has not been done, the weight of evidence favors early initiation of prednisone for drug-induced AIN. Treatment regimens are varied; however, initiation therapy with 1 mg/kg of prednisone (up to 60 mg/d) for 2 to 4 weeks with a taper for 2 to 3 months is a commonly used approach. Although it is preferred to perform a kidney biopsy to confirm the diagnosis, a biopsy is not always feasible. In all cases, the approach to care needs to be individualized, with the risks and benefits of steroid therapy and kidney biopsy carefully considered.

One form of AIN that has a somewhat different management strategy is due to checkpoint inhibitor immunotherapy for cancer treatment where discontinuation of the offending agent may not be necessary or desirable. In this case, a multidisciplinary approach to the evaluation and management of the patient will be necessary.

E. Intrinsic Kidney Disease, ATI. No specific therapy exists for the treatment of ATI, although this is a widely investigated area of interest. The Kidney Precision Medicine Project consists of a number of research centers across the United States that are collaborating to bring state-of-the-art technologies together to identify critical cells, pathways, and targets for novel therapies.

F. General Management Principles for AKI
  1. **What to Avoid in AKI**
     a. **High-Dose Diuretics in Euvolemic Patients.** No data support the use of high-dose diuretics and therapy for established ATI. Furosemide and other loop diuretics are frequently used in oliguric AKI in an effort to convert it to nonoliguric AKI. Although the conversion of oliguric to nonoliguric kidney injury may simplify fluid management, clinical

trials have failed to demonstrate that the use of diuretics is associated with improved outcomes in patients with AKI. That said, a trial of loop diuretics can be attempted to manage hypervolemia among patients with AKI, particularly those with ADHF. Lack of a diuretic response to high-dose furosemide suggests that KRT may be needed for volume removal.
   b. **Renal Dose Dopamine.** Dopamine is a selective renal vasodilator. It elicits profound natriuresis and increases urine output in patients with normal kidney function. The renal selective dose is 1 to 3 µg/kg/min. No evidence suggests that renal dose dopamine is beneficial in AKI. In fact, several studies have identified deleterious effects, such as bowel ischemia and arrhythmias, and thus, dopamine is not to be used as specific therapy for AKI.
   c. **Nephrotoxic Drugs.** Potentially nephrotoxic drugs and agents should be avoided in AKI, because they may perpetuate the kidney injury. These agents and drugs include NSAIDs, cyclosporine, tacrolimus, aminoglycosides, radiocontrast agents, and amphotericin B.
   d. **Volume Overload.** The amount of IVF necessary for critically ill patients is unknown, and IVFs must be given judiciously in the setting of AKI, especially if the patient is oliguric. In patients with acute lung injury, conservative fluid management improves outcomes without increasing the development of nonpulmonary organ failures such as the kidney. In general, IVFs should not contain potassium. It is now well documented that the development of fluid overload in patients with AKI is associated with increased mortality. Although it is currently unknown whether excess fluid administration itself is harmful, or whether fluid overload is a marker of severity of illness, a fluid conservative strategy is a reasonable approach to patients with AKI.
2. **Supportive Therapy in AKI**
   a. **Drug Dosages.** Drug dosages should be adjusted based on the measured or best estimate of CrCl, not merely on serum creatinine. Certain medication doses also must be adjusted if the patient with AKI is receiving dialysis (intermittent hemodialysis [IHD] or continuous KRT [CKRT]).
   b. **Nutritional Support.** AKI is a hypercatabolic state associated with increased protein breakdown. Nitrogen balance is extremely negative, especially in AKI associated with sepsis, postsurgery, and multiorgan dysfunction syndrome. Renal factors contributing to the negative nitrogen balance include uremia, acidosis, parathyroid hormone abnormalities, inadequate protein intake, and protein losses. If supplemental nutrition is provided, enteral feeding is the preferred method of nutritional support, although it is not always possible. The use of parenteral nutrition remains controversial, and randomized controlled clinical trials have yet to demonstrate a benefit in acutely ill patients with AKI. A total energy intake of 20 to 30 kcal/kg/d is recommended in any stage of AKI. The following protein intake is recommended: 0.8 to 1.0 g/kg/d of protein in noncatabolic AKI patients without need for dialysis, 1.0 to 1.5 g/kg/d in patients with AKI on KRT, and up to a maximum of 1.7 g/kg/d in patients on CKRT and in hypercatabolic patients.
3. **Kidney Replacement Therapy (KRT)**
   Modalities of KRT available for patients with AKI:
   a. **Intermittent Hemodialysis (IHD).** IHD is typically performed for 4 hours a session and is the same form of dialysis used in patients with end-stage kidney disease. IHD is typically used in otherwise stable patients who can tolerate rapid fluid removal (e.g., 1 L/h). IHD is mandatory in ambulatory patients. In this form of dialysis, the patient is connected to a dialysis machine for 4 hours at a time, daily or every

second day. Fluid removal and urea clearance for the day is achieved during the period of a few hours. Rapid removal of solutes and fluids may cause hemodynamic instability. The technique requires a double-lumen catheter, tubing, a HD machine (blood pump, dialysate generation system, dialysate pump, and alarms and safety monitoring devices), a dialysis membrane, and a dialysis nurse. It is strongly recommended that delivered dialysis dose be assessed in patients with AKI by quantifying urea removal (Kt/V). The 2012 KDIGO AKI guidelines recommend that the target level of clearance per session range between a Kt/V of 1.2 to 1.4, which is typically achievable in a 4-hour session.

b. **Continuous Kidney Replacement Therapy (CKRT).** CKRT is performed continuously, daily for 24 hours a day. Currently, four main types of CKRT are used: SCUF, CVVH, continuous venovenous hemodialysis (CVVHDF), and continuous venovenous hemodiafiltration (CVVHDF). In CKRT, the goal is for the patient to undergo continuous dialysis for 24 hours a day. In practice, interruptions in dialysis for patient procedures, radiologic testing, and dialysis membrane clotting are frequent and reduce the amount of time the patient is actually receiving dialysis. CKRT is commonly used for patients who are hemodynamically unstable (e.g., patients with shock who are on multiple vasopressors). Because the removal of solutes and fluid is slow and continuous, hemodynamic instability and hypotensive episodes are reduced. Minimization of hypotension theoretically avoids the perpetuation of kidney injury, although there is controversy on whether or not CKRT is associated with improved kidney outcomes versus IHD. CKRT requires a double-lumen catheter (the same catheter that is used for IHD), tubing, a simple blood pump with safety devices, sterile replacement fluid, volumetric pumps to control replacement and ultrafiltration rate, continuous anticoagulation, and a high-flux dialysis membrane. An ICU nurse typically monitors this therapy.

c. **Prolonged Intermittent Kidney Replacement Therapy (PIKRT).** PIKRT is a hybrid form of KRT that is performed for a longer period of time than IHD and a shorter time than CKRT in an acute care setting. A common length of treatment is 12 hours but may range widely. Machines used for either IHD or CKRT may be used depending on the expertise and resources of the institution. This form of KRT is appealing as it allows for mobilization of patients, time for procedures, and less intensive nursing requirements. It is often a bridge therapy in critically ill patients between CKRT and IHD.

d. **Peritoneal dialysis** is uncommonly used as a mode of acute dialysis therapy for AKI in the United States despite the fact that it is not technically difficult and can be used with minimally trained staff. It may be an option in locations where IHD or CKRT is not available. It can be used in patients with minimally increased catabolism without an immediate or life-threatening indication for dialysis. It is ideal for patients who are hemodynamically unstable. For short-term dialysis, a rigid dialysis catheter is inserted into the peritoneum, through the anterior abdominal wall, 5 to 10 cm below the umbilicus. Exchanges of 1.5 to 2.0 L of standard peritoneal dialysis solutions are infused into the peritoneum. The major risks are bowel perforation during insertion of the catheter and peritonitis. Acute peritoneal dialysis offers the same potential advantages to the pediatric patient that CKRT offers to the adult with AKI.

4. **Starting a Patient on KRT**
    a. **Indications.** In general, the indications to start KRT in AKI are not specific and should be individualized by nephrology consultation. Common indications to start KRT include: (1) refractory fluid overload

not responding to diuretics, (2) hyperkalemia (plasma potassium concentration >6.5 mEq/L) or rapidly rising potassium levels, (3) signs of uremia, such as pericarditis, neuropathy, or an otherwise unexplained decline in mental status, (4) metabolic acidosis (pH <7.2), and (5) certain alcohol and drug intoxications. The initiation of KRT depends on the entire clinical picture, not just the presence or absence of certain factors. In the absence of other specific indications, KRT is often initiated when the BUN reaches 80 to 100 mg/dL and is expected to continue to rise. A useful clinical test to assess the likelihood of needing KRT is the **furosemide stress test**. In this test, intravenous furosemide is given and the urine output is assessed for the next 2 hours. The dose of furosemide is either 1 mg/kg in patients who have not recently furosemide or 1.5 mg/kg who have not recently received furosemide. Euvolemic patients with stage 1 or 2 AKI are the appropriate patient population. Urine output of less than 200 mL over 2 hours after administration of furosemide indicates furosemide stress test (FST) unresponsiveness and predicts a high likelihood of needing KRT.

b. **Modality**: Intermittent versus continuous. Many nonrandomized studies have compared IHD and CKRT. Prospective randomized studies comparing IHD with CKRT are difficult to carry out because patients who are hemodynamically unstable and cannot tolerate IHD are almost always started on CKRT. Alternatively, confining a mobile patient to bed to receive CKRT may be unethical. Therefore, any randomization may be biased. CKRT is believed to be the modality of choice in very ill patients, and IHD is used in less ill patients. Although PIKRT is commonly used in critically ill patients. At present, IHD, PIKRT, and CKRT are generally regarded as equivalent methods for the treatment of AKI. The modality choice should be made in consultation with a nephrologist and tailored for the individual patient. The decision may also depend on facility-specific issues, such as experience, nursing resources, and technical proficiency. The cost of CKRT is greater than that of IHD and SLED. A day of CKRT is roughly equivalent to one HD treatment. Therefore, drug-dosing adjustments must be made in CKRT. At present, indications for CKRT in AKI include hemodynamic instability, brain injury, raised intracranial pressure, cerebral edema, hypercatabolism, and severe fluid overload (Table 12-11).

c. **Vascular access.** The primary vascular sites used for insertion of temporary dialysis catheters are the internal jugular or femoral vein. The internal jugular access is required in patients who are mobile, and the right internal jugular vein is preferred over the left due to a lower rate of

TABLE 12-11   Potential Indications for CKRT Versus IHD in AKI

Hemodynamic instability
Brain injury
Raised intracranial pressure
Cerebral edema
Hypercatabolism
Severe fluid overload

AKI, acute kidney injury; CKRT, continuous kidney replacement therapy.

central stenosis. Femoral access is indicated when the cardiopulmonary condition of the patient limits attempts at thoracic catheterization; it is useful in bedridden patients. The subclavian vein may be used if other access sites are unavailable; however, use of subclavian catheters entails a risk of stenosis or thrombosis of the subclavian vein or its branches.
   d. **KRT dose.** Two large randomized studies, the Acute Renal Failure Trial Network (ATN) and the RENAL study, have demonstrated that intensive dialysis does not improve mortality compared with conventional dialysis. In the ATN study, no mortality benefit was observed for intensive dialysis (IHD hemodialysis or sustained low-efficiency [daily] dialysis [SLEDD] 6 days a week, or CVVHDF at 35 mL/kg/h) versus conventional dialysis (IHD thrice weekly or CVVHDF at 20 mL/kg/h). In the ATN study, the achieved target clearance goals for IHD were 1.2 to 1.4 Kt/V urea per treatment, suggesting that this level of clearance be maintained in patients receiving IHD. In the RENAL study, CKRT at a dose of 40 mL/kg/h did not have a mortality benefit compared with CKRT at a dose of 25 mL/kg/h. Thus, the 2012 KDIGO AKI recommendations indicate that the effluent volume for CKRT should be 20 to 25 mL/kg/h; however, it should be noted that CKRT is often interrupted in ICU patients (e.g., for procedures) and that higher effluent volumes may need to be prescribed.
   e. **Timing.** Large-scale clinical trials have demonstrated that earlier initiation of KRT (in the absence of urgent indications) does not offer a survival benefit in AKI and is associated with numerous complications (e.g., hypophosphatemia). The, the timing of KRT initiation is based on the entire clinical picture versus any particular time point.
G. **Prognosis of AKI.** "How badly injured is the kidney?" The severity of AKI should be based not only on serum creatinine elevation and urine output. Newer developments for determining the severity of the AKI include measurement of urinary biomarkers, furosemide stress test, and renal angina index. In the future means for determining risk progression may include e-alert systems, machine-learning algorithms, and artificial intelligence for AKI recognition and monitoring.

SUGGESTED READINGS

Abdelhafez M, Nayfeh T, Atieh A, et al. Diagnostic performance of fractional excretion of sodium for the differential diagnosis of acute kidney injury a systematic review and meta-analysis. *Clin J Am Soc Nephrol.* 2022;17:785–797.

Choudhury D, Ahmed Z. Drug-associated renal dysfunction and injury. *Nat Clin Pract Nephrol.* 2006;2:80–91.

Dursun B, Edelstein CL. Acute renal failure—core curriculum. *Am J Kidney Dis.* 2005;45:614–618.

Edelstein CL, Faubel S. Biomarkers in acute kidney injury. In: Edelstein CL, ed. *Biomarkers of Kidney Disease.* Academic Press; 2017:241–303.

Edelstein CL, Schrier RW. Pathophysiology of ischemic acute renal injury. In: Coffman TM, Falk RJ, Molitoris BA, Neilson EG, Schrier RW, eds. *Schrier's Diseases of the Kidney.* Wolters Kluwer/Lippincott Williams & Wilkins; 2013:826–867.

Faubel S, Patel NU, Lockhart ME, Cadnapaphornchai MA. Renal relevant radiology: use of ultrasonography in patients with AKI. *Clin J Am Soc Nephrol.* 2014;9(2):382–394.

Gaudry S, Hajage D, Benichou N, et al. Delayed versus early initiation of renal replacement therapy for severe acute kidney injury: a systematic review and individual patient data meta-analysis of randomized clinical trials. *Lancet.* 2020;395(10235):1506–1515.

González E, Gutiérrez E, Galeano C, et al. Early steroid treatment improves the recovery of renal function in patients with drug-induced acute interstitial nephritis. *Kidney Int.* 2008;73(8):940.

Griffin BR, Faubel S, Edelstein CL. Biomarkers of drug-induced kidney toxicity. *Ther Drug Monit.* 2019;41(2):213–226.

Holditch SJ, Brown CN, Lombardi AM, Nguyen KN, Edelstein CL. Recent advances in models, mechanisms, biomarkers, and interventions in cisplatin-induced acute kidney injury. *Int J Mol Sci.* 2019;20(12):3011.

KDIGO. Clinical practice guidelines for acute kidney injury. *Kidney Int.* 2012;2(Suppl 1):1–141.

Koyner JL, Davison DL, Brasha-Mitchell E, et al. Furosemide stress test and biomarkers for the prediction of AKI severity. *J Am Soc Nephrol.* 2015;26(8):2023–2031.

Lameire N, Van Biesen W, Vanholder R. The changing epidemiology of acute renal failure. *Nat Clin Pract Nephrol.* 2006;2:364–377.

Legrand M, Bell S, Forni L, et al. Pathophysiology of COVID-19-associated acute kidney injury. *Nat Rev Nephrol.* 2021;17(11):751–764.

Levine Z, Vijayan A. Prolonged intermittent kidney replacement therapy. *Clin J Am Soc Nephrol.* 2023;18(3):383–391.

Ostermann M, Bellomo R, Burdmann EA, et al. Controversies in acute kidney injury: conclusions from a Kidney Disease: Improving Global Outcomes (KDIGO) Conference. *Kidney Int.* 2020;98(2):294–309.

Nejat M, Pickering JW, Devarajan P, et al. Some biomarkers of acute kidney injury are increased in pre-renal acute injury. *Kidney Int.* 2012;81(12):1254–1262.

Pepin M-N, Bouchard J, Legault L, et al. Diagnostic performance of fractional excretion of urea and fractional excretion of sodium in the evaluations of patients with acute kidney injury with or without diuretic treatment. *Am J Kidney Dis.* 2007;50(4):566–573.

RENAL Replacement Therapy Study Investigators; Bellomo R, Cass A, Cole L, et al. Intensity of continuous renal-replacement therapy in critically ill patients. *N Engl J Med.* 2009;361(17):1627–1638.

Thomas ME, Blaine C, Dawnay A, et al. The definition of acute kidney injury and its use in practice. *Kidney Int.* 2015;87(1):62–73.

Ostermann M, Zarbock A, Goldstein S, et al. Recommendations on acute kidney injury biomarkers from the acute disease quality initiative consensus conference. A consensus statement. *JAMA Netw Open.* 2020;3(10):e2019209.

Weisbord SD, Gallagher M, Jneid H, et al. Outcomes after angiography with sodium bicarbonate and acetylcysteine. *N Engl J Med.* 2018;378:603–614.

The Patient With Chronic Kidney Disease

Katherine Rizzolo, Michel Chonchol

Patients with kidney failure, or end-stage kidney disease (ESKD) have decreased quality of life and high morbidity and mortality. Overall, the prevalence of kidney failure continues to grow in the United States, and the incidence of kidney failure and mortality rates for people with kidney failure have slowed. Between 2010 and 2019, incidence of kidney failure increased in total number from 94,466 to 134,862, though the total adjusted incidence rate fell by 7.6%. The prevalence of kidney failure increased between 2000 and 2020, reaching a peak of 808,330 in 2019, before decreasing in 2020. Overall, all-cause mortality for people with kidney failure decreased 13% between 2010 and 2019, with an increase in mortality in 2020 due to the COVID-19 pandemic.

This chapter presents an overview of the current recommendations designed to slow the progression of chronic kidney disease (CKD); to optimize the medical management of comorbid medical conditions, such as cardiovascular disease (CVD), diabetes, and lipid disorders; and decrease the complications secondary to progression of kidney disease including hypertension, anemia, and mineral-bone disease. These recommendations include those outlined by KDIGO, a global organization that develops and implements evidence-based clinical practice guidelines.

I. Definition and Staging of CKD

CKD is defined as abnormalities of kidney structure or function present for at least 3 months, with implications for health. CKD is defined on basis of cause, glomerular filtration rate (GFR) categories, and albuminuria. The cause of CKD is based on the presence or absence of systemic disease, location within the kidney, and/or presumed pathologic findings. These criteria include:

A. Markers of kidney damage such as albuminuria (albumin excretion rate >300 mg/24 hours or albumin creatinine ratio >30 mg/g), urine sediment abnormalities, electrolyte or other abnormalities due to tubular disorders, abnormalities detected on pathology, structural abnormalities detected by imaging, or history of kidney transplantation.

B. Decreased GFR of less than 60 mL/min/1.73 m^2, as eGFR categories are defined along the basis of eGFR numeric ranges. However, the degree of severity is mitigated by albuminuria, for example, a person with an eGFR >90 mL/min/1.73 m^2 and albuminuria of >300 mg/g or >30 mg/mmol would be considered high risk for progression in kidney disease.

C. The staging of CKD is useful because it endorses a model in which primary physicians and specialists share responsibility for the care of patients with CKD. This classification also offers a common language for patients and the practitioners involved in the treatment of CKD.

1. **Measurement of GFR.** An essential requirement for the classification and monitoring of CKD is the measurement or estimation of GFR. The current guideline-recommended approach utilizes eGFR as the initial test for GFR evaluation, and cystatin C can be utilized for confirmatory testing. Serum creatinine is not an ideal marker of GFR, because it depends on skeletal muscle mass and is both filtered at the glomerulus and secreted by the proximal tubule.

a. **Creatinine Clearance (CrCl)** is known to overestimate GFR by as much as 20% in healthy individuals and even more in patients with CKD. Estimates of GFR based on 24-hour CrCl require timed urine collections, which are difficult to obtain and often involve errors in collection. Classic methods for measurements of GFR, including the gold standard inulin clearance, are cumbersome, require an intravenous infusion and timed urine collections, and are not clinically feasible. In adults, the normal GFR based on inulin clearance and adjusted to a standard body surface area of 1.73 m^2 is 127 mL/min/1.73 m^2 for men and 118 mL/min/1.73 m^2 for women, with a standard deviation of approximately 20 mL/min/1.73 m^2. After age 30, the average decrease in GFR is 1 mL/min/1.73 m^2/yr.
b. **Creatinine-Based Equations.** Given the difficulties with 24-hour urine estimates, the GFR is commonly estimated from serum concentrations of filtration markers. Creatinine-based equations are widely utilized by automated clinical laboratories, and incorporate demographic variables inherent to non-kidney causes of creatinine changes.
    i. **Cockcroft–Gault equation** was developed to predict CrCl, but has been used to estimate GFR:

    $$\text{CrCl} = \frac{(140 - \text{age})(\text{weight in kg})}{(\text{Serum creatinine})(72)} \times 0.85 \text{ if female} \qquad 13\text{-}1$$

    Cockcroft–Gault was based on age, weight, height, and was developed with 249 White men. As such, it has been noted to be a poor estimator of kidney function in women and non-White populations. Cockcroft–Gault is widely used for the estimate of CrCl for pharmaceutical dosing, but is no longer commonly used for GFR estimation.
    ii. **The modification of diet in renal disease (MDRD) study equation** was derived on the basis of data from a large number of patients with a wide variety of kidney diseases and GFRs up to 90 mL/min/1.73 m^2 and predicts GFR as measured by using an accepted method (urinary clearance of iodine 125 [^{125}I]-iothalamate). MDRD included a wider cohort of non-White and female patients, and its included values include race, age, sex, height, and weight:

    $$\begin{aligned}\text{GFR}(\text{mL/minute}/1.73\,\text{m}^2) = {} & 186 \times \text{serum creatinine (SCR)}^{-1.154} \\ & \times (\text{age})^{-0.203} \\ & \times (0.742 \text{ if female}) \\ & \times (1.210 \text{ if African American})\end{aligned} \qquad 13\text{-}2$$

    The calculations can be made using available web-based and downloadable medical calculators (www.kidney.org/professionals/KDOQI/gfr_calculator.cfm).

    The limitation of MDRD is that is not as accurate with higher degree of GFR and tends to overestimate CKD 1 and 2. In addition, MDRD did not contain patients with diabetic kidney disease or people over age 70.
    iii. **CKD-epidemiology equation (CKD-EPI)** was derived from a larger, more diverse sample set to accommodate these limitations. CKD EPI is the most accurate in predicting mortality and prognosis of CKD, and is generally recommended for use. At the writing of this textbook chapter, creatinine-based equations—either CKD EPI or MDRD—remain widely used by most automated laboratories. However, creatinine has its limitations, especially for those with high or low muscle mass with acute or chronic illness.

c. **Cystatin C–Based Equations.** Cystatin C is an endogenous glomerular filtration marker less affected by muscle mass. Cystatin C has been shown to be a better marker than creatinine in estimating prognosis of CKD. Cystatin C–based eGFR has previously demonstrated increased risks of all-cause and cardiovascular deaths that were not detected with creatinine-based calculations of eGFR. Further, a cystatin C equation has been developed utilizing the CKD-EPI equation. Indeed, cystatin C when combined with creatinine may help provide more accurate eGFR estimates.

In 2020, the use of creatinine-based equations came under scrutiny due to its use of race. Race was initially included in the equations because previous studies showed Black participants on average had a higher creatinine level compared with non-Black participants. However, the inclusion of race, a social construct, as a biologic variable in calculating eGFR ignores diversity within racial groups, and has been associated with worsening inequities in kidney disease between racial groups. As such, multiple institutions have eliminated race from eGFR equations, which can lead to a greater degree of inaccuracies in measuring GFR. In 2021, a race-free eGFR equation using cystatin C was unbiased across racial groups while a race-free eGFR equation utilizing creatinine and cystatin C was found to be most synonymous with measured GFR. These equations require further implementation before use, but hold promise to developing an accurate and equitable measurement of eGFR.

II. Prevalence of CKD

More than one in seven people are estimated to have CKD. CKD awareness remains low—90% of adults with CKD are unaware they have CKD. Worldwide, CKD affects an estimated 700 million people around the world, a prevalence of 9.1%. In the United States, the National Health and Nutrition Examination Survey (NHANES) data from 2003 to 2018 found the prevalence of CKD between 2003 and 2018 is around 13.3%, and has not substantially changed. However, prevalence of CKD differs by race, gender, age, and socioeconomic status. For example, women are more likely to have CKD compared to men (14% compared with 12%), non-Hispanic Black adults have a higher risk compared to non-Hispanic White adults (16% compared with 13%), people over 65 years of age (38%) compared with those between 45 and 64 (12%), and those between 18 and 44 (6%).

CKD has many risk factors, such as diabetes, hypertension, obesity, and metabolic syndrome. In addition, communicable disease burden of human immunodeficiency virus (HIV), hepatitis C and C, malaria, schistosomiasis, and tuberculosis may drive CKD prevalence in low and middle-income countries. In addition, lifestyle factors such as smoking, nephrotoxin exposure (including nonsteroidal anti-inflammatory drugs [NSAIDs], analgesics, heavy metals, certain traditional medicines), and social factors such as lower socioeconomic status (affecting access to healthy food pollution, and access to care) also affect CKD incidence and progression.

III. Mechanism of Kidney Disease Progression

Despite the many diseases that can initiate kidney injury, a limited number of common pathways are available for kidney disease progression. A general theme of many of these pathways is that adaptive changes in the nephron lead to maladaptive consequences. Multiple large trials have shown that higher proteinuria was associated the faster progression to kidney failure. Increased glomerular capillary flow and pressure leading to proteinuria are independent predictors of kidney disease. Proteinuria is toxic to the kidney and instigates a large number of pathways leading to glomerular, interstitial, and tubular damage mitigating progression of kidney dysfunction. In glomerular disease, nephron loss leads to heightened glomerular capillary pressure, which directly increases glomerular permeability to protein, ultimately causing podocyte effacement and loss of the slit basement membrane, and also leads to mesangial matrix deposition. Overall, while many noncystic diseases are glomerular in origin, the degree of tubulointerstitial disease predicts progression, which is most likely to predominant mechanism of progression in nonproteinuric disease.

IV. Risk Factors for Progression to ESKD

The risk and rate of progression are affected by severity of disease corroborated by an individual's demographics, clinical factors, and access to care. The progression of CKD is not always linear; it may be affected by factors causing acute kidney injury (such as infections, dehydration, nephrotoxins). The Chronic Renal Insufficiency Cohort (CRIC) is an ongoing longitudinal study of 5,500 adults with CKD focusing on elucidating risk factors for progression to CKD. Risk Factors for progression are described as follows and in Table 13-1, along with treatment options.

A. Clinical Factors
1. **Proteinuria.** The quantity of protein excreted in the urine is one of the strongest predictors of kidney disease progression and response to antihypertensive therapy in almost all studies of CKD.
2. **Biopsy Findings.** An important risk factor, especially for most glomerular diseases, is the extent of tubulointerstitial disease on kidney biopsy.
3. **Underlying Disease Care.** Control of underlying disease, such as glycemic control for people with diabetes, hypertensive management, as well as disease-specific therapy such as immunosuppressive agents for lupus nephritis, or controlling cyst growth for patients with polycystic kidney disease.
4. **Comorbid Conditions.** Comorbid conditions, such as CVD, metabolic syndrome, obstructive urinary diseases also affect disease progression.

B. Sociodemographic and Economic Factors
1. **Gender.** Females have higher incidence of CKD, but 28% lower risk of progressing to kidney failure compared with males. The etiology of this difference is unclear, but the effect of estrogen has been proposed.
2. Racial and ethnic minoritized individuals have a higher risk of progression to kidney failure: for Black people, the risk is 3.8 times that of non-Hispanic White people, and for Hispanic people the risk is 2.1 times. This risk is significantly mitigated by adjustment for sociodemographic variables such as age, sex, income, education, neighborhood-level factors, and clinical characteristics.

C. Behavioral Factors
1. **Healthy Lifestyle.** Smoking is associated with CKD progression. Physical activity has not shown strong correlations, though those meeting the American Heart Association physical activity guidelines had a lower risk of death.
2. **Diet.** Higher sodium intake and lower potassium intake are associated with elevated blood pressure; those with high sodium intake (over 195 mmol in 24 hours) are more likely to experience CKD progression. Increased potassium intake has been shown to lower blood pressure, but has not been shown to lower CKD progression. An inverse relationship has been shown between healthy dietary scores and risk of CKD progression, especially with those utilizing a Mediterranean diet.

D. Genetic Factors
1. The APOL1 gene has been implicated in higher risk of CKD progression among individuals with African ancestry. Independent of diabetes or hypertension, Black individuals with high-risk APOL1 group have been shown to have more rapid eGFR decline compared to White individuals.
2. Other genetic factors, such as polycystic kidney disease, medullary cystic kidney disease have varying degrees of risk of progression.

TABLE 13-1 Risk Factor Management Recommendations and Treatment Options

Risk Factor	Recommendation	Treatment Options
Clinical Risk Factors		
Hypertension	Goal BP <130/80	ACEi/ARB first line if proteinuria or diabetes CCB or thiazide second line
Albuminuria	Initiate antialbuminuric medications for albumin/creatinine ratio >300 mg/24 h	ACEi/ARB if hypertensive and/or diabetic SGLT2i if diabetic or additional therapy MRA if normal potassium
Diabetes	Goal individualized HbA1c between 6.5% and 8%	Metformin if eGFR >30 mL/min/1.73 m^2 SGLT2i if eGFR >20 mL/min/1.73 m^2 GLP-1 RA if needed Additional lipid management and BP control
Cardiovascular risk	Address individual risk factors	Secondary prevention when appropriate (ASA, beta blockers)
Sequelae of CKD		
Metabolic acidosis	Maintain levels >18 mEq/L	Sodium bicarbonate or high alkaline diet if bicarbonate <18 mEq/L
Anemia	Maintain HgB between 10 and 11.5	Initiate ESA if HgB <10 Consider iron therapy if evidence of iron deficiency
Mineral-bone disease	Maintain phosphorus and calcium within normal range PTH above the upper limit of normal should be evaluated for modifiable factors	Individualized therapy including phosphate binders, PTH analogs, active and inactive vitamin D.
Lifestyle Factors		
Smoking	Smoking cessation	
Obesity	Maintain a healthy BMI between 20 and 25 kg/m^2	
Diet	Maintain salt intake <2 g/d Low protein intake for CKD 4 and 5 0.8 g/kg/d	
Exercise	150 min of moderate-intensity physical activity per week	
Dyslipidemia	Use of lipid-lowering medications for all patients >50 and those with clinical risk factors age 18–50	

Regarding prediction of CKD progression, the Kidney Failure Risk Equation (kidneyfailurerisk.com) is the most well-validated risk prediction tool for progression to CKD. The equation utilizes urine protein, sex, age, and eGFR values to predict 2- and 5-year probability of developing kidney failure for a patient with CKD stage 3 to 5.

V. Slowing Progression to ESKD

A. Antihypertensive Therapy. Poorly controlled hypertension is associated with higher risk of progression and poor cardiovascular outcomes. There is ample evidence supporting blood pressure reduction in people with CKD. A subanalysis of the 2015 Systolic Blood Pressure Intervention (SPRINT) trial with people with CKD stages 3 to 4 demonstrated that an intensive blood pressure treatment target (systolic BP <120 mmHg) compared to standard treatment (systolic BP <140 mmHg) improved risk of all-cause mortality, albeit with a higher risk of AKI. However, SPRINT did not show a difference in eGFR in the complete cohort between cohorts. As such, blood pressure target goals at the writing of this text chapter differ depending on organization. For example, the American College of Cardiology/American Heart Association recommended a target of 130/80 mmHg. KDIGO's 2021 Clinical Practice Guideline for the Management of Blood Pressure in CKD recommends a systolic target of less than 120 mmHg for patients with CKD when standardized office readings are possible- a reflection of the overall findings of the SPRINT trial.

Renin–angiotensin–aldosterone system (RAAS) inhibition is first line for patients with proteinuria, the data is less clear in nonproteinuric disease. For patients without proteinuria or for those with proteinuria already receiving RAAS inhibition, per the American College of Cardiology, calcium channel blockers and thiazide diuretics are considered first-line medications, and beta blockade may be first line in patients with coronary artery disease and heart failure. Thiazide diuretics have traditionally been replaced with a loop diuretic under an eGFR of 30 mL/min/1.73 m^2, however, the 2021 CLICK trial demonstrated chlorthalidone, in combination with a standardized regimen of ACE inhibitor, beta-blocker, calcium channel blocker, and loop diuretics use in stage 4 CKD is safe and effective at reducing blood pressure, and may help in proteinuria reduction as well.

B. Reduction in Proteinuria. Multiple studies have demonstrated that reduction in proteinuria and lower levels of residual proteinuria can reduce eGFR decline. As such, proteinuria reduction is a mainstay of CKD treatment, via RAAS inhibition, SGLT2 inhibition, or mineralocorticoid antagonism.

1. **RAAS inhibition.** RAAS inhibitors are the first line for patients with hypertension and proteinuria due to their well-established effects of reducing progression to CKD and lower all-cause mortality. These agents are useful in diabetic kidney disease as they prevent the rise the intraglomerular pressure, release of aldosterone and RAAS—preventing downstream sequelae such as fluid and sodium retention. Multiple studies in diabetic nephropathy have demonstrated angiotensin-converting enzyme (ACE) inhibitors and angiotensin receptor blockers (ARB) are effective medications in reducing risk of kidney disease progression. In nondiabetic nephropathy, The African American Study of Kidney Disease and Hypertension (AASK) trial, whose target population was Black people with hypertensive nephrosclerosis, demonstrated that ACEi showed more favorable outcomes compared with beta blockers or calcium channel blockers.

   RAAS inhibition can reduce the risk of kidney failure in advanced CKD, though at the risk of hyperkalemia or eGFR decline. Several retrospective trials, including post hoc analysis of REIN and RENAAL, demonstrated the benefits of RAAS inhibition was not dependent on eGFR. The 2022 STOP-ACE trial, the first prospective, multicenter randomized trial examining discontinuation of ACEi in CKD stage 4 and 5 did not find any benefit by stopping ACEi or ARB, though the discontinuation arm had a higher risk of cardiovascular events and risk of needing kidney replacement therapy. Dual RAAS blockade is not recommended, due to the increased risk of hyperkalemia and AKI.

2. **SGLT2 (Sodium-Glucose Transport Protein 2) Inhibition.** SGLT2 inhibitors block proximal tubule resorption of glucose, mediating glucosuria,

and with it, natriuretic effects on glomerular hyperfiltration via tubuloglomerular feedback. Multiple studies have demonstrated reduction of risk of progression of kidney disease and reduction in proteinuria for patients with albuminuria and type II diabetes without CKD. The first study of SGLT2i in patients with CKD, the DAPA CKD trial, enrolled patients with diabetic kidney disease or nondiabetic proteinuric CKD down to an eGFR of 25 mL/min/1.73 m^2 and demonstrated a 39% relative risk reduction in the primary composite outcome, and a 34% reduction in risk of long term dialysis and a 31% reduction in all-cause mortality. EMPA Kidney examined the risk of progression in kidney failure among patients with CKD down to a eGFR of 20 mL/min/1.73 m^2 (with or without diabetes and with or without albuminuria) and showed 28% risk reduction of kidney failure progression or death from cardiovascular causes.

3. **Mineralocorticoid Antagonism.** The 2020 FIDELIO study examining use of finerenone, a novel nonsteroidal aldosterone antagonist, in patients with proteinuria and diabetic nephropathy, including lower levels of albumin/creatinine (between 30 and 300 mg/g) in the setting of eGFR <60 mL/min/1.73 m^2 and documented diabetic nephropathy. Finerenone was able to reduce the progression of diabetic kidney disease in patients on maximal ACEi or ARB. The risk of decline in eGFR or ESKD was significantly reduced in this population, hazard ratio 0.82 (0.73–0.93, $P = .0001$). While FIDELIO focused on patient with stage 3 or 4 CKD and frank albuminuria, the 2021 FIGARO study included earlier CKD stages—patient with type II diabetes and early stage (1 or 2) CKD with severely increase albuminuria, or stage 2 to 4 CKD with moderate albuminuria. Finerenone did reduced the risk of composite cardiovascular outcomes (mostly via hospitalization in heart failure) and did not meet its secondary kidney outcome (kidney failure, eGFR decrease of 40%, or kidney-related death)—however, it did show decreased progression to kidney failure.

4. **GLP-1 Receptor Agonists.** GLP-1 receptor agonists are a novel diabetes medication with evidence of slowing eGFR decline and proteinuria. The AWARD-7 trial showed dulaglutide over 1 year slowed GFR decline in patients with diabetes, CKD 3 or 4, and a urine albumin creatinine ratio >300 mg/g.

5. **Lifestyle Modifications**
    a. **Glycemic Control.** Multiple studies have demonstrated the benefits of intensive glycemic control in slowing eGFR decline and reduction in albuminuria. A large meta-analysis demonstrated intensive glycemic control is associated with 20% reduced risk in incident kidney disease <30 mL/min/1.73 m^2, urine albumin >300 mg/g, kidney failure, or death.
    b. **Weight Loss and Exercise.** Weight loss may confer some benefit in slowing eGFR decline and proteinuria. A post hoc analysis of the LOOK-Ahead trial showed weight loss conferred a 31% risk reduction in incident high-risk CKD 3 or 4 with proteinuria. Exercise has not been prospectively evaluated to improve CKD progression, but is felt to mitigate both obesity and hypertension.
    c. **Diet:** KDIGO recommends 2 g of sodium or less for patients with CKD and hypertension, and protein restriction to <1.3 g/kg for patients with CKD 3, and 0.8 g/kg for patients with CKD 4 or 5. Plant-based diets may help with reducing progression of CKD3-5 due to low endogenous acid load, which may help manage metabolic complications of CKD. Further, restricting potassium has not demonstrated significant risk of hyperkalemia, and may deprive patients of the potential beneficial effects of these foods.
    d. **Smoking Cessation:** The relationship between smoking and CKD progression has been shown—while no prospective trial has demonstrated

that smoking cessation reduces the risk of CKD progression, smoking cessation improves blood pressure and cardiovascular risk.

VI. Managing Complications of CKD

A. Anemia. Anemia associated with CKD is typically a normocytic normochromic anemia. 50% of predialysis people with CKD have some degree of anemia. The sequelae of anemia in CKD can cause fatigue and shortness of breath due to impaired oxygen activity and left ventricular hypertrophy. Several mechanisms underpin pathogenesis of anemia in CKD, including deficiency in erythropoietin (EPO) in response to reduced hemoglobin level, absolute and functional iron deficiency, and reduced erythrocyte lifespan. Causes of EPO deficiency may be considered when the severity of anemia is disproportionate to eGFR, iron deficiency is present, or there is evidence of leukopenia or thrombocytopenia.

There is variability in the hemoglobin levels defining anemia. KDIGO defines anemia as a hemoglobin less than 13 g/dL in males and 12.0 g/dL in females. However, there has been considerable debate surrounding the therapeutic target range for patients with CKD or kidney failure. Targeting hemoglobin ranges near normal range has shown increased risks of thromboembolic risk, stroke, or death. Treatment options include:

1. **Erythropoiesis Stimulating Agent (ESA).** ESAs, such as recombinant EPO, can be administered intravenously or subcutaneously. Adverse effects of ESAs include a modest increase in blood pressure, increased risk of thromboembolic events, and enhancement of tumor growth in people with malignancy. As such, the lowest possible doses of ESAs should be used whenever possible. Causes of ESA failure in CKD patients—defined by KDIGO as lack of increase in hemoglobin after one month of weight-based treatment—include infection or inflammation and concomitant iron deficiency, in addition to underdosing. KDIGO recommends against starting an ESA with a hemoglobin level ≥10 g/dL (100 g/L) and not be used to maintain a level ≥11.5 g/dL (100 g/L).

2. **Iron Treatment.** Iron deficiency in CKD is defined as absolute (transferrin saturation <20%, ferritin <100 ng/mL) or functional (transferrin saturation <20%, ferritin <500 ng/mL). The underlying etiology of functional iron deficiency is felt to be secondary to increased levels of hepcidin, which regulates iron homeostasis. For CKD patients who are not on dialysis, KDIGO recommends the route of iron administration (oral versus intravenous) depending on the severity of iron deficiency, availability of venous access, response to prior oral iron therapy, side effects with prior iron therapy, patient compliance, and cost. Oral versus IV iron are safe and efficacious, though IV iron had a faster and higher rise in hemoglobin and both therapies improve anemia in patients with CKD 3 without statistical difference. However, the IV iron group has a higher risk of cardiovascular events in these studies, requiring early termination of the study. The main issue with traditional oral iron therapies (including ferric sulfate, ferrous fumarate, ferrous gluconate) has been plagued with limited absorption and gastrointestinal side effects. More recent formulations of oral iron including ferric citrate (a phosphate binder) with an improved side effect profile.

3. **HIF Stabilizers.** HIF (hypoxia inducible factor) stabilizers competitively inhibit HIF prolyl hydroxylases—leading to increased endogenous EPO production. These oral drugs (including roxadustat, vadadustat, and daprodustat) have shown efficacy and safety in nondialysis CKD and in phase III trials comparing HIF stabilizers to ESAs, HIF stabilizers were inferior to ESA in nondialysis patients with CKD. Currently, one HIF stabilizer (daprodustat) is approved only in patients receiving dialysis.

B. Mineral and Bone Disease. As the kidney is responsible for serum calcium and phosphorous regulation, compensation for nephron loss can affect levels of parathyroid hormone (PTH), fibroblast growth factor 23 (FGF23), and decrease calcitriol levels in order to normalize calcium and phosphorous levels in those with CKD as early as stage 2. At later stages of CKD, these compensatory mechanisms can fail, leading to a spectrum of disorders collectively termed CKD Mineral and bone disorder. This can include (1) abnormalities of calcium, phosphorous, PTH, or vitamin D metabolism, (2) changes in bone turnover and growth, leading to disorders including osteitis fibrosa, osteomalacia, adynamic bone disease, osteopenia among others, (3) vascular and tissue calcification. To treat and prevent sequelae of mineral bone disease, levels of phosphorous, calcium, PTH, and alkaline phosphate activity should be monitored starting at CKD stage 3a.

1. **Calcium.** In early stages of CKD, calcium levels are maintained through elevation in PTH. Decreased calcitriol levels lead to decreased intestinal absorption of calcium. Many patients have a net positive calcium balance due to decreased calcium excretion in the kidney. KIDGO recommends calcium be maintained in the normal range, via calcium-based binders (in the case of hypocalcemia) or vitamin D analogues.
2. **Vitamin D.** Many patients with CKD have decreased $1,25(OH)_2D$ levels, which is further decreased through suppression of 1-alpha hydroxylase activity via increased phosphorous and FGF-23 levels. Vitamin D deficiency can be mitigated with 25(OH) supplementation, and management of secondary hyperparathyroidism usually requires the use of calcitriol, as well as other $1,25(OH)_2D_2$ analogs.
3. **Phosphorous.** Phosphorous control is impaired at a GFR at 60 mL/min/1.73 m^2 and maintained through increases in FGF-23 and PTH. Around a GFR of 30 mL/min/1.73 m^2, this compensatory mechanism is overwhelmed, and hyperphosphatemia may result. Hyperphosphatemia leads to inhibition of calcitriol synthesis, stimulating PTH release and secondary hyperparathyroidism. KIDGO recommends phosphorous levels be maintained at normal levels (between 3.5 and 5.5 mg/dL). Phosphate can be controlled through diet, though this may be insufficient to control, especially at later stages of CKD. Phosphorous binders can aid in phosphorous control; commonly used binders include calcium-based binders (calcium acetate and calcium carbonate) or non–calcium-based binders (sevelamer, lanthanum carbonate, ferric citrate).
4. **PTH.** PTH levels initially rise in response to hyperphosphatemia in early CKD. KDIGO recommends that PTH levels in patients requiring kidney replacement therapy be maintained between <2 and >9 times the assay reference limits, as levels outside this have shown an effect on mortality. PTH can be maintained through correction of modifiable factors, via regulation of calcium and phosphorous (through oral calcium, nutritional vitamin D, $1,25(OH)_2D_2$ analogs), correction of vitamin D and calcitriol deficiency, and suppression of PTH with calcimimetics or parathyroidectomy.

C. Acid–Base Control. Acidosis is common in almost all forms of CKD. The main mechanism responsible for the acidosis is a decrease in total ammonia excretion, leading to a decrease in net hydrogen secretion and a fall in serum bicarbonate. This net positive acid balance results in dissolution of bone, ultimately worsening uremic osteodystrophy. Other adverse consequences of metabolic acidosis include protein malnutrition and the suppression of albumin synthesis. Treatment of acidosis with oral bicarbonate therapy may help prevent some of the bone disease of chronic uremia and may slow down kidney disease progression. Treatment with alkaline-rich plant-based diets also has demonstrated benefits comparable with sodium bicarbonate. However, multiple studies have not demonstrated significant effect of maintaining higher bicarbonate levels (bicarbonate >22 mmol/L). As such, KDIGO recommends dietary or pharmacologic treatment to avoid severe acidosis (bicarbonate <18 mmol/L).

D. Accumulation of Uremic Toxins. Spherical carbon absorbent AST-120 has been utilized in some areas to reduce systemic toxic absorption via the gastrointestinal tract. While early studies demonstrated some efficacy in delaying CKD progression, this has not been demonstrated in additional randomized control trials, and is currently not recommended by KDIGO.

VII. Managing Cardiovascular Comorbidity

CKD patients with an eGFR less than 60 mL/min/1.73 m^2 are more likely to die from CVD than are expected to progress to ESKD. The CKD population has a higher incidence of traditional cardiovascular risk factors, including diabetes, hypertension, and dyslipidemias, and in addition has multiple novel risk factors including but not limited to oxidative stress, inflammation, endothelial dysfunction, mineral bone disease, and cardiovascular calcification. In addition, overwhelming scientific evidence has shown that decreased GFR and proteinuria are independent risk factors for CVD. CVD in CKD can be characterized via left ventricular hypertrophy, vascular calcification, and vascular noncompliance. Consensus exists in the nephrology community that the CKD population should undergo aggressive risk factor management. This includes strict control of BP and lipids, as well as smoking cessation, exercise. KDIGO clinical practice guidelines on the management of dyslipidemias in CKD have recommended adults ≥50 years with an eGFR <60 mL/min/1.73 m^2 be treated with a statin or statin/ezetimibe combination, or for those with an eGFR >60 mL/min/1.73 m^2, a statin alone. For those between the ages 18 and 49 with CKD, a statin may be initiated in those with diabetes mellitus, known coronary disease, prior ischemic stroke, or an estimated 10-year incidence of cardiovascular event (death or nonfatal myocardial infarction) about 10%.

VIII. When to Refer to a Nephrologist

Several studies have shown that delayed referral to a nephrologist is common and is associated with adverse consequences, including greater morbidity and mortality, more severe uremia, increased use of percutaneous vascular access with associated morbidity, reduced use of the preferred arteriovenous fistula for vascular access, restricted patient choice of treatment modality, prolonged and more costly hospitalization at initiation of dialysis, and higher rates of emotional and socioeconomic problems. An early referral allows the patient to develop an effective relationship with a multidisciplinary team consisting of a nephrologist, vascular surgeon, nurse, dietitian, social worker, and mental health professional. This relationship allows for a more informed consideration by patients of kidney replacement options including transplantation, initiation of kidney replacement therapy to maintain optimal patient health, timely placement of a dialysis access, supervision of dietary modification, and support services regarding unmet psychological, social, and financial needs. A nephrologist should participate in the care of patients with a GFR of less than 30 mL/min/1.73 m^2.

SUGGESTED READINGS

Agarwal R, Sinha AD, Cramer AE, et al. Chlorthalidone for hypertension in advanced chronic kidney disease. *N Engl J Med*. 2021;385(27):2507–2519.

Al Kribria GM, Crispen R. Prevalence and trends of chronic kidney disease and its risk factors among US adults: an analysis of NHANES 2003–18. *Prev Med Rep*. 2020;20:101193.

Appel LJ, Wright JT Jr, Greene T, et al; African American Study of Kidney Disease and Hypertension Collaborative Research Group. Long-term effects of renin-angiotensin system-blocking therapy and a low blood pressure goal on progression of hypertensive chronic kidney disease in African Americans. *Arch Intern Med*. 2008;168(8):832–839.

Bakris GL, Agarwal R, Anker SD, et al; FIDELIO-DKD Investigators. Effect of finerenone on chronic kidney disease outcomes in type 2 diabetes. *N Engl J Med*. 2020;383(23):2219–2229.

Bhandari S, Mehta S, Khwaja A, et al; STOP ACEi Trial Investigators. Renin-angiotensin system inhibition in advanced chronic kidney disease. *N Engl J Med*. 2022;387(22):2021–2032.

Chertow GM, Pergola PE, Farag YMK, et al; PRO2TECT Study Group. Vadadustat in patients with anemia and non-dialysis-dependent CKD. *N Engl J Med.* 2021;384(17):1589–1600.

Cheung AK, Rahman M, Reboussin DM, et al; SPRINT Research Group. Effects of intensive BP control in CKD. *J Am Soc Nephrol.* 2017;28(9):2812–2823.

Clegg DJ, Hill Gallant KM. Plant-based diets in CKD. *Clin J Am Soc Nephrol.* 2019;14(1):141–143.

Cockcroft DW, Gault MH. Prediction of creatinine clearance from serum creatinine. *Nephron.* 1976;16(1):31–41.

Fried LF, Emanuele N, Zhang JH, et al; VA NEPHRON-D Investigators. Combined angiotensin inhibition for the treatment of diabetic nephropathy. *N Engl J Med.* 2013;369(20):1892–1903.

Hannan M, Ansari S, Meza N, et al; CRIC Study Investigators; Chronic Renal Insufficiency Cohort (CRIC) Study Investigators. Risk factors for CKD progression: overview of findings from the CRIC study. *Clin J Am Soc Nephrol.* 2021;16(4):648–659.

He J, Mills KT, Appel LJ, et al; Chronic Renal Insufficiency Cohort Study Investigators. Urinary sodium and potassium excretion and CKD progression. *J Am Soc Nephrol.* 2016;27(4):1202–1212.

Heerspink HJL, Stefánsson BV, Correa-Rotter R, et al; DAPA-CKD Trial Committees and Investigators. Dapagliflozin in patients with chronic kidney disease. *N Engl J Med.* 2020;383(15):1436–1446.

Hu EA, Coresh J, Anderson CAM, et al; CRIC Study Investigators. Adherence to healthy dietary patterns and risk of CKD progression and all-cause mortality: findings from the CRIC (chronic renal insufficiency cohort) study. *Am J Kidney Dis.* 2021;77(2):235–244.

Hultin S, Hood C, Campbell KL, Toussaint ND, Johnson DW, Badve SV. A systematic review and meta-analysis on effects of bicarbonate therapy on kidney outcomes. *Kidney Int Rep.* 2021;6(3):695–705.

Levey AS, Bosch JP, Lewis JB, Greene T, Rogers N, Roth D. A more accurate method to estimate glomerular filtration rate from serum creatinine: a new prediction equation. Modification of Diet in Renal Disease Study Group. *Ann Intern Med.* 1999;130(6):461–470.

Levey AS, Stevens LA, Schmid CH, et al; CKD-EPI (Chronic Kidney Disease Epidemiology Collaboration). A new equation to estimate glomerular filtration rate. *Ann Intern Med.* 2009;150(9):604–612.

Look AHEAD Research Group. Effect of a long-term behavioural weight loss intervention on nephropathy in overweight or obese adults with type 2 diabetes: a secondary analysis of the Look AHEAD randomised clinical trial. *Lancet Diabetes Endocrinol.* 2014;2(10):801–809.

Madias NE. Metabolic acidosis and CKD progression. *Clin J Am Soc Nephrol.* 2021;16(2):310–312.

McClellan W, Aronoff SL, Bolton WK, et al. The prevalence of anemia in patients with chronic kidney disease. *Curr Med Res Opin.* 2004;20(9):1501–1510.

Mende CW. Chronic kidney disease and SGLT2 inhibitors: a review of the evolving treatment landscape. *Adv Ther.* 2022;39(1):148–164.

Neal B, Wu Y, Feng X, et al. Effect of salt substitution on cardiovascular events and death. *N Engl J Med.* 2021;385(12):1067–1077.

Parsa A, Kao WHL, Xie D, et al; CRIC Study Investigators. APOL1 risk variants, race, and progression of chronic kidney disease. *N Engl J Med.* 2013;369(23):2183–2196.

Pitt B, Filippatos G, Agarwal R, et al; FIGARO-DKD Investigators. Cardiovascular events with finerenone in kidney disease and type 2 diabetes. *N Engl J Med.* 2021;385(24):2252–2263.

Ricardo AC, Yang W, Sha D, et al; CRIC Investigators. Sex-related disparities in CKD progression. *J Am Soc Nephrol.* 2019;30(1):137–146.

Ruggenenti P, Cravedi P, Remuzzi G. The RAAS in the pathogenesis and treatment of diabetic nephropathy. *Nat Rev Nephrol.* 2010;6(6):319–330.

Schulman G, Berl T, Beck GJ, et al. Randomized placebo-controlled EPPIC trials of AST-120 in CKD. *J Am Soc Nephrol.* 2015;26(7):1732–1746.

System USRD. *2022 USRDS Annual Data Report: Epidemiology of Kidney Disease in The United States.* National Institutes of Health, National Institute of Diabetes and Digestive and Kidney Diseases; 2020.

Tangri N, Grams ME, Levey AS, et al; CKD Prognosis Consortium. Multinational assessment of accuracy of equations for predicting risk of kidney failure: a meta-analysis. *JAMA.* 2016;315(2):164–174.

The EMPA-KIDNEY Collaborative Group; Herrington WG, Staplin N, Wanner C, et al. Empagliflozin in patients with chronic kidney disease. *N Engl J Med.* 2023;388(2):117–127.

Tuttle KR, Lakshmanan MC, Rayner B, et al. Dulaglutide versus insulin glargine in patients with type 2 diabetes and moderate-to-severe chronic kidney disease (AWARD-7): a multicentre, open-label, randomised trial. *Lancet Diabetes Endocrinol.* 2018;6(8):605–617.

14. The Patient Receiving Chronic Kidney Replacement With Dialysis

Natalie Beck, Seth Furgeson

Maintenance dialysis is a treatment for patients with advanced chronic kidney disease (CKD). While dialysis cannot duplicate many functions of a normal kidney, the goals of dialysis are to remove toxins that are normally cleared by the kidney and to maintain euvolemia. Ideally, chronic dialysis will improve the signs and symptoms of uremia and allow patients to return to predialysis functional status. There are two major types of dialysis: hemodialysis (HD; performed in a dialysis unit or at home) and peritoneal dialysis (PD; almost always done at home). There are no well-performed prospective clinical trials comparing the two modalities, so the choice of modality depends on patient preference, treatment availability, or possible contraindications to either modality.

In the United States, there has been a steady increase in the incidence and prevalence of end-stage kidney disease (ESKD) over the last 20 years (Fig. 14-1), with the exception of 2020 at which time the incident and prevalence rates decreased; this is felt to be a result of the devastation of the COVID-19 pandemic on patients with CKD. Although utilization of PD is increasing, the United States Renal Data System (USRDS) reported that in 2020 approximately 84% of patients in the United States used HD as their initial modality. Worldwide, approximately 89% of patients with ESKD who are treated with dialysis utilize HD as opposed to 11% who use PD.

I. Indications for Initiating Dialysis

Starting a patient on dialysis is associated with dramatic changes in the patient's lifestyle and is frequently associated with medical complications, especially related to vascular access. It is therefore important to thoroughly assess the risks and benefits of initiating dialysis. In general, life-threatening conditions such as severe hyperkalemia, severe volume overload, or uremic pericarditis will mandate prompt initiation of dialysis. Less severe symptoms such as mild cognitive changes associated with uremia warrant dialysis initiation if the patient has appropriate dialysis access (e.g., arteriovenous fistula [AVF] for HD or catheter for PD). If the patient does not have access, the benefits of dialysis must be weighed against the risks of a temporary HD catheter including infection. In some health care settings, urgent start PD is an option but should generally not be used as the initial modality when a life-threatening dialysis indication is present.

Ideally, dialysis should be initiated before life-threatening symptoms develop. Possible indications for initiating dialysis are listed in Table 14-1. The most recent guideline recommendations for dialysis initiation come from Kidney Disease: Improving Global Outcomes (KDIGO) and suggest initiating dialysis when symptoms or signs of kidney failure develop, blood pressure (BP) or volume status is uncontrolled, or nutritional status deteriorates.

Although most patients with a severely depressed glomerular filtration rate (GFR; <10 mL/min) will have some complications of kidney failure, there is no specific GFR that mandates dialysis initiation. Possible benefits of starting dialysis earlier (GFR >10 mL/min) include preventing malnutrition and improving volume status. While observational studies have had conflicting results regarding the benefits of starting dialysis early, there has only been one controlled study to test the

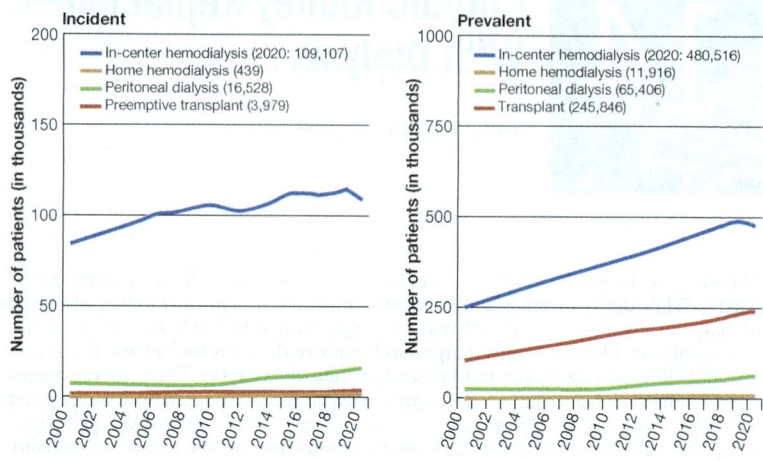

Figure 14-1. Incident and prevalent end-stage kidney disease (ESKD) counts in the United States by modality. (Adapted from the 2022 United States Renal Data System Annual Data Report.)

timing of dialysis initiation in patients with CKD. The Initiating Dialysis Early and Late (IDEAL) study randomized 828 adults to early-start dialysis (GFR 10 to 14 mL/min) or late-start dialysis (GFR 5 to 7 mL/min). The primary outcome was death from any cause. In the intention-to-treat analysis, there was no difference in the primary endpoint between the two groups. After a follow-up of 3.6 years, both groups had a mortality rate of over 35%. There was also no difference in secondary outcomes (cardiovascular events, infections) between the groups. In the study, the treating physician could initiate dialysis with a GFR above 7 mL/min if it was felt to be warranted and most patients in the late start group did start

TABLE 14-1 Potential Indications for Dialysis Initiation in CKD
Volume overload refractory to diuretics
Resistant hypertension
Pleuritis or pericarditis
Peripheral neuropathy
Encephalopathy
Malnutrition
Nausea, vomiting, or anorexia
Uremic bleeding
Metabolic acidosis
Hyperkalemia
Severe hyperphosphatemia
Severe hypocalcemia

TABLE 14-2 Comparison of Hemodialysis to Peritoneal Dialysis

Hemodialysis	Peritoneal Dialysis
Performed by medical staff (in center HD)	Performed by patient or caregiver
Intermittent	Daily
Requires travel to dialysis unit (in center HD)	Done at home
Requires vascular access	Requires peritoneal catheter
Needles used to access AVF or AVG	No needles required
May require dietary potassium restriction	No dietary potassium restriction

above this threshold. It should also be noted that the estimated GFR difference (by the Modification of Diet in Renal Disease [MDRD] equation) between the groups was small: 9.0 mL/min in the early group versus 7.2 mL/min in the late group. While the IDEAL study does not support routinely starting dialysis in patients with a GFR between 10 and 15 mL/min, it did show that most patients develop a need for dialysis soon after their GFR falls below 10 mL/min.

Education regarding dialysis is an essential part of predialysis care. Patients should understand the difference between HD and PD (Table 14-2). Patients should also be well informed regarding all possible options including kidney transplant and palliative care. Some patients with significantly reduced life expectancy (severe comorbidity or elderly patients) may not live longer with dialysis and may have a reduction in quality of life with dialysis. One study found that elderly patients requiring skilled nursing facility (SNF) placement after dialysis initiation had a 6-month mortality rate of 39%. Of those who survived at 6 months, 37% required long-term nursing home care but, of those who were discharged from SNF care, 75% remained functionally impaired. The decision to initiate dialysis in patients with a reduced life expectancy should be a collaborative one between the patient, nephrologist, and family members.

II. Hemodialysis

A. Hemodialysis Procedure. HD is the most common dialysis modality used in the United States. It is usually performed at an outpatient dialysis unit but can also be done at home. HD at dialysis units is typically performed thrice weekly with each treatment lasting close to 4 hours. Some patients receive longer nocturnal sessions at dialysis units. Home dialysis patients do shorter treatments more frequently (five or six times weekly, known as short daily dialysis) or nocturnal treatments.

During the HD procedure, blood is rapidly moved through an extracorporeal circuit. Blood is removed by a needle or through a catheter port and enters the dialysis filter (Fig. 14-2). The dialysis filter contains thousands of hollow tubes with a semipermeable membrane. On the outside of the tube is the dialysate moving in a countercurrent fashion (Table 14-3). Solutes in the blood (high concentration) move into the dialysate (low concentration) by diffusion. Blood is then returned via a separate venous needle or port. In a process known as ultrafiltration, fluid is removed by applying hydrostatic pressure across the dialysis membrane.

Conventional HD has many advantages. With modern filters, the treatment provides rapid and effective removal of small-molecular-weight solutes over a few hours. HD machines allow for precise control of ultrafiltration, allowing providers to prescribe a specific amount of fluid removal. In dialysis centers,

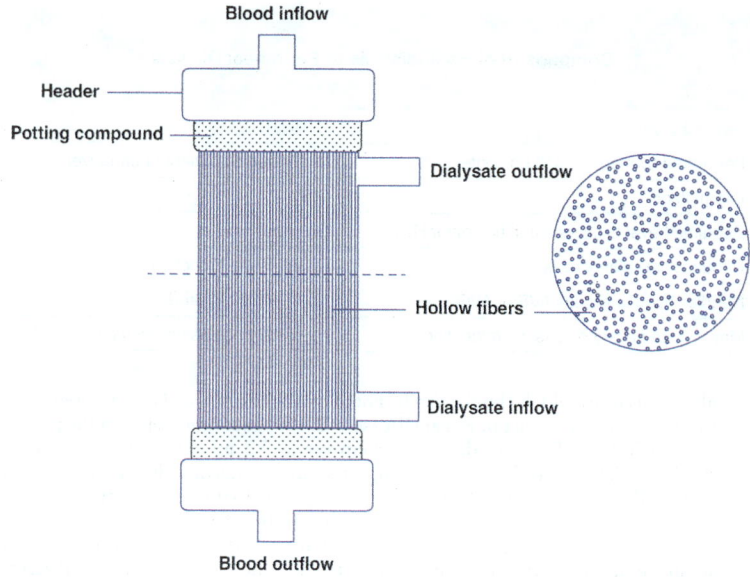

Figure 14-2. Schematic of a dialysis filter. (From Bieber SD, Himmelfarb J. Hemodialysis. In: Coffman TM, Falk RJ, Molitoris BA, Neilson EG, Schrier RW, eds. *Schrier's Diseases of the Kidney*. Vol II, 9th ed. Lippincott Williams & Wilkins, 2013:2473–2505.)

patients have trained health care professionals perform the treatment for them and the total treatment time is roughly 12 hours/wk. However, in-center HD does have some limitations. Since it is an intermittent treatment, fluid removal is not physiologic and often necessitates removing large volumes of fluid during a short period of time. HD is also not very effective at removing larger molecules or solutes that are protein-bound. Some of these limitations can be mitigated with home hemodialysis due to the longer total treatment time per week.

B. Hemodialysis Access. To perform HD regularly, it is necessary to have a dialysis access through which blood can circulate at a fast flow rate. The preferred access for HD is an AVF. AVFs are created by surgical anastomoses of an artery

TABLE 14-3 Comparison of Standard Dialysate Solutions

	Hemodialysis	Peritoneal Dialysis
Sodium	135–140 mEq/L	132 mEq/L
Potassium	2, 3 mEq/L	0 mEq/L
Calcium	2.5, 3 mEq/L	2.5, 3.5 mEq/L
Magnesium	0.5–1 mEq/L	0.5 mEq/L
Base	25–40 mEq/L (bicarbonate)	40 mEq/L (lactate)
Glucose	100 mg/dL	1.5%, 2.5%, 4.25% (dextrose)

to a vein, usually in the arm. AVFs have the lowest rate of both infectious and noninfectious complications and, on average, can be used longer than other types of accesses. However, AVFs take time to mature (at least 6 to 8 weeks but up to 6 to 9 months), can require multiple interventions to become functional, and sometimes fail to ever become suitable for dialysis. Prior to creation of an AVF, mapping of the upper extremity veins is usually done with ultrasound to measure vein diameter and can detect central stenoses. As recommended in the Kidney Disease Outcomes Quality Initiative (K/DOQI) guidelines, the AVF should ideally be placed distally in the nondominant arm. However, since the success of an AVF depends on the size of the vein, if the forearm veins are less than 3 mm, then a nondominant upper arm fistula would be the second choice.

Arteriovenous grafts (AVGs) are synthetic grafts that are connected to the artery and vein. AVGs can be used more quickly, sometimes as early as 2 to 3 weeks after placement. AVGs also have a higher primary success rate. However, AVGs fail sooner than AVFs due to neointimal hyperplasia, require frequent interventions to maintain patency, and have a higher infection risk due to prosthetic material. AVGs should ideally be placed in the arms but can be placed in the thigh if there are no suitable arm veins.

Finally, dual-lumen central venous catheters (CVCs) can be used for dialysis. CVCs are most often placed in the internal jugular vein and can be used immediately for dialysis. Subclavian CVCs should be avoided as they are associated with a high risk of subclavian stenosis, a complication that causes morbidity and usually will prevent future dialysis access in the ipsilateral arm. CVCs intended for use for more than a few days are tunneled under the skin to decrease the rate of infection but regardless, CVCs have a much higher infection rate than AVFs or AVGs and also have a high rate of dysfunction.

Since AVFs are the preferred access yet take time to mature, patients with stage 4 CKD should be referred for fistula placement prior to starting dialysis. Accesses are preferably placed in the nondominant arm; therefore, preserving the nondominant arm from needle sticks, peripheral intravenous (IV) lines, and peripherally inserted central catheters (PICCs) is important in patients with CKD. In patients with limited life expectancy, AVGs or CVCs may be preferred for dialysis access.

C. Hemodialysis Complications. HD is associated with numerous complications. There are both infectious and noninfectious complications of the vascular access. Infectious complications are relatively common in HD patients and lead to significant morbidity. Most commonly, HD patients develop bloodstream infections with gram-positive bacteria, such as *Staphylococcus aureus* and coagulase-negative staphylococci. In addition to appropriate antibiotic therapy, the dialysis catheter needs to be removed in patients with *S. aureus* bacteremia. AVFs and AVGs can develop stenosis near the venous anastomoses or in central veins. Venous stenosis can lead to arm swelling, difficulty with cannulation, and prolonged bleeding after dialysis. Stenoses are usually treated with percutaneous angioplasty.

During the first few dialysis treatments, patients starting dialysis may develop the disequilibrium syndrome, characterized by headache, somnolence, and rarely seizures or coma. It is thought that disequilibrium syndrome is due to cerebral edema after a rapid decrease in plasma osmolality; it is rarely seen if the initial dialysis treatments are short and done with low blood flows. HD also commonly causes hypotension which is associated with rapid ultrafiltration rates and/or autonomic dysfunction. A newly appreciated complication of dialysis is the development of silent myocardial ischemia (MI) and myocardial stunning during the treatment which over time likely contribute to the significant cardiovascular morbidity and mortality seen in dialysis patients. Very rare but potentially fatal complications of the dialysis procedure are air emboli and anaphylaxis.

III. Peritoneal Dialysis

A. PD Procedure. PD is usually done by the patient or caregiver at home and is designed to be a continuous therapy. To perform PD, a catheter is tunneled through the subcutaneous portion of the abdominal wall into the peritoneal cavity. The location at which the catheter penetrates the skin of the anterior abdominal wall is known as the exit site. Prepackaged sterile dialysate is infused into the peritoneal cavity and allowed to dwell there for a period of several hours. Peritoneal dialysate has a high osmotic (or oncotic) pressure due to the presence of dextrose or icodextrin (a starch). The electrolyte concentration of dextrose-based solutions is presented in Table 14-3. Therefore, fluid moves from the mesenteric capillaries to the peritoneal cavity by osmosis. Solutes move down their concentration gradient by diffusion and are also removed with fluid by convection. The dialysate and ultrafiltrate are then drained from the peritoneal cavity and fresh dialysate is instilled. There are two main types of PD. Continuous ambulatory PD (CAPD) is a manual therapy whereby the patient generally performs three to four manual exchanges of dialysate daily. Automated PD (APD) uses a cycler machine to instill and drain dialysate many times throughout the night. When a dwell of dialysate is left in the peritoneum during the day, this is known as continuous cycling PD (CCPD). When patients use the cycler to perform exchanges at night but no fluid is left in the peritoneal cavity during the day, the treatment is known as nocturnal intermittent PD (NIPD.) NIPD is commonly used for patients with significant residual kidney function who may not need a day dwell.

PD is the preferred dialysis modality in some countries due to its lower cost. It often provides the patient with more freedom and autonomy than does HD. However, the patient is responsible for performing the exchanges, taking vital signs, weighing themselves, and determining the proper dextrose concentrations for their dwells (thereby affecting their fluid removal). Although some patients on HD maintain employment, PD may make it easier to continue working due to an uninterrupted day when performing APD. Fluid removal is also more gradual and continuous than with HD, potentially making PD more tolerable from a hemodynamic standpoint. As it does not require vascular access, PD may be easier to perform than HD in a patient without adequate veins.

B. Complications of PD. PD is usually not associated with bloodstream infections. However, patients can develop exit site or tunnel infections or infectious peritonitis. Exit site infections present with pain at the exit site, erythema, and purulent drainage. The most common organisms associated with exit site infections are coagulase-negative Staphylococcus, *S. aureus*, and *Pseudomonas aeruginosa*. Unless the patient has a history of *Pseudomonas* exit site infection, initial treatment can be directed against gram-positive organisms and tailored depending on culture data. Tunnel infections (which can occur with or without an exit site infection) can present with tenderness or fluid collection along the subcutaneous path of the catheter and require prolonged antibiotic treatment. Peritonitis is diagnosed if the patient meets two out of three diagnostic criteria: abdominal pain, cloudy PD fluid with white blood cells >100 cells/L and >50% neutrophils, or positive Gram stain or culture of PD fluid. Empiric antibiotic treatment of peritonitis requires coverage for both gram-positive and gram-negative bacteria until a pathogen is identified and antibiotic therapy can be tailored. When treating peritonitis, antibiotics can be instilled into the peritoneal dialysate fluid and dwell in the abdomen for a period of hours, which in many cases can allow for treatment in the home and avoid the need for IV access. Most cases of bacterial peritonitis resolve with antibiotic therapy. Peritoneal catheters may need to be removed if there is a concurrent exit site infection or relapsing peritonitis (repeat episode with same bacteria). Fungal peritonitis can be brought on by overgrowth from antibiotic use so it is recommended to give antifungal prophylaxis whenever PD patients take a course of antibiotics. Patients with fungal peritonitis should always have the catheter removed.

Due to increased intra-abdominal pressure, PD can cause inguinal or abdominal wall hernias. As a result, patients who have a hernia will need to have it repaired prior to initiating PD. Patients with diaphragmatic disruption may have PD fluid enter the pleural space leading to pleural effusions. Standard peritoneal dialysate solutions do not contain potassium; this allows for liberalization of dietary potassium compared to patients on HD, but can sometimes result in hypokalemia (see Table 14-2 for comparison of HD and PD dialysate composition). Since PD contains hypertonic dextrose, patients typically receive a moderate carbohydrate load with therapy which can cause hyperglycemia in the diabetic patient. Finally, catheter problems such as kinking or malposition can lead to problems with dialysis and may require surgical correction.

IV. General Issues Related to Care of Chronic Dialysis Patients
A. Dialysis Dose. A major goal of dialysis is to eliminate uremic signs and symptoms. If patients continue to have uremic symptoms on dialysis, the dose should be increased to improve removal of uremic solutes. On HD, the dose can be intensified by increasing the dialysis time, blood flow rate (within limitations of the access), or surface area of the dialysis filter. On PD, the major modifications that increase dialysis dose are increasing dwell volumes or adding exchanges. In the absence of uremic symptoms, measuring urea clearance with dialysis offers a way to monitor dialysis dose. Urea is used as the primary measurement since it is an easily measured small molecule and is a surrogate for uremic toxins. The two most common equations measuring dialysis dose for HD are urea reduction ratio (URR), shown in Table 14-4, and Kt/V urea, a unitless value that represents urea clearance over time normalized to the volume of distribution. Kt/V can be estimated from many different equations where URR can be easily calculated at the bedside. However, the URR measurement does not consider changes in body volume that occur with HD. PD adequacy is typically measured by calculating the weekly standardized Kt/V urea.

Though observational studies have suggested that higher urea clearance is associated with improved mortality, these findings have not been borne out in the few randomized controlled trials testing two or more different doses of dialysis. The HEMO study randomized 1,846 patients on thrice-weekly HD to standard or high-dose dialysis. The standard-dose group received on average 190-minute dialysis treatments three times a week while the high-dose group received 219 minutes per treatment. After a follow-up of over 2 years and despite good separation in Kt/V between the two groups, there was no difference in mortality and both groups had an average yearly mortality of over 16%. The Adequacy of PD in Mexico (ADEMEX) trial randomized 965 patients to continue a standard PD prescription or increase the dose of PD to achieve a prespecified weekly clearance threshold. At 2 years, there was no survival

TABLE 14-4 Calculation of Urea Reduction Ratio

$$\frac{\text{Predialysis BUN} - \text{postdialysis BUN}}{\text{Predialysis BUN}} \times 100\%$$

BUN, blood urea nitrogen.

advantage with high-dose PD and both groups had mortality rates greater than 30%. However, fewer patients with high-dose PD developed uremic symptoms. Based on observational data and interventional studies, some guidelines recommend that in-center HD patients achieve minimum single-pool Kt/V of 1.4, home hemodialysis patients have a standardized weekly (std) Kt/V of 2.1, and that PD patients have a minimum std Kt/V of 1.7.

B. Cardiovascular Health. In the United States, the majority of the patients on dialysis die from cardiovascular causes, such as acute myocardial infarction, sudden cardiac death, and congestive heart failure. Unfortunately, reducing cardiovascular mortality has been hampered by the lack of evidence-based therapies. Two large studies randomizing dialysis patients to statins or placebo have not shown a mortality benefit. Since left ventricular hypertrophy (LVH) and volume overload are present in the majority of incident patients, it is possible that improved fluid control can prevent worsening cardiac function. Achieving euvolemia requires both fluid removal with dialysis and patient adherence to a low-salt diet. The Frequent Hemodialysis Network (FHN Daily) trial showed that more frequent dialysis may lead to regression of LVH.

As there are no interventional studies supporting a specific goal BP in dialysis patients, the ideal BP for a dialysis patient is not known. Clinical practice is dictated by extrapolating results from the general and CKD populations. Data from observational studies in dialysis patients can be helpful but unfortunately, observational studies have shown conflicting results regarding BP control and cardiovascular mortality. This is partly due to high variability of BP readings in HD patients depending on the timing of the measurement. In fact, ambulatory BP monitors predict mortality better in dialysis patients than measurements taken during dialysis. To achieve BP control, maintaining euvolemia is crucial; however, despite achieving euvolemia, many patients will require antihypertensive medications.

C. Mineral Bone Disorder. Abnormalities in mineral metabolism begin long before the patient starts dialysis. Increases in circulating parathyroid hormone (PTH) and the phosphaturic hormone fibroblast growth factor 23 (FGF-23) often occur in patients with CKD stages 2 and 3. Serum phosphorous rises and serum calcium decreases later in the course of CKD. These biochemical changes are associated with changes in bone metabolism. Elevated PTH is usually associated with high-turnover bone disease (osteitis fibrosa cystica) and can be supported by an elevated level of bone-specific alkaline phosphatase. Dialysis patients can also develop osteomalacia, a disease of defective bone mineralization sometimes associated with aluminum toxicity. Finally, low-turnover or adynamic bone disease is associated with low PTH levels and high serum calcium levels. Although blood markers can help distinguish forms of bone disease, a bone biopsy is the only definitive way to diagnose the specific abnormality in bone metabolism. It is generally accepted that maintaining a normal serum phosphorous and reducing severely elevated PTH levels will improve overall bone health.

D. Nutrition. Preventing malnutrition improves quality of life for dialysis patients and likely improves mortality. Dialysis patients are at risk for malnutrition due to enhanced muscle breakdown, inadequate caloric intake, and protein losses due to dialysis itself. A comprehensive assessment of nutritional status includes serial weight measurements, serum markers (such as albumin or creatinine), questionnaires (Subjective Global Assessment), dietary interviews, anthropomorphic measurements, and possibly urine collections to measure nitrogen excretion (an estimate of daily protein intake). Low serum albumin measurements do correlate with mortality. However, serum albumin alone is not sufficiently sensitive or specific enough to diagnose protein energy malnutrition.

K/DOQI guidelines recommend that dialysis patients consume 25 to 35 kcal/kg/d depending on what is needed to maintain nutritional status.

The recommendations also state that dialysis patients should eat 1.0 to 1.2 g/kg/d of protein. There is a significant body of data demonstrating that treatment of metabolic acidosis improves nutritional status and can reduce the risk of bone demineralization. Therefore, it is important to ensure that dialysis patients maintain normal serum bicarbonate levels while also avoiding metabolic alkalosis, which may result in decreased cerebral blood flow and increased risks of cramping and hemodynamic instability.

E. Anemia. Anemia occurs in most patients on dialysis. In observational studies, anemia was associated with decreased quality of life, impaired cardiac function, and increased mortality. In the past, anemia was mainly treated with red blood cell transfusions, with risks of iron overload, sensitization to future transplants, and potential exposure to infections such as hepatitis B, hepatitis C, and HIV. Recombinant erythropoietic agents (ESAs), such as erythropoietin and darbepoetin, are now used to treat anemia and prevent blood transfusions. However, there is no data from randomized trials that ESAs improve mortality in dialysis patients. Because high doses of ESAs can cause hypertension, vascular access problems, and strokes, it is recommended that they not be used to increase the hemoglobin above 11.5 g/dL. A variety of IV iron formulations are also commonly used in dialysis patients. The newer formulations are well tolerated and help improve responsiveness to ESAs. To date, there are no long-term data concerning IV iron formulations and mortality. There are many treatment strategies for using these agents, including some that rely more heavily on IV iron. The Proactive Intravenous Iron Therapy in Haemodialysis Patients (PIVOTAL) trial demonstrated that a proactive high-dose strategy of IV iron administration compared to a reactive approach reduced ESA dosing. The trial showed no difference in adverse events such as infection; administering high dose IV iron was noninferior to reactively administering IV iron with respect to the primary outcome of nonfatal MI, stroke, hospitalization, or death.

SUGGESTED READINGS

Bowling CB, Plantinga L, Hall RS, Mirk A, Zhang R, Kutner N. Association of nondisease-specific problems with mortality, long-term care, and functional impairment among older adults who require skilled nursing care after dialysis initiation. *Clin J Am Soc Nephrol*. 2016;11(12): 2218–2224.

Cooper BA, Branley P, Bulfone L, et al; IDEAL Study. A randomized, controlled trial of early versus late initiation of dialysis. *N Engl J Med*. 2010;363(7):609–619.

Eknoyan G, Beck GJ, Cheung AK, et al; Hemodialysis (HEMO) Study Group. Effect of dialysis dose and membrane flux in maintenance hemodialysis. *N Engl J Med*. 2002;347(25):2010–2019.

FHN Trial Group; Chertow GM, Levin NW, Beck GJ, et al. The FHN Trial Group. In-center hemodialysis six times per week versus three times per week. *N Engl J Med*. 2010;363(24):2287–2300.

Himmelfarb J, Ikizler TA. Hemodialysis. *N Engl J Med*. 2010;363(19):1833–1845.

Ikizler TA, Burrowes JD, Byham-Gray LD, et al. KDOQI clinical practice guideline for nutrition in CKD: 2020 update. *Am J Kidney Dis*. 2020;76(3)(suppl 1):S1–S107.

Kidney Disease: Improving Global Outcomes (KDIGO) Anemia Work Group. KDIGO clinical practice guideline for anemia in chronic kidney disease. *Kidney Inter Suppl*. 2012;2:279–335.

Macdougall IC, White C, Anker SD, et al; PIVOTAL Investigators and Committees. Intravenous iron in patients undergoing maintenance hemodialysis. *N Engl J Med*. 2019;380(5):447–458.

Paniagua R, Amato D, Vonesh E, et al. Effects of increased peritoneal clearances on mortality rates in peritoneal dialysis: ADEMEX, a prospective, randomized, controlled trial. *J Am Soc Nephrol*. 2002;13(5):1307–1320.

Pecoits-Filho R, Okpechi IG, Donner J-A, et al. Capturing and monitoring global differences in untreated and treated end-stage kidney disease, kidney replacement therapy modality, and outcomes. *Kidney Int Suppl (2011)*. 2020;10(1):e3–e9.

Teitelbaum I. Peritoneal dialysis. *N Engl J Med*. 2021;385(19):1786–1795.

United States Renal Data System. *2022 USRDS Annual Data Report: Epidemiology of Kidney Disease in the United States*. National Institutes of Health, National Institute of Diabetes and Digestive and Kidney Diseases; 2022.

15 The Patient With a Kidney Transplant

Sixto Giusti, James Cooper, Erik Stites

I. Introduction and Epidemiology

The prevalence of end-stage kidney disease (ESKD) in the United States and developed nations is alarmingly high. According to the United States Renal Data System 2020 Annual Data Report, nearly 786,000 people in the United States are living with ESKD. The incidence of kidney failure in the United States is projected to increase 18% by 2030, owing in large part to changes in age, race distribution, obesity, and diabetes prevalence. Currently, hemodialysis, peritoneal dialysis, and kidney transplantation are the only available therapies for ESKD.

Comparisons of kidney transplant recipients to patients on dialysis awaiting transplantation have shown that kidney transplantation, in most cases, is the ideal treatment for ESRD. Advantages include longer patient survival, less morbidity, cost savings, and improved quality of life compared with dialysis. In 2021, there were approximately 25,000 kidney transplants done in the United States, with approximately 23% coming from living donors. Living kidney donation remains the most effective therapy, with an average median graft survival of approximately 19 years. Median survival for deceased donor transplants is approximately 12 years. This good news is tempered by the reality that demand for kidney transplants far exceeds the supply of available organs. Although modest increases in deceased donor transplants have occurred owing to efforts to improve recovery from expanded donors, donors with cardiac death, and donors with brain death, these increases have not kept pace with demand. With more than 139,000 patients on the kidney waiting list in 2021, the unfortunate result is that many patients will die on the waiting list before receiving a transplant.

II. Patient Selection

There are few contraindications to receiving a kidney transplant. However, patients should not receive a transplant if they have an active infection, ongoing active immunologic disease that led to kidney failure, metastatic malignancy, are unable to follow a medical regimen due to medical or psychological reasons, or are at high operative risk due to other conditions. Although there is no definite age limit to receive a kidney transplant, elderly patients (age >70) with comorbid conditions have less demonstrable survival benefits compared with dialysis and should be screened thoroughly and counseled regarding expected benefits and potential risks of transplantation.

A. Recipient Evaluation. The goals of evaluating a potential recipient should be to identify potential barriers to transplantation, identify treatable conditions that would attenuate the risk of the surgery or immunosuppression, and explain the benefits and risks. Attention is given to the cause of ESRD and its tendency to recur in kidney transplants. Comorbid conditions and the effects of immunosuppression on these conditions are considered. Patient age older than 50 years, diabetes, abnormal electrocardiogram, angina, or congestive heart failure have been demonstrated as predictors of cardiac death and nonfatal cardiac events with kidney transplantation. Noninvasive strategies such as thallium perfusion imaging and dobutamine stress echo have demonstrated the ability to predict cardiac events and may prevent high-risk patients from requiring angiography. Screening for malignancy should follow age-appropriate guidelines. In patients with malignancies, the benefits of transplantation must be weighed against the risk of malignancy recurrence in the setting of immunosuppression. Disease characteristics such as tumor type, invasiveness, and prior treatment may necessitate a 2- to 5-year remission period before transplantation. Although obesity is a risk for wound-related complications, long-term outcomes are similar to nonobese patients unless cardiovascular disease exists. Psychosocial screening is usually performed. Testing generally includes evaluation for human immunodeficiency virus (HIV) and hepatitis B and C. Imaging or functional evaluation of the kidneys and lower urinary tract may be necessary in certain patients. ABO and human leukocyte antigen (HLA) typing is performed, along with determination of serologic status for cytomegalovirus (CMV) and varicella. After a patient has been accepted as a candidate, he or she is added to the transplant waiting list, at which time initial medical screening of potential living kidney donors can take place. A patient on the waiting list for more than 1 year should be seen periodically to update his or her condition.

The candidate's blood is screened for anti-HLA antibodies using single antigen beads (SABs) while on the transplant waiting list at various intervals depending on individual program protocols. Antibodies against another individual's HLA antigen(s) are produced as a result of sensitizing events such as prior transfusion, pregnancy, and/or organ transplant. Anti-HLA antibodies detected as a result of this screening process are used to calculate the overall degree of HLA sensitization, or calculated panel reactive antibody (cPRA). If the antibodies are deemed clinically significant by the transplant center, the corresponding HLA antigen is listed as "unacceptable" for that recipient, and donor kidneys containing that antigen will not be offered. Thus, higher values of cPRA equate to fewer potential compatible donors, potentially resulting in significantly longer expected waiting times for the recipient. Current organ allocation policy gives allocation priority to highly sensitized patients to attempt to mitigate this effect. This process is known as "virtual cross-matching." See Section IV.A for more details regarding donor/recipient cross-matching.

B. Organ Donors
1. **Living Donors.** Although the risks of kidney donation are small, these risks need to be carefully explained to a potential **living donor**. Mortality is uncommon, but has occurred in 0.02% of donors (2 per 10,000). Infection, bleeding, and other postoperative complications occur in up to 15% of patients. Progression to ESRD has occurred and may be slightly more common than in the general population, however remains an infrequent consequence. Mild blood pressure elevation and proteinuria after donation have been reported in some studies but not all, and the long-term consequences are currently unclear. After ABO compatibility and a negative cross-match are assured, the donor evaluation process can begin. If there are multiple candidates, the donor with fewer HLA mismatches is usually selected. Donors are carefully screened for kidney disease to prevent the possibility of loss of function in the remaining kidney. Hypertension, proteinuria, obesity, kidney stones, and structural or functional kidney disease are all relative contraindications to donation depending on severity. Testing for latent diabetes mellitus with a glucose tolerance test may be performed if there is a family history or perceived risk of future diabetes. When recipients are affected by hereditary disorders such as polycystic kidney disease or hereditary nephritis, the condition must be ruled out in related donors either clinically or with genetic testing. If a donor is thought to be acceptable, imaging of the kidneys is performed with computed tomographic (CT)

angiography or other modalities, allowing the team to assess for structural or vascular anomalies and suitability for laparoscopic donation.
2. **Deceased Donors.** A deceased donor must also be evaluated. The presence of metastasis, unknown cause of death, HIV, or widespread infection precludes donation. Donors with hepatitis C are sometimes accepted for hepatitis C–positive recipients. A combination of factors such as hypertension, advanced age, elevated serum creatinine, oliguria, or dependence on pressor support may exclude a donor. Preimplantation biopsies can be performed on an individual basis when there is concern about the function of a donor kidney. Each deceased donor is classified by the **kidney donor profile index** (KDPI), which is a composite score of a variety of donor factors that correlate with expected graft survival. The KDPI score is on a scale of 0% to 100% with a higher score correlated with greater risk of decreased graft survival. Despite higher risk of graft failure, high KDPI kidneys (>85%) still provide a survival advantage relative to remaining on dialysis for selected populations. They are commonly used in recipients with characteristics associated with poor dialysis survival such as advanced age or diabetes. In **donation after cardiac death** (DCD), organs are recovered from a donor who has undergone cardiac death after a period of circulatory arrest, usually in the setting of a withdrawal of care in the hospital. Although longer warm ischemia times lead to an increase in delayed graft function (DGF), DCD kidneys have similar long-term survival and function when compared with kidneys from brain-dead donors (DBD).

C. Predictors of Outcome. Recipient factors, donor factors, and donor/recipient compatibility all influence long-term graft survival. Recipients who are younger, have low levels of PRA, have spent less time on dialysis, and who are employed or college-educated have superior graft survival. Race and ethnicity may affect graft survival for both donors and recipients, with non-Black donor kidneys and non-Black, non-Hispanic recipients of grafts having the longest graft survival. Kidneys from living-related or unrelated donors survive longer on average than deceased donor kidneys, as do kidneys from younger compared with older donors. As described above, KDPI is composite score of multiple donor factors that correlate with expected graft survival. Finally, factors of donor and recipient compatibility also affect outcomes: better HLA matching, negative immunologic cross-matching, CMV serologic status matching, and equivalent donor/recipient body mass index all have positive effects on long-term graft survival.

III. Immunology and Pharmacotherapy

A. Immunology. A basic review of the mechanisms of immune recognition and response to an allograft is helpful to better understand the patient who has undergone kidney transplantation as well as the pharmacologic agents used to prevent allograft rejection.

1. **Major Histocompatibility Complex.** Cells in the tissues of mammals, birds, and bony fish express major histocompatibility complex (MHC) surface molecules, which are crucial for the immune system to be able to recognize and respond to a foreign antigen. In humans, these MHC molecules are located on the short arm of chromosome 6 and encode proteins termed the *HLAs*. MHC molecules serve two basic functions: they identify self from nonself and coordinate the T-cell receptor (TCR) recognition of the antigen–MHC complex. The MHC molecules are divided into two groups: class I and class II. MHC class I molecules appear on the surface of all nucleated cells and are known as *HLA-A, B,* and *C.* MHC class II molecules appear on antigen-presenting cells (APCs) and are termed *HLA-DR, DP,* and *DQ*. One MHC *haplotype* is inherited from each parent as a locus containing each of the six genetically linked HLA molecules. A "zero-antigen

mismatched kidney" has no mismatches in either locus for HLA-A, -B, and -DR, although mismatches may be present at HLA-C, -DP, -DQ, or at other minor antigens. Although advances in immunosuppression have narrowed advantages for well-matched transplants, a two-haplotype identical transplant from a family member or a zero-antigen mismatched deceased donor transplant confers a graft survival benefit compared with transplants with lesser degrees of matching.

2. **Antigen-Presenting Cells.** APCs are distributed in a ubiquitous manner in body tissues and allow T-cells to recognize foreign antigens. Monocytes, macrophages, dendritic cells, and activated B-cells can all serve as APCs. Either by phagocytosis or through surface immunoglobulin (Ig) (B-cells), APCs capture foreign antigens, degrade and process them into peptides, and express these foreign peptides on MHC class II surface molecules. Through TCR interactions and various downstream events, the T-cell is then able to coordinate an immune response to this foreign antigen.

3. **T-Cells.** T-cells are processed in the thymus and are central to cellular immunity and allograft recognition and rejection. These properties make them a common target of drugs designed to prevent rejection. Central to the immune response is the ability of the T-cell to recognize foreign antigens through a surface TCR. These receptors recognize antigens through either indirect or direct pathways. The *indirect pathway* involves TCR recognition of a foreign (nonself) MHC antigen that has been shed from the graft and is presented by a self-MHC molecule located on an APC surface. The *direct pathway* involves TCR recognition of an intact foreign MHC antigen present on the surface of a *donor* APC that has been shed from the graft. This latter phenomenon occurs only in alloimmune responses and is responsible for the majority of TCR recognition in acute graft rejection at a frequency of 100:1 compared with indirect recognition.

    There are two major classes of T-cells: T-helper cells which express CD4 surface molecules ($CD4^+$), and cytotoxic T-cells which express CD8 ($CD8^+$). $CD4^+$ cells recognize MHC class II molecules on the surface of APCs, whereas $CD8^+$ cells are restricted to recognition of MHC class I. $CD4^+$ cells are activated after recognition of a foreign antigen (e.g., foreign MHC from a kidney transplant). They then initiate an immune response to foreign peptides by secreting cytokines important in B-cell proliferation and activation and cytotoxic T-cell activation. $CD8^+$ T-cells kill cells bearing foreign antigen through the use of cytotoxic molecules such as perforins, granzymes, and Fas, which triggers apoptosis in the targeted cell. Regulatory T-cells (Treg) are a recently described T-helper cell subset that suppress the activation and proliferation of $CD4^+$ and $CD8^+$ T-cells and have been implicated in allograft tolerance.

4. **T-Cell and APC Interactions.** T-cells and APCs have a number of important interactions central to allograft recognition and rejection. *Signal 1* is the term for initial binding of the T-cell to the APC through interactions between the TCR/CD3 complex and foreign peptide expressed in MHC. Signal 1 is a calcium-dependent process and results in calcineurin activation. Although signal 1 alone will cause anergy, the addition of **signal 2**, also known as *costimulation*, will lead to an immune response. The best-understood costimulation signal is between CD28 on the T-cell surface and B7 on the APC surface. CD28/B7 activation leads to intracellular signaling, interleukin 2 (IL-2) production, and T-cell activation. While CD28 is expressed on resting T-cells, the T-cell surface molecule cytotoxic T lymphocyte antigen-4 (CTLA-4) Ig is expressed only on activated T-cells. CTLA-4 binds preferentially to B7 and eventually inactivates the immune response, thereby providing potent negative feedback. Another

costimulatory molecule, CD40, is found on APCs and activated B-cells, and binds to CD40 ligand (CD40L) on T-cells. The CD40/CD40L pathway is important in Ig production and class switching by B-cells.
5. **B-Cells.** B-cells develop at multiple sites of the body, including the liver, spleen, and lymph nodes. In response to T-cell allorecognition-induced activation and proliferation signaling, B-cells produce antibodies that are specific to foreign MHC antigens. When these antibodies are specific to donor antigens they are termed donor-specific antibodies (DSA). Antibody-mediated cellular cytotoxicity occurs via complement fixation and subsequent cell lysis. B-cells and antibodies are important in allograft rejection, with the potential to cause hyperacute rejection (immediate allograft destruction due to preformed antibodies), as well as acute and chronic antibody-mediated rejection (due to either preformed or de novo DSA).

B. **Pharmacotherapy.** In the 1960s and 1970s, the first transplant immunosuppressive agents consisted of steroids and azathioprine. Since that time the number of available immunosuppressive agents has increased greatly. Agents can be used for *desensitization* therapy prior to transplant, *induction* therapy at the time of transplant, *maintenance* therapy to prevent rejection of the allograft, or the treatment of *acute rejection*. There is a large degree of overlap between indications, and many agents are used "off-label." Commonly used agents, their mechanism of action, and common toxicities appear in Table 15-1. Desensitization is discussed separately (see Section IV.A).
1. **Agents Used for Induction**
   a. **Basiliximab:** Chimeric murine/human monoclonal antibody that binds to the IL-2 receptor on activated T-cells, inhibiting IL-2-induced T-cell activation and proliferation without depleting T-cell populations. It is given as 20 mg intravenous (IV) infusions at the time of transplant and 4 days later and is 75% humanized with minimal side effects.
   b. **Antithymocyte Globulin (ATG, thymoglobulin):** Polyclonal Ig preparations developed by injecting human thymic extracts into rabbits (rATG) or, less commonly, horses (Atgam) and purifying the antibodies produced. These preparations neutralize lymphocytes by multiple antibody-mediated mechanisms, with a sustained effect on proliferation, and are more effective than basiliximab in preventing acute rejection. Toxicities are related to immunosuppression, heterogeneity of preparations, allergic or anaphylactoid responses to nonhuman preparations, and cytopenias. Dosing schedules are commonly 1.5-mg/kg IV daily for 3 to 5 days but vary by center. It is generally assumed that the risk of malignancy, lymphoma in particular, increases with increasing exposure to ATG however data showing a consistent dose-dependent association is lacking.
   c. **Alemtuzumab (Campath):** Humanized monoclonal anti-CD-52 antibody that depletes both B- and T-cells. Due to its potent immunosuppressive properties, it is often used with steroid avoidance and immunosuppression-reduction protocols; however, it is also associated with profound lymphopenia, susceptibility to infection, and autoimmune syndromes. Furthermore, a change in type and timing of rejection may be seen, including monocyte-induced and humoral rejections occurring past the early posttransplant months. It is used off-label for kidney transplant induction and standard dosing has not been defined; however, 30-mg IV at the time of transplant is common.
2. **Agents Used for Maintenance**
   a. **Calcineurin Inhibitors:** Cyclosporine A (CsA) and tacrolimus (FK506) are the mainstay of maintenance immunosuppression. Both agents bind intracellular calcineurin, inhibiting translocation of transcription factor

TABLE 15-1 Commonly Used Drugs in Renal Transplantation

Class and Drugs	Mechanism	Toxicity	Indication
Calcineurin Inhibitors			
Cyclosporin	Binds cyclophilin and blocks action of calcineurin	Hypertension, hyperlipidemia nephrotoxicity, neurotoxicity, hirsutism, gingival hyperplasia	M
Tacrolimus	Binds to FKBP, inhibiting action of calcineurin	PTDM, neurotoxicity side effects similar to cyclosporine	M
TOR Inhibitors			
Sirolimus Everolimus	Binds to FKBP and inhibits mTOR effects, cytokine signaling, cell cycling, and CD28-mediated costimulation	Elevated cholesterol and triglycerides, cytopenias, acne, wound healing, pneumonitis	M, CIM
Antimetabolites			
Azathioprine	6-MP release in vivo, interferes with DNA synthesis, cell cycling	Cytopenias, diarrhea, hepatotoxic, neoplasias	M
Mycophenolate mofetil Mycophenolic acid	Inosine monophosphate dehydrogenase inhibitors, blocks de novo purine synthesis	Diarrhea, GI discomfort, cytopenias, invasive CMV	M M
Corticosteroids	Multiple sites of action; cytokine production, T-cell proliferation, leukocyte traffic, and others	HTN, PTDM, hyperlipidemia, obesity, infection, osteoporosis, AVN	I, M, CR
Belatacept	Fusion protein of human IgG and CTLA-4, inhibits CD28-mediated costimulation	PTLD: only for use in EBV-seropositive patients	M, CIM
Antibody Therapies			
Antithymocyte globulin	Rabbit polyclonal Ab against thymocytes	Allergic reaction, leukopenia	I, CR
Basiliximab	Partially humanized (75%) monoclonal Ab, same target as daclizumab		I
Alemtuzumab	Humanized monoclonal Ab against CD52 on lymphocytes and monocytes	Lymphopenia, autoimmune syndromes, infection, delayed rejection	I
IVIG	Immune modulation, multiple sites of action	Infusion reactions, headache, acute kidney injury when sucrose based	AMR, D
Rituximab	B–cell-depleting anti-CD20 monoclonal antibody	Infusion and dermatologic reactions, cytopenias	AMR, D

Ab, antibody; AMR, antibody-mediated rejection; AVN, avascular necrosis; CIM, calcineurin inhibitor minimization; CMV, cytomegalovirus; CR, cellular rejection; D, desensitization; EBV, Epstein–Barr virus; FKBP, FK binding protein; GI, gastrointestinal; HTN, hypertension; I, induction; IgG, immunoglobulin G; IVIG, intravenous immunoglobulin; M, maintenance; 6-MP, 6-mercaptopurine; PTDM, posttransplant diabetes mellitus; PTLD, posttransplant lymphoproliferative disorder; mTOR, mammalian target of rapamycin.

nuclear factor of activated T-cells (NFAT) to the nucleus and subsequent cytokine-induced cell proliferation. Cyclosporine and tacrolimus have similar side effects, but hyperlipidemia, hypertension, hirsutism, and gingival hyperplasia are more common with cyclosporine, and post-transplant diabetes mellitus (PTDM) and neurotoxicity may be more common with tacrolimus. They both have potential to cause nephrotoxicity. Dosing is adjusted according to trough blood levels and varies depending on immunosuppressive regimen (see Section V.C.1).

b. **Mammalian Target of Rapamycin Inhibitors (mTOR-Is):** Sirolimus and everolimus downregulate mTOR, inhibiting IL-2–mediated signal transduction and cell proliferation. Important toxicities include hypertriglyceridemia, hypercholesterolemia, cytopenias, pneumonitis, delayed wound healing, lymphoceles, diarrhea, and proteinuria, as well as potentiation of calcineurin inhibitor toxicity. As with calcineurin inhibitors, dosing is adjusted according to trough blood levels and varies depending on immunosuppressive regimen (see Section V.C.1).

c. **Antimetabolites:** Mycophenolate mofetil (MMF), mycophenolic acid (MPA), and azathioprine can be used in combination with calcineurin inhibitors and corticosteroids for maintenance immunosuppression. They inhibit purine synthesis and subsequent lymphocyte proliferation. MMF and MPA often cause diarrhea and gastrointestinal discomfort, can be associated with cytopenias, and may be associated with an increased risk of tissue-invasive CMV. They are dosed at 1 g (MMF) or 720 mg (MPA) twice daily. Azathioprine provides less selective lymphocyte inhibition and can be associated with cytopenias and neoplasias. It is commonly dosed at 1.5 mg/kg daily.

d. **Corticosteroids** are used during induction, as maintenance therapy, and for the treatment of acute rejection. They inhibit the immune response via a broad effect on inflammatory mediators. Their effectiveness is complicated by a variety of well-known side effects, including hypertension, glucose intolerance, weight gain, cataracts, poor wound healing, osteoporosis, and osteonecrosis. Although corticosteroid withdrawal and avoidance have been explored (see Section V.C.2), and, despite slightly higher rates of rejection, have comparable patient and graft outcomes to corticosteroid maintenance protocols. However, maintenance corticosteroids remain a mainstay of current immunosuppression in ~70% of US transplant centers.

e. **Belatacept** is a fusion protein consisting of the Fc portion of human IgG and the extracellular domain of CTLA-4 that was approved in the United States for use in kidney transplant recipients in 2011. It binds with high affinity to B7 on the APC, inhibiting CD28-mediated T-cell costimulation (signal 2, see Section III.A.4). It is used in calcineurin inhibitor–sparing protocols (see Section V.C.2) and is generally well tolerated. However, it is associated with higher rates of acute rejection, viral infection (particularly CMV), and posttransplant lymphoproliferative disorder (PTLD) relative to calcineurin-based regimens. It is only indicated in patients who are seropositive for Epstein–Barr virus (EBV; who have a lower risk of PTLD). It is only available in IV formulation and is infused once monthly during the maintenance phase (more frequently during initiation).

3. **Agents Used for Treatment of Rejection.** The pharmacologic treatment of rejection depends on the type of immune response as determined by histology from an allograft biopsy (see Section VI.B). Corticosteroids and antithymoctye globulin (described in the previous sections) are used in cell-mediated (T-cell) rejection. Intravenous immunoglobulin (IVIG), rituximab, bortezomib, and eculizumab have been used to treat antibody-mediated

(B-cell) rejection, often in combination with plasma exchange therapy. IVIG exerts immunomodulatory action via numerous mechanisms, including inhibition of cytokine activity, inhibition of T-cell activation and functionality, and inhibition of complement activation. Rituximab is a chimeric murine/human monoclonal anti-CD20 antibody that reduces populations of pre-B and mature B lymphocytes. Bortezomib is a proteasome inhibitor that reduces numbers of antibody-secreting plasma cells. Eculizumab is a monoclonal antibody that inhibits terminal C5 complement activation, thereby limiting antibody-mediated cell toxicity, and is approved for treatment of atypical hemolytic uremic syndrome. These agents, while often very effective, are all considered off-label for the indication of kidney transplant rejection, and dosing has not been standardized. Common side effects of these agents are listed in Table 15-1.
4. **Drug Interactions.** Although it is not possible to list all potential drug interactions, it is important for the clinician to be aware of general types of interactions when initiating new therapies or witnessing unexpected toxicities. In general, interactions can result from changes in absorption, metabolism, and excretion, or through additive or synergistic toxicity with agents that have similar side effects. Agents that can decrease the absorption of immunosuppressive agents include antacids, cholestyramine, and food, whereas promotility agents can increase absorption. Metabolism of tacrolimus and cyclosporine occurs through cytochrome P-450-3A4; therefore, agents that affect this system can alter calcineurin inhibitor levels or alter metabolism of the interacting agent, leading to toxicity or inadequate levels. Examples include calcium channel blockers, azole antifungals, macrolide antibiotics, and grapefruit juice, which can increase calcineurin inhibitor levels, and anticonvulsants and rifampin, which can decrease levels. Simvastatin and atorvastatin should not be used with cyclosporine due to decreased clearance and risk of myopathy and rhabdomyolysis. Allopurinol can cause severe myelosuppression when used with azathioprine and should be avoided. Cyclosporine reduces MMF exposure, and mTOR-Is can potentiate calcineurin inhibitor nephrotoxicity. Also, nonsteroidal anti-inflammatory drugs and ACE inhibitors may have additive effects on glomerular hemodynamics with calcineurin inhibitors. Although this summary is not exhaustive, cautious attention to these possibilities can prevent morbidity from drug interactions.

IV. Transplantation

A. Cross-Matching and Desensitization. Cross-matching between the recipient and donor is usually performed immediately prior to transplantation in order to minimize the risk of hyperacute and acute antibody-mediated rejection. This is accomplished using cell-based flow cytometry, solid-phase SAB assays, or a combination of these methods. If a cross-match assay is positive, a decision is made to either continue without desensitization (in the case of low-level reactivity on the SAB assay), cancel the procedure, or proceed with some form of desensitization depending on the perceived rejection risk, transplant center experience, and available resources. Desensitization protocols aim to reduce the risk of rejection by mitigating the impact of preexisting recipient DSA. They vary depending on donor organ source and degree of cross-match positivity and generally consist of therapies that are used to treat antibody-mediated rejection (Sections III.B.3 and VI.B). Transplantation across a positive cross-match generally increases the risk of rejection and graft loss even with desensitization. This is, however, associated with improved patient survival compared with remaining on dialysis.

Desensitization can be used in the setting of both living and deceased donor transplantation, however, the time constraints inherent to the deceased donor process render these therapies logistically challenging in this setting.

Two important developments over the past decade have significantly reduced the need for transplant centers to expose patients to potent and resource-intense desensitization therapy. First, the widespread availability and success of national paired exchange programs have offered a safer and more effective option for patients with a positive cross-match against a living donor. Second, the wait-list prioritization for highly sensitized patients, enacted in 2014 as part of a broader overhaul of the US kidney allocation system, has succeeded in equalizing wait times for a large majority of sensitized patients on the deceased donor waitlist. As a result, desensitization for recipients of either living or deceased donor kidneys has become an increasingly rare practice in recent years.

B. Induction. With few exceptions, kidney transplant recipients will receive a brief course of high-dose steroids at the time of transplantation, followed by a taper to either a maintenance dose or discontinuation. Either for perceived increased risk of rejection or by local protocol, antibody therapy may be given during induction. Increased risks of rejection may be seen in those with preexisting DSA, previous transplants, and African Americans. Available antibody-based therapies include ATG, IL-2 receptor antagonists, and alemtuzumab. ATG and alemtuzumab deplete the lymphocyte pool and provide more potent immunosuppression compared with IL-2 receptor antagonists, but also have more potential for toxicity (see Section III.B.1).

C. Donor Nephrectomy. A minimally invasive laparoscopic or robotic surgical approach is the standard of care for live donor nephrectomy. The left kidney is most often selected due to its longer renal vein and accessibility, however, the right kidney may be selected in various circumstances. Factors that influence this decision include anatomical variants such as multiple vessels or duplicate ureters, the presence of small stones, and size and/or functional discrepancy between the two kidneys. In the latter scenario, the donor will most often be left with the larger or higher-functioning kidney. Deceased donor kidneys are removed together with a patch of aorta and inferior vena cava as part of a multiorgan recovery. The organs are then separated and stored in hypothermic preservation solution until implantation. Pulsatile perfusion may be used; this practice varies center-to-center and region-to-region.

D. Transplant Surgery. The transplanted kidney is placed in either the right or left iliac fossa. The renal vein and artery are both connected through an end-to-side anastomosis, the donor vein usually being connected to the external iliac vein and the donor artery to the external iliac artery. The ureter is implanted into the bladder, and the bladder mucosa is pulled over the ureter to create a tunnel that prevents reflux and urine leaks. A ureteral stent is often placed at the time of surgery to ensure patency and prevent urine leaks. Lymphatics are ligated to prevent postoperative lymphocele formation. A Foley catheter is placed at the time of surgery and in most cases is removed within several days. Kidney transplantation in the absence of donor ischemia or technical complications is usually accompanied by prompt urine formation.

V. Postoperative Management

A. Immediate postoperative care of the transplant recipient involves close monitoring of urine output, fluid administration, and vital signs. Many centers use algorithms, which replace the urine output with half-normal saline or similar solution. The brisk diuresis that can ensue in a transplant recipient can cause disturbances in potassium, magnesium, calcium, and phosphorus. Elevated parathyroid hormone and FGF-23 levels along with a suddenly functioning kidney result in hypophosphatemia in a large majority of kidney recipients with good immediate graft function. Insulin requirements may increase in diabetic patients or those without prior diabetes due to the presence of steroids, calcineurin inhibitors, and improved clearance of insulin by the transplanted kidney. An uncomplicated patient with a functioning kidney can usually ambulate by postoperative day 1 or 2, and the diet can be advanced as tolerated. By postoperative day 3 or 4, the Foley catheter can be removed and the patient can be discharged if he or she is free of other complications.

B. **Surgical complications** include problems with each of the aspects of the transplant: the vascular anastomoses, urologic complications, lymphocele, and wound complications.
1. Urologic complications include urine leak, obstruction, and reflux. Routine stenting at many centers may be responsible for a decrease in the incidence of urologic complications. *Urine leak* can occur in approximately 2% of transplants. It is usually due to ureteral necrosis caused by interruption of distal ureteral blood supply but can be at the site of bladder implantation or the calyces. The clinical presentation is one of decreased urine output, pain, fever, abdominal tenderness, swelling, and a perinephric fluid collection by ultrasonography. Elevated serum creatinine values due to the peritoneal reabsorption of urine creatinine can mimic AKI. Fluid aspiration reveals a high creatinine that far exceeds the plasma creatinine. The diagnosis can be confirmed by nuclear scan or CT urography demonstrating extravasation into local tissues. Temporary Foley catheterization and ureteral stenting followed by surgical repair are the usual management. *Ureteric obstruction* can be secondary to ureteral ischemia as well as fluid collections or masses. Imaging by ultrasonography, cystogram, or other studies usually leads to a diagnosis; the obstruction can be relieved by ureteral repair, stenting, or nephrostomy. *Vesicoureteral reflux* into the transplanted ureter is less common since the introduction of submucosal tunneling of the ureter through the bladder.
2. **Arterial or venous thrombosis** is uncommon but may occur as a result of preexisting hypercoagulability or technical difficulty, and should be suspected when sudden deterioration develops in a previously functioning transplant. While venous thromboses can occasionally be reversed by surgery or thrombolysis, vascular thromboses most often lead to graft loss.
3. **Lymphocele** presents as an asymptomatic cystic fluid collection. It may, however, cause graft obstruction and reduced kidney function, pain, or lower extremity edema and deep vein thrombosis due to compression of the iliofemoral vessels. Lymphoceles are distinguished from urine leaks as fluid aspiration yields a fluid creatinine equal to serum creatinine. The aspirated fluid should also be sent for cell count and Gram stain to rule out hematoma or abscess. Lymphoceles can be aspirated but may require surgical repair if they are recurrent.
4. **Wound complications** may stem from the problems detailed earlier, or due to infection. Clinical suspicion is necessary, as immunosuppression masks the symptoms and increases the risk of wound infections. Prompt drainage and antibiotic administration are central to treatment. Wound complications are most commonly seen in obese patients.
5. **Infections** in the first postoperative month are similar to those in other postoperative patients but occur more frequently in immunosuppressed patients. Lung, urine, and wound infections and infections related to dialysis catheters are common culprits. Infections of fluid collections (lymphocele, urinoma, and hematoma) may also occur. Opportunistic and other infections are discussed in Section VI.

C. **Maintenance Immunosuppression**
1. **Conventional Therapy.** Since 1995, the available options for maintenance immunosuppression have been expanded with the introduction of MMF, tacrolimus, cyclosporine microemulsion, and sirolimus. Standard therapy in the United States consists of a calcineurin inhibitor, an antimetabolite, and corticosteroids. The calcineurin inhibitors, tacrolimus and

cyclosporine, have similar efficacy in patient and graft survival, but with slightly different toxicity profiles. Tacrolimus has also lowered both the incidence and severity of acute rejection in head-to-head comparisons. One approach is to maintain target trough levels of cyclosporine that are highest (300 ng/mL) in the first month, with gradual tapering to 150 to 250 ng/mL by 6 months and 50 to 200 ng/mL after 12 months. Similarly, target tacrolimus levels are 6 to 12 ng/mL in the first month, 5 to 8 ng/mL for months 1 to 5, and 4 to 7 ng/mL after 6 months. Target levels may need to be lower in patients receiving sirolimus, and are often individualized based on age, PRA, matching, rejection history, and the presence of infection. MMF and sirolimus have largely supplanted azathioprine in clinical use, as both result in less acute rejection. The third agent used in combination regimens is corticosteroids; they are usually tapered rapidly to 20 mg daily by 1 to 2 weeks posttransplant. They are then gradually tapered to 5 to 10 mg daily by month 6. The availability of multiple agents has allowed clinicians to choose a regimen that best fits a patient's profile of immunologic risk and perceived susceptibility to side effects. For example, patients with second transplants or poor matching who are at greater risk for rejection may be placed on tacrolimus. However, an obese patient with a family history of diabetes but with low immunologic risk may be placed on cyclosporine or chosen for a steroid withdrawal protocol in an attempt to reduce the risk of PTDM.

2. **Alternative Regimens.** The toxicities of corticosteroids and calcineurin inhibitors have led to multiple clinical trials of withdrawal and avoidance strategies. Meta-analysis of late steroid withdrawal has been associated with acute rejection and graft loss, particularly in African Americans. In contrast, trials of early withdrawal or avoidance of steroids in low-risk patients have shown promise; however, they are associated with higher rates of rejection with limited benefit in metabolic complications and lack of long-term results. Calcineurin inhibitor withdrawal/avoidance is another goal due to nephrotoxicity and other side effects. Clinical trials of belatacept, a costimulation blocker, in combination with steroids and MMF, show improved 3-year graft function despite increased acute rejection rates compared with cyclosporine-containing regimens; however, long-term graft and patient survival data are not yet available and there is a higher risk of PTLD (Section VII.C). The mTOR-Is sirolimus and everolimus have been studied in several calcineurin inhibitor avoidance strategies including avoidance, withdrawal, and conversion protocols. While results from the ELITE-Symphony study show calcineurin inhibitor avoidance using mTOR-I is associated with worse graft outcomes, studies of early (1 to 6 months) or late (>6 months) conversion or withdrawal have been more promising. However, as with belatacept, most trials of calcineurin inhibitor minimization using mTOR-Is have shown increased rates of acute rejection, and long-term improvements in patient or graft survival have not been published.

VI. Medical Complications

In addition to DGF, acute or chronic rejection, and recurrent disease, patients who have undergone kidney transplantation are susceptible to kidney failure from all the causes that affect the general population. In the initial 48 hours after transplantation, technical causes related to surgery or DGF are most common. After 48 hours, the approach to a patient with kidney dysfunction should rule out hypovolemia, medication toxicity, and urinary tract obstruction, and should attempt to uncover causes of acute tubular necrosis (ATN) such as hypotension, sepsis, or radiocontrast. Evaluation for acute rejection should take place if clear causes are not found.

A. **Delayed Graft Function.** DGF is commonly defined as the requirement for dialysis in the first 7 days after transplantation. It occurs in 20% to 30% of deceased donor transplants but is uncommon in living donor transplants. Although technical factors or other events that affect kidney function can cause DGF, it is most commonly a result of postischemic ATN, caused by donor hypovolemia or hypotension, or prolonged cold or warm ischemia during recovery and preservation. DGF adds to the cost and length of hospitalization and is associated with decreased short- and long-term graft survival. To determine the cause of graft dysfunction in the early postoperative period, a kidney ultrasonography should be performed to rule out technical causes, and the timing of kidney biopsy to rule out acute rejection should be guided by the patient's immunologic risk.

B. **Acute Rejection.** Rejection refers to an immunologic response by the recipient to the transplanted organ. There are several types of acute rejection. *Hyperacute rejection* is rare and is caused by preformed antibodies against donor antigen, leading to immediate graft destruction after perfusion. *Accelerated acute rejection* usually occurs 2 to 3 days after transplant and often is an antibody-mediated process that takes place in presensitized patients with prior transplants, transfusions, or pregnancies. Acute cellular rejection is either a T-cell or antibody-mediated response, or a combination of both, that may occur at any time, but is most common from 5 to 7 days posttransplant until 4 weeks after transplant, with a gradual lessening of risk in the first 6 months. Clinically, symptoms such as low-grade fever; a swollen, tender allograft; and oliguria are not seen commonly with modern immunosuppression. Therefore, frequent laboratory monitoring and a high index of suspicion are necessary to diagnose acute rejection. Acute rejection typically presents as a decrease in kidney function, as measured by the serum creatinine. However, rejection can occur without discernable changes in kidney function, a process referred to as *subclinical rejection*. Some centers perform routine "protocol biopsies" to evaluate for subclinical rejection and other graft abnormalities. Current regimens incorporating newer agents have lowered the incidence of acute rejection in the first year to 10% or lower, have improved 1-year deceased donor allograft survival to approximately 93%, and may be responsible for some of the improvement in long-term outcomes. The diagnosis of acute rejection requires an ultrasound-guided kidney biopsy, with application of the Banff criteria to grade the severity of rejection or disclose other pathology. Pathologic features of interstitial infiltration with lymphocytes, tubulitis, and endarteritis are seen in T-cell rejection, whereas peritubular capillary inflammation and C4d staining, circulating DSA, and tissue injury are diagnostic for antibody-mediated processes. Treatment of acute T-cell rejection is usually a 3- to 5-day course of high-dose IV steroids and/or a 5- to 10-day course of ATG for more severe rejection. Treatment of antibody-mediated rejection usually involves five or more sessions of plasma exchange followed by IVIG, and occasionally rituximab or bortezomib for more severe cases. Although most acute rejection can be reversed, its occurrence remains a powerful predictor of long-term graft survival, most notably antibody-mediated rejection or T-cell rejection involving the large vessels.

C. **Recurrent Disease.** The diagnosis of recurrent disease is guided by the clinical scenario and knowledge of which diseases tend to recur in kidney transplants. Recurrent nephritis may present as proteinuria, nephrotic syndrome, microscopic hematuria, and loss of function. It can be differentiated from other causes (chronic allograft dysfunction, *de novo* glomerular disease) by kidney biopsy. In the patient who has undergone transplantation, the important variables are the frequency of recurrence and frequency of graft loss due to recurrence. For example, type II membranoproliferative glomerulonephritis (MPGN) recurs in close to 100% of the cases and commonly leads to graft loss. Primary focal and segmental glomerulosclerosis and type I MPGN recur in 20% to 60% of patients, and also commonly may lead to graft loss. Alternatively, IgA nephropathy recurs in approximately 50% of recipients, but uncommonly causes graft loss. Systemic lupus erythematosus may also recur microscopically in kidney allografts but rarely is clinically important. Glomerular disease was the cause of 30% of all graft loss in one study, half of which was due to recurrent disease.

D. Chronic Allograft Damage. Despite a significant reduction in the incidence of acute rejection over the last several decades, long-term graft survival has improved only marginally. The most common cause of graft loss is patient death with a functioning graft, the majority of which is due to cardiovascular disease, and accounts for close to half of all cases. The remaining cases of graft loss are due to a range of both immunologic (chronic rejection) and nonimmunologic (e.g., donor organ quality, hypertension, drug toxicity) allograft injuries, the epidemiology of which has changed over time. Protocol biopsy studies of patients transplanted in the 1980s and 1990s described interstitial fibrosis/tubular atrophy (IFTA) due to calcineurin inhibitor toxicity as the dominant cause of late graft dysfunction. More recent studies have shown a much lower rate of IFTA in failed grafts, placing more emphasis on glomerular pathology and chronic antibody-mediated graft damage. Glomerular pathology can consist of recurrent primary or de novo disease, the latter often in the form of transplant glomerulopathy. This lesion is characterized by double contouring of the glomerular basement membrane with proteinuria, is often associated with glomerular C4d staining and circulating DSA, and portends a particularly poor prognosis for the graft. Chronic antibody-mediated graft damage, occasionally in the form of transplant glomerulopathy, is often due to medication nonadherence and has been reported as responsible for over 60% of graft failures. IFTA is still a pathologic finding in up to 30% of graft failures, the cause of which is usually multifactorial and can include chronic infection, rejection, drug toxicity, or glomerular disease. Chronic allograft damage is not typically a reversible disease, and treatment is patient-specific. For example, a patient with suspected calcineurin inhibitor toxicity may benefit from a reduction or withdrawal of the offending agent, whereas a patient with circulating DSA and chronic antibody-mediated rejection may benefit from increasing immunosuppressive exposure.

VII. Medical Care of the Transplanted Patient

The success of kidney transplantation and the growing population of transplant recipients are unfortunately accompanied by the complications from comorbid diseases and side effects of long-term immunosuppression. Patients often die with functioning grafts due to cardiovascular disease, infections, and malignancy, and these and other conditions contribute to a spectrum of common disorders in transplantation.

A. Infectious Diseases. In the patient who has undergone transplantation, typical signs and symptoms of infection may be absent, and coinfections are common, necessitating increased scrutiny. Infections after kidney transplantation occur in patterns that are important to recognize. Immediately after transplant, patients are at risk for common postoperative infections: wound infections, pneumonia, line, and urinary infections. The first 6 months after transplant are marked by a risk of opportunistic infections due to more intense immunosuppression, especially after antibody induction. For this reason, patients usually receive prophylaxis against *Pneumocystis jirovecii* pneumonia for at least 6 months, and for CMV for 1, 3, or 6 months depending on their risk (see next section). Some centers provide prophylaxis for fungal infections. After 6 months, the risk of opportunistic infections is lower but remains present, and

patients remain at risk for more frequent and severe infections with community-acquired pathogens. Some common pathogens and principles specific to kidney transplantation will be reviewed.
1. **Immunosuppression During Infection.** There are no clear guidelines for decreasing immunosuppression during infection. Furthermore, many infections carry an increased risk of acute rejection due to upregulation of immune surveillance and activity. In general, mild infections treated with appropriate antimicrobials can be managed without a change in immunosuppression. However, more severe infections may require decreasing or stopping antiproliferative medications (sirolimus, MMF, azathioprine) and reductions in calcineurin inhibitor dosing. Severe or life-threatening infections should include attention to the requirement for stress doses of corticosteroids, which are often adequate to decrease the risk of rejection during an illness. Reduction of immunosuppression is best done with careful monitoring of graft function along with the consultation of transplant physicians.
2. **Cytomegalovirus.** CMV is a human herpes virus that is common in the general population but usually does not lead to serious morbidity without immunosuppression. The risk of CMV infection is tied to serologic status of the donor and recipient. A potential organ recipient who has not been exposed to CMV is at risk for a primary infection if transplanted with a CMV-positive organ, a recipient who has been exposed before transplant is at risk for reactivation or superinfection, especially if receiving antibody induction, and CMV disease is uncommon in donor-negative/recipient-negative transplants. Therefore, donor-positive/recipient-negative patients and recipient-positive patients generally receive prophylaxis for CMV for 3 to 6 months, usually with valganciclovir. CMV infection leads to morbidity related directly to infection, but also increases the risk of acute rejection, graft loss, and death. Clinically, the disease often presents as low-grade fever, leukopenia and/or thrombocytopenia, and malaise. Tissue invasion can occur in 5% to 15% of infections, with syndromes of pneumonitis, hepatitis, esophagitis, and diarrhea being the most common. Polymerase chain reaction (PCR)–based testing is the most sensitive diagnostic technique, but other options exist, including biopsy of affected tissues. Standard therapy is IV ganciclovir, a nucleoside analog, although ganciclovir resistance can develop. Recently, newer antiviral agents have been approved for the treatment of CMV infection/disease that is refractory to treatment with above-mentioned agents; these include maribavir (IV) and letermovir (PO).
3. **BK Virus Nephropathy (Polyomavirus).** BK polyomavirus (BKPyV) is a small DNA virus that establishes lifelong infection in the renal tubular and uroepithelial cells of most of the world's population. For the majority, infection is quiescent and benign. However, in kidney transplant recipients BKPyV can reactivate and lead to BKPyV-associated nephropathy (BKPyVAN). In patients who have undergone kidney transplantation, BKPyV may cause a syndrome of decreased kidney function and interstitial nephritis, which appears clinically and pathologically similar to acute rejection. BKPyVAN is a risk factor for premature allograft loss. Because discovery at the time of BKPyVAN may be too late to prevent graft loss, current practices emphasize preemptive screening for BK viremia using PCR-based testing. Immunohistochemical techniques and the presence of viral inclusions can be used to confirm the diagnosis through kidney biopsy. It is important to suspect BKPyVAN when presumed acute rejection does not respond to steroids or occurs after 6 months, as increasing the intensity of immunosuppression may lead to graft loss. The mainstay of management is decreasing the intensity of immunosuppression, which may stabilize

BKV-related kidney dysfunction but increase the risk of acute rejection. IVIG, cidofovir, and leflunomide have been used anecdotally with varying success in subjects with ongoing viremia or declining kidney function despite immunosuppression reduction.

4. **Hepatitis B and C.** The incidence of hepatitis B in patients with ESKD has been declining due to immunization, isolation techniques, screening of transfused blood, decreased need for blood transfusion, and the implementation of infection control measures within dialysis units. For hepatitis B, patients with antigenemia usually receive evaluation and liver biopsy before transplant, as antiviral therapies may be more effective before transplantation. Hepatitis C virus infection has been declining as well in ESKD for similar reasons. Data suggest that hepatitis C infection increases the risk of graft loss, death, and PTDM. The advent of newer antiviral therapy for Hepatitis C with fewer side effects allows patients to receive preventive therapy and avoid liver-related morbidity, mortality, and extrahepatic manifestations. In addition, these newer antiviral agents have allowed the use of HCV NAT+ organs in patients without hepatitis C with the rationale of starting antiviral therapy shortly after transplantation, increasing the pool of potential donors for patients on the kidney transplant waitlist.

5. **Human Immunodeficiency Virus.** HIV infection was historically a contraindication to transplantation, but successful kidney transplantation is now more common in patients free of opportunistic infections with undetectable viral replication and sustained CD4 counts greater than 200. For reasons that are not completely understood, HIV+ kidney recipients experience acute rejection at rates up to fourfold higher compared with HIV-negative patients. Protease inhibitors can significantly increase calcineurin inhibitor exposure, and frequent monitoring for appropriate dose titration is essential when used together.

6. **Other Infections.** Urinary infections are common after kidney transplantation and pyelonephritis of the transplanted kidney can lead to decreased kidney function. Pulmonary infections from both common and uncommon pathogens are the most common cause of tissue-invasive infection. Although the list of pathogens affecting patients is too long to mention, differential diagnosis should include fungal diseases such as *Cryptococcus*, *Candida*, endemic fungi, mycobacterial disease, nocardia, *P. jirovecii*, *Clostridium difficile*–associated diarrhea, viral pathogens, and others.

7. **Immunization.** Potential transplant recipients should receive immunization against influenza, pneumococcus, hepatitis B, and varicella if they are seronegative. After transplant, many centers wait for 3 to 6 months before any immunizations because of theoretic risks of stimulating the immune system and increasing the risk of rejection. Also, the vaccines may be less effective in this time period. The oral polio, typhoid, varicella, yellow fever, and Bacillus Calmette–Guérin (BCG) vaccines are live vaccines that are contraindicated after kidney transplant due to their ability to cause disease in immunocompromised hosts. However, the live measles–mumps–rubella (MMR) vaccine can be given after 6 months if indicated. Vaccination for influenza, pneumococcus, hepatitis A and B, and tetanus/diphtheria should be given as indicated. All potential kidney transplant candidates should be offered COVID-19 vaccination to prevent severe outcomes related to COVID-19. Vaccination against human papillomavirus (HPV) is appropriate in transplant candidates who have an indication based upon recommendations for the general population.

B. **Cardiovascular Disease.** Cardiovascular disease is the most common cause of death in patients with a functioning allograft. Ischemic coronary artery disease, congestive heart failure, and left ventricular hypertrophy are all more common in patients with kidney disease, and cerebrovascular disease is another important cause of morbidity and mortality. Therefore, efforts at improving outcomes after kidney transplantation have been appropriately shifted to focus on cardiovascular risks. Efforts at preventing cardiovascular events begin with pretransplant evaluation, risk stratification, and intervention when necessary. After transplantation, attention is given to modification of existing risk factors and careful evaluation and treatment of new symptoms or disease.

1. **Hypertension.** Since the introduction of calcineurin inhibitors, hypertension has been present in 70% to 90% of patients after kidney transplant. Hypertension not only represents a modifiable cardiovascular risk factor but also is correlated with graft loss. Clinicians should aim for a target blood pressure below 130/80 mmHg as indicated by current recommendations for patients with chronic kidney disease. The choice of agents after kidney transplantation is controversial and complicated by interpretation of fluctuations in kidney function that occur with diuretics, ACE inhibitors, and angiotensin receptor blockers (ARBs). In general, β-blockers and dihydropyridine calcium channel blockers are used in the early posttransplant period due to their lack of drug interactions and effects on kidney function. Many patients require diuretics because of salt retention due to corticosteroids, calcineurin inhibitors, and other blood pressure medication. ACE inhibitors and ARBs are often avoided early after transplantation due to effects on renal hemodynamics and serum creatinine.

2. **Hyperlipidemia.** Lipid abnormalities occur in at least 50% of transplant recipients and represent an important modifiable cardiovascular risk factor. Hypertriglyceridemia, high low-density lipoprotein, and low high-density lipoprotein often occur as part of a metabolic syndrome that is common after transplantation. Corticosteroids, calcineurin inhibitors, and sirolimus may all play important roles in worsening lipid profiles. Despite concerns about rhabdomyolysis due to drug interactions, there is now prospective data from randomized controlled trials indicating that statins (specifically, fluvastatin) may prevent cardiac death and nonfatal myocardial infarction after kidney transplantation without effects on graft survival. Other therapies such as niacin, fibrates, omega-3 fatty acids, and binding resins have been used as well. As always, attention to drug interactions must be given, especially regarding the risk of rhabdomyolysis (statins, fibrates, and calcineurin inhibitors) and decreased or enhanced absorption (binding resins and ezetimibe).

3. **Diabetes Mellitus**
   a. **Background.** Diabetes is a major independent risk factor for cardiovascular disease, is present in 30% to 40% of patients before transplant, and develops after transplant in 2.5% to 35% of nondiabetic patients depending on pretransplant risk factors and the immunosuppressive regimen. Complications from diabetes have important effects on patient outcomes, leading to cardiovascular and infectious morbidity, renal allograft loss, and decreased function, as well as decreased patient survival. In patients with diabetes preceding transplant, control may be worsened by corticosteroids, calcineurin inhibitors, and the decreased half-life of endogenous and exogenous insulin due to improved kidney function. Rigorous control of diabetes is likely to decrease diabetic complications, based on accumulated evidence in other populations. A glycosylated hemoglobin target of 6.5 to 7.0 is likely to be associated with improved outcomes.
   b. **Posttransplant Diabetes Mellitus.** PTDM, also called *new-onset diabetes after transplantation*, complicates a substantial percentage of kidney transplants and is associated with poorer patient outcomes. Risks

for PTDM include increasing age, obesity, family history of diabetes, African American or Hispanic race/ethnicity, hepatitis C infection, and abnormal glucose tolerance. Corticosteroids have well-known adverse effects on insulin resistance, and calcineurin inhibitors are diabetogenic, likely due to a combination of β-cell toxicity and promotion of insulin resistance. Fasting plasma glucose should be routinely monitored after transplant because the incidence of PTDM is high. Prevention of diabetes through weight loss and exercise in patients at risk should be attempted, and treatment of new-onset diabetes should follow established guidelines.
4. **Other Cardiovascular Risk Factors.** Smoking is obviously an important modifiable cardiovascular risk factor, and evidence is accumulating that smoking also influences deterioration of kidney function and is a risk for graft loss. At any stage in the transplant process, counseling, formal smoking cessation programs, and pharmacologic agents should be offered to encourage smoking cessation. Anemia is present in many patients both before and after transplant and may be under-recognized and undertreated. Anemia is correlated with left ventricular hypertrophy and cardiovascular disease; therefore, diagnosis and treatment based on cause is probably appropriate.

C. **Malignancy.** Malignancy is an important complication of immunosuppression, probably due to its effects on immune surveillance of abnormal tumor cell populations and viral-mediated cancers. The intensity of immunosuppression, including exposure to antilymphocyte antibodies, is an important factor in determining risk of malignancy. Nonmelanoma skin cancers, especially squamous cell carcinomas (SCC), have a particularly high incidence and aggressiveness in transplant patients compared with the general population. mTOR-Is have been shown to decrease subsequent SCC in patients with at least one prior event, and conversion from calcineurin inhibitor–based therapy to an mTOR-I may be warranted in this population. Transplant recipients are counseled to avoid the sun, use protective sunscreens and clothing, and see a dermatologist at least once yearly. After skin cancers, posttransplant lymphoproliferative disorders are the next most common malignancy. These lymphomas are associated with EBV infection and usually contain EBV DNA. Risks are increased after T–cell-depleting antibody therapies. These malignancies are often managed with reduction in immunosuppression, but aggressive tumors, particularly when monoclonal, may require systemic chemotherapy. Similarly, women are at increased risk for cervical SCC related to HPV infection and require yearly Pap smears with increased frequency of surveillance and attention if there are any abnormalities. Vulvar, perineal, and anogenital cancers are also more frequent after transplantation. Hepatitis B and C may lead to hepatocellular carcinoma, and Kaposi sarcoma, caused by human herpes virus 8, is another viral-mediated cancer that affects transplant recipients. Renal cell carcinoma occurs in 4% of transplant candidates, perhaps due to acquired cystic kidney disease. Screening native kidneys for disease has been advocated. Other solid tumors, such as breast, lung, and colon cancer, show modest elevation in risk compared with the general population. Given the risks of malignancy in transplantation, age-appropriate screening should occur before placement on the waiting list and should continue for the patient's lifetime.

D. **Bone Disease**
1. **Preexisting Bone Disease.** The clinical picture after kidney transplantation is often complicated by the presence of preexisting bone disease. Most commonly, secondary hyperparathyroidism leads to osteitis fibrosa, imparting a risk of bone loss and fracture. Other causes of preexisting bone disease include adynamic (low turnover) bone disease, aluminum-related

osteomalacia, and β_2-microglobulin-associated arthropathy. Furthermore, diabetic patients have decreased bone mineral density compared with other populations.
2. **Posttransplant Bone Disease.** It is well established that up to 9% of bone density is lost in the first 6 to 12 months after transplantation. Furthermore, osteopenia and osteoporosis are present in a substantial number of patients who have undergone transplantation after long-term follow-up. Kidney transplant recipients carry an increased risk of fracture of 3% to 4% per year for the first 3 years after transplant, declining somewhat after that time. Fracture risk is increased in both males and females and is particularly increased in older females. There are many contributing factors to the milieu that support bone loss. Steroids are known to induce osteopenia and osteoporosis through effects on calcium absorption and excretion, aggravation of secondary hyperparathyroidism, hypogonadism, and effects on bone turnover. Cyclosporine, secondary hyperparathyroidism, renal phosphate wasting, uremia, and gonadal hormones are other contributing factors to bone loss. Another syndrome affecting transplant recipients is avascular osteonecrosis, especially of the femoral head, which is associated with steroid use. Patients present with bone pain but may be asymptomatic. Often patients require operative intervention including replacement of the affected joint.
3. **Management.** The timing and frequency of measuring bone mineral density is not well defined but should be performed at some established interval due to the risk of fractures. Control of secondary hyperparathyroidism before transplant is important. After transplant, calcium and vitamin D supplements are recommended unless hypercalcemia is present. Parathyroidectomy is usually reserved for patients with symptomatic or persistent hypercalcemia or with persistent (greater than 1 to 2 years) hyperparathyroidism. Cinacalcet has been used with some success in posttransplant hyperparathyroidism. Trials of bisphosphonates have been shown to reduce bone loss especially when given immediately after transplant, but indications are not defined and concerns remain regarding promotion of adynamic bone disease. Weight-bearing exercise is a low-cost intervention that should be recommended for all patients.

E. **Hematologic Disease.** Hematologic disorders are common after transplantation and have multifactorial origins. Anemia and posttransplant erythrocytosis (PTE) are common and are covered in the subsequent text. Leukopenia and thrombocytopenia are often seen as complications of antiproliferative medication, CMV other viral infections, or any of a number of primary diseases.
1. **Anemia.** Anemia is common after kidney transplantation, occurring in 30% to 40% of patients in some series. Furthermore, it has been correlated with an increased risk of cardiovascular events and death and therefore may be an important prognostic factor. It is more common in the early posttransplant period but is also present in high frequency in patients with decreased kidney function. An obvious factor involved in the presence of anemia is decreased production of erythropoietin, especially when graft function is impaired. Iron deficiency, ACE inhibitors, ARBs, MMF, and azathioprine have also been associated with anemia after transplantation. Recurrent or de novo hemolytic uremic syndrome can be a dramatic cause of anemia and graft loss and may be associated with calcineurin inhibitors and other medications. Although prospective data are needed, it seems prudent to correct anemia depending on the underlying etiology, including administration of erythropoietin to those with chronic kidney disease stages III to V.
2. **Posttransplant Erythrocytosis.** PTE is defined as persistently elevated hemoglobin and hematocrit levels that occur following kidney transplantation and persist for more than 6 months in the absence of thrombocytosis,

leukocytosis, or another potential cause of erythrocytosis. PTE occurs in 8% to 15% of kidney transplant recipients. Most clinicians use a hematocrit threshold of 51% for diagnosis. The etiology of the disorder is not clear, but erythropoietin- and nonerythropoietin-dependent mechanisms have been implicated. It is more common in smokers, those without acute rejection episodes, and patients with diabetes. This condition can usually be managed by treatment with ACE inhibitors or ARBs. Occasionally, phlebotomy may be necessary if the hematocrit cannot be lowered below 56%.

F. Pregnancy. Years of experience in kidney transplantation have allowed some understanding of pregnancy after transplantation. Most women are counseled to avoid pregnancy for some time after the transplant, usually 6 months to 2 years. Fertility is improved after transplantation, and attention should be given to contraception. In mothers at high risk for primary CMV infection, pregnancy should probably be delayed until an antibody response has occurred and viremia has cleared. Kidney function, if normal at the time of conception, is probably not adversely affected during pregnancy. However, the risk of a pregnancy-related deterioration in kidney function is increased when renal insufficiency is present. Glucose intolerance may also complicate pregnancy, leading to gestational diabetes or increased insulin requirements in those with diabetes. Immunosuppression should be maintained at levels similar to nonpregnant women, but levels should be checked frequently as changes in pharmacokinetics are unpredictable. Prednisone is unlikely to be teratogenic, and calcineurin inhibitors and azathioprine have minimal to small risks. MMF is teratogenic and contraindicated in pregnancy, and women planning for pregnancy should be converted to azathioprine at least 3 months prior to attempting conception. mTOR-Is have limited experience in pregnancy. Fetal outcomes after kidney transplantation include a significant risk of preterm delivery (50%) and growth restriction (40%), but these outcomes may be more closely related to decreased kidney function than the transplant per se. After delivery, breastfeeding may not be recommended in patients taking calcineurin inhibitors, but discussion of the risks and benefits should occur on an individual basis.

SUGGESTED READINGS

Cooper JE. Evaluation and treatment of acute rejection in kidney allografts. *Clin J Am Soc Nephrol.* 2020;15(3):430–438.

Ekberg H, Tedesco-Silva H, Demirbas A, et al; ELITE-Symphony Study. Reduced exposure to calcineurin inhibitors in renal transplant. *N Engl J Med.* 2007;357(25):2562–2575.

Halloran PF. Immunosuppressive drugs for kidney transplantation. *N Engl J Med.* 2004;351(26):2715.

Kidney Disease: Improving Global Outcomes (KDIGO) Transplant Work Group. KDIGO clinical practice guideline for the care of kidney transplant recipients. *Am J Transplant.* 2009;(9 Suppl 3): S1–S155.

Poggio ED, Augustine J, Arrigain S, Brennan DC, Schold JD. Long-term kidney transplant graft survival-making progress when most needed. *Am J transplant.* 2021;21(8):2824–2832.

Wojciechowski D, Wiseman A. Long-term immunosuppression management: opportunities and uncertainties. *Clin J Am Soc Nephrol.* 2021;16(8):1264–1271.

Wolfe RA, Ashby VB, Milford EL, et al. Comparison of mortality in all patients on dialysis, patients on dialysis awaiting transplantation, and recipients of a first cadaveric transplant. *N Engl J Med.* 1999;341(23):1725–1730.

16 The Patient With Kidney Disease and Hypertension in Pregnancy

Maitreyee Gupta, Prasoon Verma, Silvi Shah

In most instances, pregnancy in women with kidney disorders is successful, provided kidney function is well preserved and hypertension is absent.

I. The Kidney Function and Blood Pressure in Normal Pregnancy

The anatomy and function of the kidneys and lower urinary tract are altered during gestation. Physiologic alterations in volume homeostasis and blood pressure (BP) control also occur, and recognizing this is a prerequisite for the appropriate interpretation of data from pregnant patients with kidney disease or hypertension (Table 16-1).

A. Anatomic and Functional Changes in Urinary Tract. Kidney length increases by approximately 1 cm during normal gestation. The major anatomic alterations of the urinary tract during pregnancy, however, are seen in the collecting system, where calyces, renal pelves, and ureters dilate often giving the erroneous impression of obstructive uropathy. The dilation is accompanied by hypertrophy of ureteral smooth muscle and hyperplasia of its connective tissue, but whether bladder reflux is more common in gravidas is unclear. The cause of the ureteral dilation is disputed. Some researchers favor hormonal mechanisms, whereas other researchers believe that it is obstructive in origin. Clearly, as pregnancy progresses, the assumption of a supine or upright posture may cause ureteral obstruction when the enlarged uterus entraps the ureters at the pelvic brim (Fig. 16-1). These morphologic changes result in stasis in the urinary tract and a propensity of pregnant women with asymptomatic bacteriuria to develop pyelonephritis, especially in women with a history of prior urinary tract infection (UTI).

Acceptable norms of kidney size increase should be by 1 cm if estimated during pregnancy or the immediate puerperium, and reductions of renal length noted several months postpartum need not be attributed to renal disease. Rarely, ureteral dilation is of sufficient magnitude to cause a "distension" syndrome (characterized by abdominal pain, and on occasion small increments in serum creatinine levels presenting in late gestation; these resolve with the placement of ureteral stents). Also, because dilation of the ureters may persist until the 12th postpartum week, elective ultrasonographic, or radiologic examination of the urinary tract should be deferred, if possible, until after this time.

B. Renal Hemodynamics. The changes in renal hemodynamics in gestation are the most striking and clinically significant of all the urinary tract alterations of pregnancy.

1. **Glomerular filtration rate (GFR) and renal plasma flow (RPF)** increase to levels 30% and 50%, respectively, above nongravid values during pregnancy. Increments in GFR that are already present during the early days after conception reach a maximum during the first trimester. The basis for the increase in GFR and RPF is unknown. Animal studies suggest that renal vasodilation (mediated by nitric oxide [NO]) leading to increased glomerular plasma flow is a contributing, but not the sole, factor. RPF is greatest at midgestation, declining somewhat in the third trimester. The increase in GFR has important clinical implications. Because creatinine production is unchanged during pregnancy,

TABLE 16-1 Renal Changes in Normal Pregnancy

Alteration	Manifestation	Clinical Relevance
Increased renal size	Renal length approximately 1 cm greater on radiographs	Postpartum decreases in size should not be mistaken for parenchymal loss
Dilation of pelves, calyces, and ureters	Resembles hydronephrosis on renal ultrasonography or intravenous pyelography (more marked on right)	Not to be mistaken for obstructive uropathy; elective evaluation should be deferred to the 12th postpartum week; upper urinary tract infections are more virulent; retained urine leads to collection errors
Increased renal vasodilation	Glomerular filtration rate and renal plasma flow increase 35–50%	Serum creatinine and urea nitrogen values decrease during normal gestations; protein, amino acid, and glucose urinary excretion all increase
Changes in acid–base metabolism	Renal bicarbonate threshold decreases	Serum bicarbonate is 4–5 µmol/L lower in normal gestation
Renal water handling	Osmoregulation altered	Serum osmolality decreases 10 mOsm/L (serum sodium decreases 5 mEq/L) during normal gestation
—	Osmotic thresholds for thirst and AVP decrease; the metabolic clearance of AVP increases markedly; high levels of vasopressinase circulating	Increased metabolism of AVP may cause transient diabetes insipidus in pregnancy

AVP, arginine vasopressin.

increments in its clearance result in decreased serum levels. Using the Hare method, one group of investigators observed that true serum creatinine, which averaged 0.67 mg/dL in nongravid women, decreased to 0.46 mg/dL during gestation (to convert to SI units [µmol/L], multiply serum creatinine [mg/dL] by 88.4). In studies that also measured creatinine chromogen (which yielded results resembling those reported in most clinical laboratories), values were 0.83 mg/dL in nonpregnant women and decreased to 0.74, 0.58, and 0.53 mg/dL in the first, second, and third trimester of pregnancy, respectively. Therefore, values considered normal in nongravid women may reflect decreased kidney function during pregnancy. For example, in gravid women, concentrations of serum creatinine exceeding 0.8 mg/dL or of serum urea nitrogen that are greater than 13 mg/dL suggest the need for additional evaluation of kidney function.

2. **Other Consequences of the Increased Renal Hemodynamics.** Increased GFR and RPF also alter urinary solute content. For example, excretion of glucose, most amino acids, and several water-soluble vitamins increases, and these increments in the nutrient content of urine may be a factor in the enhanced susceptibility of gravidas to UTIs. Urinary protein excretion also increases during gestation, and excretion up to 300 mg/d may still be normal.

C. **Acid–Base Regulation in Pregnancy.** Renal acid–base regulation is altered during gestation. The bicarbonate threshold decreases, and early morning urines are often more alkaline than those in the nongravid state. Pregnant women hyperventilate and their P_{CO_2} averages only 30 mmHg. The mild alkalosis (arterial

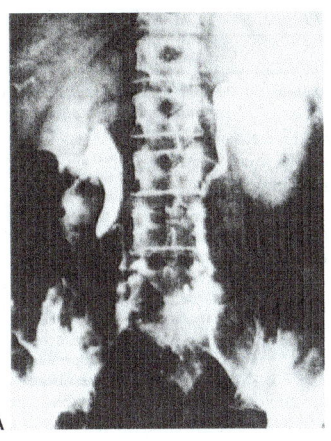 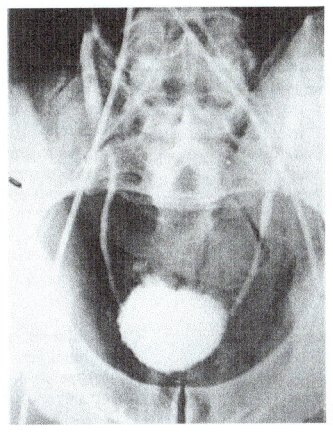

Figure 16-1. Intravenous pyelogram. **A:** Ureteral dilation of pregnancy. The right ureter is sharply cut off at the pelvic brim where it crosses the iliac artery (the iliac sign). **B:** Relationship between the ureters and iliac arteries can be demonstrated in postmortem studies. Note the iliac sign at the pelvic brim on the right. (Used with permission of Radiology society of North America, from Dure-Smith P. Pregnancy dilation of the urinary tract. *Radiology*. 1970;96:545; permission conveyed through Copyright Clearance Center, Inc.)

pH averages 7.44) found in pregnancy is in accord with this view. Plasma bicarbonate concentrations decrease approximately 4 μmol/L, averaging 22 μmol/L. This change most likely represents a compensatory renal response to hypocapnia. Because steady-state P_{CO_2} and HCO_3 levels are already diminished, pregnant women are, in theory, at a disadvantage when threatened by sudden metabolic acidosis (e.g., lactic acidosis in preeclampsia, diabetic ketoacidosis, or acute kidney injury [AKI]); however, they respond with appropriate increments in urinary titratable acid and ammonia after an acid load, and proton regeneration is already evident at blood pH levels higher than those in similarly tested nonpregnant women. Finally, when managing gravidas with pulmonary disorders, it should be noted that a P_{CO_2} of 40 mmHg, normal in nonpregnant women, signifies considerable carbon dioxide retention in pregnancy.

D. Water Excretion. After conception, a rapid decrease in plasma osmolality levels of 5 to 10 mOsm/kg below that of nongravid subjects occurs. If this decrease occurred in a nonpregnant woman, she would cease secreting antidiuretic hormone and enter a state of water diuresis; however, gravidas maintain this new osmolality, diluting and concentrating urine appropriately when the woman is subjected to water loading or dehydration. This suggests a resetting of the osmoreceptor system, and, indeed, clinical studies demonstrate that the osmotic thresholds for both thirst and arginine vasopressin (AVP) release are decreased in pregnant women. Furthermore, the plasma of pregnant women contains large quantities of a placental enzyme (vasopressinase) capable of destroying substantial quantities of AVP in vitro; moreover, the metabolic clearance of AVP hormone is increased fourfold after midgestation. The changes in osmoregulation and AVP metabolism may be responsible for two unusual syndromes of transient diabetes insipidus that complicate pregnancy. One, in which polyuria is responsive to both AVP and deamino-8-D-arginine vasopressin (dDAVP), probably occurs in women with unapparent partial central diabetes insipidus whose disease is brought to the fore by the increment in hormonal disposal rates during late gestation. The other disorder, in which the marked polyuria continues despite large doses of AVP, is responsive to dDAVP, an analog resistant to inactivation by vasopressinase. These gravidas may have excessively high circulating levels of this aminopeptidase enzyme due to increased activation.

E. Volume Regulation. Most healthy women gain approximately 12.5 kg during the first pregnancy and 1 kg less during subsequent pregnancies. Most of the increment is fluid, with total body water increasing from 6 to 8 L, 4 to 6 L of which is extracellular. Plasma volume increases by 50% during gestation, with the largest rate of increment occurring during midpregnancy, whereas increments in the interstitial space are greatest in the third trimester. A gradual cumulative retention of approximately 900 mEq of sodium occurs in pregnancy; this is distributed between the products of conception and the maternal extracellular space. These alterations in maternal intravascular and interstitial compartments produce apparent hypervolemia, yet the gravida's volume receptors sense these changes as normal. Therefore, when salt restriction or diuretic therapy limits this physiologic expansion, maternal responses resemble those in salt-depleted nonpregnant women. This is one compelling reason for the reluctance to recommend sodium restriction or diuretics during pregnancy. Pregnant women are now advised to salt their food to taste, and some researchers believe that a liberal sodium intake is beneficial during gestation. Another physiologic adaptation that appears to influence sodium balance during pregnancy is the marked stimulation of the renin–angiotensin–aldosterone system. Aldosterone levels are markedly increased during pregnancy, despite normal BP and normal potassium balance. It is likely that the increased aldosterone secretion is a compensatory mechanism to counteract the increase in sodium excretion that would be expected as a result of the large increase in GFR and RPF. Arterial vasodilation that causes relative arterial underfilling, as occurs in pregnancy, is known to stimulate the renin–angiotensin–aldosterone system. Moreover, increases in aldosterone balance the natriuretic effects of the large increases in progesterone during pregnancy.

F. Blood Pressure Regulation. Mean BP starts to decrease early in gestation, with diastolic levels in midpregnancy averaging 10 mmHg less than measurements postpartum. In later pregnancy, BP increases, gradually approaching nonpregnancy values near term. Because cardiac output rises quickly in the first trimester and remains relatively constant thereafter, the decrease in pressure is due to a marked decrement in systemic vascular resistance. The slow rise toward nonpregnant levels after a midtrimester nadir is interesting because it demonstrates that increasing vasoconstrictor tone is a feature of late gestation in healthy women as well as in women in whom preeclampsia is developing. The cause of the decrease in systemic vascular resistance during pregnancy is obscure. Studies of arterial compliance in pregnancy demonstrate early rises, perhaps due to alterations in vessel ground substance. Elevations of plasma estrogen and progesterone to concentrations that may relax smooth muscle occur, and increments in vasodilating prostaglandins and relaxin are also present during gestation. Hormonally mediated increases in endothelial NO production may also contribute to the vasodilation in pregnancy. With the lower BP, the levels of all components of the renin–angiotensin system are increased during pregnancy. Exaggerated hypotensive responses to converting enzyme inhibition in normal gravidas suggest that the increased renin–angiotensin system in pregnancy is a normal physiologic response to decreased BP and increased sodium excretion.

Lack of awareness of the fluctuation in BP during normal gestation may lead to diagnostic errors. For example, women with mild essential hypertension often experience a decrease in BP during early pregnancy, and BP may even approach normal levels. They may then be erroneously labeled preeclamptic in the last trimester, when frankly elevated pressures occur.

G. Mineral Metabolism. Serum calcium levels decrease in pregnancy, in conjunction with a decrease in circulating albumin concentrations. Ionized calcium levels, however, remain in the normal nonpregnant range. Striking changes relating to calcium regulatory hormones also occur during normal pregnancy. Production of 1,25-dihydroxyvitamin D_3 increases as early as the first trimester, reaching circulating levels that are approximately twice the nonpregnant values. Gastrointestinal absorption of calcium increases, resulting in an "absorptive hypercalciuria," with 24-hour urine excretion often exceeding 300 mg/d (in appropriately nourished individuals). Intact parathyroid hormone levels are lower during normal pregnancy.

II. Clinical Evaluation of Kidney Function in Pregnancy

A. Examination of the Urine. The association of proteinuria with eclampsia was first noted in the 1840s, and the science of prenatal care advanced dramatically when physicians began to systematically examine the urine of gravidas, primarily for albuminuria. In certain instances, kidney disease is first uncovered by the detection of excessive protein excretion or microscopic hematuria during a routine prenatal evaluation.

Healthy nonpregnant women excrete considerably less than 100 mg of protein in the urine daily, but due to the relative imprecision and variability of testing methods used in hospital laboratories, proteinuria is not considered abnormal until it exceeds 150 mg/d. During pregnancy, protein excretion increases, and excretion up to 300 mg/d may still be normal. On occasion, a healthy gravida can excrete more than that amount. In pregnancy, the gold standard for evaluation of abnormal proteinuria is the 24-hour urine protein measurement. A 24-hour protein excretion of greater than 300 mg is abnormal in pregnancy and correlates with a urine dipstick 1+ protein measurement. Although commonly used to detect proteinuria, urine dipstick testing is susceptible to error due to variations in urine concentration; therefore, if the level of suspicion is high, 24-hour urine testing should be performed.

Few attempts have been made to quantitate the urine sediment in pregnancy. The excretion of both red and white blood cells may increase during normal gestation, and one to two red blood cells per high-power field is acceptable in a urinalysis.

B. Kidney Function Tests. The clearance of endogenous creatinine, the most satisfactory approximation of GFR in nongravid subjects, is equally useful for assessing kidney function in gravidas. Gravidas, as well as nonpregnant women, show little variation (approximately 10% per day) in urinary creatinine excretion and, presumably, in creatinine production, which in a given woman is similar both during and after gestation. The lower limit of normal creatinine clearance during gestation should be 30% greater than the average of 110 to 115 mL/min for nongravid women. Calculation of GFR by serum creatinine-based formulae is confounded by increasing maternal weight which is not muscle weight, and neither Modification of Diet in Renal Disease (MDRD) nor Cockroft–Gault GFR estimates have been validated in pregnancy.

Acid excretion and urinary concentration and dilution are similar in gravid and nonpregnant women. Therefore, tests such as ammonium loading (rarely indicated in gestation) give values similar to those in nongravid women. When examining urinary diluting ability, the clinician should be aware that supine posture can interfere with this test. Therefore, studies to detect minimal urinary osmolal concentrations should be performed with the patient lying on her side. However, although lateral recumbency is the required position for prenatal measurement of most renal function parameters, this posture interferes with tests of concentration. For example, a urine osmolality that was 800 mOsm/kg after overnight dehydration may decrease to 400 mOsm/kg within 1 hour through fluid mobilization from the extremities during bed rest, thereby resulting in volume-induced inhibition of AVP secretion, a mild osmotic diuresis, or both. These observations demonstrate the importance of upright posture, such as quiet sitting, when maximum urinary concentration is measured in pregnancy.

Detection of AKI in pregnancy is confounded by the physiologic lowering of serum creatinine due to glomerular hyperfiltration in pregnancy. The diagnosis of AKI is not standardized in clinical practice due to inconsistency in the definition of pregnancy-related AKI and nonvalidation of Kidney Disease Improving Outcomes guidelines, and Acute Kidney Injury Network (AKIN) criteria in pregnant women. Attention should be paid to trends in serum creatinine levels in pregnancy, and even small changes in creatinine may be sensitive, picking up early kidney injury in specific clinical settings. The timing of onset of AKI by trimester may point toward underlying etiology. Hyperemesis gravidarum and septic abortions are common in first trimester; while second and third-trimester AKI causes are specific to the complications of preeclampsia, hemolysis, elevated liver enzymes, low platelet count (HELLP) syndrome, acute fatty liver of pregnancy, thrombotic microangiopathies and placental abruption. Evaluation of urinalysis, urine microscopy, comprehensive metabolic panel coagulation panel, and appropriate serologic work-up will help narrow the etiology of AKI. Serum complement levels can be elevated in pregnancy because of increased synthesis and can complicate the diagnosis of lupus nephritis. Kidney ultrasound helps post obstructive cause of AKI, but in pregnancy, pathologic obstruction should be differentiated from physiologic ureteral dilation. Common causes of AKI in the second and third trimesters such as preeclampsia, HELLP syndrome, atypical hemolytic syndrome, acute fatty liver of pregnancy, and lupus nephritis can have overlapping features and require detailed evaluation. Kidney biopsy should be considered when lab evaluation of AKI is nondiagnostic, and a definitive diagnosis will facilitate specific treatment options that outweigh the risk of biopsy.

C. Role of Kidney Biopsy in Pregnancy. Biopsy should be considered for treatment of kidney disease that presents or aggravates during pregnancy and requires a diagnosis that will facilitate specific treatment options. Potential risk of harm must be carefully weighed against the benefits or clinical diagnosis and management during pregnancy, individual patient's clinical status, and gestational age. Indications for kidney biopsy include sudden, severe decrease in GFR or new development of nephrotic-range proteinuria, lupus flare, and in whom less-invasive means of diagnosis have failed to elucidate disease etiology. If deemed medically necessary, kidney biopsy should be performed before 30-week gestation.

The risk of bleeding increases twofold after 26 weeks of gestation, particularly if hypertension is present, as frequently is the case in the conditions for which kidney biopsy is indicated. Furthermore, technical difficulties increase after 20 to 25 weeks of pregnancy, when the lateral decubitus or the sitting position, rather than the prone position, is used to avoid compression of the inferior vena cava by the pregnant uterus. Prior studies have reported complications of macroscopic hematuria, perirenal hematoma, and the need for blood transfusion between 23 and 28 weeks of gestation, and no serious complications occurring prior to 22 weeks of gestation.

In summary, kidney biopsy may be performed safely during pregnancy specifically in the first and second trimester but should be done only if therapeutic decisions require precise diagnosis that cannot be safely postponed until the postpartum period.

III. Kidney Disease in Pregnancy

A. Asymptomatic Bacteriuria. UTI is the most common kidney problem occurring in pregnancy. The urine of gravidas supports bacterial growth better than that of nonpregnant women because of its increased nutrient content. This, as well as ureteral dilation, stasis, and occasional obstruction, would be expected to increase the susceptibility of pregnant women to UTI. Surprisingly, this is not the case and, with the exception of certain high-risk groups (diabetic patients and gravidas with sickle cell trait), the prevalence of asymptomatic bacteriuria during gestation varies between 4% and 7%, a value similar to that in sexually active nonpregnant women. The natural history of asymptomatic UTIs is, however, quite different in pregnancy. Although in the nonpregnant state, asymptomatic bacteriuria is quite benign, progression to overt cystitis or pyelonephritis occurs in up to 40% of affected gravidas. Therefore, screening all pregnant women for the presence of asymptomatic bacteriuria and treating those with positive urine cultures are important.

Pregnant women contaminate midstream urine specimens more frequently and the incidence can be reduced by the use of multiple vulval washings.

The optimum way to manage asymptomatic UTI in pregnancy has not been precisely defined. More than 90% of the uropathogens involved are aerobic gram-negative rods, usually *Escherichia coli*, and the physicians recommend a 4- to 7-day course of the antibiotic to which the cultured organism is sensitive, preferably a short-acting sulfa drug, nitrofurantoin, amoxicillin, or a cephalosporin. This approach, when combined with surveillance for recurrent bacteriuria, has been shown to be quite effective.

B. Symptomatic Bacteriuria. The clinical approach to symptomatic UTI during gestation differs from that for asymptomatic bacteriuria.

1. **Acute Pyelonephritis.** Pyelonephritis was a cause of maternal death in the preantibiotic era, and 3% of pregnant patients in a reported series developed septic shock. At one time, symptomatic UTIs complicated almost 2% of all gestations, but prenatal screening combined with rapid treatment of asymptomatic bacteriuria has reduced this incidence to approximately 0.5%. The bacteriology of these infections resembles that in asymptomatic patients (predominantly *E. coli*), and most cases present after midpregnancy. The clinical presentation of pyelonephritis in pregnancy can be dramatic. As noted in the preceding text, the disease caused maternal deaths in the preantibiotic era, and upper UTIs in gravidas are associated with exaggerated effects of endotoxemia, including shock, respiratory distress syndrome, marked kidney dysfunction, and hematologic and liver abnormalities. Symptomatic UTIs have also been implicated in the etiology of intrauterine growth restriction, prematurity, congenital anomalies, and fetal demise; however, most studies reporting these associations were not adequately controlled for potential confounders. The treatment of pyelonephritis should be aggressive and is best performed in the hospital.

    Most patients with pyelonephritis respond quickly, with defervescence within 48 to 72 hours. Once afebrile for 48 hours, oral therapy may be started and continued to complete 10 to 14 days of treatment. Continuous low-dose suppressive therapy during the remainder of pregnancy is recommended because of the high rate of recurrence. An alternative approach, frequent surveillance for recurrent infection with prompt treatment when significant bacteriuria is identified, has been claimed to be as effective as suppressive therapy.

2. **Antibiotic Use in Pregnancy.** The first-choice antibiotic for symptomatic infections changes from decade to decade because of the rapid emergence of resistant strains. The physicians continue to recommend starting treatment with cephalosporins, because a significant percentage of community-acquired *E. coli* infections are resistant to ampicillin. For routine cystitis, nitrofurantoin is often effective and is acceptable during pregnancy. Certain antibiotics cannot be used in pregnancy due to the potential fetal toxicity of agents that cross the placental barrier. (Information concerning drug safety during pregnancy is listed in the *Physicians' Desk Reference*, which is updated annually.) In brief, sulfa drugs should not be used near term, because they may precipitate kernicterus in the newborn. The antifolic acid activity of trimethoprim has been associated with anomalies such as cleft palate in animals, and this combination drug should also be avoided,

at least before midpregnancy. Fluoroquinolones cross the placenta and should be avoided if possible. Tetracyclines are contraindicated because they deposit in fetal bones and teeth and may cause severe reactions in the mother, including hepatic failure. Nitrofurantoin is contraindicated at term because of risk of hemolytic disease in the newborn.

C. Acute Kidney Injury
1. **Incidence.** Before 1970, the incidence of AKI in pregnancy severe enough to require dialytic therapy was estimated at between 1 in 2,000 and 1 in 5,000 gestations, and it represented a considerable proportion of cases reported in large series. Since then, the number of patients with AKI from obstetric causes has declined markedly attributed to the improvement of prenatal care.

   Changing trends in the epidemiology of pregnancy-related acute kidney injury have been observed over the past years with global variations in the predominant causes. Though the incidence remains higher in developing countries, this appears to be decreasing, while pregnancy-related AKI appears to be on the rise in developed countries. This is attributable to changing demographics of the pregnant population which includes older women with more preexisting comorbidities such as obesity, diabetes, chronic hypertension, chronic kidney disease (CKD), and increased rates of assisted reproduction. Whereas in developed countries, pregnancy-induced hypertensive disorders are the leading etiology, in developing countries sepsis and hemorrhage are main contributors. The frequency distribution of AKI during gestation is bimodal, with one peak early in pregnancy (12 to 18 weeks) comprising most of the cases associated with septic abortion, and a second peak between gestational week 35 and the puerperium, primarily due to preeclampsia, sepsis, and bleeding complications, especially placental abruption.

   The changing pattern of the etiology of pregnancy-related AKI is apparent, with a decline in AKI in early pregnancy due to abortion and puerperal sepsis-related causes but an increase in the frequency of hypertensive disorders, thrombotic microangiopathies, and postpartum-associated AKI.

   Overall, the rate of AKI during pregnancy-related hospitalizations has been reported to be 0.08%. In the United States, a higher likelihood of AKI during pregnancy-related hospitalizations was seen in 2015 (OR 2.20; 95% CI 1.89–2.55) than in 2006; in older women aged 36 to 40 years (OR 1.49; 95% CI 1.36–1.64) and 41 to 49 years (OR 2.12; 95% CI 1.84–2.45) than in women aged 20 to 25 years; in Blacks (OR 1.52; 95% CI 1.40–1.65) and Native Americans (OR 1.45; 95% CI 1.10–1.91) than in Whites, and in diabetic women (OR 4.43; 95% CI 4.04–4.86) than in those without diabetes. In addition, pregnancy-related hospitalizations with AKI were associated with a higher likelihood of inpatient mortality (OR 13.50; 95% CI 10.47–17.42) and cardiovascular events (OR 9.74; 95% CI 9.08–10.46) than were pregnancy-related hospitalizations with no AKI. Pregnancy-related AKI remains a serious complication and has been associated with increased maternal and fetal mortality.

2. **Causes.** AKI in pregnancy can be induced by any of the disorders leading to kidney failure in the general population, such as acute tubular necrosis (ATN). Early in pregnancy, the most common problems are prerenal disease due to hyperemesis gravidarum, and ATN resulting from a septic abortion. Several different disorders can lead to AKI later in pregnancy including preeclampsia (discussed in Section VI.A) and HELLP syndrome (Table 16-2).

   a. **Thrombotic Microangiopathy (TMA).** TMA is characterized by fibrin and platelet aggregates in the microvasculature, particularly in the kidney and the brain. Histologic features include endothelial cell swelling, accumulation of protein in the endothelial cell layer, and sometimes splitting of the glomerular basement membrane.

TABLE 16-2 Causes of Acute Kidney Injury in Pregnancy and Differentiating Features

	Preeclampsia With Severe Features	HELLP Syndrome	Acute Fatty Liver of Pregnancy (AFLP)	Hemolytic Uremic Syndrome (HUS)	Thrombotic Microangiopathic Purpura (TTP)	Lupus Nephritis
Timing of gestation	>20 wk, commonly in 3rd trimester	>20 wk	Near term	Near term and worsens postpartum	Second and Third trimesters	Any trimester
Presenting features	Hypertension, non-specific symptoms like headache, abdominal pain, visual changes	Hypertension, abdominal pain, jaundice	Nausea, vomiting, abdominal pain, jaundice, headache	Fever	Neurologic involvement and fever	Other symptoms of lupus flare like rash, arthralgias, fever
Supportive Laboratory tests	Elevated sFLT/PIGF ratio; may have thrombocytopenia, elevated transaminases, and urine with proteinuria	Hemolysis with schistocytes, low platelets, elevated transaminases	Elevated bilirubin, transaminases, disseminated intravascular coagulation is common, low fibrinogen, hypoglycemia	Severe hemolysis and thrombocytopenia (>20,000/mm³), urine with nondysmorphic RBC and proteinuria	Severe hemolysis and thrombocytopenia (<2,000/mm³), ADAMTS13 <5%	Hypocomplementemia, elevated dsDNA, urine with proteinuria and dysmorphic RBC, casts
Treatment	Delivery	Delivery	Delivery	Eculizumab	Plasma exchange	Immunosuppression

sFLT, Soluble fms like tyrosine kinase; PlGF, placental growth factor; ADAMTS13, a disintegrin and metalloproteinase with a thrombospondin type 1 motif, member 13.

TMA affecting primarily the kidney is termed hemolytic uremic syndrome (HUS), whereas TMA characterized by profound thrombocytopenia and neurologic disturbances is called thrombotic thrombocytopenic purpura (TTP). TTP is caused by an acquired or inherited disorder of a metalloproteinase ADAMTS13 that cleaves ultralarge multimers of von Willebrand factor, whereas HUS is caused by dysregulation and uncontrolled activation of the complement system.

An important and difficult differential diagnosis is that of AKI in late pregnancy in association with microangiopathic hemolytic anemia and thrombocytopenia. Pregnancy is considered to be a risk factor for TTP/HUS. However, whether the pathogenesis of these disorders in pregnancy is similar to that in nonpregnant individuals is unclear. TTP/HUS is rare in pregnancy, and must be distinguished from the HELLP variant of preeclampsia, a much more common condition. The distinction of these syndromes is important for therapeutic and prognostic reasons, but considerable overlap exists in their clinical and laboratory features. Features that may be helpful in making the diagnosis include timing of onset and the pattern of laboratory abnormalities, which in TTP may include decreased levels of a von Willebrand cleaving protease. Preeclampsia typically develops in the third trimester, with only a few cases developing in the postpartum period, usually within a few days of delivery. TTP usually occurs antepartum, with many cases developing in the second trimester, as well as the third. HUS is usually a postpartum disease. Symptoms may begin antepartum, but most cases are diagnosed postpartum.

Preeclampsia is much more common than TTP/HUS, and it is usually preceded by hypertension and proteinuria. Kidney failure is unusual even with severe cases, unless significant bleeding or hemodynamic instability, or marked disseminated intravascular coagulation (DIC) occurs. In some cases, preeclampsia develops in the immediate postpartum period, and when thrombocytopenia is severe, it may be indistinguishable from HUS. However, preeclampsia spontaneously recovers, whereas HUS only infrequently improves.

In contrast to TTP/HUS, preeclampsia may be associated with mild DIC and prolongation of prothrombin and partial thromboplastin time. Another laboratory feature of preeclampsia/HELLP syndrome that is not usually associated with TTP/HUS is marked elevations in liver enzymes. The presence of fever is more consistent with a diagnosis of TTP than preeclampsia or HUS. The main distinctive features of HUS are its tendency to occur in the postpartum period and the severity of the associated kidney failure. Treatment of preeclampsia/HELLP syndrome is delivery and supportive care. More aggressive treatment is rarely indicated. Treatment of TTP/HUS includes plasmapheresis, eculizumab, and other modalities used in nonpregnant patients with these disorders, although clinical trials of these modalities in pregnancy have not been performed.

b. **Renal Cortical Necrosis.** Renal cortical necrosis occurs in 1.5% to 2% of all causes of AKI in developed countries and in 3% to 7% of all causes of AKI in developing countries. The primary inciting events for renal cortical necrosis are obstetric complications (septic abortions, abruptio placenta, and DIC). Affected patients typically present with oliguria or anuria, hematuria, and flank pain. Ultrasonography or computed tomographic scanning may demonstrate hypoechoic or hypodense areas in the renal cortex. Most patients require chronic dialysis, but 20% to 40% have partial recovery of kidney function.

c. **Acute Pyelonephritis.** Some pregnant women may develop AKI in association with pyelonephritis.

d. **Acute fatty liver of pregnancy** (fatty infiltration of hepatocytes without inflammation or necrosis) is a rare complication of pregnancy that is associated with significant AKI. Women with this disorder often complain of anorexia and occasionally abdominal pain in the third trimester. Clinical features suggesting preeclampsia, including hypertension and proteinuria, are not uncommon. Laboratory test results reveal elevations in liver enzymes, hypoglycemia, hypofibrinogenemia, and prolonged partial thromboplastin time. Delivery is indicated, and most patients improve shortly afterward.

e. **Urinary Tract Obstruction.** Pregnancy is associated with dilation of the collecting system, which is not usually associated with kidney dysfunction. Rarely, complications such as large uterine fibroids, which may enlarge in the setting of pregnancy, can lead to obstructive uropathy. Uncommonly, acute urinary tract obstruction in pregnancy is induced by a kidney stone. Diagnosis can usually be made by ultrasonography. Often the stones pass spontaneously, but occasionally cystoscopy is necessary for insertion of a stent to remove a fragment of stone and relieve obstruction, particularly if there is sepsis or a solitary kidney.

3. The **management** of AKI occurring in gestation or immediately postpartum is similar to that in nongravid subjects (see Chapter 12: The Patient with Acute Kidney Injury), but several points peculiar to pregnancy deserve emphasis. Because uterine hemorrhage near term may be concealed and blood loss underestimated, any overt blood loss should be replaced early. Hemodialysis has been successfully used in patients with obstetric-related AKI. Because urea, creatinine, and other metabolites that accumulate in uremia traverse the placenta and are associated with adverse fetal outcomes, dialysis should be undertaken early, with the aim of maintaining the blood urea nitrogen at approximately 50 mg/dL. Excessive fluid removal should be avoided, because it may contribute to hemodynamic compromise, reduction of uteroplacental perfusion, and premature labor. Some obstetricians and perinatologists recommend continuous fetal monitoring during hemodialysis treatments, starting at midpregnancy.

D. Pregnancy in Women With Preexisting Kidney Disease. The current approach to management of pregnancy in women with CKD is primarily based on retrospective studies (Table 16-3).

1. **Prognosis.** Counseling and managing women with CKD is based on the following general approach: Fertility and ability to sustain an uncomplicated pregnancy relate to the stage of CKD, BP, and proteinuria.

    a. **Degree of Impaired Kidney Function.** Patients are arbitrarily considered in three categories: preserved or mildly impaired kidney function (serum creatinine less than 1.5 mg/dL), moderate kidney insufficiency (creatinine 1.5 to 3.0 mg/dL), and severe kidney insufficiency (creatinine higher than 3 mg/dL).

    Pregnancy is associated with a higher risk of adverse maternal and fetal outcomes in the presence of moderate or severe kidney dysfunction because up to 40% of pregnancies in the former category are complicated by either difficult-to-control hypertension or sudden decline in GFR, which may not reverse after delivery. An even higher incidence of serious maternal problems occurs when kidney insufficiency is severe. This is especially true for women receiving dialytic therapy, in which fewer than 50% of the gestations succeed, and problems of extreme prematurity plague many of those who do.

    b. **Hypertension.** The BP level at the time of gestation is an important prognostic index. When kidney disease and hypertension coexist, the gestation is more likely to be complicated by preeclampsia and worsening of

TABLE 16-3	Summary of Pregnancy in Women With Preexisting Kidney Disease
Disease	**Comments**
Chronic glomerulonephritis and focal and segmental glomerular sclerosis (FSGS)	Increased incidence of high blood pressure, usually later in gestation, but usually no adverse effect results if kidney function is preserved and hypertension is absent before gestation; some cases of exacerbation in pregnancy have been reported in women with immunoglobulin A nephropathy, membranoproliferative glomerulonephritis, and FSGS
Systemic lupus erythematosus	Controversial: prognosis is most favorable if disease is in remission 6 mo or more before conception
Vasculitis	Case reports of granulomatosis with polyangiitis suggest acceptable outcomes if disease is in remission and kidney function is normal; scleroderma and polyarteritis may be associated with severe and accelerated hypertension during pregnancy
Diabetic nephropathy	Increased frequency of infections; high incidence of heavy proteinuria and hypertension near term; optimal time for pregnancy is when kidney function is normal, hypertension absent, and albuminuria is <300 mg/d
Vesicoureteral reflux	Bacteriuria in pregnancy may lead to exacerbation; urinary infection is common
Polycystic kidney disease	Fewer complications when function is preserved and hypertension is absent; however, the incidence of preeclampsia is increased
Urolithiasis	Ureteral dilation and stasis do not seem to affect natural history, but infections can be more frequent; stents have been successfully placed during gestation
Previous urologic surgery	Urinary tract infection is common with urinary diversion, and kidney function may undergo reversible decrease; cesarean section might be necessary to avoid disruption of the continence mechanism if artificial sphincters or neourethras have been constructed
After nephrectomy, solitary pelvic kidneys	Pregnancy is well tolerated; might be associated with other malformations of the urogenital tract; dystocia occurs rarely with a pelvic kidney

GN, glomerulonephritis.

Generalizations are for women with only mild kidney dysfunction (serum creatinine level less than 1.5 mg/dL) and without hypertension at conception.

kidney function. Women with well-controlled BP and only mild kidney dysfunction may have relatively uncomplicated pregnancies; however, they must be closely followed in clinic.

- **E. Proteinuria.** Urinary protein excretion, which increases in normal pregnancy, may increase markedly in pregnant women with underlying parenchymal kidney disease. In one large series, one-third of the patients with preexisting kidney disease developed nephrotic-range proteinuria during gestation. These increments may reflect worsening of the underlying kidney disease.
    1. **Renal Hemodynamics.** Gravidas with kidney disorders with only minimal kidney dysfunction usually experience increments in GFR during gestation,

although levels do not reach those seen in healthy pregnant women. Therefore, a decrement in serum creatinine level early in pregnancy is a good prognostic sign. If serum creatinine levels before conception exceed 1.5 mg/dL, decrements during gestation are less common, and, as noted, the prognosis of such pregnancies is more guarded.
F. **Glomerulonephritis.** Glomerulonephritis in women of childbearing age includes immunoglobulin (Ig) a nephropathy, focal and segmental glomerulosclerosis, membranoproliferative glomerulonephritis, minimal change nephritis, and membranous nephropathy. Data is lacking regarding the prognosis for pregnancy with histologic subtype. Rather, when kidney function is normal and hypertension and proteinuria are absent, prognosis is good.
G. **Collagen Vascular Disease**
  1. **Lupus Nephritis.** The effect of gestation in women with lupus erythematosus who have kidney involvement is difficult to evaluate, in part because of the unpredictable course of the disease regardless of pregnancy. Activity of the disease in the 6 months before conception is often a useful prognostic guide (the longer the remission the better the outlook). Although most pregnancies, in the presence of preserved function, proceed uneventfully or are accompanied by only transient functional declines, in approximately 10%, gestation appears to cause permanent kidney damage and accelerate the kidney disease. Also, placental transmission of maternal autoantibodies is associated with an increased frequency of spontaneous abortion in these women, and certain anticytoplasmic antibodies such as anti-Sjögren syndrome antigen (ASS-A/Ro) cause a neonatal lupus syndrome characterized by congenital heart block, transient cutaneous lesions, or both. Women with systemic lupus erythematosus (SLE) have a high incidence of detectable levels of antiphospholipid antibodies (anticardiolipin antibodies and lupus anticoagulant). High titers of these antibodies are associated with several complications of pregnancy, including spontaneous fetal loss, hypertensive syndromes indistinguishable from preeclampsia, and thrombotic events including deep vein thrombosis, pulmonary embolus, myocardial infarction, and strokes. Also, pregnant women with circulating antiphospholipid antibodies can manifest a rare form of rapid kidney failure postpartum, associated with glomerular thrombi. Therefore, women with SLE should be screened for antiphospholipid antibodies early in gestation. The therapeutic approach when gravidas manifests antiphospholipid antibodies is disputed, and many would not treat asymptomatic patients who manifest low titers. However, when titers are elevated (more than 40 GPL IgG antiphospholipid level), most authorities prescribe aspirin (80 to 325 mg/d). Heparin in combination with aspirin is recommended for patients with a history of thrombotic events and may also be advisable when titers are higher than 80 GPL.

  A flare of lupus nephritis may be difficult to distinguish from preeclampsia when a woman with a history of lupus develops worsening kidney function, proteinuria, and hypertension. Elevation in liver enzymes and new-onset severe hypertension is more consistent with preeclampsia. Hypocomplementemia, and severe nephritic syndrome without hypertension, are more consistent with lupus nephritis. Often, a flare of nephritis in the third trimester appears to trigger "superimposed preeclampsia," and improvement in BP and proteinuria occurs only after delivery. However, in the presence of abnormal serologic testing, it is often reasonable to treat worsening proteinuria and AKI with increased prednisone in the hope that it will improve, particularly if the fetus is immature. However, close maternal and fetal surveillance is of utmost importance, and delivery should be considered in the setting of obvious signs of HELLP syndrome, accelerating hypertension and/or progression of kidney disease, and other signs of worsening maternal condition.

2. Pregnancy in patients with other **vasculitis** has only rarely been reported. Successful pregnancies in women with granulomatosis with polyangiitis have been reported. Women may be treated with corticosteroids, azathioprine, cyclosporine, and intravenous immunoglobulin with safety. Cyclophosphamide is contraindicated in pregnancy. Such pregnancies are high risk and should be managed by a multidisciplinary team, and when possible women should be advised to wait until their disease is in remission before contemplating pregnancy.

H. **Diabetic Nephropathy.** Diabetes is one of the most common medical disorders encountered during pregnancy, and most cases are due to gestational diabetes. Preexisting diabetes poses significant risks to pregnancy. Many younger women with pregestational diabetes have type 1 diabetes, and if their disease has been present for 10 to 15 years, they may show early signs of diabetic nephropathy. Women with microalbuminuria rather than macroalbuminuria, well-preserved kidney function, and normal BP have a good prognosis for pregnancy, although they are at increased risk for transient proteinuria, preeclampsia, and urinary infection. Women with type 1 diabetes with microalbuminuria and normal kidney function and normotension should be encouraged *not* to postpone pregnancy because of the worse prognosis once overt nephropathy develops. Few studies of pregnancy and nephropathy associated with type 2 diabetes are available. However, the limited evidence suggests similar outcomes to individuals with type 1 diabetes.

The effects of gestation in diabetic patients with overt nephropathy are similar to those in women with other forms of kidney parenchymal disease. Prognosis is determined by the degree of hypertension and kidney function impairment.

I. **Nephrotic-Range Proteinuria during Pregnancy.** A common cause of nephrotic-range proteinuria (more than 3.5 g/d) in late pregnancy is preeclampsia. Other causes of nephrotic syndrome, including membranous nephropathy, proliferative or membranoproliferative glomerulonephritis, minimal change disease, diabetic nephropathy, amyloidosis, and focal segmental glomerulosclerosis, have been described in gravidas. The risks and benefits of kidney biopsy during pregnancy have already been mentioned.

Diuretic therapy for treating edema should be used cautiously during pregnancy, particularly when BP is not elevated. The concern is that intravascular volume depletion might impair uteroplacental perfusion. Exceptions to this, however, are women with hypertension, in whom diuretics may be necessary to control BP.

Prognosis in most nephrotic gravidas with preserved function is good; however, there is evidence to suggest that fetal outcome may be worse in the setting of significant and sustained maternal proteinuria. Focal segmental glomerulosclerosis, a frequent cause of nephrotic syndrome in women of childbearing age, is a disease in which the natural history during gestation remains disputed. Some claim pregnancy leads to irreversible functional loss and hypertension-sustained postpartum; others find the natural history of this entity in pregnancy similar to that of most other disorders.

J. **Management of Glomerular Disease in Pregnancy.** General management strategies for glomerular disease are discussed below.
  1. Prepregnancy: The planning of pregnancy when preexisting kidney disease is quiescent or well-controlled enhances successful outcomes. It involves active contraception counseling, changes to nonteratogenic medications, and educating patients about the need for heightened surveillance and complications.
  2. During Pregnancy: The BP target is <140/90 mmHg. Serial renal function, proteinuria, and markers of disease activity are essential, as is increased fetal monitoring via biophysical profile, placental Dopplers, and growth scans. Low-dose aspirin has been shown to reduce the incidence of preeclampsia. Venous thromboembolism prophylaxis is advocated in patients with risk factors such as nephrotic syndrome, previous clotting events, and

high body mass index. For any maternal or fetal decompensation, immediate delivery is planned. Corticosteroid administration should be performed for fetal lung maturation at least 24 hours and up to 7 days before anticipated delivery <34 weeks gestation.
3. Postpartum: Breastfeeding is encouraged. Continued surveillance for active glomerulonephritis and calcineurin drug level check with dose adjustment is required. Venous thromboembolism prophylaxis is continued for 6 weeks postpartum if needed.

K. **Tubulointerstitial Disease**
  1. **Vesicoureteral Reflux (VUR).** Reflux nephropathy due to VUR may cause CKD in young women. A prospective study of 54 pregnancies in 46 women with reflux nephropathy found that preeclampsia occurred in 24% and was more common in women with hypertension. Nine (18%) experienced deterioration in kidney function during pregnancy, and those with preexisting reduced kidney function were at greater risk. One-third of the infants were delivered preterm, and 43% had VUR. These high-risk women should be screened with urine cultures and treated promptly when infections are present with consideration to suppressive antibiotic therapy for the duration of pregnancy in some cases.
  2. **Adult dominant polycystic kidney disease** may remain undetected in gestation. Careful questioning of gravidas for a family history of kidney problems and ultrasonography may lead to its earlier detection. Patients with minimal functional impairment have few complications but are at increased risk for preeclampsia. They are also prone to UTIs, so it may be prudent to culture their urines more frequently. Hypertension usually accompanies or antedates the onset of functional deterioration, and pregnancy in such gravidas is more hazardous.

    Some women with autosomal dominant polycystic kidney disease have cysts in their livers that may enlarge with repeated pregnancy and with oral contraceptive use. A high incidence of cerebral aneurysms also occurs in certain affected families. When aware of such family clustering, usually identified by a history of subarachnoid hemorrhages among relatives, the patient should undergo screening using magnetic resonance angiography. If an aneurysm is detected, neurosurgical consultation should be obtained, and the obstetrician may wish to avoid natural labor. All these patients should undergo genetic counseling before pregnancy to ensure they know that 50% of their offspring are at risk. Finally, predicting the fetal outcome using molecular probes on cells cultured from the amniotic fluid is possible.
  3. **Solitary Kidneys.** Women with solitary kidneys appear to tolerate gestation well. However, if the nephrectomy was performed for nephrolithiasis or chronic pyelonephritis, the remaining kidney may be infected. Patients with these conditions must be carefully scrutinized by frequent examination and culture of the urine throughout pregnancy and in the puerperium.

L. **Pelvic kidneys** may be associated with other malformations of the urogenital tract of the mother. In addition, dystocia may occur when the kidney is in the true pelvis.

M. **Urolithiasis and Hematuria.** The prevalence of urolithiasis in gestation varies between 0.03% and 0.35% in the Western hemisphere. Many of the stones contain calcium, and some are infective in origin. A survey of 148 gestations in 78 nonselected stone formers suggests that pregnancy has little influence on the course of stone disease (although women with renal calculi may have an increased incidence of spontaneous abortions). It should be noted that most of the reported series focuses on women whose calculi are mainly of the noninfective variety, and little is known of the natural history of the more serious infected struvite stones during gestation. In any event, UTI in the presence of nephrolithiasis requires prompt and prolonged treatment (3 to 5 weeks), followed by suppressive therapy through the immediate puerperium, because the calculus may represent a nidus of infection resistant to sterilization.

Experience with cystinuria in pregnancy is limited, but most women with this disease also do well in gestation. D-Penicillamine as used in these patients appears to have no adverse effects on the mother or fetus.

Renal calculi are among the most common causes of abdominal pain (of nonobstetric origin) requiring hospitalization during gestation, and when complications suggest the need for surgical intervention, pregnancy should not be a deterrent to radiologic examination. If the stone obstructs the ureter, intervention with ureteral stenting, percutaneous nephrostomy, or, rarely, surgery is indicated. Spontaneous gross or microscopic hematuria occasionally complicates an otherwise uneventful gestation. The differential diagnosis includes all causes of hematuria in nongravid patients (see Chapter 1: The Nephrology Consult), but frequently, no etiology is demonstrable, and the bleeding subsides postpartum. It has been suggested that these events are due to the rupture of small veins around the dilated renal pelvis. Hematuria may or may not occur in subsequent gestations. In any event, investigation of the hematuria can often be deferred until after delivery, and noninvasive techniques such as ultrasonography and magnetic resonance imaging help arrive at such decisions.

IV. Kidney Transplantation

A. Menstruation and fertility resume in most women from 1 to 12 months after a kidney transplant. Pregnancy is not uncommon following kidney transplantation and the risk to mother and baby is much lower in this population than in pregnant patients on dialysis. The 2009 Kidney Disease: Improving Global Outcomes (KDIGO) Clinical Practice Guideline recommends delaying pregnancy until at least the first-year posttransplant. However, pregnancy in transplant patients remains at high risk for maternal and fetal complications. Most pregnancies (greater than 90%) that proceed beyond the first trimester succeed. Rates of preeclampsia and cesarean sections are significantly higher. A recent comprehensive meta-analysis by Shah et al. of various worldwide registries, single-center studies, and case series through 2017, representing 6,712 pregnancies in 4,174 kidney transplant recipients, noted live-birth rate of 72.9% (95% CI 70.0–75.6). induced abortions (12.4%; 95% CI 10.4–14.7), miscarriages (15.4%; 95% CI 13.8–17.2), stillbirths (5.1%; 95% CI 4.0–6.5), ectopic pregnancies (2.4%; 95% CI 1.5–3.7), preeclampsia (21.5%; 95% CI 18.5–24.9), gestational diabetes (5.7%; 95% CI 3.7–8.9), pregnancy induced hypertension (24.1%; 95% CI 18.1–31.5), cesarean section (62.6, 95% CI 57.6–67.3), and preterm delivery was 43.1% (95% CI 38.7–47.6). The mean maternal age was 29.6 years, the mean gestational age was 34.9 weeks, the mean birth weight was 2,470 g, and the mean interval between transplant and pregnancy was 3.7 years. About a quarter of the women developed preeclampsia, and this rate was almost sixfold higher compared to the general US population (21% vs. 3.8%). The cesarean section rate was twofold higher, about 60% to 77%. Several factors can contribute to the onset of hypertension after kidney transplantation, including the type of immunosuppressive therapy (calcineurin inhibitors and corticosteroids), allograft function, obesity, and the presence of a native kidney (increased production of renin). Fetal complications, kidney allograft dysfunction, or preeclampsia are common indications of early iatrogenic delivery.

Despite the higher incidence of preterm delivery and lower birth weight, long-term studies show that children born to transplant recipients develop normally.

Best practice guidelines have outlined criteria for considering pregnancy in kidney transplant recipients, and it is suggested that those contemplating pregnancy should meet the following:
- Stable kidney function with no recent rejection or ongoing infections
- Absent or minimal proteinuria (less than 0.5 g/d)
- Normal BP or well-controlled hypertension
- Serum creatinine less than 1.5 mg/dL
- Drug therapy: prednisone 15 mg daily or less, azathioprine 2 mg/kg or less, cyclosporine or tacrolimus
- Time of conception is 1 to 2 years after transplantation, according to American Society of Transplantation, and >2 years per European best practice guidelines. (European best practice guidelines for renal transplantationSection IV: Long-term management of the transplant recipient. IV.10. Pregnancy in renal transplant recipients, 2002.)

Calcineurin inhibitors remain the standard of care immunosuppression among kidney transplant recipients and are safe to be used during pregnancy. Due to pharmacokinetic changes in pregnancy, calcineurin inhibitor levels must be monitored at least monthly. Tacrolimus is measured in whole blood and due to the anemia and hypoalbuminemia in pregnancy, whole blood levels may decrease without a significant decrease in unbound tacrolimus, which is the relevant "free" level. Free tacrolimus levels are not available outside of research settings. Hence, targeting slightly lower tacrolimus levels during pregnancy with close monitoring and adjustment is recommended during mid–late pregnancy to avoid supratherapeutic exposure with "normal" appearing tacrolimus levels.

Mycophenolate mofetil has been reported to be teratogenic and is associated with ear and other deformities including hypoplastic nails, short fingers, cleft palate, and Tetralogy of Fallot in humans. This drug should be discontinued at least 6 weeks before conception, and women should be switched to azathioprine if indicated. Sirolimus causes delayed ossification in animal studies, and although successful live-born human outcomes have been reported, it should be used during pregnancy until more data are available. Finally, data from the National Transplantation Pregnancy Registry and the European Dialysis and Transplant Association suggest that in women with stable, near normal kidney function in the absence of risk factors, pregnancy rarely negatively affects the graft, although there may be minor increases in serum creatinine postpartum compared with prepregnancy creatinine. On the other hand, women with significantly reduced kidney allograft function antepartum are at risk for irreversible deterioration after delivery, as observed with CKD in native kidneys. Pregnancy is a state of immunologic tolerance associated with decreased immune activity of lymphocytes, which creates tolerance to the fetus and may benefit the kidney allograft. However, the fetus does provide antigenic stimulus. Pregnancy may pose a risk of rejection due to the risk of sensitization and also due to alterations in previously stable immunosuppressive regimens. Kidney biopsy is the gold standard for diagnosis of rejection. The availability of noninvasive biomarkers (genomic or donor-derived cell-free DNA techniques) might be useful in kidney transplant recipients with advanced pregnancy or high risk for biopsy complications; however, these have not been studied in pregnant kidney transplant recipients. Treatment for rejection is dependent on biopsy findings (antibody-mediated rejection vs. acute cellular rejection), the presence of donor-specific antibodies, and a history of infections. The consensus opinion is that corticosteroids and intravenous immunoglobulins are safe treatments for acute rejection, but the safety of antilymphocyte globulins and rituximab in pregnancy is unknown.

V. Dialysis

Pregnant women on chronic dialysis for end-stage renal disease are at a high risk of maternal and fetal complications including miscarriage, stillbirth, medical pregnancy interruption, arterial hypertension, preeclampsia, anemia, polyhydramnios, intrauterine growth restriction, small-for-gestational-age infants, preterm birth and the need for neonatal intensive care. Fertility is reduced in patients undergoing dialysis due to disruption of the hypothalamic gonadal axis leading to anovulation. Since the first reported case of successful pregnancy in a hemodialysis patient in the 1970s, there has been an increase in the number of pregnancies in recent years, reflecting improvement in prognosis with more intensified hemodialysis regimens (longer duration, use of high flux membranes, nocturnal therapy), and increased clearance, increased use of erythropoietin, change in counseling practices and intensive fetal monitoring. Live birth rates in pregnant women on hemodialysis in the United States have improved, from 37% in the 1980s to 52% in the 1990s, to currently greater than 80% with intensive dialysis and improvements in obstetric and neonatal care. However, the rate of pregnancy complication rate remains high due to kidney failure, advanced maternal age, and other comorbidities such as hypertension and diabetes. A meta-analysis by Piccoli et al. established the association between dialysis schedule and pregnancy outcomes in 574 pregnancies from 2000 to 2014. The hours of dialysis per week were significant for preterm deliveries (<37 gestational weeks: P-value = .044) and for small gestational age (P-value = .017). The authors also reported a lower incidence of small for gestational age on hemodialysis versus peritoneal dialysis (31% vs. 66.7%; P = .015). Another landmark study compared 22 pregnancies prospectively supported by intensive dialysis in Toronto from 2000 to 2013 to a cohort of 70 pregnancies from the American Registry for Pregnancy in Dialysis Patients. The Canadian cohort received significantly more dialysis (43 ± 6 vs. 17 ± 5 h/wk) and had a live birth rate of 82% versus 53% in the US cohort. When stratified by dialysis time, the live birth rate was 48% in women receiving 20 hours of hemodialysis per week or less and 85% in women receiving 36 hours of dialysis per week or more. The duration of pregnancy was longer in the Canadian cohort at 36 weeks compared to 27 weeks in US patients, with trends toward higher birth weights. A predialysis midweek serum blood urea nitrogen level <35 mg/dL can be a threshold for dialysis dose adjustment during pregnancy especially to improve fetal outcomes.

A recent systematic review by Baouche et al. of published studies between 2010 and 2020 on pregnant women on dialysis, including 2,754 pregnancies, reported a live birth rate of 71.4% and the following rates of pregnancy complications—16.9% spontaneous miscarriages, 5.2% therapeutic abortions, 8.3% stillbirths, 7.6% neonatal deaths, and 15.3% perinatal deaths. The fetal birth weight ranged from 590 to 3,500 g and preterm birth was the main, most common complication in all studies, ranging from 50% to 100%, with median gestational age ranging from 25.2 to 36 weeks. Intrauterine growth restriction was present in 5.9% and small-for-gestational-age in 18.9% of babies.

The hemodialysis prescription must include a minimum of 20 hours, with hemodialysis duration increasing to 36 hours/wk for women with no residual kidney function. The dry weight should be regularly reevaluated with an increase of about 0.5 kg/wk in the second and third trimester. Heparinization should be minimized to prevent obstetric bleeding. Dialysate bicarbonate should be decreased to 25 mEq/L, in keeping with the expected lower bicarbonate levels of pregnancy. If peritoneal dialysis is being used, decreasing exchange volumes by increasing exchange frequency or cycler use is recommended. Protein intake should be increased from 1.5 to 1.8 g/kg/d. Antihypertensive therapy should be adjusted for pregnancy by discontinuing angiotensin-converting enzyme (ACE) inhibitors and angiotensin receptor blockers (ARBs) ideally in the preconception

TABLE 16-4 Management of Pregnant Women on Dialysis

Medication Management
Discontinue ACE inhibitors and ARBs
Low-dose aspirin as prophylaxis for prevention of preeclampsia
Dialysis
Intensity hemodialysis duration ≥36 h if no residual function, goal BUN <35 mg/L
Dialysate bath with potassium at 3 mEq/L
Hypertension and Volume
BP <140/90 mmHg and avoid dialytic hypotension
Dry weight adjustment of approximate increase by 0.5 kg/mo during second and third trimester
Nutrition
Daily protein intake of 1.5–1.8 g/kg/d
Anemia
Erythropoietin to hemoglobin target of 10–11 g/dL
Folic acid 5 mg/d
Iron to maintain optimal stores
Obstetric management
Early (8–9 wk) ultrasound assessment of gestational age, and then monthly till delivery per discretion of maternal–fetal medicine

period since they carry risks of teratogenicity and fetotoxicity. Calcium inhibitors such as nifedipine and other antihypertensive drugs such as labetalol and methyldopa can be prescribed to reach arterial pressure targets <140/90 mmHg. Anemia should be treated with supplemental iron, folic acid, and erythropoietin. Erythropoietin is safe in pregnancy, and pregnancy-related erythropoietin resistance may require a dose increase of approximately 50% to maintain hemoglobin target levels of 10 to 11 g/dL. Owing to placental 25-hydroxyvitamin D3 conversion decreased supplemental vitamin D may be required and should be guided by levels of vitamin D, parathyroid hormone, calcium, and phosphorus. Magnesium supplementation may be needed to maintain serum magnesium level at 5 to 7 mg/dL (2 to 3 mmol/L). Low-dose aspirin should be started as prophylaxis by the end of the first trimester to prevent preeclampsia. Obstetrical monitoring should include an initial ultrasound assessment at 8 to 9 weeks of gestation and normal first-trimester ultrasonography at 11 to 14 weeks, followed by 20 weeks and then monthly, First trimester screening for aneuploidy should be standard, but pregnancy-associated plasma protein A is increased in hemodialysis patients and can be less sensitive to detect genetic trouble (Table 16-4).

VI. Hypertensive Disorders of Pregnancy

Hypertension during gestation remains a major cause of morbidity and death in both mother and child.

A. As per the American College of Obstetrics and Gynecology (ACOG) guidelines 2022, hypertensive disorders of pregnancy can be classified into four groups depending on the onset of hypertension and the presence of target organ involvement: preeclampsia, chronic hypertension, gestational hypertension, and superimposed preeclampsia on chronic hypertension.

1. **Preeclampsia.** Preeclampsia, which affects between 2% and 7% of pregnant women, is defined by systolic BP of 140 mmHg or more or diastolic BP of 90 mmHg or more on two occasions at least 4 hours apart or systolic BP of 160 mmHg or more or diastolic BP of 110 mmHg or more confirmed within a short interval after 20 weeks of gestation in a woman with previously normal BP, and proteinuria of 300 mg or more per 24-hour urine collection, protein/creatinine ratio of 0.3 mg/dL or more, or dipstick reading of 2+.
2. **Chronic Hypertension.** Chronic hypertension is defined by hypertension (systolic BP ≥140 mmHg and/or diastolic BP ≥90 mmHg) diagnosed or present before pregnancy or at least two occasions before 20 weeks of gestation. If hypertension is diagnosed de-novo during pregnancy and persists for more than 12 weeks postdelivery, it is also considered chronic hypertension.
3. **Chronic Hypertension With Superimposed Preeclampsia.** Women with a history of chronic hypertension is at increased risk for developing superimposed preeclampsia, associated with adverse maternal and fetal outcomes.
4. **Gestational hypertension** is defined by the new onset of systolic BP ≥140 mmHg and/or diastolic BP ≥90 mmHg on at least two occasions 4 hours apart detected for the first time after 20 weeks of gestation and the absence of proteinuria.

   The physician should be aware that on rare occasions convulsions and hypertension may develop after delivery. The so-called late postpartum eclampsia (hypertension and convulsions 48 hours to weeks after delivery) is poorly understood and is treated by hospitalization, magnesium sulfate, and supportive care. Recent studies suggest that hypertension during pregnancy is associated with an increased risk of cardiovascular disease, kidney disease, and diabetes. This is true for all types of hypertensive disorders of pregnancy.

B. **Pathophysiology of Preeclampsia.** Preeclampsia is a syndrome, the manifestations of which affect many organ systems, including the brain, liver, kidney, blood vessels, and placenta (Fig. 16-2). The placenta may be critically involved in the genesis of preeclampsia, and failure of cytotrophoblast invasion of the uterine spiral arteries is one of the earliest changes in this disorder. Therefore, these vessels do not undergo the expected transformation into the dilated blood vessels characteristic of normal placentation. The reason for the failure of the trophoblast to invade the uterine spiral arteries is obscure. Research has focused on the abnormal modulation of cytotrophoblast adhesion molecules, integrins, and abnormal vascular endothelial growth factor (VEGF) receptor–ligand interactions. The abnormal placentation leading to the maternal syndrome of preeclampsia is believed to occur early in pregnancy (10 to 20 weeks of gestation). Finally, a growing body of evidence has implicated the production of antiangiogenic factors such as sFlt-1 and endoglin in the genesis of preeclampsia. Women with preeclampsia have been found to have increased circulating levels of a soluble, splice variant of a receptor for VEGF called *sFlt-1*. sFlt-1 is believed to be released from the placenta into the maternal blood, and by binding to VEGF causes decreased bioavailability of VEGF, maternal vascular endothelial cell dysfunction, and the characteristic clinical features such as hypertension and proteinuria. Experimental administration of sFlt-1 and endoglin to pregnant rats recapitulates the classic renal histologic findings of glomerular endotheliosis. The mediators of hypertension in preeclampsia are not clearly understood. Evidence suggests that vasoconstriction results from a complex interplay of hormonal and vascular alterations. The renin–angiotensin system is stimulated in normal pregnancy and relatively suppressed in women with preeclampsia. However, patients with preeclampsia are more sensitive to the pressor effects of angiotensin II, and therefore this

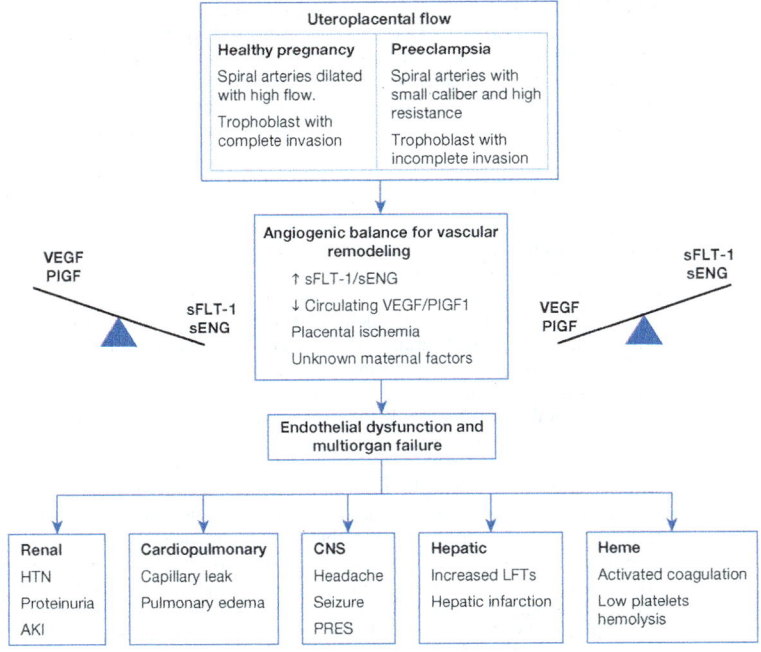

Figure 16-2. Pathophysiology of preeclampsia.

pressor peptide may play a role in their elevated BP. Aldosterone levels are also lower in preeclamptic women than in women with normal pregnancies, although still higher than nonpregnant levels.

Alterations in vascular endothelial cell function are important features of the pathophysiology of preeclampsia. Endothelial cells produce a variety of substances important in modulating vascular tone and coagulation (e.g., NO, prostacyclin, and endothelin). Animal studies of gestational hypertension as well as clinical studies in women suggest that decreased NO and prostacyclin, and increased endothelin, in addition to antiangiogenic factors mentioned earlier, are both sequelae and contributory factors leading to vasoconstriction, platelet aggregation, and increased intravascular coagulation and, finally, the maternal clinical manifestations of preeclampsia.

In one variant of preeclampsia, HELLP syndrome, coagulation abnormalities, and liver dysfunction predominate, and few patients can present without hypertension and proteinuria. This syndrome is life-threatening, and early recognition is critical. The pathogenesis of the eclamptic convulsion is poorly understood. Vasospasm, ischemia, and local hemorrhage may all play a role. The importance of hypertension per se in the genesis of seizures is debated because convulsions may be observed in women whose BP is only mildly elevated.

C. Kidney Function and Morphology in Preeclampsia
1. **GFR and RPF.** Both GFR and RPF decrease in preeclampsia. The decrements approximate 25% in most instances so that the GFR of preeclamptic women often remains above pregravid values. However, in rare instances, large decreases in function may occur and, on occasion, lead to acute tubular or cortical necrosis.

2. **Uric Acid.** Changes occur in the renal handling of urate in preeclampsia. A decrease in the clearance of uric acid, accompanied by increments in blood levels of this solute, may occur weeks before any clinical signs of the disease appear. In pregnancy, serum urate levels above 4.5 mg/dL are suspect (to convert to SI units [μmol/L], multiply mg/dL by 59.48). The level of hyperuricemia also correlates with the severity of the preeclamptic renal lesion, as well as with fetal outcome.
3. Increased **proteinuria**, which may be mild, moderate, or heavy, is a feature of preeclampsia, and protein excretion in the nephrotic range is associated with greater fetal loss.
4. **Calcium.** Studies have demonstrated that calcium handling by kidneys is altered in preeclampsia and that in contrast to normotensive gravidas, or those with chronic or transient hypertension, patients with preeclampsia demonstrate marked hypocalciuria. The basis for this abnormality is unknown. Levels of 1,25 vitamin D are lower, and parathyroid hormone is higher when compared with normal pregnancy.
5. Preeclampsia is accompanied by a characteristic histologic lesion: **glomerular capillary endotheliosis** (Fig. 16-3). In women diagnosed clinically as preeclamptic, this lesion is present in only approximately 85% of biopsies obtained from primiparas and considerably fewer biopsies from multiparas. The remaining patients have evidence of nephrosclerosis or another parenchymal disease. Glomerular endotheliosis is characterized by swollen glomerular capillary endothelial cells with the appearance of a "bloodless glomerulus." Some claim that preeclampsia is a cause of focal glomerular sclerosis, but others believe preeclampsia lesions to be completely reversible, with the presence of focal glomerular sclerosis reflecting preexisting nephrosclerosis or primary kidney disease. Women with glomerular endotheliosis alone tend to have uneventful subsequent gestations, but when focal glomerular sclerosis or alterations in the renal vessels are present, hypertension is more likely to recur in later pregnancies.

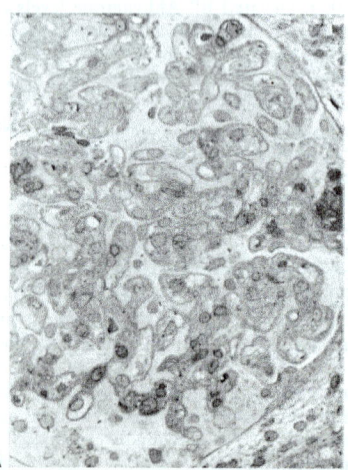 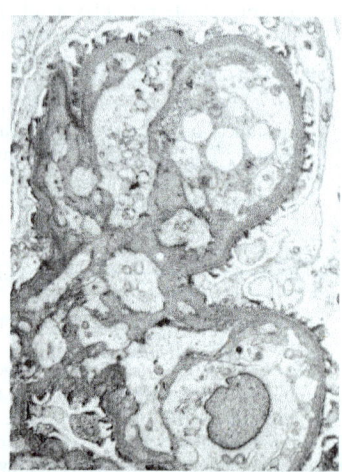

Figure 16-3. A: Electron micrograph demonstrating complete capillary obliteration by a swollen endothelial cell. Note, however, that the basement membrane is normal and the epithelial foot processes are intact. **B:** Micrograph showing glomerulus from a preeclamptic kidney. Swollen endothelial and mesangial cells that display prominent vacuolization encroach on the capillary lumina. (Courtesy of B. H. Spargo, M.D.)

D. Management of Preeclampsia
1. Delivery of the placenta is the only definitive treatment for preeclampsia, which prevents the disease's progression and its associated complications. The delivery timing should be individualized and depends on the gestational age, BP, and maternal and fetal complications.
2. **Treatment of the Eclamptic Convulsion.** Several large clinical trials have demonstrated that magnesium sulfate is superior to other anticonvulsants for preventing recurrent eclamptic convulsions and for primary prevention of eclampsia in women with preeclampsia. The usual protocol is to administer a loading dose of 4 g magnesium sulfate, infused over 15 minutes, followed by a sustaining infusion of 1 to 2 g/h to achieve plasma levels of 2 to 4 μmol/L. Because the incidence of convulsion is highest in the immediate puerperium, it is common practice to begin magnesium sulfate immediately after delivery and continue it for 24 hours.

E. Prevention of Preeclampsia. Many strategies have been investigated in well-conducted clinical trials (including thousands of women) of antiplatelet therapy, nutritional supplementation, and antioxidant vitamins for the prevention of preeclampsia. These trials and subsequent meta-analyses demonstrate a benefit (10% to 15% reduction in relative risk) for low-dose aspirin for the prevention of preeclampsia and meaningful adverse maternal and fetal outcomes. With respect to nutritional strategies, calcium supplementation appears to have a small benefit in women ingesting a baseline low-calcium diet and not much benefit in women ingesting a normal calcium diet. To date, antioxidant supplementation with vitamins C and E has not shown benefit in three large randomized controlled trials.

F. The Hypertensive Patient Without Preeclampsia. Pregnancies in women with chronic hypertension are associated with increased maternal and fetal risks. Complications include superimposed preeclampsia, placental abruption, acute tubular and cortical necrosis, intrauterine growth restriction, and fetal death. Such events seem to correlate with the age of the gravida and the duration of hypertension. Therefore, most of these complications occur in women older than 30 years or with evidence of end-organ damage. Women with chronic hypertension often have reductions in BP by midpregnancy, so their blood pressure may not exceed that observed in normotensive pregnant women. The failure of this decrement to occur, or increases in BP in early- or midtrimester pregnancy, indicates a guarded prognosis for the gestation. Fetal outcome is poorer in hypertensive women with superimposed preeclampsia than in previously normotensive women with this complication, and the combination of chronic hypertension and preeclampsia increases the risk of cerebral hemorrhage.

G. The treatment guidelines for hypertensive disorders in pregnancy have been slow to change over the decades, unlike hypertension guidelines for the general population, despite growing evidence of immediate and long-term cardiovascular risks. The reason for this had been question of benefit from BP normalization treatment in pregnant women, fueled by theoretical concerns for fetal well-being from reduction in utero-placental perfusion and risks of in utero exposure to antihypertensive medication. Current guidelines now address emerging evidence that reducing BP treatment goals in pregnancy may reduce maternal severe hypertension without increasing the risk of pregnancy loss, high-level neonatal care, or overall maternal complications.
1. In the Chronic Hypertension and Pregnancy (CHAP) Study, an open-label, multicenter, randomized trial, 2,408 pregnant women with singleton gestation and mild chronic hypertension were enrolled before 23 weeks of gestation and randomized to receive antihypertensive therapy at a threshold of 140/90 mmHg versus no treatment until severe hypertension (defined by

systolic BP ≥160 or diastolic BP ≥105) developed. The study found a reduced risk of the primary composite outcome (preeclampsia with severe features, medically indicated preterm birth at less than 35 weeks of gestation, placental abruption, or fetal or neonatal death) (30.2% vs. 37.0%; adjusted risk ratio [RR], 0.82; 95% CI 0.74–0.92; P <.001). The incidence of birthweight less than the 10th percentile was similar in the groups (11.2% in the active-treatment group and 10.4% in the control group; adjusted RR, 1.04; 95% CI 0.82–1.31; P = .76), as were serious maternal and neonatal complications (2.1% and 2.8%; RR, 0.75; 95% CI 0.45–1.26), and 2.0% and 2.6% (RR, 0.77; 95% CI 0.45–1.30), respectively. American College of Gynecology recommends utilizing 140/90 mmHg as the threshold for initiation or titration of medical therapy for chronic hypertension in pregnancy rather than the previously recommended threshold of 160/110 mmHg. In addition, the baseline risk of fetal growth restriction in patients with chronic hypertension warrants a third-trimester ultrasound assessment of fetal growth.

2. **Antihypertensive Therapy.** The effectiveness of antihypertensive agents must be balanced with risks to the fetus. Earlier medications during pregnancy were classified under five letter risk categories (A, B, C, D, or X). As per the US Food and Drug Administration (FDA), these categories are no longer used, and specific drug information should be checked at the US FDA website under pregnancy and lactation registries (https://www.fda.gov/consumers/free-publications-women/medicine-and-pregnancy). The drugs of choice for treating hypertension during pregnancy include methyldopa, beta-blockers, and calcium channel blockers. ACE inhibitors, ARBs, and direct renin inhibitors are contraindicated during pregnancy. For the treatment of hypertension, the selection of an antihypertensive regimen and its route of administration depends on the expected time of delivery. Tables 16-5 and 16-6 summarize current knowledge on the use of antihypertensive drugs in pregnancy.

TABLE 16-5	Guidelines for Treating Severe Hypertension Near Term or During Labor

Regulation of blood pressure
Blood pressure threshold for initiating treatment ≥160/110 mmHg for acute hypertension
Drug therapy
Labetalol, administered intravenously, is an effective and safe agent for preeclamptic hypertension; start with 20 mg and repeat the dose every 20 min, up to 300 mg, until desired blood pressure is achieved; side effects include headache
Hydralazine administered intravenously may also be used; start with low doses (5 mg as an intravenous bolus), then administer 5 to 10 mg every 20–30 min to avoid precipitous decreases in pressure; side effects include tachycardia and headache
Calcium channel blockers (*long acting*) have been used, oral drug
Avoid using *sodium nitroprusside*, because fetal cyanide poisoning has been reported in animals
Prevention of convulsions
Parenteral *magnesium sulfate* is the drug of choice for preventing eclamptic convulsions; therapy should be continued for 12–24 hours postpartum, because one-third of women with eclampsia have convulsions during this period

TABLE 16-6. Antihypertensive Drugs Used to Treat Chronic Hypertension in Pregnancy

α_2-Adrenergic receptor agonists
Methyldopa is the most extensively used drug in this group. Its safety and efficacy are supported by evidence from randomized trials and a 7.5-yr follow-up study of children born to mothers treated with methyldopa
β-Adrenergic receptor antagonists
Fetal growth retardation has been reported with atenolol. Fetal bradycardia can occur, and animal studies suggest that the fetus' ability to tolerate hypoxic stress may be compromised
α-Adrenergic receptor and β-adrenergic receptor antagonists
Labetalol appears to be as effective as methyldopa, but no follow-up studies of children born to mothers given labetalol have been carried out, and concern about maternal hepatotoxicity still exists
Calcium channel blockers
Several small studies and reviews suggest that both dihydropyridines (long acting) and verapamil and diltiazem are safe and effective in pregnancy
Direct-acting vasodilators
Hydralazine is frequently used as adjunctive therapy with methyldopa and **α-Adrenergic receptor and** β-adrenergic receptor antagonists. Rarely, neonatal thrombocytopenia has been reported. The experience with *minoxidil* is limited, and this drug is not recommended
Angiotensin-converting enzyme (ACE) inhibitors
Captopril causes fetal death in diverse animal species, and several ACE inhibitors have been associated with oligohydramnios and neonatal renal failure when administered to humans; do not use at any time in pregnancy
Angiotensin II receptor blockers
These drugs have not been used in pregnancy; in view of the deleterious effects of blocking angiotensin II generation with ACE inhibitors, angiotensin II receptor antagonists are also considered to be contraindicated in pregnancy
Diuretics
Diuretics may be used in women with salt-sensitive hypertension and/or renal disease; attempts should be made to use the lowest possible dose and avoid volume depletion

VII. Acknowledgment

Acknowledgment to prior authors–Phyllis August, Diana I. Jalal, and Judy Blaine.

Disclosure

Silvi Shah is supported by the K23 career development award, under award number 1K23HL151816-01A1, National Heart, Lung, and Blood Institute (NHLBI), National Institutes of Health (NIH). The content is solely the responsibility of the authors and does not necessarily represent the official views of the NIH. The funders of the study had no role in study design; collection, analysis, and interpretation of data; writing the report; and the decision to submit the report for publication.

SUGGESTED READINGS

Armenti VT, Radomski JS, Moritz MJ, et al. Report from the National Transplantation Pregnancy Registry (NTPR): outcomes of pregnancy after transplantation. *Clin Transpl.* 2004; 103–114. ·

August P, Mueller FB, Sealey JE, Edersheim TG. Role of renin-angiotensin system in blood pressure regulation in pregnancy. *Lancet.* 1995;345(8954):896–897.

Bajpai D, Popa C, Verma P, Dumanski S, Shah S. Evaluation and management of hypertensive disorders of pregnancy. *Kidney360.* 2023;4(10):1512–1525.

Baouche H, Jais JP, Meriem S, et al. Pregnancy in women on chronic dialysis in the last decade (2010–2020): a systematic review. *Clin Kidney J.* 2022;16(1):138–150.

Cadnapaphornchai MA, Ohara M, Morris KG, et al. Chronic NOS inhibition reverses systemic vasodilation and glomerular hyperfiltration in pregnancy. *Am J Physiol Renal Physiol.* 2001; 280(4):F592–F598.

Chapman AB, Johnson AM, Gabow PA. Pregnancy outcome and its relationship to progression of renal failure in autosomal dominant polycystic kidney disease. *J Am Soc Nephrol.* 1994;5(5): 1178–1185.

Chapman AB, Zamudio S, Woodmansee W, et al. Systemic and renal hemodynamic changes in the luteal phase of the menstrual cycle mimic early pregnancy. *Am J Physiol.* 1997;273(5 Pt 2): F777–F782.

Chen HH, Lin HC, Yeh JC, Chen CP. Renal biopsy in pregnancies complicated by undetermined renal disease. *Acta Obstet Gynecol Scand.* 2001;80(10):888–893.

Clowse ME, Magder L, Witter F, Petri M. Hydroxychloroquine in lupus pregnancy. *Arthritis Rheum.* 2006;54(11):3640–3647.

Conde-Agudelo A, Villar J, Lindheimer M. World Health Organization systematic review of screening tests for preeclampsia. *Obstet Gynecol.* 2004;104(6):1367–1391.

Conrad KP, Debrah DO, Novak J, Danielson LA, Shroff SG. Relaxin modifies systemic arterial resistance and compliance in conscious, nonpregnant rats. *Endocrinology.* 2004;145(7):3289–3296.

Davison JM, Sheills EA, Philips PR, Barron WM, Lindheimer MD. Metabolic clearance of vasopressin and an analogue resistant to vasopressinase in human pregnancy. *Am J Physiol.* 1993; 264(2 Pt 2):F348–F353.

Davison JM, Shiells EA, Philips PR, Lindheimer MD. Serial evaluation of vasopressin release and thirst in human pregnancy. Role of human chorionic gonadotrophin in the osmoregulatory changes of gestation. *J Clin Invest.* 1988;81(3):798–806.

Derksen RH, Bruinse HW, de Groot PG, Kater L. Pregnancy in systemic lupus erythematosus: a prospective study. *Lupus.* 1994;3(3):149–155.

Duley L. Evidence and practice: the magnesium sulphate story. *Best Pract Res Clin Obstet Gynaecol.* 2005;19(1):57–74.

Duley L, Henderson-Smart DJ, Knight M, et al. Antiplatelet agents for preventing preeclampsia and its complications. *Cochrane Database Syst Rev.* 2004;(1):CD004659.

Erkan D. The relation between antiphospholipid syndrome-related pregnancy morbidity and non-gravid vascular thrombosis: a review of the literature and management strategies. *Curr Rheumatol Rep.* 2002;4(5):379–386.

Fakhouri F, Vercel C, Fremeaux-Bacchi V. Obstetric nephrology: AKI and thrombotic microangiopathies in pregnancy. *Clin J Am Soc Nephrol.* 2012;7:2100–2106.

Fesenmeier MF, Coppage KH, Lambers DS, Barton JR, Sibai BM. Acute fatty liver of pregnancy in 3 tertiary care centers. *Am J Obstet Gynecol.* 2005;192(5):1416–1419.

Gammill HS, Jeyabalan A. Acute renal failure in pregnancy. *Crit Care Med.* 2005;33(Suppl 10): S372–S384.

Haase M, Morgera S, Budde K, et al. A systematic approach to managing pregnant dialysis patients—the importance of an intensified haemodiafiltration protocol. *Nephrol Dial Transplant.* 2006;20(11):2537–2542.

Hladunewich MA, Hou S, Odutayo A, et al. Intensive hemodialysis associates with improved pregnancy outcomes: a Canadian and United States cohort comparison. *J Am Soc Nephrol.* 2014;25(5):1103–1109.

Hofmeyr GJ, Atallah AN, Duley L, et al. Calcium supplementation during pregnancy for preventing hypertensive disorders and related problems. *Cochrane Database Syst Rev.* 2006;(3): CD001059.

Holley JL, Reddy SS. Pregnancy in dialysis patients: a review of outcomes, complications, and management. *Semin Dial.* 2003;16(5):384–388.

Kaimal AJ, Gandhi M, Pettker CM, Simhan H. Clinical guidance for the integration of the findings of the Chronic Hypertension and Pregnancy (CHAP) Study. ACOG (2022). Accessed August 1, 2023.

Available at: https://www.acog.org/clinical/clinical-guidance/practice-advisory/articles/2022/04/clinical-guidance-for-the-integration-of-the-findings-of-the-chronic-hypertension-and-pregnancy-chap-study

Khan KS, Wojdyla D, Say L, Gülmezoglu AM, Van Look PF. WHO analysis of causes of maternal death: a systematic review. *Lancet*. 2006;367(9516):1066–1074.

Le Ray C, Coulomb A, Elefant E, Frydman R, Audibert F. Mycophenolate mofetil in pregnancy after renal transplantation: a case of major fetal malformations. *Obstet Gynecol*. 2004;103 (5 Pt 2):1091–1094.

Maynard S, Min JY, Merchan J, et al. Excess placental soluble fms-like tyrosine kinase 1 (sFlt1) may contribute to endothelial dysfunction, hypertension, and proteinuria in preeclampsia. *J Clin Invest*. 2003;111:649–658.

McKay DB, Josephson MA. Pregnancy in recipients of solid organs—effects on mother and child. *N Engl J Med*. 2006;354(12):1281–1293.

McKay DB, Josephson MA, Armenti VT, et al; Women's Health Committee of the American Society of Transplantation. Reproduction and transplantation: report on the AST Consensus Conference on Reproductive Issues and Transplantation. *Am J Transplant*. 2005;5(7):1592–1599.

National High Blood Pressure Education Program Working Group. National High Blood Pressure Education Program Working Group report on high blood pressure in pregnancy. *Am J Obstet Gynecol*. 2000;183:S1–S22.

Piccoli GB, Minelli F, Versino E, et al. Pregnancy in dialysis patients in the new millennium: a systematic review and meta-regression analysis correlating dialysis schedules and pregnancy outcomes. *Nephrol Dial Transplant*. 2016;31(11):1915–1934.

Prakash J, Kumar H, Sinha DK, et al. Acute renal failure in pregnancy in a developing country: twenty years of experience. *Ren Fail*. 2006;28(4):309–313.

Richman K, Gohh R. Pregnancy after transplantation: a review of registry and single-center practices and outcomes. *Nephrol Dial Transplant*. 2012;27:3428–3434.

Rossing K, Jacobsen P, Hommel E, et al. Pregnancy and progression of diabetic nephropathy. *Diabetologia*. 2002;45(1):36–41.

Ruiz-Irastorza G, Lima F, Alves J, et al. Increased rate of lupus flare during pregnancy and the puerperium: a prospective study of 78 pregnancies. *Br J Rheumatol*. 1996;35(2):133–138.

Rumbold AR, Crowther CA, Haslam RR, et al. Vitamins C and E and the risks of preeclampsia and perinatal complications. *N Engl J Med*. 2006;354(17):1796–1806.

Shah S, Gupta A. Hypertensive disorders of pregnancy. *Cardiol Clin*. 2019;37(3):345–354.

Shah S, Meganathan K, Christianson AL, Harrison K, Leonard AC, Thakar CV. Pregnancy-related acute kidney injury in the united states: clinical outcomes and health care utilization. *Am J Nephrol*. 2020;51(3):216–226.

Shah S, Venkatesan RL, Gupta A, et al. Pregnancy outcomes in women with kidney transplant: metaanalysis and systematic review. *BMC Nephrol*. 2019;20(1):24.

Shah S, Verma P. Overview of pregnancy in renal transplant patients. *Int J Nephrol*. 2016;2016:4539342.

Sinkey RG, Battarbee AN, Bello NA, Ives CW, Oparil S, Tita ATN. Prevention, diagnosis, and management of hypertensive disorders of pregnancy: a comparison of international guidelines. *Curr Hypertens Rep*. 2020;22(9):66.

Smith WT, Darbari S, Kwan M, O Reilly-Green C, Devita MV. Pregnancy in peritoneal dialysis: a case report and review of adequacy and outcomes. *Int Urol Nephrol*. 2005;37(1):145–151.

Sturgiss SN, Wilkinson R, Davison JM. Renal reserve during human pregnancy. *Am J Physiol*. 1996;271(1 Pt 2):F16–F20.

Taber-Hight E, Shah S. Acute kidney injury in pregnancy. *Adv Chronic Kidney Dis*. 2020;27(6):455–460.

Tita AT, Szychowski JM, Boggess K, et al; Chronic Hypertension and Pregnancy (CHAP) Trial Consortium. Treatment for mild chronic hypertension during Pregnancy. *N Engl J Med*. 2022;386(19):1781–1792.

Wiles K, Chappell L, Clark K, et al. Clinical practice guideline on pregnancy and renal disease. *BMC Nephrol*. 2019;20(1):401.

Yadav A, Salas MAP, Coscia L, et al. Acute kidney injury during pregnancy in kidney transplant recipients. *Clin Transplant*. 2022;36(5):e14668.

17. The Patient With Hypertension

Ruth Campbell, Seth Furgeson

I. Definition and Classification of Hypertension

The definition of hypertension is somewhat arbitrary because blood pressure (BP) is not distributed bimodally in the population. Instead, the distribution of BP readings in the population is unimodal, and an arbitrary level of BP must be defined as the threshold above which hypertension can be diagnosed. The correlation between the levels of systolic BP (SBP) and diastolic BP (DBP) and cardiovascular risk has long been recognized. It has become clear that in patients older than 50 years, SBP of more than 140 mmHg is a much more important cardiovascular disease risk factor than DBP. Increasing BP clearly has an adverse effect on mortality over the entire range of recorded pressures, even those generally considered to be in the normal range. The goal of identifying and treating high BP is to reduce the risk of cardiovascular disease and associated morbidity and mortality. The 2017 American College of Cardiology/American Heart Association (ACC/AHA) guidelines have established updated criteria for the diagnosis and classification of BP in adult patients (Table 17-1). The optimal BP in an individual who is not acutely ill is lower than 120/80 mmHg. Individuals with an SBP of 120 to 129 mmHg or a DBP of ≤80 mmHg should be considered as having elevated BP; these patients require health-promoting lifestyle modifications to prevent cardiovascular disease. Patients with elevated BP have twice the risk of developing hypertension as those with lower values. These patients with elevated BP should be rechecked annually to exclude the development of hypertension. Hypertension is defined as an SBP of 130 mmHg or greater or a DBP of 80 mmHg or greater, or by virtue of the patient taking antihypertensive medications. The stage of hypertension (stage 1 or 2) is determined by the levels of both SBP and DBP (see Table 17-1). This classification should be based on the average of two or more BP readings at each of two or more visits after the initial BP screening. When SBP and DBP fall into different categories, the higher category should be selected to classify the individual's BP.

II. Epidemiology of Hypertension

Data from the National Health and Nutrition Examination Survey (NHANES) indicate that approximately 28% of the adult population in the United States has hypertension, a number that has remained relatively stable over the last decade. According to the same study, prevalence of hypertension increases sharply with age. The increasing burden of hypertension is not only the result of the increased size of the population, but also reflects the increased prevalence of obesity and the overall aging of the population. Data from the Framingham Heart Study indicate that even individuals who are normotensive at 55 years have a 90% lifetime risk of developing hypertension. Many hypertensive patients have a positive family history of parental hypertension. The mode of inheritance is complex and probably polygenic in most instances. Black men and women have a twofold higher prevalence of hypertension (30%) than White men and women (15%) in a sampling of almost 18,000 American adults aged 48 to 75 years in the NHANES data. Prevalence appears to be equal in men and women in most surveys. Obese individuals have significantly more hypertension than nonobese individuals. In childhood, obesity is a major cause of hypertension. More than one-half of the adult population is overweight (body mass

TABLE 17-1 Classification of Blood Pressure (BP) for Adults[a]

BP Classification[b]	Systolic BP (mmHg)[c]		Diastolic BP (mmHg)[c]
Normal	<120	and	<80
Elevated blood pressure	120–129	and	<80
Stage 1 hypertension	130–139	or	80–89
Stage 2 hypertension	≥140	or	≥90

[a]Adults aged 18 years and older.
[b]Classification should be based on the mean of two or more properly measured seated blood pressure readings obtained on each of two or more office visits.
[c]When systolic and diastolic BP fall into different categories, classify based on the higher category.

index [BMI] of 25 to 29.9) or obese (BMI ≥ 30). Data from NHANES III show that among men and women, Whites, Blacks, and Mexican Americans, the prevalence of hypertension and the mean levels of SBP and DBP increase as BMI increases at ages younger than 60 years. Overall, the prevalence of hypertension in obese adults is 41.4% for men and 37.8% for women; compared with 14.9% for men and 15.2% for women with BMI ≤ 25. Further proof of the significant relationship between body weight and BP is found in the observation that BP falls with even modest weight reduction. The intake of dietary salt (sodium chloride) has significant effects on BP, especially in patients with other factors predisposing to the development of hypertension, such as advancing age, obesity, adult-onset diabetes, positive family history of hypertension, Black race, or underlying renal disease. Numerous epidemiologic studies have shown that the dietary intake of salt correlates with the average BP in a population. Northern Japanese fishermen who ingest 450 mEq of sodium daily have a 40% prevalence of hypertension. In contrast, indigenous Alaskan populations and the Yanomani Indians in Brazil and Venezuela, who have dietary intake of 1 mEq of sodium daily, do not develop hypertension at any age. Intersalt, an international epidemiologic study, examined the relation between dietary sodium intake (based on 24-hour urinary sodium excretion) and BP in more than 10,000 individuals aged 20 to 59 years from 52 countries around the world. The results demonstrate a significant correlation between median SBP and DBP and dietary sodium intake. More recently, the Effect of Salt Substitution on Cardiovascular Events and Deaths (SSaSS) study revealed that in over 20,000 Chinese patients, both the reduction in dietary salt and the addition of potassium reduced SBP, and reduced risk of stroke, major cardiovascular events, and death from any cause compared to regular salt alone. These observations can be explained based on the role of abnormal renal sodium handling in the pathogenesis of hypertension, which is discussed in Section IV. The therapeutic implications of these observations include dietary sodium restriction as part of nonpharmacologic therapy and the recommendation of thiazide diuretics as first-line drug therapy for the treatment of hypertension in most patients. Despite the known cardiovascular risks of untreated hypertension and the widespread availability of effective pharmacologic treatment, the identification and effective control of hypertension remain a significant public health problem in the United States. According to the most recent NHANES data, there have been gradual improvements in hypertension control. Overall, hypertension prevalence decreased from 47% to 41.7% from 2013 to 2014, but recently increased to 45.4% from 2017 to 2018. However, this increase may reflect the changes to the definitions for hypertension. The continued high prevalence of hypertension and hypertension-related complications such as stroke, cardiovascular complications, heart failure, and end-stage renal disease (ESRD) represents a major public health challenge.

III. Cardiovascular Disease Risk

The relationship of BP to cardiovascular risk is continuous and independent of other cardiovascular risk factors. Beginning at 115/75 mmHg and across the entire BP range, each increment of 20/10 mmHg doubles the risk of cardiovascular disease. The overall risk of cardiovascular morbidity and mortality in patients with hypertension is determined not only by the stage of hypertension but also by the presence of other risk factors, such as smoking, hyperlipidemia, and diabetes, and by the existence of target organ damage (Table 17-2). The major target organs affected by hypertension are the heart, peripheral vasculature, central nervous system, kidney, and the eye. Most of the consequences of hypertension are the result of progressive vascular injury. Hypertension accelerates atherosclerotic vascular disease and aggravates the deleterious effects of diabetes, smoking, and hyperlipidemia on the aorta and its major branches. Atherosclerotic disease results in significant morbidity from myocardial infarction (MI), atherothrombotic cerebral infarction, peripheral vascular disease with claudication, and renal disease due to ischemia or cholesterol embolization. Hypertensive renal disease may result from hypertension-induced vasculitis in the setting of malignant hypertension or more insidious renal injury from long-standing essential hypertension with benign hypertensive nephrosclerosis. Hypertension is also an important cofactor in the progression of other renal diseases, especially diabetic nephropathy. Hypertension may also cause cerebrovascular disease in the form of lacunar infarction or intracerebral hemorrhage. Left ventricular hypertrophy (LVH) and congestive heart failure (CHF), often due to isolated diastolic dysfunction, are the result of the heightened peripheral vascular resistance (afterload) imposed by systemic hypertension. In clinical trials, antihypertensive therapy has been associated with significant reductions in the incidence of stroke (35% to 40%), MI (20% to 25%), and heart failure (50%). In the setting of preexisting cardiovascular disease or target organ damage, treatment of nine patients would prevent one death.

IV. Pathogenesis of Hypertension

A large body of experimental data has demonstrated the importance of the kidney in the pathogenesis of hypertension. To date, each of the genetic causes of hypertension that have been elucidated has been shown to relate to an abnormality of renal sodium handling. For example, Liddle syndrome results from enhanced distal tubular sodium reabsorption due to an abnormality in sodium channels in the distal nephron. Cross-transplant experiments in hypertensive and normotensive rat strains validate the importance of the kidney in the pathogenesis of hypertension, because the presence or absence of hypertension depends on the donor source of the kidney.

Guyton hypothesis states that the most important and fundamental mechanism in determining the long-term control of BP is the renal fluid–volume feedback mechanism. In simple terms, through this basic mechanism, the kidneys regulate arterial pressure by altering renal excretion of sodium and water, thereby controlling circulatory volume and cardiac output. Changes in BP, in turn, directly influence the renal excretion of sodium and water, thereby providing a negative feedback mechanism for the control of extracellular fluid (ECF) volume, cardiac output, and BP. For instance, an increase in systemic BP will lead to an increase in sodium excretion, a process known as pressure natriuresis. The hypothesis is that derangements in this renal fluid–volume pressure control mechanism are the fundamental cause of virtually all hypertensive states (Fig. 17-1). In every hypertensive state, an underlying abnormality exists in the intrinsic natriuretic capacity of the kidney, so that the daily salt intake cannot be excreted at a normal BP, and

TABLE 17-2 Cardiovascular Risk Factors and Target Organ Damage

Modifiable Risk Factors	Fixed Risk Factors	Target Organ Damage
Unhealthy diet	Age (older than 55 yrs for men, older than 65 yrs for women)	Retinopathy
Cigarette smoking	Family history of premature cardiovascular disease (men younger than 55 yrs or women younger than 65 yrs)	Left ventricular hypertrophy
Overweight or obesity	Microalbuminuria or estimated GFR <60 mL/min	Congestive heart failure
Physical inactivity	Obstructive sleep apnea	Coronary artery disease
Dyslipidemia		Peripheral arterial disease
Diabetes mellitus		

Adapted from Whelton PK, Carey RM, Aronow WS. 2017 ACC/AHA/AAPA/ABC/ACPM/AGS/APhA/ASH/ASPC/NMA/PCNA Guideline for the prevention, detection, evaluation, and management of high blood pressure in adults: executive summary: a report of the American College of Cardiology/American Heart Association Task Force on Clinical Practice Guidelines. *Hypertension.* 2018;6:1269–1324 and Chobanian AV, Bakris GL, Black HR, et a. The seventh report of the Joint National Committee on prevention, detection, evaluation and treatment of high blood pressure. The JNC 7 Report. *JAMA.* 2003;289:2560–2572.

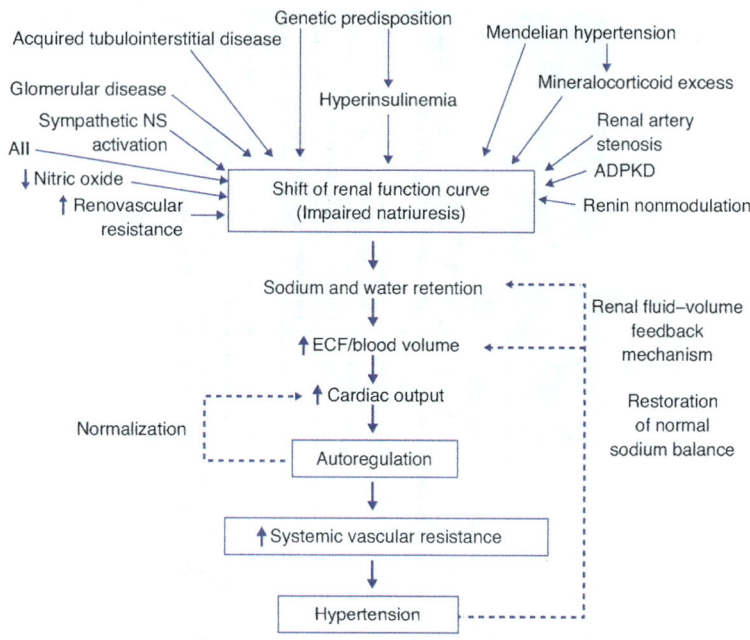

Figure 17-1. Abnormal renal sodium handling in the pathogenesis of hypertension (Guyton hypothesis). In the setting of essential hypertension, primary renal disease, mineralocorticoid excess, or insulin resistance with hyperinsulinemia, a defect in the intrinsic natriuretic capacity of the kidney is present that prevents sodium balance from being maintained at a normal level of BP. Initially, this impairment in natriuresis leads to increases in extracellular fluid (ECF) volume and cardiac output. However, this hemodynamic state is short lived. Circulatory autoregulation occurs to maintain normal perfusion of the tissues, resulting in an increase in the systemic vascular resistance (SVR). The increase in SVR leads to systemic hypertension. With pressure-induced natriuresis, the renal fluid–volume feedback mechanism returns sodium balance, ECF volume, and cardiac output to normal. Systemic hypertension can be conceptualized as an essentially protective mechanism that prevents life-threatening fluid overload in the setting of reduced renal natriuretic capacity. Normal salt balance and fluid volume are maintained but at the expense of systemic hypertension. (ADPKD, autosomal dominant polycystic kidney disease; NS, nervous system; AII, angiotensin II.) (From Jalal DI, Nolan CR, Schrier RW. The kidney in hypertension. In: Schrier RW, ed. *Renal and Electrolyte Disorders*. 8th ed. Wolters Kluwer; 2018:275–324.)

the development of hypertension is necessary to induce a pressure natriuresis that allows the kidney to excrete the daily salt intake. Normal sodium balance and ECF volume are maintained but at the expense of systemic hypertension. The underlying cause for the abnormality in the natriuretic capacity depends on the etiology of hypertension. In essential hypertension, some underlying abnormality increases renal avidity for sodium. In patients with obesity and insulin resistance (metabolic syndrome), hyperinsulinemia increases proximal tubular sodium reabsorption. Increased angiotensin II levels and sympathetic nervous system activity also enhance sodium reabsorption. Mineralocorticoids enhance distal tubular sodium reabsorption. Renal parenchymal disease causes nephron loss, resulting in a natriuretic defect. Abnormalities in renal endothelin or nitric oxide levels may also impair natriuresis. Guyton hypothesis states that this decreased natriuretic capacity of the kidney initially leads to renal salt and water retention, ECF volume expansion, and increased cardiac output with hypertension. This phase of volume expansion and high cardiac output is short lived. In the setting of high cardiac output, autoregulatory vasoconstriction of each vascular bed matches the blood flow to the metabolic requirements of the tissues. This phenomenon of circulatory autoregulation leads to an increase in systemic vascular resistance (SVR). Therefore, hypertension that was initially caused by high cardiac output becomes high-SVR hypertension.

The development of hypertension represents a protective mechanism, because it induces the kidney to undergo a pressure natriuresis and diuresis, thereby restoring normal salt balance and returning ECF volume to normal. This mechanism explains why an underlying problem with sodium excretion, as in salt-sensitive hypertension, is manifest as high-SVR hypertension without evidence of overt fluid overload. In the absence of pressure natriuresis, patients with a primary disorder in sodium retention would progressively develop overt fluid overload and consequences such as pulmonary edema. This explains why thiazide diuretics are an important first-line BP medication. Thiazides block sodium reabsorption by inhibiting the NaCl cotransporter in the distal tubule. The sustained antihypertensive effect of thiazides, however, is mediated through a reduction in SVR, rather than through chronic volume depletion and a reduction of cardiac output. In fact, thiazides do not cause a large, sustained decrease in intravascular volume or negative sodium balance when used for the treatment of hypertension. Within a few days to weeks of the initiation of therapy with thiazide diuretics, salt balance returns toward normal, and total body sodium and intravascular volume return toward pretreatment levels. This seeming paradox can be understood in the context of Guyton hypothesis regarding the pathogenesis of hypertension, whereby the development of systemic hypertension through an increase in SVR is conceptualized as an essential protective mechanism to maintain normal fluid volume in various disease states in which daily sodium load cannot be excreted at a normal BP.

Support for this hypothesis is found in animal models of mineralocorticoid-induced hypertension. To substantiate the role of direct pressure-induced natriuresis in the regulation of sodium balance in mineralocorticoid hypertension, Hall et al. compared the systemic BP and natriuretic effect of aldosterone infusion in a dog model in which the renal perfusion pressure was either allowed to increase or mechanically servocontrolled to maintain renal artery pressure at normal levels. In the intact animal, continuous aldosterone infusion caused a transient period of sodium and water retention with a mild increase in BP. This sodium retention lasted only a few days, however, and was followed by an escape from the sodium-retaining effects of aldosterone and a restoration of normal sodium balance. In contrast, when the renal perfusion pressure was servocontrolled to maintain normal renal perfusion pressure during aldosterone infusion, no aldosterone escape occurred, and a relentless increase in sodium and water retention occurred, accompanied by severe hypertension, edema, ascites, and pulmonary edema. When the servocontrol device was removed and the renal perfusion pressure was allowed to rise to the systemic level, a prompt natriuresis and diuresis ensued, with the restoration of sodium balance and a fall in BP. These observations highlight the pivotal role of BP in the regulation of renal sodium and water excretion. Moreover, the observation that abnormal renal sodium handling is central in the pathogenesis of all forms of hypertension provides a sound pathophysiologic rationale for the Eight Joint National Committee (JNC 8) recommendation regarding thiazide-type diuretics as one of the first-line antihypertensive agents in most patients.

V. Diagnostic Evaluation of Hypertension

Detection of hypertension begins with proper measurement of BP at each health care encounter. Repeated BP measurements are used to determine whether initial

TABLE 17-3 Measuring Blood Pressure at Home

1. **Setting up to measure**
   - Avoid using any stimulants (caffeine, tobacco, food, or exercise)
   - Empty bladder
   - Rest calmly without talking for ~5 min
   - Remove clothing covering the site of cuff placement
2. **Measuring**
   - Sit with feet uncrossed and flat on the floor
   - Rest arm on table at heart's height
   - Place cuff on bare arm
   - Avoid talking during blood pressure monitoring
3. **Follow-up**
   - Repeat measurement twice, with 5 min of calm rest in between each measurement

Adapted from Whelton PK, Carey RM, Aronow WS. 2017 ACC/AHA/AAPA/ABC/ACPM/AGS/APhA/ASH/ASPC/NMA/PCNA Guideline for the prevention, detection, evaluation, and management of high blood pressure in adults: executive summary: a report of the American College of Cardiology/American Heart Association Task Force on Clinical Practice Guidelines. *Hypertension.* 2018;6:1269–1324 and TargetBP.org (AMA and AHA).

elevations persist and require prompt attention or have returned to normal values and require only periodic surveillance. BP measurement should be standardized as follows: After at least 5 minutes of rest, the patient should be seated in a chair with the back supported, feet flat on the floor, and one arm bared and supported at heart level (Table 17-3). The patient should refrain from smoking or ingesting caffeine for 30 minutes before the examination. For an appropriately sized cuff, the bladder should encircle at least 80% of the arm. Many patients require a large adult cuff. Measurements should ideally be taken with either a validated oscillometric device or a manual, calibrated auscultatory sphygmomanometer. When using an auscultatory device, the first appearance of sound (phase 1) is used to define SBP. The disappearance of sound (phase 5) is used to define DBP. The BP should be confirmed in the contralateral arm and repeat measurements should be taken 1 to 2 minutes apart. Measurement of BP outside of the physician's office may provide some valuable information regarding the diagnosis and treatment of hypertension. Self-measurement is useful in distinguishing sustained hypertension from "white coat hypertension," a condition in which the patient's pressure is consistently elevated in the clinician's office but normal at other times. Self-measurement may also be used to assess the response to antihypertensive medications and as a tool to improve patient adherence to treatment. Ambulatory monitoring is useful for the evaluation of suspected white coat hypertension, apparent drug resistance, hypotensive symptoms with antihypertensive medications, and episodic hypertension. However, ambulatory BP measurement is not indicated for the routine evaluation of patients with suspected hypertension. In elderly patients, the possibility of **pseudohypertension** should always be considered in the diagnostic evaluation of possible hypertension. Pseudohypertension is a condition in which the indirect measurement of arterial pressure using a cuff sphygmomanometer is artificially high in comparison to direct intra-arterial pressure measurement. Failure to recognize pseudohypertension can result in unwarranted and sometimes frankly dangerous treatment. Pseudohypertension can result from Monckeberg medial calcification or advanced atherosclerosis with widespread calcification of intimal plaques. In these entities, stiffening of the arterial wall may prevent its collapse by externally applied pressure, resulting in artificially high indirect BP

TABLE 17-4	Common Etiologies of Secondary Hypertension
Obstructive sleep apnea	
Drug-induced hypertension (Table 17-7)	
Chronic kidney disease	
Primary hyperaldosteronism	
Renal artery stenosis	
Chronic steroid use or Cushing syndrome	

Adapted from Whelton PK, Carey RM, Aronow WS. 2017 ACC/AHA/AAPA/ABC/ACPM/AGS/APhA/ASH/ASPC/NMA/PCNA Guideline for the prevention, detection, evaluation, and management of high blood pressure in adults: executive summary: a report of the American College of Cardiology/American Heart Association Task Force on Clinical Practice Guidelines. *Hypertension*. 2018;6:1269–1324 and Chobanian AV, Bakris GL, Black HR, et al. The seventh report of the Joint National Committee on prevention, detection, evaluation and treatment of high blood pressure. The JNC 7 Report. *JAMA*. 2003;289:2560–2572.

readings affecting both systolic and diastolic measurements. The presence of a positive Osler maneuver, in which the radial or brachial artery remains palpable despite being made pulseless by proximal inflation of a cuff above systolic pressure, is an important physical examination finding that should suggest the diagnosis. Roentgenograms of the extremities frequently reveal calcified vessels. The diagnosis can only be made definitively by a direct measurement of intra-arterial pressure. Patients with pseudohypertension are often elderly and therefore may have a critical limitation of blood flow to the brain or heart, such that inappropriate BP treatment may precipitate life-threatening ischemic events.

The initial history and physical examination of patients with documented hypertension should be designed to assess lifestyle, identify other cardiovascular risk factors, and identify the presence of target organ damage that may affect prognosis and impact treatment decisions (see Table 17-2). Although the majority of hypertensive patients have essential (primary) hypertension without a clearly definable etiology, the initial evaluation is also designed to screen for identifiable causes of secondary hypertension (Table 17-4). A medical history should include information about prior BP measurements, to assess the duration of hypertension, and details about adverse effects from any prior antihypertensive therapy. History or symptoms of coronary heart disease, CHF, cerebrovascular disease, peripheral vascular disease, or renal disease should be carefully evaluated. Symptoms suggesting unusual secondary causes of hypertension should be queried, such as weakness (hyperaldosteronism) or episodic anxiety, headache, diaphoresis, and palpitations (pheochromocytoma). Information regarding other risk factors, such as diabetes, tobacco use, hyperlipidemia, physical activity, and any recent weight gain, should be obtained. Dietary assessment regarding the intake of salt, alcohol, and saturated fat is also important. Detailed information should be sought regarding all prescription and over-the-counter medication use, including herbal remedies and illicit drugs, some of which may raise BP or interfere with the effectiveness of antihypertensive therapy. For example, nonsteroidal anti-inflammatory drugs impair the response to virtually all antihypertensive agents and increase the risk of hyperkalemia or renal insufficiency with angiotensin-converting enzyme (ACE) inhibitor therapy. Stimulants such as cocaine, ephedra, amphetamines, and anabolic steroids can raise BP. A family history of hypertension, diabetes, premature cardiovascular disease, or renal disease should be sought. A psychosocial history is important to identify family situation, working conditions, employment status, educational level, and sexual dysfunction that may influence adherence to antihypertensive treatment.

Physical examination should include the measurement of height and weight and calculation of BMI (weight in kilogram divided by the square of height in meters). Funduscopic examination is important to identify striate hemorrhages, cotton wool spots, and papilledema, the characteristic findings of hypertensive neuroretinopathy (HNR), which are indicative of the presence of malignant hypertension. Documentation of the presence of arteriosclerotic retinopathy (e.g., arteriolar narrowing, arteriovenous crossing changes, changes in light reflexes) is less important, given its lack of prognostic significance with regard to the potential long-term cardiovascular complications of hypertension. Examination of the neck for carotid bruits, distended neck veins, and thyromegaly is important. Cardiac examination should include investigation for abnormalities of rate or rhythm, murmurs, and third or fourth heart sounds. The lungs should be examined for rales and evidence of bronchospasm. Abdominal examination should include auscultation for bruits (an epigastric bruit present in both systole and diastole suggests renal artery stenosis), abdominal or flank masses (polycystic kidney disease), or increased aortic pulsation (abdominal aortic aneurysm). Peripheral pulses should be examined for quality and bruits. The lower extremities should be examined for edema. A neurologic screening examination is used to identify prior cerebrovascular events. Routine laboratory tests are recommended before the initiation of antihypertensive therapy to identify other risk factors and screen for the presence of target organ damage. These routine tests include blood chemistry (sodium, potassium, creatinine, fasting glucose), lipid profile (total cholesterol, low-density lipoprotein, and high-density lipoprotein [HDL] cholesterol), and a complete blood cell count. Creatinine clearance should be estimated using the chronic kidney disease epidemiology (CKD-Epi) formula. A urinalysis is used to identify proteinuria or hematuria that would suggest the presence of underlying primary renal disease. A 12-lead electrocardiogram is used to identify left atrial enlargement, LVH, or prior MI. Optional tests, depending on the clinical situation, include 24-hour creatinine clearance, 24-hour urine protein or a spot urine protein to creatinine ratio, serum uric acid, glycosylated hemoglobin, and thyroid function tests. An echocardiogram to identify the presence of LVH may be useful in selected patients to determine the clinical significance of labile hypertension. Most patients with hypertension have primary (essential) hypertension in which no clearly definable underlying etiology is apparent.

In contrast, a wide variety of uncommon conditions can lead to so-called **secondary hypertension**, some of which are potentially amenable to surgical correction (see Table 17-4). Secondary causes of hypertension include underlying chronic kidney disease (CKD), primary hyperaldosteronism (PHA), pheochromocytoma, renovascular hypertension due to fibromuscular dysplasia or atherosclerotic renal artery stenosis, coarctation of the aorta, and Cushing syndrome. Secondary causes of hypertension amenable to surgical intervention are so uncommon that extensive diagnostic testing is not warranted. Secondary hypertension should be considered when the patient has onset of hypertension at an early age (younger than 30 years) or late age (older than 55 years); inadequate BP control in a compliant patient on a three-drug regimen which includes a diuretic (resistant hypertension); previously well-controlled hypertension becomes uncontrolled in a compliant patient; hematuria or proteinuria (underlying renal disease) or elevated serum creatinine (renal disease or ischemic nephropathy due to bilateral renal artery stenosis). The initial history, physical examination, and routine laboratory tests are usually all that is required to evaluate for the possibility of secondary hypertension. Normal estimated creatinine clearance and urinalysis are usually sufficient to exclude underlying renal disease as a secondary cause of hypertension.

Detection of abdominal or flank masses may indicate polycystic kidney disease, a diagnosis that can be confirmed with ultrasound. Although routine screening of all patients with hypertension for PHA is not warranted, in a patient with drug-resistant hypertension or significant hypokalemia induced by low-dose diuretic therapy, the possibility of PHA should be considered. In this regard, patients with resistant hypertension due to PHA often have a dramatic BP response following the initiation of a mineralocorticoid antagonist (spironolactone or eplerenone). Assessment for any delay or diminution of pulses in the lower extremities, or a discrepancy between arm and leg BP can be used to screen for coarctation of the aorta. A careful assessment of a history of episodic hypertension, associated with headache, palpitations, diaphoresis, and pallor, is all that is usually required to screen for pheochromocytoma. The routine measurement of serum or urine catecholamines is not warranted. Likewise, evaluation for truncal obesity and abdominal purple striae is all that is usually required to screen for Cushing syndrome; therefore, routine measurement of serum cortisol or cortisol suppression testing is unnecessary. Renal artery stenosis should be considered both in patients with known peripheral arterial disease and patients <35 years old with sudden increase in BP, a potential manifestation of fibromuscular dysplasia.

Obstructive sleep apnea (OSA) is an important treatable cause of hypertension. Clues to the presence of OSA include morbid obesity, daytime hypersomnolence, headache, snoring, or fitful sleep. The diagnosis can be confirmed with a sleep study to document apneic episodes. Appropriate treatment with a continuous positive airway pressure device may result in a significant reduction in BP.

VI. Treatment of Hypertension

A. Goals of Treatment. The goal of treating hypertension is the reduction of cardiovascular and renal morbidity and mortality. Because SBP correlates best with target organ damage and mortality, the primary focus should be on achieving the SBP goal. In general, the ACC/AHA guidelines recommend a goal of treatment is an SBP less than 130 mmHg and a DBP less than 80 mmHg.

B. Nonpharmacologic Treatment. Lifestyle modification is recommended in the management of all individuals with hypertension, even in those who require antihypertensive drug treatment. All patients should be encouraged to adopt the lifestyle modifications outlined in Table 17-5, especially if they have additional cardiovascular risk factors such as hyperlipidemia or diabetes. Modest weight reduction of as little as 4 kg (10 lb) significantly reduces BP. In addition to the positive effects on overall health, regular aerobic exercise is associated with a significant reduction in BP.

Changes in diet can have significant effects on BP. Dietary sodium intake in the form of sodium chloride (NaCl; table salt) has a strong epidemiologic link to hypertension. Meta-analysis of clinical trials indicates that the limitation of dietary sodium intake to 75 to 100 mEq/d lowers BP over a period of several weeks to a few years. The restriction of sodium intake has been shown to reduce the need for antihypertensive medication, reduce diuretic-induced renal potassium wasting, lead to regression of LVH, and prevent renal stones through a reduction in renal calcium excretion. The average American dietary sodium intake is in excess of 150 mEq/d, most of which (75%) is derived from processed foods. Moderation of sodium intake to a level of less than 100 mEq/d (2.4 g of sodium or 6 g of sodium chloride) is recommended for the nonpharmacologic treatment of hypertension.

The Dietary Approaches to Stop Hypertension (DASH) study group compared a diet rich in fruits and vegetables to a control diet in patients with mild diastolic hypertension (DBP >95 mmHg). The DASH diet lowered both SBP and DBP significantly in this population. A follow-up study, the DASH-sodium study, randomized patients with stage 1 hypertension to the DASH diet or a control diet. Within each group, patients were randomized to three levels of sodium intake. Sodium reduction decreased BP and the DASH diet decreased

TABLE 17-5 Nonpharmacologic Approaches to Manage Hypertension

Recommendation	Approximate SBP Reduction
Weight loss	5–20 mmHg/10 kg loss
1,000 mg/d reduction in dietary sodium	2–8 mmHg
Follow DASH diet. Eat fruits, vegetables, and whole grains. Choose foods low in saturated fat such as low-fat dairy products, fish, poultry, and beans. Limit sugary drinks and foods.	8–14 mmHg
Increase dietary potassium to 3,500–5,000 mg/d dietary potassium	4–5 mmHg
Regular aerobic physical activity (90–150 min/wk) or resistance training	4–9 mmHg
Limit alcohol intake to no more than two drinks per day in men (>60–70 kg), and no more than one drink per day in women and lighter-weight men (<60 kg) (a drink is defined as 1-oz or 30-mL ethanol per day)	2–4 mmHg

DASH, Dietary Approaches to Stop Hypertension; SBP, systolic blood pressure.

Adapted from Whelton PK, Carey RM, Aronow WS. 2017 ACC/AHA/AAPA/ABC/ACPM/AGS/APhA/ASH/ASPC/NMA/PCNA Guideline for the prevention, detection, evaluation, and management of high blood pressure in adults: executive summary: a report of the American College of Cardiology/American Heart Association Task Force on Clinical Practice Guidelines. *Hypertension.* 2018;6:1269–1324.

Chobanian AV, Bakris GL, Black HR, et al. The seventh report of the Joint National Committee on prevention, detection, evaluation and treatment of high blood pressure. The JNC 7 Report. *JAMA.* 2003;289:2560–2572. National Heart, Lung, and Blood Institute. *DASH Eating Plan.* Updated December 29, 2021. Accessed August 2, 2024. https://www.nhlbi.nih.gov/education/dash-eating-plan

BP at all levels of sodium intake. Patients in the low-sodium DASH group had an SBP that was 8 mmHg lower than patients in the high-sodium control group, a change similar to that seen with antihypertensive agents.

Excessive intake of ethanol is an important risk factor for high BP, and it can lead to resistant hypertension. Ethanol intake should be limited to not more than 30 mL (1 oz) per day in men and 15 mL (0.5 oz) per day in women and lighter-weight men. Smoking cessation and reductions in dietary fat and cholesterol are also recommended to reduce the overall cardiovascular risk. Although caffeine may acutely raise BP, tolerance to this effect develops quickly. Most epidemiologic studies have found no direct relationship between caffeine intake and BP.

C. **Pharmacologic Treatment of Hypertension.** The decision to treat hypertension with medications after the failure of lifestyle modifications to adequately control BP, or initially as an adjunct to lifestyle modifications, is based on the severity (stage) of hypertension and an assessment of the risk of cardiovascular morbidity, given the presence of other cardiovascular risk factors and preexisting target organ damage or cardiovascular disease (see Table 17-2). Reducing BP with drugs clearly decreases cardiovascular morbidity and mortality regardless of age, gender, race, stage of hypertenson, or socioeconomic status. Benefits have been demonstrated for stroke, coronary events, heart failure, progression of primary renal disease, prevention of progression to malignant hypertension, and all-cause mortality. Numerous clinical trials have demonstrated that lowering BP with several classes of drugs, including thiazide-type diuretics, ACE inhibitors, angiotensin receptor blockers (ARBs), β-blockers, and calcium channel blockers (CCBs), reduces all the complications of hypertension.

If therapy with one agent is begun, the recommendation of the JNC 8 is that in the general population in non-Black patients with essential hypertension, with or without diabetes, should be treated with an ACE inhibitor or ARB (but not both), CCB or thiazide-type diuretic (Fig. 17-2). In the general Black population, with or without diabetes, initial management should include either a thiazide-type diuretic or a CCB. These recommendations are based on several long-term studies, the largest of which is the pivotal Antihypertensive and Lipid-Lowering Treatment to Prevent Heart Attack Trial (ALLHAT). ALLHAT studied 41,000 patients over 55 years old with stage 1 or 2 hypertension and with at least one other cardiovascular risk factor. The patients received first-line treatment with chlorthalidone (thiazide-type diuretic), doxazosin (selective α-blocker), amlodipine (CCB), or lisinopril (ACE inhibitor). In this study, 47% of patients were women, 35% were Black, 19% were Hispanic, 36% were diabetic, and the mean BMI was approximately 30. The doxazosin arm was terminated prematurely because of excess risk of CHF. After a mean follow-up of 4.9 years, neither the primary clinical outcome (fatal coronary heart disease or nonfatal MI) nor the secondary outcomes of all-cause mortality, combined coronary heart disease, peripheral arterial disease, cancer, or ESRD had occurred more often in the chlorthalidone group than in the amlodipine or lisinopril groups.

It should be noted that in ALLHAT and most clinical trials, achievement of the desired BP goal often requires treatment with two or more antihypertensive agents. According to the JNC 8, addition of a second drug from the same class should be implemented when use of a single drug in optimal doses fails to adequately control BP.

D. **Treatment of Hypertension in Patients with Diabetes.** Several large clinical trials have demonstrated that control of hypertension in patients with diabetes reduces diabetic complications and improves outcomes (Table 17-6). The United Kingdom Prospective Diabetes Study Group (UKPDS) compared tight BP control (SBP <150 mmHg) to control (SBP >180 mmHg) in 1,148 patients

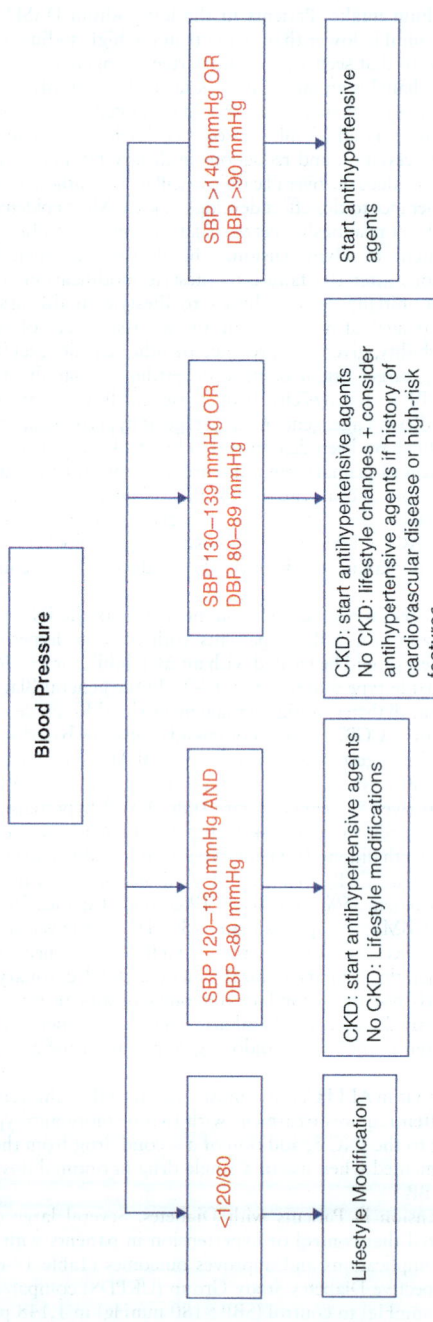

Figure 17-2. Initial approach to hypertension treatment. The decision to start antihypertensive agents can be made based on the value of blood pressure readings and the presence of CKD. Since patients with CKD have a higher rate of cardiovascular events, recent guidelines advocate treating to a BP of <120/80 mmHg. In the general population, for patients with a BP between 130 and 140/80–89 mmHg, the decision to start antihypertensive agents can be made by assessing the overall risk of cardiovascular events for the patient. (Adapted from: Whelton PK, Carey RM, Aronow WS. 2017 ACC/AHA/AAPA/ABC/ACPM/AGS/APhA/ASH/ASPC/NMA/PCNA Guideline for the prevention, detection, evaluation, and management of high blood pressure in adults: executive summary: a report of the American College of Cardiology/American Heart Association Task Force on Clinical Practice Guidelines. *Hypertension.* 2018;6:1269–1324 and KDIGO Blood Pressure Work Group. KDIGO 2021 Clinical practice guideline for the management of blood pressure in chronic kidney disease. *Kidney Int.* 2021;99(Suppl):S1–S87.)

TABLE 17-6	Evidence-Based Drug Recommendations for Comorbid Conditions
Underlying Condition	Drug Classes
Chronic kidney disease	ACE inhibitor, ARB, aldosterone antagonist
Congestive heart failure with reduced ejection fraction	Diuretic, β-blocker, ACE inhibitor, ARB, aldosterone antagonist
High coronary disease risk	Diuretic, β-blocker, ACE inhibitor, CCB
Ischemic heart disease	β-Blocker, ACE inhibitor, CCB, aldosterone antagonist
Recurrent stroke prevention	Diuretic, ACE inhibitor, ARB

with diabetes and hypertension. Those in the lower BP group had fewer diabetic complications (retinopathy) and fewer diabetes-related deaths. The ADVANCE trial was a placebo-controlled study comparing perindopril-indapamide to placebo in over 11,000 diabetic patients. Patients mainly had an average entry SBP of 145 mmHg. The drug therapy was associated with a decrease in microvascular and macrovascular events, as well as all-cause mortality.

At the recommendation of the JNC 8, the initial therapy for the general non-Black population, with diabetes, includes ACE inhibitors or ARBs (but not both), CCBs, or thiazide-type diuretics. In the general Black population, with diabetes, initial management should include either a thiazide-type diuretic or a CCB. Support for this comes from studies such as the UKPDS and ADVANCE trials, which used ACE inhibitors (captopril or perindopril), atenolol, and indapamide. In ALLHAT, diabetic patients had no significant difference in the primary outcome (fatal coronary heart disease or nonfatal MI) whether they were treated with amlodipine, lisinopril, or chlorthalidone. A subgroup analysis from ALLHAT of Black patients with or without diabetes showed that the thiazide-type diuretic had significantly better outcomes with cerebrovascular, heart failure, and combined cardiovascular outcomes, compared to ACE inhibitors. CCBs were comparable to the thiazide-type diuretic in these outcomes, except for in the category of heart failure, in which the thiazide-type diuretic was preferable. However, in all patients with diabetes and proteinuria, the 2018 American Diabetes Association (ADA) supports the initial use of ACE inhibitors or ARB.

The appropriate goal BP in diabetics has been the subject of many large trials. Early studies, such as the Appropriate Blood Pressure Control in Diabetes (ABCD) and the Hypertension Optimal Trial (HOT) showed that intensive BP control (<130/80 or DBP <80 mmHg, respectively) in hypertensive diabetic patients had a significant decrease in mortality and number of cardiovascular events, respectively. The ABCD trial additionally showed that in normotensive diabetic patients, intensive BP control slowed retinopathy, decreased albuminuria, and was associated with fewer cerebrovascular events. Importantly, in the ABCD trial, significantly fewer MIs occurred in patients with diabetes allocated to initial therapy with the ACE inhibitor enalapril compared to those receiving CCB therapy. These results indicate that intensive BP control reduces all-cause mortality in diabetic patients and that ACE inhibitor therapy should be preferred over CCB as part of the multidrug regimen often required for intensive treatment of hypertension in diabetic patients.

More intensive control was evaluated in The Action to Control Cardiovascular Risk in Diabetes (ACCORD) BP trial, which randomized 4,733 diabetic patients at high cardiovascular risk to two different BP goals—SBP of 120 versus 140 mmHg. After 4 years, there was no difference in the primary endpoint of death. However, the lower BP group did have a lower rate of strokes but a higher rate of adverse events, such as hypotension and elevation in serum creatinine.

Thus, less than 130/80 mmHg, as in the ABCD study, may be optimal in diabetic patients, a recommendation reflected in the AHA/ACC guidelines.

E. Treatment of Hypertension in Patients with Cardiac Disease. LVH is an independent risk factor for subsequent cardiovascular disease. Regression of LVH occurs with aggressive BP management using all classes of drugs except direct-acting vasodilators such as hydralazine and minoxidil. The Losartan Intervention for Endpoint Reduction in Hypertension (LIFE) trial compared losartan to atenolol in over 9,000 patients with electrocardiogram evidence of LVH. Both therapies caused regression in LVH, but the losartan group had significantly greater reduction in LVH as compared to the atenolol group. Ischemic heart disease is a common form of target organ damage in hypertension. In patients with hypertension and stable angina pectoris, the treatment regimen should include an ACE-inhibitor or ARB or β-blocker should be used. If needed, a dihydropyriodine (DHP) CCB or thiazide-type diuretic can be added. In patients with acute coronary syndromes (unstable angina or acute MI), hypertension should be treated initially with β-blockers and ACE inhibitors, with the addition of other agents such as thiazide diuretics as needed for BP control. In the chronic BP management of post-MI patients, β-blockers, ACE inhibitors, and aldosterone receptor antagonists have proven to be of the highest benefit. In patients with ischemic heart disease, low-dose aspirin therapy and intensive lipid-lowering therapy are also indicated. Heart failure represents another special hypertensive patient population; it can occur in the setting of either systolic or diastolic dysfunction. In patients with heart failure with reduced ejection fraction (HFrEF), ACE inhibitors, β-blockers and aldosterone receptor blockers (spironolactone or eplerenone), and sodium-glucose transporter-1 (SGLT1) inhibitors are recommended as part of guideline-directed medical therapy, along with potent loop diuretics as needed for fluid overload. Use of non-DHP CCBs is not recommended in HFrEF.

F. Treatment of Hypertension in the Elderly. The treatment of elderly patients with predominant systolic hypertension should follow the same treatment algorithm. In the Systolic Hypertension in the Elderly Program (SHEP) trial, a double-blind placebo-controlled trial of low-dose chlorthalidone in patients older than 60 years with isolated systolic hypertension (SBP greater than 160 mmHg with DBP less than 90 mmHg), the relative risks (RRs) of stroke, left ventricular failure, nonfatal MI or fatal coronary heart disease, and the requirement for coronary artery bypass grafting were all significantly reduced in the active treatment group. The Hypertension in the Very Elderly Trial (HYVET) studied patients over 80 years of age. Over 3,000 patients were assigned to either indapamide-perindopril or placebo with a target SBP in the treatment group of less than 150 mmHg. The primary endpoint was stroke and fatal stroke; the treatment group had a 30% reduction in stroke, 39% reduction in fatal stroke, and 20% reduction in rate of death from any cause. These results are reflected in the JNC 8 recommendations that patients ≥60 years old be treated to a target BP of SBP <150 mmHg and DBP <90 mmHg.

More recently, the Systolic Blood Pressure Intervention Trial (SPRINT) evaluated intensive in a subset of elderly nondiabetic patients >75 years of age, and included patients determined to be "frail," but excluded those in skilled nursing facilities or those with a baseline standing SBP <110 mmHg after 1 minute. Patients were randomized to either standard treatment (SBP <140 mmHg) versus intensive treatment (SBP <120 mmHg.) The intensive group had a 34% reduction in cardiovascular events and a 33% reduction in total mortality, including in those deemed to be frail. Adverse events, including orthostatic hypotension and falls, were similar between the two groups. However, of note, the median SBP achieved in the intensive group after 6 months was 121.2 mmHg. In line with this, the 2017 AHA/ACC recommendations suggest that in noninstitutionalized community-dwelling patients ≥65 years old, target BP should be <130/80 mmHg. While BP goals should be individualized in the elderly population (especially those with high medical comorbidity and limited life expectancy), a prudent goal would be <130/80 mmHg for noninstitutionalized patients ≥65 years old.

G. Treatment of Hypertension in Patients with Metabolic Syndrome. The metabolic syndrome is a clustering of clinical and biochemical characteristics related to insulin resistance and hyperinsulinemia. It is characterized by hypertension, central obesity, dyslipidemia (high triglycerides and low HDL cholesterol levels), and elevated glucose levels. Long-term studies comparing different antihypertensive classes solely in hypertensive patients with metabolic syndrome have not been done. In the past, concerns have often been raised that diuretics should not be used as first-line therapy for hypertension because they have unfavorable effects on insulin sensitivity and increase the risk of new-onset diabetes, thereby having the potential to adversely affect cardiovascular and renal outcomes. A retrospective analysis of ALLHAT compared different antihypertensive classes in patients with metabolic syndrome. In study participants with metabolic syndrome, at 4 years of follow-up, the incidence of newly diagnosed diabetes (fasting glucose greater than 126 mg/dL) was 17.1% for chlorthalidone, 16.0% for amlodipine ($P = .49$ vs. chlorthalidone), and 12.6% for lisinopril ($P <.05$ vs. chlorthalidone). For those without metabolic syndrome, the rate of newly diagnosed diabetes was 7.7% for chlorthalidone, 4.2% for amlodipine, and 4.7% for lisinopril ($P <.05$ for both drugs vs. chlorthalidone). Among participants with metabolic syndrome, the RRs for the primary outcome (fatal coronary heart disease or nonfatal MI) and the secondary cardiovascular outcomes were not different for amlodipine versus chlorthalidone. In participants with metabolic syndrome, outcomes were superior with chlorthalidone versus lisinopril for heart failure (RR 1.31; 95% CI, 1.04–1.64) and for the combined cardiovascular disease endpoint (coronary heart disease, stroke, treated angina, and heart failure; RR, 1.19; 95% CI, 1.07–1.32). However, meta-analyses have found that the use of ACE inhibitor or ARB is actually protective of developing incident diabetes. More recently, the SPRINT trial (which evaluated intensive vs. standard SBP control, <120 mmHg or <140 mmHg, respectively) looked at the development of either incident diabetes or impaired fasting glucose (glucose 100 to 126 mg/dL) in each arm of the trial. While there was no significant increase in development of diabetes, the intensive arm was associated with a higher risk of impaired fasting glucose.

H. Treatment of Hypertension in Patients with CKD. The Kidney Disease Improving Global Outcomes (KDIGO) 2021 recommendations regarding BP control in kidney disease were recently released. In patients with HTN and CKD, regardless of proteinuria, KDIGO recommends targeting a BP <120/80 mmHg. These recommendations stem from the SPRINT trial. In SPRINT, patients were included if they were ≥50 years old, with an SBP of 130 to 180 mmHg and increased cardiovascular risk (which was defined as having underlying CKD, or an ASCVD score >15% or age were ≥75 years old). They were stratified to either an intensive BP control (SBP <120 mmHg) or standard BP control (SBP <140 mmHg). Of the patients evaluated, 2,646 patients had CKD, with a mean GFR of 48 mL/min/1.73 m² (those with a GFR of <20 mL/min/1.73 m² were excluded.) Patients were also excluded if they were diabetic or if they had >1 g/d of proteinuria. The intensive BP control group had significantly lower rates of MI, stroke, and composite cardiovascular events. In patients with CKD, there was no significant difference between treatment groups for worsening of albuminuria, 50% reduction in GFR, or need for starting dialysis. However, within the CKD subset, the mean SBP achieved in the intensive group was 123 mmHg. In addition, the intensive group also had significantly more hypotension, AKI, and electrolyte abnormalities. The KDIGO guidelines and the SPRINT trial differ from AHA/ACC guidelines, which recommend a BP goal of <130/80 for patients with CKD and HTN.

In patients with nonproteinuric CKD, initial therapy consists of agents from the first-line regimen as recommended by JNC 8 (i.e., ACE inhibitors, ARBs, CCBs, or thiazide-type diuretics). In patients with proteinuric CKD, whether diabetic or not, initial therapy should be with ACE inhibitor or an ARB (but not both), regardless of race.

Treating proteinuric patients with ACE inhibitors or ARBs has significant experimental and clinical support. Since ACE inhibitors and ARBs decrease efferent arteriolar tone, they should decrease intraglomerular hypertension. In the Benazepril trial, patients already in reasonable BP control were randomized to treatment with benazepril or placebo. Patients on benazepril had a greater reduction in BP and a 25% reduction in protein excretion. The risk of progression to a primary endpoint (doubling of serum creatinine or progression to dialysis) was reduced by 53% in the benazepril-treated patients. The benefits of ACE inhibitor therapy were seen mainly in patients with chronic glomerular diseases or diabetic nephropathy, whereas there was no benefit in patients with polycystic kidney disease or other CKD excreting less than 1 g of protein per day. These are settings in which hemodynamically mediated factors may not be as important in disease progression. In the Ramipril Efficacy in Nephropathy (REIN) trial, patients with nondiabetic renal disease were randomized to ramipril or placebo plus other antihypertensive therapy as needed to achieve DBP below 90 mmHg. The trial was terminated prematurely among patients excreting more than 3 g protein per day because of a significant benefit of ACE inhibitor treatment with regard to ameliorating the rate of decline of renal function. Although the final results of the African American Study of Kidney Disease (AASK) trial showed no difference among the drug treatment groups in the rate of decline of GFR, the ramipril group had a 22% reduction in risk of the composite endpoint (reduction in GFR by more than 50% from baseline, ESRD, or death). In the REIN-2 trial, dihydropyridine CCB failed to provide renoprotection in patients with nondiabetic renal disease, despite further reduction of BP from that obtained with fixed doses of ACE inhibitors. The non-DHP CCBs (diltiazem and verapamil) have antiproteinuric effects, whereas the DHPs (amlodipine and nifedipine) have been shown to increase proteinuria in some studies. This paradox may be explained by the varied effects of the different classes of CCBs on renal autoregulation. In this regard, dihydropyridines cause preferential afferent arteriolar dilation, which allows more of the systemic pressure to be transmitted to the glomerulus, thereby increasing glomerular pressure and limiting their antiproteinuric effect. If this BP goal is not achieved after initial therapy with an ACE inhibitor or an ARB, a diuretic should be added to the regimen. Addition of a diuretic is logical therapy given the central role of impaired natriuresis in the pathogenesis of hypertension in the setting of CKD. Originally, thiazide diuretics were thought to be less beneficial in advancing CKD, but this has been changed based on the recent Chlorthalidone for Hypertension in Advanced CKD (CLICK) trial. This trial showed that in patients with advanced CKD, chlorthalidone use decreased

SBP by ~10 to 12 mmHg compared to placebo in patients with an average GFR of 23 mL/mg/1.73 m^2.

I. **Treatment of the Patient With Resistant Hypertension.** Resistant hypertension is defined as a failure to reach BP <130/80 mmHg in an adherent patient treated with a first-line three-drug regimen that are max-doses and include a diuretic. Providers must first ensure that the patient has resistant hypertension by following all of the steps above regarding the diagnosis of hypertension (Section V). Truly resistant hypertension should prompt an investigation for underlying potentially treatable forms of secondary hypertension (see Table 17-4). Table 17-7 outlines other causes of resistant hypertension. Treatment of resistant hypertension is detailed in Figure 17-3 and involves the addition of a mineralocorticoid receptor antagonist (MRA), such as spironolactone or eplerenone. Experimental therapies like renal denervation have also shown promise as a treatment for resistant hypertension. Renal denervation is performed via percutaneous catheterization of the renal arteries, and studies (such as RADIANCE II) have shown this technique can significantly decrease BP, even when patients are not on antihypertensives. However, at this time, this

TABLE 17-7 Causes of Resistant Hypertension
Improper blood pressure (BP) measurement (use of inadequately sized BP cuff in obese patients)
Pseudohypertension in elderly individuals
White coat (office) hypertension
Volume overload or pseudotolerance
Excess dietary sodium intake
Fluid retention from underlying renal disease
Inadequate diuretic therapy (failure to use loop diuretic with advanced CKD)
Noncompliance
Patient nonadherence with therapy due to ignorance, cost, or side effects
Physician noncompliance (inadequate drug dosage or failure to include diuretic in regimen)
Drug induced
Nonsteroidal anti-inflammatory agents or cyclooxygenase 2 inhibitors
Cocaine, amphetamines, or other illicit drugs
Sympathomimetics (decongestants or anoretic agents)
Oral contraceptives
Adrenal steroids
Erythropoietin
Licorice
Over-the-counter dietary supplements (ephedra, ma huang, bitter orange)
Excessive alcohol consumption
Identifiable secondary causes of hypertension (Table 17-4)

Resistant hypertension

Def: uncontrolled hypertension despite optimized dosing of 3 antihypertensives of different classes (including a diuretic.)

Rule out other causes of uncontrolled blood pressure

- Noncompliance with medications
- Causes of BP (smoking, NSAID use, uncontrolled obstructive sleep apnea, high salt diet, sedentary lifestyle)
- Eval for secondary causes of HTN, if appropriate: primary hyperaldosteronism, pheochromocytoma, renal artery stenosis

---

Pharmacologic management of resistant hypertension

1. Ensure use of first–line antihypertensives that are optimally dosed (i.e. on max tolerated dose and use of medications with long half life)
    - ACE inhibitors or ARB
    - Diuretics – thiazides (chlorthalidone, HCTZ)
    - DHP CCBs – amlodipine, nifedipine

2. Mineralocorticoid receptor antagonists
    - Spironolactone, eplerenone

3. Beta blockers
    - Carvedilol

4. Alpha blockers, clonidine, vasodilators
    - Doxazosin, prazosin (alpha blockers)
    - Hydralazine, minoxidil (vasodilators)

Figure 17-3. Approach to treating resistant hypertension. BP, blood pressure; NSAID, nonsteroidal anti-inflammatory drug; HTN, hypertension; ACE, angiotensin-converting enzyme; ARB, aldosterone receptor blocker; DHP CCBs, dihydropyridine calcium channel blockers; HCTZ, hydrochlorothiazide.

technique has yet to be FDA-approved in the United States. Consultation with a hypertension specialist should be considered if the BP goal cannot be achieved.

VII. Hypertensive Crises

A. Definition of Hypertensive Crises. The vast majority of hypertensive patients are asymptomatic for many years until complications due to atherosclerosis, cerebrovascular disease, or CHF supervene. In a minority of patients, this "benign" course is punctuated by a hypertensive crisis. A hypertensive crisis is defined as the turning point in the course of an illness at which acute management of the elevated BP plays a decisive role in the eventual outcome. The haste with which the BP must be controlled varies with the type of hypertensive crisis. However, the crucial role of hypertension in the disease process must be identified, and a plan for managing the BP successfully implemented if the patient's outcome is to be optimal. The absolute level of the BP is clearly not the most important factor in determining the existence of a hypertensive crisis. For example, in children, pregnant women, and other previously normotensive individuals in whom mild to moderate hypertension develops suddenly, a hypertensive crisis

TABLE 17-8	Spectrum of Hypertensive Crises

Malignant hypertension (*hypertensive neuroretinopathy present*)

Hypertensive encephalopathy (*occurs with either malignant or severe benign hypertension*)

Nonmalignant ("benign") hypertension with acute complications (*acute end-organ dysfunction in the absence of hypertensive neuroretinopathy*)
   Acute hypertensive heart failure (pulmonary edema due to acute diastolic dysfunction)
   Acute coronary syndromes
      Acute myocardial infarction
      Unstable angina
   Acute aortic dissection
   Central nervous system catastrophe
      Hypertensive encephalopathy
      Intracerebral hemorrhage
      Subarachnoid hemorrhage
      Severe head trauma
   Catecholamine excess states
      Pheochromocytoma crisis
      Monoamine oxidase inhibitor–tyramine interactions
      Antihypertensive drug withdrawal syndromes
      Phenylpropanolamine overdose
   Preeclampsia and eclampsia
   Active bleeding (including postoperative bleeding)
   Poorly controlled hypertension in patients requiring emergency surgery
   Severe postoperative hypertension
      Post-coronary artery bypass hypertension
      Post-carotid endarterectomy hypertension
   Scleroderma renal crisis
   Autonomic hyperreflexia in quadriplegic patients

Adapted from Nolan CR. Malignant hypertension and other hypertensive crises. In: Schrier RW, ed. *Diseases of the Kidney and Urinary Tract*. 8th ed. Lippincott Williams & Wilkins; 2007:1370–1436.

can occur at a BP level that is normally well tolerated by adults with chronic hypertension. Furthermore, in adults with mild to moderate hypertension, a crisis can occur with the onset of acute end-organ dysfunction involving the heart or brain. Table 17-8 outlines the spectrum of hypertensive crises.

B. Malignant hypertension is a clinical syndrome characterized by a marked elevation of BP with widespread acute arteriolar injury (hypertensive vasculopathy). Fundoscopy reveals HNR with flame-shaped hemorrhages, cotton wool spots (soft exudates), and sometimes papilledema (Fig. 17-4, Table 17-9). Regardless of the severity of BP elevation, in the absence of HNR, malignant hypertension cannot be diagnosed. HNR is therefore an extremely important clinical finding, indicating the presence of a hypertension-induced arteriolitis that may involve the kidneys, heart, and central nervous system. With malignant hypertension, a rapid and relentless progression to ESRD occurs if effective BP control is not

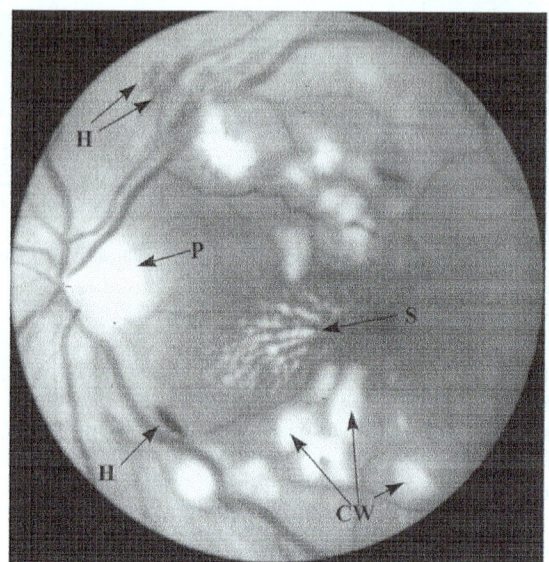

Figure 17-4. Hypertensive neuroretinopathy in malignant hypertension. Fundus photograph in a 30-year-old man with malignant hypertension demonstrates all the characteristic features of hypertensive neuroretinopathy, including striate hemorrhages (*H*), cotton wool spots (*CW*), papilledema (*P*), and a star figure at the macula (*S*).

implemented. Mortality can result from acute hypertensive heart failure, intracerebral hemorrhage, hypertensive encephalopathy, or complications of uremia. Malignant hypertension represents a hypertensive crisis; adequate control of BP clearly prevents these morbid complications.

C. **Hypertensive Crises Due to Nonmalignant Hypertension With Acute Complications.** Even in patients with benign hypertension, in whom HNR is absent, a hypertensive crisis may be diagnosed based on the presence of concomitant acute end-organ dysfunction (see Table 17-8). Hypertensive crises due to nonmalignant hypertension with acute complications include hypertension accompanied by hypertensive encephalopathy, acute hypertensive heart failure, acute aortic dissection, intracerebral hemorrhage, subarachnoid hemorrhage, severe head trauma, acute MI or unstable angina, and active bleeding. Poorly controlled hypertension in a patient requiring surgery increases the risk of intraoperative cerebral or myocardial ischemia and postoperative acute renal failure. Severe postoperative hypertension, including post-coronary artery bypass hypertension and post-carotid endarterectomy hypertension, increases the risk of postoperative bleeding, hypertensive encephalopathy, pulmonary edema, and myocardial ischemia. The various catecholamine excess states can cause a hypertensive crisis with hypertensive encephalopathy or acute hypertensive heart failure. Preeclampsia and eclampsia represent hypertensive crises that are unique to pregnancy. Scleroderma renal crisis is a hypertensive crisis in which failure to adequately control BP (with a regimen that includes an ACE inhibitor) results in rapid and irreversible loss of renal function. Hypertensive crises can also occur in quadriplegic patients due to autonomic hyperreflexia induced by bowel or bladder distension. The sudden onset of hypertension can lead to hypertensive encephalopathy or acute pulmonary edema.

TABLE 17-9	Classification of Hypertensive Retinopathy

Retinal Arteriosclerosis and Arteriosclerotic Retinopathy (Characteristic of Benign Hypertension)
Arteriolar narrowing (focal or diffuse)
Arteriovenous crossing changes
Broadening of the arteriolar light reflex
Copper or silver wiring changes
Perivasculitis
Solitary round retinal hemorrhages
Hard exudates
Central or branch venous occlusion

Hypertensive Neuroretinopathy (Sine Qua Non of Malignant Hypertension)
Generalized arteriolar narrowing
Striate (flame-shaped hemorrhages)[a]
Cotton wool spots (soft exudates)[a]
Bilateral papilledema[a]
Star figure at the macula

[a]These features distinguish retinal arteriosclerosis (benign hypertension) from hypertensive neuroretinopathy (malignant hypertension).

Adapted with permission from Nolan CR. Malignant hypertension and other hypertensive crises. In: Schrier RW, ed. *Diseases of the Kidney and Urinary Tract*. 8th ed. Lippincott Williams & Wilkins; 2007:1370–1436.

D. Treatment of Malignant Hypertension. Malignant hypertension must be treated expeditiously to prevent complications such as hypertensive encephalopathy, acute hypertensive heart failure, and renal failure. The traditional approach to patients with malignant hypertension has been the initiation of potent parenteral agents. In general, parenteral therapy should be used in patients with evidence of acute end-organ dysfunction (hypertensive encephalopathy or pulmonary edema) or those unable to tolerate oral medications. Nitroprusside, nicardipine, or intravenous (IV) labetalol are the treatments of choice for patients requiring parenteral therapy. Nicardipine is a parenteral CCB. Although it has a longer onset of action and a longer half-life than nitroprusside, there are fewer adverse reactions and lower risks of toxicity compared to nitroprusside. In general, reducing the mean arterial pressure by 10% to 20% within the first hour, and by an additional 5% to 15% over the next 24 hours (or to a range of <180/120 in the first hour and a 24-hour goal of <160/100 to 110 mmHg.) If no evidence of vital organ hypoperfusion is apparent during the initial reduction, the BP can gradually be lowered to less than 140/90 mmHg over a period of 12 to 36 hours. An exception to this rule is in the setting of acute aortic dissection, in which the goal is to reduce the SBP <100 to 120 mmHg within the first hour. Oral antihypertensive agents should be initiated as soon as possible to minimize the duration of parenteral therapy, and typically, patients will require combination therapy. The infusion can be weaned as the oral agents become effective. The cornerstone of initial oral therapy should be arteriolar vasodilators, such as long-acting CCBs, which can be used in combination with oral medications that can be continued long-term, such as ACE inhibitors or ARBs. Alternatively, β-Blockers can be used to control reflex tachycardia, and a diuretic must be initiated within a few days to prevent salt and water retention in response to vasodilator therapy when the patient's dietary salt intake increases. Diuretics may not be necessary as a part of initial parenteral therapy, because patients with malignant hypertension often present with volume depletion due to pressure-induced natriuresis. Although many patients with malignant hypertension definitely require initial parenteral therapy, some patients may not yet have evidence of cerebral or cardiac dysfunction or rapidly deteriorating renal function and therefore do not require instantaneous control of BP. These patients can often be managed with an intensive oral regimen, again using first-line agents that can be continued outpatient, such as CCBs (such as nifedipine) in combination with either a β-blocker or ACE inhibitor or ARB, with the goal to bring the BP under control within 12 to 24 hours. After the immediate crisis has resolved and the hypertension has been controlled with initial parenteral therapy, oral therapy, or both, lifelong surveillance of BP is mandatory. If control lapses, malignant hypertension can recur even after years of successful antihypertensive therapy. Triple therapy with a diuretic, a β-blocker, and a vasodilator is often required to maintain satisfactory long-term BP control.

E. Treatment of Other Hypertensive Crises. Nicardipine can be used for the management of virtually all hypertensive crises outlined in Table 17-8, including in pregnancy, with malignant hypertension, hypertensive encephalopathy, intracerebral hemorrhage, perioperative hypertension, catecholamine-related hypertensive crises, and acute aortic dissection (in combination with β-blockers). Nicardipine should not be used for acute heart failure. Sodium nitroprusside can also be used for the majority of these hypertensive crises but is not the preferred agent due to risk of toxicities and limitations. Nitroprusside increases cyclic guanosine monophosphate (cGMP) at the level of the arteriolar smooth muscle, causing vasodilation and a decrease in SVR. Nitroprusside is rapidly metabolized to cyanide, which is then converted to thiocyanate in the liver and excreted by the kidneys. Toxicity can occur when nitroprusside is used in higher doses (>10 mcg/kg/min for >10 minutes) or when it is used in the setting of kidney or liver dysfunction. It also cannot be used in pregnancy. Because of this, it is not the preferred agent if other agents are available. IV labetalol is also an appropriate treatment for most hypertensive crises. Intravenous nitroglycerin may also be useful in patients with concomitant myocardial ischemia, because it dilates intracoronary collaterals.

F. Treatment of Severe Uncomplicated Hypertension in the Acute Care Setting. The benefits of acute reduction in BP in the setting of true hypertensive crisis are obvious (Fig. 17-5). Fortunately, true hypertensive crises are relatively rare events that never affect the vast majority of hypertensive patients. Much more common than true hypertensive crisis is the patient who presents with markedly elevated BP (greater than 180/100 mmHg) in the absence of HNR (malignant hypertension) or acute end-organ damage that would signify a true crisis. This entity, known as *severe uncomplicated hypertension*, is very common in the emergency department or other acute care settings. Of patients with severe uncomplicated hypertension, 60% are entirely asymptomatic and present for prescription refills or routine BP checks, or are found to have elevated pressure during routine physical examinations. The other 40% present with nonspecific findings such as headache, dizziness, or weakness in the absence of evidence of acute end-organ dysfunction.

In the past, this entity was referred to as *urgent hypertension*, reflecting the erroneous notion that an acute reduction of BP over a few hours before discharge from the acute care facility was essential to minimize the risk of short-term complications from severe hypertension. Commonly used treatment regimens included oral clonidine loading or sublingual nifedipine. However,

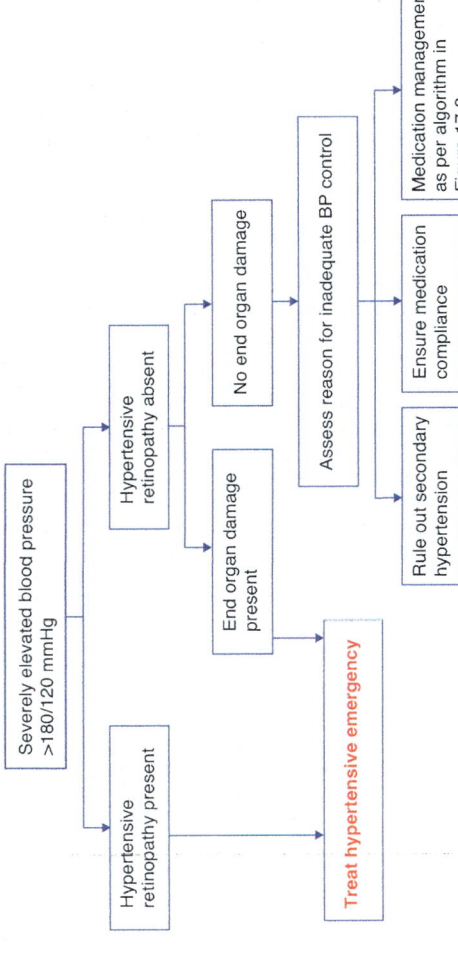

Figure 17-5. Algorithm for treatment of severe hypertension. (Used with permission of John Wiley & Sons, from Nolan CR. Hypertensive crises. In: Schrier RW, ed. *Atlas of Diseases of the Kidney*. Vol. 3. Current Medicine; 1999; permission conveyed through Copyright Clearance Center, Inc.)

the practice of acute BP reduction in severe uncomplicated hypertension is no longer considered the standard of care. The Veterans Administration Cooperative Study of patients with severe hypertension included 70 placebo-treated patients who had an average DBP of 121 mmHg at entry. Among these untreated patients, 27 experienced morbid events at a mean of 11 (±2) months of follow-up. However, the earliest morbid event occurred after 2 months. These data suggest that in patients with severe uncomplicated hypertension in which severe hypertension is not accompanied by evidence of malignant hypertension or acute end-organ dysfunction, eventual complications due to stroke, MI, or heart failure tend to occur over a time frame of months to years rather than hours to days. Although the long-term control of BP can clearly prevent these eventual complications, a hypertensive crisis cannot be diagnosed, because no evidence indicates that the acute reduction of BP results in an improvement in short- or long-term prognosis. Although the acute reduction of BP in patients with severe uncomplicated hypertension using sublingual nifedipine or oral clonidine loading was once the de facto standard of care, this practice was often an emotional response on the part of the treating physician to the dramatic elevation of BP, or it was motivated by the fear of medicolegal repercussions in the unlikely event of a hypertensive complication occurring within hours to days. Observing and documenting the dramatic fall in BP is a satisfying therapeutic maneuver, but no scientific basis for this approach exists. No literature supports the notion that some goal level of BP reduction must be achieved before the patient with severe uncomplicated hypertension leaves the acute care setting. In fact, the acute reduction of BP is often counterproductive, because it can produce untoward side effects that render the patient less likely to comply with long-term drug therapy. Instead, the acute therapeutic intervention should focus on tailoring an effective, well-tolerated maintenance antihypertensive regimen, with patient education regarding the chronic nature of the disease process and the importance of long-term compliance and medical follow-up. If the patient has simply run out of medicines, reinstitution of the previously effective drug regimen should suffice. If the patient is thought to be compliant with an existing drug regimen, a sensible change in the regimen, such as an increase in a suboptimal dosage of an existing drug or the addition of a drug of another class, is appropriate. In this regard, the addition of a low dose of a thiazide diuretic as a second-step agent to existing monotherapy with ACE inhibitor, ARB, CCB, β-blocker, or central α-agonist is often remarkably effective. Another essential goal of the acute intervention should be to arrange suitable outpatient follow-up within a few days. A gradual reduction of BP to normotensive levels over a few days to a week should be accomplished in conjunction with frequent outpatient visits to modify the drug regimen and reinforce the importance of lifelong compliance with therapy. Although less dramatic than the acute reduction of BP in the acute care setting, this type of approach to the treatment of chronic hypertension is more likely to prevent long-term hypertensive complications and recurrent episodes of severe uncomplicated hypertension.

SUGGESTED READINGS

Acute Infarction Ramipril Efficacy (AIRE) Study Investigators. Effects of ramipril on mortality and morbidity of survivors of acute myocardial infarction with clinical evidence of heart failure. *Lancet.* 1993;342:821–828.

Agadoa LY, Appel L, Bakris GL, et al. Effect of ramipril versus amlodipine on renal outcomes in hypertensive nephrosclerosis: a randomized controlled trial. *JAMA.* 2001;285:2719–2728.

Agarwal R, Sinha AD, Cramer AE, et al. Chlorthalidone for hypertension in advanced chronic kidney disease. *New Engl J Med.* 2021;385:2507–2519.

ALLHAT Collaborative Research Group. Major cardiovascular events in hypertensive patients randomized to doxazosin versus chlorthalidone: the antihypertensive and lipid-lowering to prevent heart attack trial (ALLHAT). *JAMA*. 2000;238:1967–1975.

ALLHAT Officers and Coordinators for the ALLHAT Collaborative Research Group. Major outcomes in high-risk hypertensive patients randomized to angiotensin-converting enzyme inhibitor, calcium channel blocker versus diuretic. *JAMA*. 2002;288:2981–2997.

Appel LJ, Moore TJ, Obarzanek E, et al. A clinical trial of the effects of dietary patterns on blood pressure. DASH Collaborative Research Group. *New Engl J Med*. 1997;336(16):1117–1124.

Appel LJ, Wright JT Jr, Greene T, et al. Intensive blood-pressure control in hypertensive chronic kidney disease. *New Engl J Med*. 2010;363(10):918–929.

Azizi M, Saxena P, Wang Y, et al. Endovascular ultrasound renal denervation to treat hypertension: The RADIANCE II randomized clinical trial. *JAMA*. 2023;329:651–661.

Beckett NS, Peters R, Fletcher AE, et al. Treatment of hypertension in patients 80 years of age or older. *New Engl J Med*. 2008;358(18):1887–1898.

Black HR, Davis B, Barzhay J, et al. Metabolic and clinical outcomes in nondiabetic individuals with the metabolic syndrome assigned to chlorthalidone, amlodipine, or lisinopril as initial treatment for hypertension. A report for the Antihypertensive and Lipid-Lowering Treatment to Prevent Heart Attack Trial (ALLHAT). *Diabetes Care*. 2008;31:353–360.

Black HR, Elliott JW, Grandits G, et al. Principal results of the controlled onset verapamil investigation of cardiovascular end points (CONVINCE) trial. *JAMA*. 2003;289:2073–2082.

Brenner BM, Copper ME, de Zeeuq D, et al. Effects of losartan on renal and cardiovascular outcomes in patients with type 2 diabetes and nephropathy (RENAAL). *N Engl J Med*. 2001;345:861–869.

Capricorn Investigators. Effect of carvedilol on outcome after myocardial infarction in patients with left-ventricular dysfunction: the CAPRICORN randomized trial. *Lancet*. 2001;357:1358–1390.

Cohn J, Tognoni G. A randomized trial of the angiotensin receptor blocker valsartan in chronic heart failure (ValHEFT). *N Engl J Med*. 2001;345:1667–1675.

Cushman WC, Evans GW, Byington RP, et al. Effects of intensive blood-pressure control in type 2 diabetes mellitus. *New Engl J Med*. 2010;362(17):1575–1585.

Dahlof B, Devereux RB, Kjeldsen SE, et al. Cardiovascular morbidity and mortality in the Losartan Intervention for Endpoint Reduction in Hypertension Study (LIFE). *Lancet*. 2002;359:995–1003.

Egan BM, Zhao Y, Axon RN. US trends in prevalence, awareness, treatment, and control of hypertension, 1988–2008. *JAMA*. 2010;303(20):2043–2050.

Estacio RO, Jeffers BW, Hiatt WH, Biggerstaff SL, Gifford N, Schrier RW. The effect of nisoldipine as compared with enalapril on cardiovascular outcomes in patients with non-insulin dependent diabetes mellitus and hypertension. *N Engl J Med*. 1998;338:645–652.

GISEN (Cruppo Italiano di Studi Epidemiologici in Nefrologia) Group. Randomized placebo-controlled trial of effect of ramipril on decline in glomerular filtration rate and risk of terminal renal failure in proteinuric, non-diabetic nephropathy (REIN). *Lancet*. 1997;349:1857–1863.

Guyton AC, Manning RD, Norman RA, Montani JP, Lohmeier TE, Hall JE. Current concepts and perspectives of renal volume regulation in relationship to hypertension. *J Hypertens*. 1986;4(Suppl 4):S49–S56.

Hall JE, Granger JP, Smith MJ, Premen AJ. Role of renal hemodynamics and arterial pressure in aldosterone "escape". *Hypertension*. 1984;6(Suppl 1):I183–I192.

Hansson L, Zanchetti A, Carruthers SG, et al. Effects of intensive blood-pressure lowering and low-dose aspirin in patients with hypertension: principal results of the Hypertension Optimal Treatment (HOT) randomized trial. HOT Study Group. *Lancet*. 1998;351(9118):1755–1762.

Heart Outcomes Prevention Evaluation Study Investigators. Effects of an angiotensin-converting-enzyme inhibitor, ramipril on cardiovascular events in high-risk patients (HOPE). *N Engl J Med*. 2000;342:145–153.

Intersalt Cooperative Research Group. Intersalt: an international study of electrolyte excretion and blood pressure. Results for 24 hour urinary sodium and potassium excretion. *Br Med J*. 1988;297:319–330.

Jamerson K, Weber MA, Bakris GL, et al. Benazepril plus amlodipine or hydrochlorothiazide for hypertension in high-risk patients. *New Engl J Med*. 2008;359(23):2417–2428.

James PA, Oparil S, Carter BL. 2014 evidence-based guideline for the management of high blood pressure in adults: report from the panel members appointed to the Eighth Joint National Committee (JNC 8). *JAMA*. 2014;311:507–520.

KDIGO Blood Pressure Work Group. KDIGO 2021 Clinical practice guideline for the management of blood pressure in chronic kidney disease. *Kidney Int*. 2021;99(Suppl):S1–S87.

Kober L, Torp-Pedersen C, Carlsen JE, et al. Trandolapril Cardiac Evaluation (TRACE) study group. A clinical trial of the angiotensin-converting enzyme inhibitor trandolapril in patients with left ventricular dysfunction after myocardial infarction. *N Engl J Med.* 1995;333: 1670–1676.

Lewis EJ, Hunsicker LG, Bain RP, et al. The effect of angiotensin-converting enzyme inhibitor on diabetic nephropathy: the Collaborative Study Group (Captopril trial). *N Engl J Med.* 1993; 329:1456–1462.

Lewis EJ, Hunsicker LG, Clarke WR, et al. Renoprotective effect of the angiotensin-receptor antagonist irbesartan in patients with nephropathy due to type 2 diabetes (INDT). *N Engl J Med.* 2001;345:851–860.

Lifton RP, Gharavi AG, Geller DS. Molecular mechanisms of human hypertension. *Cell.* 2001; 104:545–556.

Mancia G, Fagard R, Narkiewicz K, et al. 2013 ESH/ESC guidelines for the management of arterial hypertension: the Task Force for the Management of Arterial Hypertension of the European Society of Hypertension (ESH) and of the European Society of Cardiology (ESC). *Eur Heart J.* 2013;34(28):2159–2219.

Maschia G, Alberti D, Janin G, et al. Effect of the angiotensin-converting-enzyme inhibitor benazepril on the progression of chronic renal insufficiency. *N Engl J Med.* 1996;334:939–945.

Neal B, Wu Y, Xiangxian F, et al. Effect of salt substitution on cardiovascular events and death. *N Engl J Med.* 2021;385:1067–1077.

Nolan CR. Hypertensive crises. In: Schrier RW, ed. *Atlas of Diseases of the Kidney*, Vol. 3. Current Medicine; 1999:8.1–8.30.

Nolan CR. Malignant hypertension and other hypertensive crises. In: Schrier RW, ed. *Diseases of the Kidney and Urinary Tract*. 7th ed. Lippincott Williams & Wilkins; 2001:1513–1592.

Nolan CR, Schrier RW. The kidney in hypertension. In: Schrier RW, ed. *Olyte Disorders*. 6th ed. Lippincott Williams & Wilkins; 2003:341–400.

Okin PM, Devereux RB, Jern S, et al. Regression of electrocardiographic left ventricular hypertrophy by losartan versus atenolol: the Losartan Intervention for Endpoint reduction in Hypertension (LIFE) Study. *Circulation.* 2003;108(6):684–690.

Packer M, Coats AJ, Fowler MB, et al. Effect of carvedilol on survival in severe chronic heart failure (COPERNICUS). *N Engl J Med.* 2001;344:1651–1658.

Pitt B, Remme W, Zannad F, et al. Eplerenone, a selective aldosterone blocker, in patients with left ventricular dysfunction after myocardial infarction (EPHESUS). *N Engl J Med.* 2003;348:1309–1321.

Pitt B, Zannad F, Remme WJ, et al. Randomized Aldactone Evaluation Study Investigators. The effect of spironolactone on morbidity and mortality in patients with severe heart failure (RALES). *N Engl J Med.* 1999;341:709–717.

PROGRESS Collaborative Study Group. Randomised trial of perindopril-based blood pressure lowering regimen among 6105 individuals with previous stroke or transient ischaemic attack. *Lancet.* 2001;358:1033–1041.

Ruggenenti P, Perna A, Loriga G, et al. Blood pressure control for renoprotection in patients with non-diabetic renal disease (REIN-2): mulicentre, randomised controlled trial. *Lancet.* 2005;365:939–946.

Sacks FM, Svetkey LP, Vollmer WM, et al. Effects on blood pressure of reduced dietary sodium and the Dietary Approaches to Stop Hypertension (DASH) diet. DASH-Sodium Collaborative Research Group. *New Engl J Med.* 2001;344(1):3–10.

Sarnak MJ, Greene T, Wang X, et al. The effect of a lower target blood pressure on the progression of kidney disease: long-term follow-up of the Modification of Diet in Renal Disease study. *Ann Intern Med.* 2005;142(5):342–351.

Schrier RW, Estacio R, Esler A, Mehler P. Effects of aggressive blood pressure control in normotensive type 2 diabetic patients on albuminuria, retinopathy and strokes. *Kidney Int.* 2002;61: 1086–1097.

Schrier RW, Estacio RO, Mehler PS, Hiatt WR. Appropriate blood pressure control in hypertensive and normotensive type 2 diabetes mellitus: a summary of the ABCD trial. *Nat Clin Pract Nephrol.* 2007;3:428–438.

SHEP Cooperative Research Group. Prevention of stroke by antihypertensive treatment in older persons with isolated systolic hypertension. Final results of the Systolic Hypertension in the Elderly Program (SHEP). *JAMA.* 1991;265:3255–3264.

SPRINT Research Group. A randomized trial of intensive versus standard blood-pressure control. *N Engl J Med.* 2015;373:2103–2116.

SOLVD Investigators. Effect of enalapril on survival in patients with reduced left ventricular ejection fractions and congestive heart failure. *N Engl J Med.* 1991;325:293–302.

UK Prospective Diabetes Study Group. Efficacy of atenolol and captopril in reducing risk of macrovascular and microvascular complications in type 2 diabetes: UKPDS 39. *Br Med J.* 1998;317:713–720.

Whelton PK, Barzilay J, Cushman WC, et al. Clinical outcomes in antihypertensive treatment of type 2 diabetics, impaired fasting glucose concentration and normoglycemia. Antihypertensive and Lipid-Lowering Treatment to Prevent Heart Attack Trial (ALLHAT). *Arch Intern Med.* 2005;165:1401–1409.

Whelton PK, Carey RM, Aronow WS. 2017 ACC/AHA/AAPA/ABC/ACPM/AGS/APhA/ASH/ASPC/NMA/PCNA Guideline for the prevention, detection, evaluation, and management of high blood pressure in adults: executive summary: a report of the American College of Cardiology/American Heart Association Task Force on Clinical Practice Guidelines. *Hypertension.* 2018;6:1269–1324.

Wing LMH, Reid CM, Ryan P, et al. Second Australian National Blood Pressure Study Group. A comparison of outcomes with angiotensin-converting-enzyme inhibitors and diuretics for hypertension in the elderly (ANBP2). *N Engl J Med.* 2003;348:583–592.

Wright JT Jr, Harris-Haywood S, Pressel S, et al. Clinical outcomes by rate in hypertensive patients with and without the metabolic syndrome. Antihypertensive and Lipid-Lowering Treatment to Prevent Heart Attack Trial (ALLHAT). *Arch Intern Med.* 2008;168:207–217.

18. The Patient With Diabetes and Chronic Kidney Disease

L. Parker Gregg, Sankar Navaneethan

The prevalence of diabetes mellitus is rising, affecting over a third of patients with chronic kidney disease (CKD). In addition to the management of CKD and its corollary considerations such as electrolyte abnormalities, metabolic acidosis, and anemia, there are some special considerations in the management of patients with both diabetes and kidney disease. This chapter will provide an overview of the epidemiology, diagnostic considerations, and management of patients with diabetes and CKD, consistent with the Kidney Disease Improving Global Outcomes (KDIGO) 2022 Clinical Practice Guidelines for the management of diabetes in CKD and the American Diabetes Association (ADA) 2023 Standards of Care in Diabetes (Table 18-1).

I. Epidemiology of Diabetes and CKD

A. **The diagnosis of diabetes** can be made based on a fasting plasma glucose level ≥126 mg/dL, a 2-hour plasma glucose level ≥200 mg/dL during an oral glucose tolerance test, a hemoglobin A1c (HbA1c) ≥6.5%, or a random plasma glucose ≥200 mg/dL in the setting of symptoms of hyperglycemia or hyperglycemic crisis. Diabetes can be classified into several heterogeneous categories:
  1. **Type 1 diabetes mellitus (T1DM)** is an autoimmune disease characterized by destruction of the pancreatic β-cells. This leads to a deficiency of insulin.
  2. **Type 2 diabetes mellitus (T2DM)** is a state of inadequate insulin secretion in the setting of insulin resistance.
  3. **Additional causes of diabetes** include monogenic syndromes, exocrine pancreatic disorders, drug-induced diabetes (including after organ transplantation), and gestational diabetes mellitus.

B. **Diabetes and CKD are frequently comorbid.** The prevalence of diabetes has been rising among individuals with and without CKD. By some estimates, diabetes is approximately three times as prevalent among those with CKD as those without (51.1% vs. 18.6% according to the US Renal Data System). The prevalence of CKD among patients with diabetes is also approximately three times higher than among patients without diabetes. From 2017 to 2020, the prevalence of CKD was 38.0% among those with diabetes, compared to 10.4% among those without diabetes.

C. **Diabetic kidney disease is defined as** CKD attributed to diabetes mellitus. It is important to note that not all kidney disease in patients with diabetes is caused by the pathogenic microvascular effects of elevated blood glucose on the kidney. CKD is typically a clinical diagnosis in a patient with a urinary albumin to creatinine ratio ≥30 mg/g and/or a progressive reduction in estimated glomerular filtration rate (eGFR). Patients with diabetes and concomitant CKD of other underlying causes may be misclassified as having diabetic kidney disease in the absence of confirmation of an alternative diagnosis. Consequently, the term diabetic kidney disease is not used by KDIGO as it is considered confusing, and they instead refer to patients with diabetes and CKD.

D. **The clinical course of diabetic kidney disease** can be variable, but often involves albuminuria and progressive decline in eGFR. Microscopic hematuria and nephrotic range proteinuria can both be seen in patients with diabetic

TABLE 18-1 Guideline Recommendations for the Management of Patients With Diabetes and CKD

Metric	ADA[a]	KDIGO[b]	ESC and EASD[c]
Year	2023	2022	2019
Glycemic control			
HbA1c target	<7.0% for most adults (A) <8.0% for those with greater anticipated harms of a more stringent target (B)	Individualized, <6.5% to <8.0% (1C)	<7.0% (IA) Individualized by duration of diabetes, comorbidities, and age (IC)
Preferred glucose-lowering agents	Metformin (A) SGLT2 inhibitor or GLP-1 RA (A)	SGLT2 inhibitor for eGFR ≥20 (1A) Metformin for eGFR ≥30 (1B) GLP-1 RA after SGLT2 inhibitor and metformin (1B)	SGLT2 inhibitor for eGFR 30–89 (IB) or GLP-1 RA if eGFR >30 (IIaB)
Lifestyle			
Physical activity	Moderate-to-vigorous intensity, ≥150 min/wk (B for T2DM, C for T1DM)	Moderate intensity, ≥150 min/wk (1D)	Moderate-to-vigorous intensity, ≥150 min/wk (IA)
Weight management	Achieve and maintain ≥5% weight loss for most people with overweight or obesity (B)	Consider advising patients with obesity, diabetes, and CKD to lose weight (ungraded)	Reduced calorie intake is recommended for lowering excessive body weight (IA)
Protein intake	0.8 g/kg body weight/d for nondialysis CKD (A) Higher levels of protein intake for patients on dialysis (B)	0.8 g protein/kg body weight/d for nondialysis CKD (2C) 1.0–1.2 g protein/kg body weight/d for dialysis-dependent kidney disease (ungraded)	Less protein is recommended (ungraded)
Sodium intake	<2,300 mg/d (B)	<2,000 mg/d (2C)	<2,300 mg/d (IA)
Other			
Blood pressure target	<130/80 mmHg (B)	<120 mmHg (per KDIGO 2021 Clinical Practice Guideline for Management of Blood Pressure in CKD, 2B)	Systolic blood pressure <130 mmHg (IA) Diastolic blood pressure <80 mmHg (IC)
Albuminuria reduction	RAAS blockade if UACR 30–299 (B) and ≥300 (A) and/or eGFR <60 (A)	RAAS blockade (1B)	RAAS blockade (IA)

(continued)

TABLE 18-1	Guideline Recommendations for the Management of Patients With Diabetes and CKD (Continued)		
Metric	ADA[a]	KDIGO[b]	ESC and EASD[c]
Cardiovascular risk reduction	SGLT2 inhibitor for eGFR ≥20 and UACR ≥200 (A) or <200 (B) SGLT2 inhibitor, GLP-1 RA, or nonsteroidal MRA (if eGFR ≥25) (A)	SGLT2 inhibitor (1A) GLP-1 RA (1B) Nonsteroidal MRA if eGFR ≥25, normal K⁺ level, and UACR ≥30 despite RAAS inhibition (2A)	SGLT2 inhibitor (IA) GLP-1 RA (IA)
Slow CKD progression	SGLT2 inhibitor for eGFR ≥20 and UACR ≥200 (A) or <200 (B)	SGLT2 inhibitor (1A) GLP-1 RA (ungraded)	SGLT2 inhibitor (IB) GLP-1 RA (IIaB)

[a]Evidence is graded as A (clear or supportive evidence from well-conducted, generalizable, adequately powered randomized controlled trials), B (supportive evidence from well-conducted cohort or case-control studies), C (supportive evidence from poorly controlled or uncontrolled studies or conflicting evidence with the weight of the evidence supporting the recommendation), or E (expert consensus or clinical experience).

[b]Recommendations are graded as level 1 (recommended) or level 2 (suggested). Quality of evidence is graded as A (high), B (moderate), C (low), or D (very low).

[c]Recommendations are classified as I (recommended or indicated), IIa (should be considered), IIb (may be considered), and III (not recommended). Levels of evidence include A (derived from multiple randomized trials or meta-analyses), B (derived from a single randomized trial or large nonrandomized studies), and C (consensus of opinion).

ADA, American Diabetes Association; EASD, European Association for the Study of Diabetes; eGFR, estimated glomerular filtration rate in mL/min/1.73 m²; ESC, European Society of Cardiology; GLP-1 RA, glucagon-like peptide-1 receptor agonist; HbA1c, hemoglobin A1c; KDIGO, Kidney Disease Improving Global Outcomes; MRA, mineralocorticoid receptor antagonist; RAAS, renin-angiotensin-aldosterone system; SGLT2 inhibitor, sodium-glucose co-transporter 2 inhibitor; T1DM, type 1 diabetes mellitus; T2DM, type 2 diabetes mellitus; UACR, urine albumin-to-creatinine ratio in mg/g.

kidney disease. In earlier stages of diabetic kidney disease, hyperfiltration can lead to an increase in eGFR that can delay diagnosis if not carefully considered by clinicians.

1. **The glomerular filtration rate (GFR)** frequently may be normal or elevated early in the course of diabetic kidney disease due to glomerular hypertrophy and hyperfiltration (Fig. 18-1A). Glomerular hyperfiltration is associated with progression of albuminuria and GFR decline. Other patients may have a lesser degree of hyperfiltration early in their course. The rate of GFR decline varies between individuals from slow to rapid, and some individuals may develop a stabilization of their GFR.
2. **The degree and trajectory of albuminuria** similarly varies widely between individuals and often evolves over time (Fig. 18-1B). Albuminuria may progress or regress during the course of the disease. Some individuals reach nephrotic range proteinuria, while others may never develop albuminuria at all.
3. The timeline and features of disease may also differ notably between individuals with T1DM and T2DM (Table 18-2). In patients with T2DM, diabetic kidney disease can occur with or without a history of long-standing diabetes, albuminuria, or retinopathy. In patients with T1DM, the presence of retinopathy is much more closely associated with diabetic kidney disease.

II. Diagnosis of Diabetic Kidney Disease

A. Patients with T2DM and CKD are frequently presumed to have kidney disease attributable to diabetes. However, performing the appropriate diagnostic

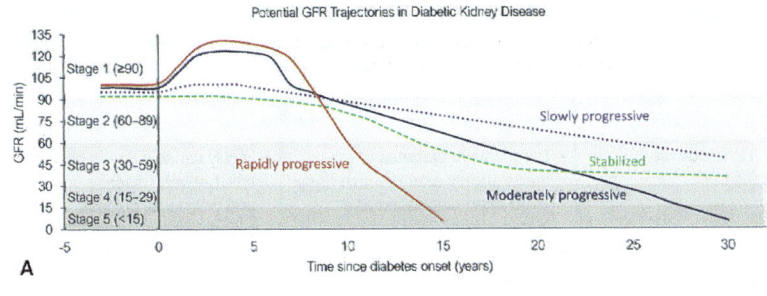
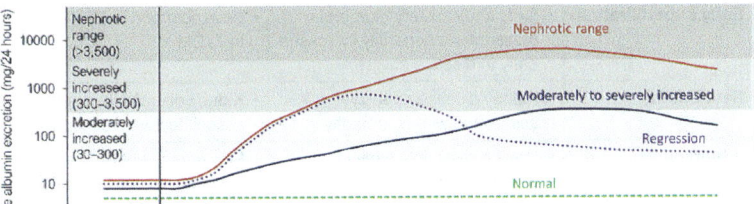

Figure 18-1. Clinical progression of diabetic kidney disease. There are many potential clinical trajectories of GFR (**A**) and albuminuria (**B**) after the development of diabetes. In some patients, GFR may be normal or increased early after the onset of diabetes due to glomerular hypertrophy, increased intraglomerular pressure, and hyperfiltration. The rate of progression of GFR decline is variable between individuals and may range from gradual to rapid. Some individuals may have stabilization of their GFR, while others continue to decline until reaching kidney failure requiring kidney replacement therapy. Urinary albumin excretion may range from normal (<30 mg/24 hours) to nephrotic range (>3,500 mg/24 hours). The degree of albuminuria may worsen over the course of the disease, may stabilize, or may regress, particularly with the introduction of proteinuria-lowering therapies. Although a higher degree of albuminuria is generally considered a risk factor for more rapid decline of GFR, some individuals may have progressive GFR decline in the absence of albuminuria.

workup to identify patients in whom an alternative diagnosis may explain their kidney disease is important to appropriately manage CKD.

B. **Evaluating patients for other causes of kidney disease** is important for establishing the correct diagnosis. For patients with cellular casts in their urine, nephrotic syndrome, rapid worsening of eGFR or albuminuria, gross hematuria, or clinical signs and symptoms of an alternative diagnosis (e.g., systemic lupus erythematosus, etc.), additional assessment should be completed. A serologic workup including antinuclear antibodies, complement levels, antinuclear cytoplasmic antibodies, antiglomerular basement membrane antibodies, serum protein electrophoresis, serum free light chains with immunofixation, human immunodeficiency virus, hepatitis C virus, and hepatitis B virus should be completed to evaluate for alternative diagnoses.

C. **Kidney biopsy** should be considered if the patient's clinical presentation does not seem fully explained by diabetic kidney disease or if the serologic workup or history and physical examination increase clinical suspicion of an alternative diagnosis.

1. **Indications for kidney biopsy** include, but are not limited to, nephrotic-range proteinuria (particularly in the setting of short duration of diabetes or history

TABLE 18-2. Key Differences in Diabetic Kidney Disease Between Patients With T1DM and T2DM

Characteristic	Features in T1DM	Features in T2DM
Time course	• Diagnosis of diabetes often made shortly after disease onset • More often diagnosed at a younger age • More predictable timeline of disease development and progression	• Highly variable due to elapsed time between disease onset and diagnosis, disease severity, comorbidities • Age-related GFR decline needs to be considered when interpreting lab results
Early hyperfiltration	• GFR and capillary glomerular pressure are generally increased early in disease course	• Less common in T2DM than in T1DM
Retinopathy	• Kidney disease strongly associated with retinopathy	• Kidney disease less strongly associated with retinopathy
Albuminuria	• May be reversible early in disease course	• May or may not be present • Is not specific for diabetic kidney disease • Can be reversible early in disease course • May progress over the course of the disease and can rise to nephrotic range
Kidney biopsy findings	• Interstitial fibrosis and tubular atrophy follow glomerular lesions and may be less severe	• Arteriosclerosis is common • Microscopic findings are more heterogeneous • Chronic tubulointerstitial injury may exceed glomerulopathy in severity
Blood pressure	• Blood pressure can be normal or high (more likely to rise as kidney disease progresses)	• Comorbid hypertension is common

GFR, glomerular filtration rate; T1DM, type 1 diabetes mellitus; T2DM, type 2 diabetes mellitus.

of mild or well-controlled diabetes), rapid decline in kidney function, new escalation of proteinuria, the presence of hematuria, acute kidney injury, lack of diabetic retinopathy in the case of patients with T1DM, or signs or symptoms of an alternative diagnosis. Kidney biopsy is particularly important to pursue if distinguishing between items on the differential diagnosis may impact the management of the patient.

2. **Common biopsy findings** of diabetic kidney disease include:
   a. **Mesangial expansion** is typically present and can be diffuse due to the accumulation of mesangial matrix. In more advanced disease, round nodular hypercellular matrix may develop in the mesangium.
   b. **Segmental glomerulosclerosis** is common in later stages of disease.
   c. **Interstitial fibrosis and tubular atrophy** typically develop after glomerular lesions in patients with T1DM. In patients with T2DM, this can be heterogeneous and may be more severe than the glomerular findings.

d. **Immunofluorescence microscopy** frequently shows diffuse linear IgG and albumin. Patients with advanced disease may have nonspecific segmental staining for IgM, C3, and C1q.
e. **Electron microscopy** typically shows diffuse basement membrane thickening in the glomeruli and tubules. Podocyte foot processes may be effaced in advanced disease. There is typically no immune complex deposition in diabetic kidney disease.
3. Approximately 40% to 50% of patients with diabetes undergoing kidney biopsy have findings attributable to a disease other than diabetes, such as glomerulosclerosis, IgA nephropathy, etc. Factors associated with higher likelihood of diabetic kidney disease include the presence of diabetic retinopathy and higher levels of proteinuria, whereas hematuria, well-controlled hemoglobin A1c, a duration of diabetes less than 5 years, and a clinical course more consistent with an acute kidney injury are more associated with alternative diagnoses.

III. Glycemic Monitoring and Targets

A. Early glycemic control targeting lower HbA1c levels is associated with lower long-term microvascular complications in patients with T2DM, including albuminuria >30 mg/d or >300 mg/d.
B. **Glycemic monitoring** typically occurs *via* HbA1c measurement in accordance with major society guidelines. Patients are also instructed to monitor their fingerstick blood glucose levels at home to better guide the management of glycemic control.
   1. HbA1c represents the average glycemic control over approximately the preceding 3-month span of time.
      a. **The frequency of HbA1c monitoring** depends on the stability of glycemic control. In patients with stable glycemic control who have met their target HbA1c, this should be monitored at least biannually. For individuals who have not achieved target HbA1c, this should be monitored at least every 3 months. HbA1c should also be monitored in any individual for whom treatment has been modified.
      b. **There are some pitfalls to HbA1c.** In patients with advanced kidney disease, decreased red blood cell life span, recent red blood cell transfusion, or use of erythropoietin-stimulating agents may lead to falsely low HbA1c levels. Patients with other conditions that alter red blood cell turnover such as hemolytic anemia, glucose-6-phosphate dehydrogenase deficiency, or pregnancy may also have a falsely low HbA1c. Furthermore, HbA1c represents an "average" glucose control and does not provide insight into hypoglycemia or variability in blood glucose levels.
   2. **Home blood glucose monitoring** is necessary in addition to HbA1c to guide medication titration. KDIGO guidelines suggest this as a means to optimize glycemic control and avoid hypoglycemic episodes.
      a. **Fingerstick blood glucose monitoring** is useful for self-management of T2DM and guides insulin dosing when administered on a sliding scale.
      b. **Continuous glucose monitoring** provides a more comprehensive and detailed assessment than can be obtained from HbA1c or fingerstick blood glucose monitoring. Continuous glucose monitors report additional metrics such as "time in range" and "time below range" (i.e., hypoglycemia) that are associated with complications of diabetes. The ADA recommends targeting a "time in range" of >70% and a "time below range" of 4% for many adults, but these recommendations vary for individuals with increased risk for hypoglycemia.
C. **Glycemic targets** vary between guideline-writing organizations. The ADA recommends an individualized HbA1c target of <7.0% for most patients but allows for a goal as relaxed as <8.0% for those with advanced CKD, known

microvascular complications of T2DM, limited life expectancy, high risk of hypoglycemia, patient preference, or lack of resources and support system. KDIGO recommends an individualized target HbA1c between <6.5% and <8.0%, based on similar factors. These guidelines are generally based on the benefits of intensive glucose control seen for microvascular complications of diabetes, balanced with the increased risk of hypoglycemia and death seen with intensive blood glucose control in patients with kidney disease in the action to control cardiovascular risk in diabetes (ACCORD) trial.

IV. Lifestyle counseling should be offered to patients with T2DM and CKD, per the KDIGO guidelines.
  A. **Diet** is a complex phenomenon that is affected by cultural, socioeconomic, social, health, and personal factors. It is complex to change, and shared decision-making is key to counseling patients about diet. Dietary recommendations for patients with T2DM and CKD focus on eating an individualized diet rich in plant-based foods, such as vegetables, fruits, whole grains, fiber, legumes, and nuts. Consumption of processed meats, refined carbohydrates, and sweetened beverages should be low.
  1. **Intake of <2,000 mg of sodium per day** is recommended to decrease blood pressure and the risk of cardiovascular disease, stroke, and CKD progression.
  2. **Protein intake of 0.8 g of protein per kg of body weight for day** is recommended for patients not receiving dialysis, and 1.0 to 1.2 g of protein per kg of body weight per day for patients on dialysis.
  B. **Moderate-intensity physical activity for at least 150 minutes per week** has known health benefits. Lower levels of physical activity are associated with increased risk of atherosclerotic cardiovascular disease (ASCVD) and death. Individualized recommendations for physical activity should take into account the patient's age, comorbidities, access to resources, and preferences to incorporate both exercise intensity and type of exercise in a plan that will work for the patient.
  C. **Weight loss** counseling for patients with obesity, diabetes, and CKD should be considered, as this may decrease albuminuria and blood pressure. Achieving recommended body weight has also been shown to complement pharmacologic therapy for glycemic control in patients with T2DM.
  D. **Smoking cessation** has numerous well-known health benefits and is a key part of lifestyle recommendations for patients with T2DM and CKD who use tobacco products.

V. Pharmacologic management in patients with diabetes and CKD aims to achieve individualized glycemic target, achieve individualized blood pressure target, and reduce ASCVD risk. A summary of the KDIGO 2022 clinical practice guideline recommendations for the pharmacologic management of patients with T1DM and CKD is shown in Figure 18-2A, and for patients with T2DM and CKD is shown in Figure 18-2B. The guiding principle behind the recommendations is that patients should preferentially receive agents that improve cardiovascular and kidney outcomes (Table 18-3).
  A. **Glycemic Control in Patients With T1DM**
  1. **Early glycemic control targeting lower HbA1c levels** is associated with lower long-term microvascular complications in patients with T1DM. In the diabetes control and complications trial (DCCT), intensive therapy aimed at achieving a goal HbA1c <6.05% reduced the incidence of albuminuria ≥30 mg/d or ≥300 mg/d, eGFR <60 mL/min/1.73 m^2, and hypertension compared to standard therapy at the time, which entailed preventing symptomatic hyperglycemia and hypoglycemia with one or two daily injections of insulin.
  2. **Insulin** is the primary medical therapy for glycemic control in patients with T1DM. The pathophysiology of T1DM centers around a primary

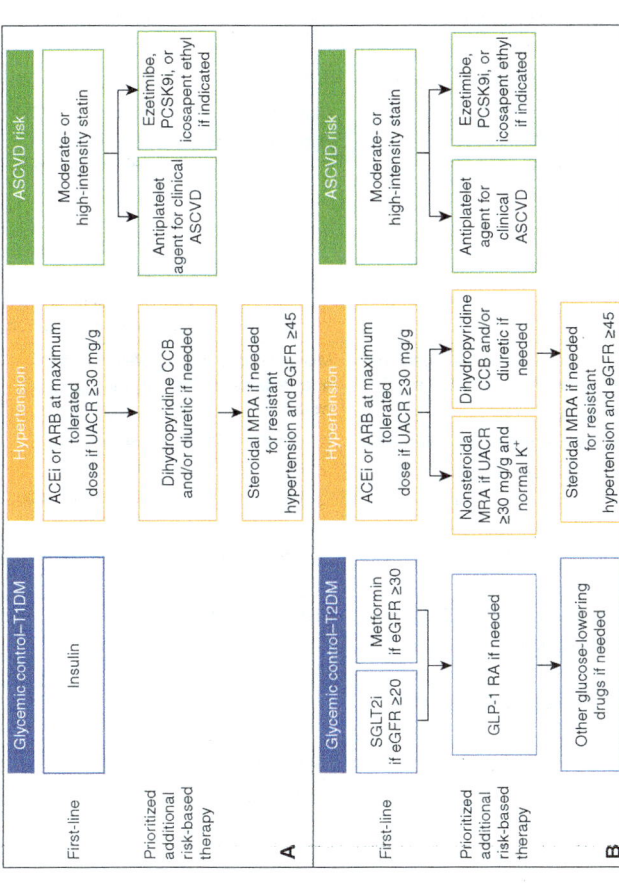

Figure 18-2. Summary of KDIGO 2022 Clinical Practice Guideline recommendations for pharmacologic management in patients with CKD and T1DM (**A**) and T2DM (**B**). Abbreviations: ACEi, angiotensin-converting enzyme inhibitor; ASCVD, atherosclerotic cardiovascular disease; ARB, angiotensin receptor blocker; CCB, calcium channel blocker; eGFR, estimated glomerular filtration rate (in mL/min/1.73 m²); GLP-1 RA, glucagon-like peptide-1 receptor agonist; MRA, mineralocorticoid receptor antagonist; PCSK9i, proprotein convertase subtilisin/kexin type 9 inhibitor; SGLT2i, sodium-glucose co-transporter 2 inhibitor; UACR, urine albumin-to-creatinine ratio.

TABLE 18-3 Medication Classes for Glycemic Control in Patients With Diabetes and CKD

Medication Class	Indications for Chronic Use	Contraindications	Additional Benefits
Metformin	Preferred agent for glycemic control in T2DM and CKD Polycystic ovary syndrome Antipsychotic-induced weight gain	eGFR <30 Acute or chronic metabolic acidosis Hypersensitivity	Weight loss Cardiovascular prevention
SGLT2 inhibitor	Preferred agent for glycemic control in T2DM and CKD Heart failure Proteinuria	eGFR <20 Dialysis Hypersensitivity	Weight loss Slowing of CKD progression AKI prevention Decrease in albuminuria Cardiovascular prevention Modest blood pressure reduction
GLP-1 RA	Preferred second-line agent for glycemic control in T2DM and CKD Obesity Cardiovascular disease prevention Nonalcoholic steatohepatitis Polycystic ovary syndrome	Multiple endocrine neoplasia syndrome type 2 Hypersensitivity	Weight loss Cardiovascular prevention Prevention of albuminuria Slowing of CKD progression
DPP4 inhibitor	Glycemic control in T2DM	Hypersensitivity	
TZD	Glycemic control in T2DM Nonalcoholic steatohepatitis	Class III or IV heart failure Hypersensitivity	
Sulfonylurea	Glycemic control in T2DM	Diabetic ketoacidosis T1DM Hypersensitivity	
Insulin	Glycemic control in T2DM Glycemic control in T1DM Gestational diabetes	Hypersensitivity	

AKI, acute kidney injury; CKD, chronic kidney disease; DPP4 inhibitor, dipeptidyl peptidase-4 inhibitor; eGFR, estimated glomerular filtration rate (in mL/min/1.73 m^2); GLP-1 RA, glucagon-like peptide-1 receptor agonist; SGLT2 inhibitor, sodium-glucose co-transporter-2 inhibitor; T1DM, type 1 diabetes mellitus; T2DM, type 2 diabetes mellitus; TZD, thiazolidinedione.

deficiency of insulin, rather than a resistance to insulin as is more commonly seen in T2DM. Most patients with T1DM require multiple daily injections of long- and short-acting insulin or a continuous infusion of insulin to achieve glycemic control.

TABLE 18-4	Considerations for Pharmacologic Agents for Glycemic Control in Patients With T2DM and CKD	
Medication Class	**Dose Adjustment in CKD**	**Kidney Pharmacokinetics**
Metformin	Reduce dose for eGFR 30–45 At eGFR <45 do not initiate treatment	Cleared by the kidneys so elimination half-life is prolonged in CKD
SGLT2 inhibitor	Reduce dose for eGFR <30	Largely excreted in the urine either unchanged or as metabolites
GLP-1 RA	None	Minimally cleared by the kidneys
DPP4 inhibitor	None for linagliptin Saxagliptin, sitagliptin decrease dose for eGFR <45 Alogliptin decrease dose for eGFR <60	Linagliptin minimally cleared by the kidneys Saxagliptin, sitagliptin, alogliptin largely excreted by the kidneys
TZD	None	Low to moderate degree of renal excretion
Sulfonylurea	Conservative dosing	Largely excreted in the urine
Insulin	Dose adjust as needed to target glycemic control	Moderate degree of renal metabolism

CKD, chronic kidney disease; DPP4 inhibitor, dipeptidyl peptidase-4 inhibitor; eGFR, estimated glomerular filtration rate (in mL/min/1.73 m^2); GLP-1 RA, glucagon-like peptide-1 receptor agonist; SGLT2 inhibitor, sodium-glucose co-transporter-2 inhibitor; T2DM, type 2 diabetes mellitus; TZD, thiazolidinedione.

B. Glycemic Control in Patients With T2DM
1. **Indications, contraindications, and dosing** of medications for glycemic control in T2DM have important caveats to consider in patients with CKD (Table 18-4).
2. **Metformin** is in the biguanide class of medications for T2DM and is considered first line for glycemic control in patients with T2DM and CKD with an eGFR ≥30 mL/min/1.73 m^2. In clinical trials, metformin reduced mortality by 36% compared to conventional therapy with diet control alone. It has a lower risk of hypoglycemia than sulfonylureas or insulin. It also decreases cardiovascular risk compared to other medications. The dose should be decreased and treatment should not be initiated in individuals with eGFR <45 mL/min/1.73 m^2. It should be discontinued in individuals with an eGFR <30 mL/min/1.73 m^2 due to an elevated risk of developing lactic acidosis.
3. **Sodium-glucose co-transporter-2 (SGLT2) inhibitors** include canagliflozin, dapagliflozin, empagliflozin, ertugliflozin, and sotagliflozin. They are recommended in patients with T2DM and CKD with an eGFR ≥20 mL/min/1.73 m^2 by both the ADA and KDIGO to reduce cardiovascular events and the progression of kidney disease.
   a. **The mechanism of action of** these oral medications is to inhibit sodium and glucose reabsorption via the SGLT2 cotransporter in the proximal tubule of the nephron. Due to downstream effects likely related in part to increased tubuloglomerular feedback, these agents decrease intraglomerular pressure, albuminuria, and oxidative stress.

b. **They have favorable impact on long-term cardiovascular and kidney outcomes.** In large clinical trials, they consistently decreased the risk of cardiovascular events, CKD progression, and acute kidney injury in patients with and without CKD.
c. **Adverse effects** include diabetic ketoacidosis, lower extremity amputation, and urogenital infections including mycotic infections.
d. **Contraindications** for initiating therapy include hypersensitivity, an eGFR <20 mL/min/1.73 m^2, or dialysis-dependence. Treatment may be continued for those with CKD whose eGFR decreases from ≥20 to <20 mL/min/1.73 m^2 but should be discontinued at the time of dialysis initiation.

4. **Glucagon-like peptide-1 receptor agonists (GLP-1 RAs)** are injectable agents that include dulaglutide, liraglutide, lixisenatide, and semaglutide. The ADA recommends GLP-1 RAs for patients with T2DM and CKD for cardiovascular risk reduction. KDIGO recommends the use of GLP-1 RAs in patients with T2DM and CKD who have not achieved their glycemic target despite use of an SGLT2 inhibitor and metformin (in the absence of contraindications to these).
   a. **The mechanism of action** of this class is to enhance glucose-dependent endogenous insulin secretion by stimulating the incretin hormone pathway. They also increase the sensation of satiety and slow gastric emptying.
   b. **Indications for GLP-1 RAs** include glycemic control, weight loss, and cardiovascular and kidney protection in patients with T2DM.
   c. **They have kidney and cardiovascular protective effects.** In clinical trials, GLP-1 RAs have had favorable impact on cardiovascular events, albuminuria, and the progression of CKD.
   d. **Adverse effects** include discomfort with subcutaneous injection; dose-dependent gastrointestinal symptoms such as nausea, vomiting, and diarrhea; and increased heart rate. The risk of hypoglycemia is low with GLP-1 RAs but can be higher in individuals concomitantly treated with a sulfonylurea or insulin.
   e. **Contraindications** include concomitant medullary thyroid cancer, multiple endocrine neoplasia type 2 (MEN-2), or a history of acute pancreatitis.

5. **Other Glucose-Lowering Drugs**
   a. **Insulin** is a potent glucose-lowering therapy. Long-acting basal insulin and short-acting prandial insulin are often required to achieve adequate glycemic control in patients who require insulin therapy. Per the KDIGO guidelines, it may be a more suitable treatment for individuals who need potent glucose-lowering, who have an eGFR <15 mL/min/1.73 m^2, or who are on dialysis. It is a less suitable medication when prioritizing avoiding injections, avoiding hypoglycemia, weight loss, or cost. Insulin may have a longer half-life in patients with advanced CKD due to decreased metabolism and clearance by the kidneys.
   b. **Dipeptidyl peptidase-4 (DPP4) inhibitors** include alogliptin, linagliptin, saxagliptin, and sitagliptin. KDIGO lists DPP4 inhibitors as more suitable medications for individuals who want to avoid hypoglycemia or injections, but less suitable for prioritizing low cost or potent glucose-lowering effect.
   c. **Sulfonylureas** include glipizide, glimepiride, and glyburide. KDIGO recommends these as more suitable medications for prioritizing low cost or avoiding injections, but less suitable for avoiding hypoglycemia, weight loss, or for use in patients with eGFR <15 mL/min/1.73 m^2 or on dialysis.
   d. **Thiazolidinediones (TZDs)** include pioglitazone and rosiglitazone. KDIGO lists TZDs as a more suitable choice for achieving low cost,

in individuals with eGFR <15 mL/min/1.73 m² or on dialysis, and to avoid injections or hypoglycemia. They are considered less suitable for achieving weight loss, for use in heart failure, or a potent glucose-lowering effect.
- **C. Hypertension** is prevalent in approximately 58% to 70% of patients with diabetes and CKD.
    1. **Blood pressure targets** vary by guideline organization. The KDIGO 2021 Blood Pressure in CKD Guideline recommends a systolic blood pressure target <120 mmHg using standardized blood pressure measurements for patients with nondialysis CKD. The Kidney Disease Outcomes Quality Initiative (KDOQI) commentary on the KDIGO guideline recommends a systolic blood pressure <130 mmHg in patients with diabetes and CKD. The American College of Cardiology/American Heart Association (ACC/AHA) 2017 guidelines recommend a goal blood pressure <130/80 mmHg for patients with CKD. The Eighth Joint National Committee (JNC8) recommended a target of <140/90 mmHg.
    2. **Renin-angiotensin-aldosterone system (RAAS) blockade** with an angiotensin-converting enzyme inhibitor (ACEi) or angiotensin receptor blocker (ARB) is considered first-line treatment for hypertension for patients with a urine albumin-to-creatinine ratio ≥30 mg/g. Reduction of albuminuria is one of the cornerstones of decreasing cardiovascular risk in patients with diabetes and CKD. RAAS blockade with ACEi or ARB is a critical intervention to decrease albuminuria, decrease cardiovascular risk, and slow the progression of CKD in patients with diabetes.
        a. **There is an expected dip in the eGFR** after initiation or dose escalation of an ACEi or ARB due to hemodynamic effects in the glomerulus. Creatinine and eGFR should be checked 2 to 4 weeks after initiation or dose increase. It is acceptable for the serum creatinine to increase by up to 30% and continue treatment. If the serum creatinine increases by >30% in the absence of an alternative explanation or if mitigation strategies fail to improve eGFR, ACEi or ARB treatment should be discontinued or reduced to the previously tolerated lower dose.
        b. **Dual therapy with both an ACEi and an ARB is not recommended.** Trials showed that combined ACEi and ARB therapy did not improve cardiovascular outcomes but did increase the risk of hyperkalemia and acute kidney injury.
    3. **Additional medications** for hypertension are indicated based on comorbidities or to achieve blood pressure target.
        a. **Thiazide or loop diuretics** may be indicated for patients with volume overload or heart failure.
        b. **Beta blockers** are indicated for patients with heart failure with reduced ejection fraction.
        c. **Calcium channel blockers** may be indicated for patients with Raynaud's.
    4. **Mineralocorticoid receptor antagonists (MRAs)** are indicated for the management of hypertension that is not at goal despite maximally tolerated doses of three antihypertensive agents.
        a. **Steroidal MRAs** such as spironolactone or eplerenone are indicated for patients with resistant hypertension and an eGFR ≥45 mL/min/1.73 m². These agents are also indicated for the treatment of heart failure and hyperaldosteronism in this patient population.
        b. **Nonsteroidal MRAs** such as finerenone have been shown to have cardiovascular and kidney benefits for patients with T2DM. KDIGO recommends their use for patients with T2DM and CKD with an eGFR ≥25 mL/min/1.73 m², a urine albumin-to-creatinine ratio ≥30 mg/g despite use of other first-line treatments, and a serum potassium level

within normal limits. These can be added to maximum tolerated dose of an ACEi or ARB and an SGLT2 inhibitor. Potassium should be regularly monitored on these agents to assess for hyperkalemia.

   i. **Cardiovascular protective effects** of finerenone compared to placebo in patients with CKD and T2DM were studied in the Finerenone in Reducing Kidney Failure and Disease Progression in Diabetic Kidney Disease (FIDELIO-DKD) and Finerenone in Reducing Cardiovascular Mortality and Morbidity in Diabetic Kidney Disease (FIGARO-DKD) trials. Finerenone decreased the hazard of the composite cardiovascular outcome of death from cardiovascular causes, nonfatal myocardial infarction, nonfatal stroke, or hospitalization for heart failure compared to placebo.
   ii. **Kidney protective effects** of finerenone compared to placebo were also demonstrated in FIDELO-DKD and in the Finerenone in CKD and Type 2 Diabetes: Combined FIDELIO-DKD and FIGARO-DKD Trial Programme Analysis (FIDELITY), which was the pooled analysis of FIDELIO-DKD and FIGARO-DKD. The kidney composite outcomes of kidney failure, a sustained ≥40% or ≥57% decrease in eGFR, or renal death were lower in the finerenone group.

D. ASCVD Risk
   1. **Lipid-lowering therapy** with statins is recommended as secondary prevention in patients with cardiovascular disease or as primary prevention for patients who are ≥40 years of age with concomitant diabetes, nondialysis CKD stages 1 to 4, or kidney transplantation. Patients on chronic dialysis may continue taking a previously prescribed statin but should not initiate treatment with this.
   2. **Antiplatelet agents** such as aspirin are recommended for secondary prevention in patients with established cardiovascular disease or primary prevention in high-risk individuals (if potential benefit outweighs the risk of bleeding). Dual antiplatelet therapy is recommended for patients with acute coronary syndrome or percutaneous coronary intervention.

VI. Conclusions

The prevalence of diabetes and CKD are both rising, and increasingly these conditions affect patients concomitantly. Appropriate diagnosis of the etiology of kidney disease is critical to the management of the patient with diabetes and CKD. Important caveats to diagnostic and treatment considerations can impact clinical decision-making for patients with kidney disease. The comprehensive management of patients with diabetes and CKD includes lifestyle counseling, glycemic control, management of hypertension, and other interventions to decrease ASCVD risk, with an overarching prioritization of therapies that improve cardiovascular and kidney outcomes, including RAAS inhibitors, metformin, SGLT2 inhibitors, and GLP-1 receptor agonists.

SUGGESTED READINGS

ADVANCE Collaborative Group; Patel A, MacMahon S, Chalmers J, et al. Intensive blood glucose control and vascular outcomes in patients with type 2 diabetes. *N Engl J Med.* 2008;358(24):2560–2572.

Agarwal R, Filippatos G, Pitt B, et al; FIDELIO-DKD and FIGARO-DKD investigators. Cardiovascular and kidney outcomes with finerenone in patients with type 2 diabetes and chronic kidney disease: the FIDELITY pooled analysis. *Eur Heart J.* 2022;43(6):474–484.

Agrawal L, Azad N, Bahn GD, et al; VADT Study Group. Long-term follow-up of intensive glycaemic control on renal outcomes in the Veterans Affairs Diabetes Trial (VADT). *Diabetologia.* 2018;61(2):295–299.

Alexandrou M-E, Papagianni A, Tsapas A, et al. Effects of mineralocorticoid receptor antagonists in proteinuric kidney disease: a systematic review and meta-analysis of randomized controlled trials. *J Hypertens.* 2019;37(12):2307–2324.

Alvarez CA, Halm EA, Pugh MJV, et al. Lactic acidosis incidence with metformin in patients with type 2 diabetes and chronic kidney disease: a retrospective nested case-control study. *Endocrinol Diabetes Metab*. 2021;4(1):e00170.

Bakris GL, Agarwal R, Anker SD, et al. Effect of finerenone on chronic kidney disease outcomes in type 2 diabetes. *N Engl J Med*. 2020;383(23):2219–2229.

Bhatt DL, Szarek M, Steg PG, et al. Sotagliflozin in patients with diabetes and recent worsening heart failure. *N Engl J Med*. 2021;384(2):117–128.

Brenner BM, Cooper ME, de Zeeuw D, et al; RENAAL Study Investigators. Effects of losartan on renal and cardiovascular outcomes in patients with type 2 diabetes and nephropathy. *N Engl J Med*. 2001;345(12):861–869.

Cannon CP, Pratley R, Dagogo-Jack S, et al; VERTIS CV Investigators. Cardiovascular outcomes with ertugliflozin in type 2 diabetes. *N Engl J Med*. 2020;383(15):1425–1435.

Chemouny JM, Bobot M, Sannier A, et al. Kidney biopsy in type 2 diabetes: a multicenter cross-sectional study. *Am J Nephrol*. 2021;52(2):131–140.

Cosentino F, Grant PJ, Aboyans V, et al. 2019 ESC Guidelines on diabetes, pre-diabetes, and cardiovascular diseases developed in collaboration with the EASD. *Eur Heart J*. 2020;41(2):255–323.

Cowie MR, Fisher M. SGLT2 inhibitors: mechanisms of cardiovascular benefit beyond glycaemic control. *Nat Rev Cardiol*. 2020;17(12):761–772.

DCCT/EDIC Research Group. Effect of intensive diabetes treatment on albuminuria in type 1 diabetes: long-term follow-up of the diabetes control and complications trial and epidemiology of diabetes interventions and complications study. *Lancet Diabetes Endocrinol*. 2014;2(10):793–800.

DCCT/EDIC Research Group; de Boer IH, Sun W, Cleary PA, et al. Intensive diabetes therapy and glomerular filtration rate in type 1 diabetes. *N Engl J Med*. 2011;365(25):2366–2376.

Drawz PE, Beddhu S, Bignall ONR 2nd, et al. KDOQI US commentary on the 2021 KDIGO clinical practice guideline for the management of blood pressure in CKD. *Am J Kidney Dis*. 2022;79(3):311–327.

ElSayed NA, Aleppo G, Aroda VR, et al. 11. Chronic kidney disease and risk management: standards of care in diabetes-2023. *Diabetes Care*. 2023;46(Suppl 1):S191–S202.

ElSayed NA, Aleppo G, Aroda VR, et al. 2. Classification and diagnosis of diabetes: standards of care in diabetes-2023. *Diabetes Care*. 2023;46(Suppl 1):S19–S40.

ElSayed NA, Aleppo G, Aroda VR, et al. 6. Glycemic targets: standards of care in diabetes-2023. *Diabetes Care*. 2023;46(Suppl 1):S97–S110.

ElSayed NA, Aleppo G, Aroda VR, et al. 9. Pharmacologic approaches to glycemic treatment: standards of care in diabetes-2023. *Diabetes Care*. 2023;46(Suppl 1):S140–S157.

ElSayed NA, Aleppo G, Aroda VR, et al. Standards of care in diabetes-2023. *Diabetes Care*. 2023;46(Suppl 1):S140–S157.

Fried LF, Emanuele N, Zhang JH, et al; VA NEPHRON-D Investigators. Combined angiotensin inhibition for the treatment of diabetic nephropathy. *N Engl J Med*. 2013;369(20):1892–903.

Fu EL, D'Andrea E, Wexler DJ, Patorno E, Paik JM. Safety of sodium-glucose cotransporter-2 inhibitors in patients with CKD and type 2 diabetes: population-based US cohort study. *Clin J Am Soc Nephrol*. 2023;18(5):592–601.

Gerstein HC, Colhoun HM, Dagenais GR, et al; REWIND Investigators. Dulaglutide and cardiovascular outcomes in type 2 diabetes (REWIND): a double-blind, randomised placebo-controlled trial. *Lancet*. 2019;394(10193):121–130.

Heerspink HJL, Oshima M, Zhang H, et al. Canagliflozin and kidney-related adverse events in type 2 diabetes and CKD: findings from the randomized CREDENCE trial. *Am J Kidney Dis*. 2022;79(2):244–256 e1.

Heerspink HJL, Stefansson BV, Correa-Rotter R, et al. Dapagliflozin in patients with chronic kidney disease. *N Engl J Med*. 2020;383(15):1436–1446.

Ismail-Beigi F, Craven T, Banerji MA, et al; ACCORD trial group. Effect of intensive treatment of hyperglycaemia on microvascular outcomes in type 2 diabetes: an analysis of the ACCORD randomised trial. *Lancet*. 2010;376(9739):419–430.

James PA, Oparil S, Carter BL, et al. 2014 evidence-based guideline for the management of high blood pressure in adults: report from the panel members appointed to the Eighth Joint National Committee (JNC 8). *JAMA*. 2014;311(5):507–520.

Kidney Disease: Improving Global Outcomes Blood Pressure Work G. KDIGO 2021 clinical practice guideline for the management of blood pressure in chronic kidney disease. *Kidney Int*. 2021;99(3S):S1–S87.

Kidney Disease: Improving Global Outcomes Diabetes Work G. KDIGO 2022 clinical practice guideline for diabetes management in chronic kidney disease. *Kidney Int*. 2022;102(5S):S1–S127.

Kristensen SL, Rorth R, Jhund PS, et al. Cardiovascular, mortality, and kidney outcomes with GLP-1 receptor agonists in patients with type 2 diabetes: a systematic review and meta-analysis of cardiovascular outcome trials. *Lancet Diabetes Endocrinol.* 2019;7(10):776–785.

Laiteerapong N, Ham SA, Gao Y, et al. The legacy effect in type 2 diabetes: impact of early glycemic control on future complications (the diabetes & aging study). *Diabetes Care.* 2019;42(3):416–426.

Lazarus B, Wu A, Shin JI, et al. Association of metformin use with risk of lactic acidosis across the range of kidney function: a community-based cohort study. *JAMA Intern Med.* 2018;178(7):903–910.

Lewis EJ, Hunsicker LG, Clarke WR, et al. Renoprotective effect of the angiotensin-receptor antagonist irbesartan in patients with nephropathy due to type 2 diabetes. *N Engl J Med.* 2001;345(12):851–860.

Mann JFE, Orsted DD, Brown-Frandsen K, et al. Liraglutide and renal outcomes in type 2 diabetes. *N Engl J Med.* 2017;377(9):839–848.

Marso SP, Bain SC, Consoli A, et al; SUSTAIN-6 Investigators. Semaglutide and cardiovascular outcomes in patients with type 2 diabetes. *N Engl J Med.* 2016;375(19):1834–1844.

Marso SP, Daniels GH, Brown-Frandsen K, et al. Liraglutide and cardiovascular outcomes in type 2 diabetes. *N Engl J Med.* 2016;375(4):311–322.

McMurray JJV, Solomon SD, Inzucchi SE, et al. Dapagliflozin in patients with heart failure and reduced ejection fraction. *N Engl J Med.* 2019;381(21):1995–2008.

Navaneethan SD, Zoungas S, Caramori ML, et al. Diabetes management in chronic kidney disease: synopsis of the KDIGO 2022 clinical practice guideline update. *Ann Intern Med.* 2023;176(3):381–387.

Neal B, Perkovic V, Mahaffey KW, et al. Canagliflozin and cardiovascular and renal events in type 2 diabetes. *N Engl J Med.* 2017;377(7):644–657.

ONTARGET Investigators; Yusuf S, Teo KK, Pogue J, et al. Telmisartan, ramipril, or both in patients at high risk for vascular events. *N Engl J Med.* 2008;358(15):1547–1559.

Pandey A, Garg S, Khunger M, et al. Dose-response relationship between physical activity and risk of heart failure: a meta-analysis. *Circulation.* 2015;132(19):1786–1794.

Papademetriou V, Lovato L, Doumas M, et al; ACCORD Study Group. Chronic kidney disease and intensive glycemic control increase cardiovascular risk in patients with type 2 diabetes. *Kidney Int.* 2015;87(3):649–659.

Parving HH, Lehnert H, Brochner-Mortensen J, Gomis R, Andersen S, Arner P; Irbesartan in Patients with Type 2 Diabetes and Microalbuminuria Study Group. The effect of irbesartan on the development of diabetic nephropathy in patients with type 2 diabetes. *N Engl J Med.* 2001; 345(12):870–878.

Perkovic V, Heerspink HL, Chalmers J, et al; ADVANCE Collaborative Group. Intensive glucose control improves kidney outcomes in patients with type 2 diabetes. *Kidney Int.* 2013; 83(3):517–523.

Perkovic V, Jardine MJ, Neal B, et al; CREDENCE Trial Investigators. Canagliflozin and renal outcomes in type 2 diabetes and nephropathy. *N Engl J Med.* 2019;380(24):2295–2306.

Perkovic V, Tuttle KR, Rossing P, et al; FLOW Trial Committees and Investigators. Effects of Semaglutide on Chronic Kidney Disease in Patients with Type 2 Diabetes. *N Engl J Med.* 2024; 391(5):109–121.

Pfeffer MA, Claggett B, Diaz R, et al; ELIXA Investigators. Lixisenatide in patients with type 2 diabetes and acute coronary syndrome. *N Engl J Med.* 2015;373(23):2247–2257.

Pitt B, Filippatos G, Agarwal R, et al; FIGARO-DKD Investigators. Cardiovascular events with finerenone in kidney disease and type 2 diabetes. *N Engl J Med.* 2021;385(24):2252–2263.

Sanghavi SF, Roark T, Zelnick LR, et al. Histopathologic and clinical features in patients with diabetes and kidney disease. *Kidney360.* 2020;1(11):1217–1225.

Sattelmair J, Pertman J, Ding EL, Kohl HW 3rd, Haskell W, Lee IM. Dose response between physical activity and risk of coronary heart disease: a meta-analysis. *Circulation.* 2011;124(7): 789–795.

Stevens PE, Levin A; Kidney Disease: Improving Global Outcomes Chronic Kidney Disease Guideline Development Work Group M. Evaluation and management of chronic kidney disease: synopsis of the kidney disease: improving global outcomes 2012 clinical practice guideline. *Ann Intern Med.* 2013;158(11):825–830.

The EMPA-KIDNEY Collaborative Group; Herrington WG, Staplin N, Wanner C, et al. Empagliflozin in patients with chronic kidney disease. *N Engl J Med.* 2023;388(2):117–127.

UK Prospective Diabetes Study (UKPDS) Group. Effect of intensive blood-glucose control with metformin on complications in overweight patients with type 2 diabetes (UKPDS 34). UK Prospective Diabetes Study (UKPDS) Group. *Lancet.* 1998;352(9131):854–865.

UK Prospective Diabetes Study (UKPDS) Group. Intensive blood-glucose control with sulphonylureas or insulin compared with conventional treatment and risk of complications in patients with type 2 diabetes (UKPDS 33). *Lancet.* 1998;352(9131):837-853.

United States Renal Data System. 2022 USRDS annual data report: ckd in the general population. Accessed March 9, 2023. https://usrds-adr.niddk.nih.gov/2022/chronic-kidney-disease/1-ckd-in-the-general-population

United States Renal Data System. 2022 USRDS annual data report: identification and care of patients with CKD. Accessed March 9, 2023. https://usrds-adr.niddk.nih.gov/2022/chronic-kidney-disease/2-identification-and-care-of-patients-with-ckd

Whelton PK, Carey RM, Aronow WS, et al. 2017 ACC/AHA/AAPA/ABC/ACPM/AGS/APhA/ASH/ASPC/NMA/PCNA Guideline for the prevention, detection, evaluation, and management of high blood pressure in adults: executive summary: a report of the American College of Cardiology/American Heart Association Task Force on Clinical Practice guidelines. *Circulation.* 2018;138(17):e426-e483.

Wiviott SD, Raz I, Bonaca MP, et al; DECLARE–TIMI 58 Investigators. Dapagliflozin and cardiovascular outcomes in type 2 diabetes. *N Engl J Med.* 2019;380(4):347-357.

Zinman B, Wanner C, Lachin JM, et al. Empagliflozin, cardiovascular outcomes, and mortality in type 2 diabetes. *N Engl J Med.* 2015;373(22):2117-2128.

Zoungas S, Arima H, Gerstein HC, et al; Collaborators on Trials of Lowering Glucose (CONTROL) group. Effects of intensive glucose control on microvascular outcomes in patients with type 2 diabetes: a meta-analysis of individual participant data from randomised controlled trials. *Lancet Diabetes Endocrinol.* 2017;5(6):431-437.

Zoungas S, Chalmers J, Neal B, et al; ADVANCE-ON Collaborative Group. Follow-up of blood-pressure lowering and glucose control in type 2 diabetes. *N Engl J Med.* 2014;371(15):1392-1406.

19 The Patient With Cancer and Kidney Involvement

Mitchell H. Rosner, Amanda DeMauro Renaghan

The field of onconephrology encompasses the intersection of nephrology with oncology and highlights the important needs of patients who have cancer and kidney disease in its many forms (Fig. 19-1). These intersections are complex and are expanding and changing at a rapid rate largely due to advances in the therapies utilized to treat cancer. Examples of these include various kidney diseases associated with hematopoietic stem cell transplantation (HSCT), kidney-related effects of chemotherapeutic agents and immunotherapies, and numerous electrolyte abnormalities associated with either the cancer or its therapies. An important consideration is the intersection of chronic kidney disease (CKD) with the heightened risk for development of certain cancers (especially those of the urogenital tract) as well as its impact on therapeutic decision-making and dosing of chemotherapeutic agents. Broadly, the mission of onconephrology is to help cancer teams identify, treat, and, if possible, prevent kidney-related complications and diseases. In addition, while data are currently lacking, it is hoped that such a multidisciplinary focus will result in improved outcomes.

Incidence and Prevalence of Kidney Diseases in Patients With Cancer

Patients with cancer may develop acute kidney injury (AKI) or may have preexisting CKD (defined as abnormalities of kidney function or structure present for more than 3 months) that impacts their care or worsens during therapy. In fact, CKD is present in a substantial number of patients with cancer. This is likely due to common comorbid conditions, such as diabetes mellitus and hypertension that lead to CKD and are present in patients with cancer. In addition, CKD may be directly associated with a higher risk for certain malignancies, especially those of the urinary tract.

Two large observational studies have demonstrated that nearly 50% of patients with cancer had an estimated glomerular filtration rate (eGFR) <90 mL/min/1.73 m². More severe CKD such as stage 3 (eGFR, 30 to 59 mL/min/1.73 m²) CKD was found in 12% of cancer patients, and <1% of patients had stage 4 (eGFR, 15 to 29 mL/min/1.73 m²) CKD. In another study of 4,077 patients with various forms of cancer, 30% had an eGFR of <60 mL/min/1.73 m², and 8.3% had an eGFR of 45 mL/min/1.73 m². Thus, a substantial proportion of the cancer population had clinically significant CKD that might affect care (such as need for modified drug dosing, being excluded from receiving some therapies, or being excluded from clinical trials that often include eGFR below a certain threshold as an exclusion criteria). Other studies have shown an even higher prevalence of CKD; for instance, only 38.6% of patients with breast cancer, 38.9% of patients with lung cancer, 38.3% of patients with prostate cancer, 27.5% of patients with gynecologic cancer, and 27.2% of patients with colorectal cancer had an eGFR ≥90 mL/min/1.73 m² at the time of therapy initiation. Importantly, CKD in patients who have cancer is associated with reduced survival. Several studies have demonstrated that stage 3 or 4 CKD is associated with an approximately 12% to 27% higher risk for death compared with patients who have cancer with normal eGFR. As an example, in a cohort of 8,223 patients who had cancer, cancer-specific mortality had an adjusted hazard ratio (aHR) of 1.12 for those with an eGFR of 30 to 59 mL/min/1.73 m² (95% CI, 1.01–1.26; P = .04) and an aHR of 1.75 for those with an eGFR <30 mL/min/1.73 m² (95% CI, 1.32–2.32; P < .001).

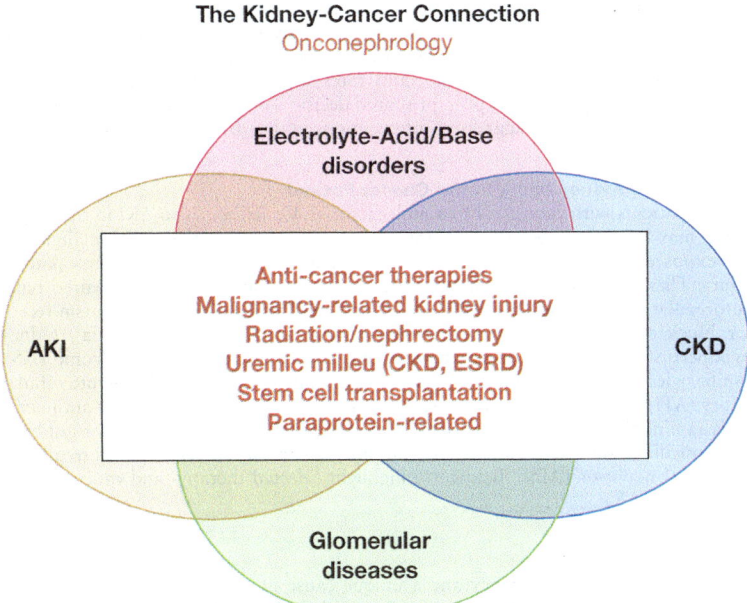

Figure 19-1. Onconephrology. Onconephrology encompasses the various forms of kidney disease that may be encountered in the patient with cancer. This may include: acute kidney injury (AKI), chronic kidney disease (CKD), and end-stage renal disease (ESRD) as well as electrolyte and acid–base disorders. These various manifestations of kidney disease may be caused by the cancer itself, anticancer therapies, or radiation, be related to a paraprotein, or occur after nephrectomy or stem cell transplantation.

The reasons for the higher mortality rate with CKD remain uncertain, but speculation is that CKD may limit options for chemotherapy and access to clinical trials. In addition, dosing of several chemotherapeutic agents is changed in CKD, and this may lower efficacy and increase the risk of side effects. Further, comorbidities associated with CKD, such as diabetes mellitus, hypertension, and heart failure, also play a large role in the excess mortality seen in this group.

AKI, as defined by the Kidney Disease Improving Global Outcomes (KDIGO) or other older AKI grading systems, is also a common occurrence in patients with cancer. For instance, in a study from Denmark of 1.2 million people, there were 37,267 patients with incident cancer between 1999 and 2006. Over a 5-year period, 27% of patients developed AKI (here, defined as an increase >50% in serum creatinine), and 7.6% of patients developed severe AKI that required dialysis. The highest risk of AKI was seen in patients with multiple myeloma (MM) and kidney and liver cancer. In another study of 163,071 patients with cancer between 2007 and 2014, AKI requiring dialysis occurred in nearly 1%, with the highest incidence in patients with MM, bladder and kidney cancer, and acute leukemia. A French study investigated the outcomes of patients who were admitted to the intensive care unit (ICU) with a solid organ malignancy and found that KDIGO stage 3 AKI occurred in 26% of patients and 24% of these patients died. The overall AKI rate (all stages) was 59% and the overall mortality rate at 90 days was 37%. The etiologies of AKI in this ICU cohort included sepsis, hypovolemia, urinary tract obstruction, hypercalcemia, and tumor lysis syndrome (TLS) (as discussed in more detail). A consistent finding is that cancer patients in the ICU who develop AKI requiring dialysis have particularly poor outcomes with mortality rates approaching 80% to 90% compared to 10% to 20% for patients without AKI. These high mortality rates in patients with cancer who develop AKI requiring dialysis should prompt shared decision-making and careful assessment of the appropriateness of aggressive interventions in this patient population.

Etiologies of Kidney Injury in the Cancer Patient

AKI in patients with cancer is often multifactorial. Contributors to AKI in this population may be patient-specific or therapy- or cancer-related. Patients with malignancy are exposed to a wide range of insults that may potentiate hemodynamic kidney injury. These include volume depletion (nausea, vomiting, diuretics), impaired renal autoregulation (angiotensin-converting enzyme inhibitors [ACEis], angiotensin receptor blockers [ARBs]), afferent arteriolar vasoconstriction (hypercalcemia), kidney hypoperfusion (cardiomyopathy, hepatorenal syndrome, nephrotic syndrome (NS), capillary leak syndrome), and administration of iodinated contrast dye. Acute tubular injury (ATI) may occur in the context of sepsis or exposure to nephrotoxic antimicrobials (aminoglycosides, amphotericin B, vancomycin). Additionally, use of antibiotics (penicillins, ciprofloxacin) and proton pump inhibitors (PPis) may lead to allergic interstitial nephritis (AIN). Below, we highlight selected therapy- and cancer-related etiologies of AKI.

Tumor Lysis Syndrome

TLS is an oncologic emergency and a unique cause of AKI in patients with cancer. The true frequency of AKI among patients with TLS is unknown and likely varies according to tumor characteristics and coexisting disorders, as well as the chemotherapeutic regimen and preventive measures used. In-hospital mortality associated with TLS approaches 21%, with nearly 70% of patients experiencing a severe complication (such as sepsis, acute respiratory failure, need for mechanical ventilation, cardiac arrest, seizure, or cerebral hemorrhage), and approximately 15% requiring dialysis. TLS typically develops after initiation of anticancer therapy, but may occur spontaneously. Nearly all hematologic and solid organ cancers have been associated with TLS, however, it is much more common in the context of chemosensitive malignancies with large tumor burdens and high proliferative rates (i.e., Burkitt lymphoma, acute lymphoblastic leukemia). Beyond traditional cytotoxic chemotherapy, TLS has been described after administration of several targeted agents (venetoclax, bortezomib, rituximab, BRAF/mitogen-activated protein kinase [MEK] inhibitors), as well after chimeric antigen receptor (CAR) T cell therapy. Importantly, underlying kidney dysfunction predisposes to the development of TLS.

TLS is caused by the release of cellular contents (intracellular electrolytes and nucleic acids) from tumor cells. The syndrome is characterized by the classic findings of hyperuricemia, hyperkalemia, and hyperphosphatemia (with associated secondary hypocalcemia). AKI in this context occurs due to a combination of (1) cytokine release with inflammatory tubular injury; (2) acute uric acid and xanthine nephropathy; and (3) acute nephrocalcinosis due to an elevated calcium-phosphate product. Tumor cell breakdown results in the release of purines, which are converted to intermediate products (i.e., hypoxanthine and xanthine) and subsequently metabolized to insoluble uric acid. Uric acid precipitates in the renal tubules, causing intratubular obstruction and the release of inflammatory mediators ("crystal-dependent pathway"). Additionally, soluble uric acid may augment kidney injury by inducing renal vasoconstriction and stimulating proinflammatory and pro-oxidative mechanisms ("crystal-independent pathway"). TLS is traditionally defined using the Cairo–Bishop criteria (see Table 19-1).

Because TLS is associated with significant morbidity and mortality, all patients with cancer should be assessed for TLS risk prior to therapy. Prophylaxis against TLS

TABLE 19-1	Cairo–Bishop Criteria for Diagnosis of Tumor Lysis Syndrome

Lab tumor lysis syndrome

≥2 of the following criteria achieved in the same 24-h period from 3 d before to 7 d after chemotherapy initiation:

- Uric acid 25% increase from baseline or ≥8.0 mg/dL
- Potassium 25% increase from baseline or ≥6.0 mEq/L
- Phosphorus 25% increase from baseline or ≥4.5 mg/dL (≥6.5 mg/dL in children)
- Calcium 25% decrease from baseline or ≤7.0 mg/dL

Clinical tumor lysis syndrome

Laboratory tumor lysis syndrome + ≥1 of the following:

- Creatinine ≥1.5 times the upper limit of normal of an age-adjusted reference range[a]
- Seizure
- Cardiac arrhythmia or sudden death

[a]Alternative causes of acute kidney injury ruled out.

Adapted from Cairo MS, Bishop M. Tumour lysis syndrome: new therapeutic strategies and classification. *Br J Haematol*. 2004;127(1):3–11.

is recommended for all patients with hematologic malignancies undergoing chemotherapy, and is also recommended for all moderate- and high-risk patients such as those with reduced eGFR, large tumor burdens, and highly chemosensitive tumors. The exact regimen for prophylaxis should be tailored to the clinical situation. TLS may be prevented by maintaining adequate glomerular filtration and high urine flow rates through the administration of intravenous saline; this allows for rapid and effective clearance of uric acid, potassium, and phosphorus. While urinary alkalinization increases uric acid solubility, this practice is no longer recommended, as it can increase calcium phosphate precipitation.

The use of a xanthine oxidase inhibitor (typically allopurinol) should be considered in patients with moderate to severe risk of TLS. Importantly, these drugs increase xanthine oxidase production, a risk factor for xanthine oxidase nephropathy, and decrease uric acid formation, with no reduction in high preexisting uric acid levels. Allopurinol should be started at least 24 to 48 hours prior to initiation of anticancer therapy. Dose reduction is recommended in patients with a creatinine clearance below 20 mL/min; caution should be used with higher doses in the setting of AKI. Side effects of allopurinol include fever, rash, eosinophilia, hypersensitivity reactions, Stevens–Johnson syndrome, hepatitis, and AIN. Febuxostat, a nonpurine analog xanthine oxidase inhibitor, may be considered in patients with a history of allopurinol intolerance.

Patients with hyperuricemia or high risk for TLS may benefit from prophylactic administration of rasburicase, a recombinant urate oxidase enzyme that converts uric acid to more soluble allantoin, rapidly lowering plasma uric acid levels. Its use is contraindicated in patients with glucose-6-phosphate dehydrogenase (G6PD) deficiency due to the risk of methemoglobinemia and hemolytic anemia. Screening for G6PD deficiency among high-risk patients is important, but may not be practical in acute settings; when prior screening is not feasible, close monitoring for methemoglobinemia and hemolytic anemia is essential.

Management of established TLS follows similar approaches to prophylaxis, including continued aggressive intravenous hydration, xanthine oxidase inhibition to prevent further uric acid production, and administration of rasburicase to rapidly lower uric acid levels. Diuretics may be used when indicated for volume overload, but are not part of initial TLS management. All patients with TLS require close monitoring. ICU admission should be considered for patients with laboratory TLS and cardiorenal comorbid conditions, as well as those with clinical TLS. Hyperuricemia is rarely an indication for renal replacement therapy (RRT) in the era of rasburicase, however, patients with TLS may require dialysis for management of volume overload, severe hyperkalemia, or severe hyperphosphatemia with refractory hypocalcemia. Continuous renal replacement therapies may be used in the treatment of TLS and have the advantage of avoiding "rebound" metabolic disturbances. For patients in whom hyperphosphatemia is the indication for dialysis, a continuous modality may be preferred due to enhanced removal of phosphate as compared with conventional hemodialysis.

Monoclonal Gammopathies and Kidney Dysfunction

Monoclonal gammopathies (paraproteinemias) are defined by the presence of monoclonal immunoglobulins (MIgs) in the plasma and/or urine that are produced by clonal plasma cells or B lymphocytes. Kidney dysfunction in patients with monoclonal gammopathies may result from abnormal deposition or activity of intact immunoglobulins or immunoglobulin fragments (i.e., light or heavy chains) in the kidney, or may be unrelated to a paraprotein (i.e., hypercalcemia, hyperuricemia, sepsis, side effects of therapy). Symptomatic MM is the most common malignant monoclonal gammopathy, with approximately 20% to 50% of patients presenting with AKI or CKD at time of diagnosis and patients with AKI experiencing higher mortality compared with patients without AKI.

While patients with MM are most prone to develop paraprotein-mediated kidney injury, patients with other malignant monoclonal gammopathies (i.e., symptomatic Waldenström macroglobulinemia and chronic lymphocytic leukemia [CLL], high-grade lymphoma) are also at risk. Additionally, there are associations of paraprotein-driven kidney diseases with monoclonal gammopathies of undetermined significance (MGUS), smoldering MM, smoldering Waldenström macroglobulinemia, monoclonal B cell lymphocytosis, and low-grade lymphoma. These diseases are broadly defined as monoclonal gammopathies of renal significance (MGRS), a group of disorders in which a nephrotoxic MIg is secreted by a *nonmalignant* or *premalignant* plasma cell or B cell clone leading to kidney damage. Despite not meeting previously defined hematologic criteria for treatment of a specific malignancy, patients with MGRS lesions are at high risk of progressive CKD, end-stage kidney disease, and recurrence of kidney disease after transplant if not identified and managed appropriately.

Clinically, patients with paraprotein-mediated kidney diseases may present with AKI, subacute decline in kidney function/CKD, proteinuria/hematuria, or electrolyte disturbances and evidence of tubular dysfunction. The diagnosis of paraprotein-mediated kidney disease is sometimes challenging. Serum protein electrophoresis (SPEP), along with serum immunofixation (SIFE) and quantification of serum free light chains (FLCs), offers a nearly 100% detection rate for MM and a 96% detection rate for amyloid light (AL) amyloidosis. Kidney biopsy should be considered in patients with unexplained kidney dysfunction and coexistent monoclonal gammopathy.

The classification of paraprotein-mediated kidney diseases is complex, and Table 19-2 describes the kidney biopsy findings and clinical presentations for various kidney lesions associated with monoclonal gammopathies. More than one pattern of kidney injury may coexist. Once the renal pathologic diagnosis is made, the next challenge is detecting a clonal cell line responsible for the production of the monoclonal protein. Treatment of MGRS is directed at the underlying plasma cell or B cell clone. If a clonal cell population is eradicated, then renal outcomes are improved. For patients who present with significant fibrosis on kidney biopsy and late-stage CKD, such as stage 4 and 5 disease and/or end-stage renal disease (ESRD), chemotherapy might not be indicated unless a kidney transplant is planned. A complete hematologic response is required before

TABLE 19-2 Selected Paraprotein-Related Kidney Diseases

Kidney Disease	Clinical Manifestations	Key Laboratory and Pathologic Findings
Cast nephropathy	Acute kidney injury, proteinuria	Tubular damage, protein-filled casts, interstitial inflammation, urine dipstick negative for albuminuria
Light chain proximal tubulopathy	Acute kidney injury, Fanconi syndrome	Tubular damage, wasting of phosphate, amino acids, glucose, and bicarbonate in varying degrees
AL/AH amyloidosis	Acute kidney injury or progressive chronic kidney disease with proteinuria +/– nephrotic syndrome	Glomerular and vascular Congo-red positive deposits, 8–12 nm randomly organized fibrils
Light chain deposition disease	Acute kidney injury or progressive chronic kidney disease with proteinuria +/– nephrotic syndrome	Deposition of pathologic light chains in glomeruli, tubules, and vasculature
Heavy chain deposition disease	Acute kidney injury or progressive chronic kidney disease with proteinuria +/– nephrotic syndrome	Deposition of pathologic heavy chains or fragments in glomeruli, tubules, and vasculature
Light and heavy chain deposition disease	Acute kidney injury or progressive chronic kidney disease with proteinuria +/– nephrotic syndrome	Deposition of pathologic light and heavy chains in glomeruli, tubules, and vasculature
Immunotactoid glomerulonephritis	Acute kidney injury or progressive chronic kidney disease with proteinuria +/– nephrotic syndrome	Glomerular deposition of protein fibrils, Congo Red negative, 20–60 nm microtubules
Fibrillary glomerulonephritis	Acute kidney injury or progressive chronic kidney disease with proteinuria +/– nephrotic syndrome	Glomerular deposition of protein fibrils, Congo Red negative, 15–20 nm random microtubules
Proliferative glomerulonephritis with monoclonal immunoglobulin deposits	Acute kidney injury or progressive chronic kidney disease with proteinuria +/– nephrotic syndrome	Glomerular protein deposition

kidney transplantation to prevent recurrence, because most patients with MGRS have a high risk of recurrent renal disease after kidney transplantation.

Light Chain Cast Nephropathy

Light chain cast nephropathy (LCCN; also known as myeloma kidney) is the most common cause of AKI in patients with MM, and is considered a "myeloma-defining event." LCCN has also been (rarely) described in patients with other malignant monoclonal gammopathies in association with high tumor burden and high light chain levels. In LCCN, large amounts of monoclonal light chains bind to Tamm–Horsfall glycoprotein (uromodulin) in the thick ascending loop of Henle, forming obstructing casts and leading to tubulointerstitial inflammation. Another key mechanism of injury is proximal tubular reabsorption of excess FLCs, leading to release of inflammatory cytokines, oxidative stress, apoptosis, and, ultimately, fibrosis. The combination of proximal tubule cell cytotoxicity, increased intraluminal tubular pressure, and tubulointerstitial nephritis lead to AKI.

Risk of LCCN is directly related to the urinary FLC concentration and the pathologic light chain's affinity for uromodulin. Importantly, binding of toxic FLCs to Tamm–Horsfall protein is enhanced in the setting of volume depletion, metabolic acidosis, increased luminal sodium and chloride concentrations (such as with loop diuretic use), hypercalcemia (by way of volume depletion, vasoconstriction, and increased urinary calcium concentration), and the administration of radiocontrast media and nonsteroidal anti-inflammatory agents.

Patients with monoclonal gammopathy and unexplained AKI should undergo quantitative testing of serum FLCs as well as SPEP and 24-hour urine protein electrophoresis (UPEP). Serum FLCs and SPEP identify the presence of pathologic FLCs, while UPEP helps to distinguish LCCN (characterized by a predominance of FLCs [nonalbumin protein] in the urine) from paraprotein-related glomerular diseases (characterized by heavy albuminuria). Although high FLC levels in both the serum and urine are consistent with AKI due to LCCN, kidney biopsy should be considered when the diagnosis is uncertain.

LCCN is an oncologic emergency and should be managed accordingly. Treatment of LCCN involves discontinuation of nephrotoxic agents, correction of hypercalcemia (if present), and intravenous hydration to augment tubular flow and treat preexisting volume depletion. The International Myeloma Working Group recommends adequate *hydration with fluids ($\geq$3 L/d, approximately 2 L/m^2/d) along with close monitoring of* fluid balance, especially in those presenting with reduced urine output and those with preexisting congestive heart failure. Loop diuretics are reserved for those who develop hypervolemia. Hemodialysis may be required in patients with persistent oliguanuria.

Because rapid reduction in serum FLC concentration is critical for improving kidney function in patients with LCCN, systemic chemotherapy should be started immediately, targeting >50% reduction of the involved FLC and an involved FLC level <50 mg/dL by the end of cycle 1. Bortezomib-based regimens are considered standard of care, supported by robust data demonstrating rapid reduction in tumor load with subsequent high overall response rates, renal response rates, and rates of dialysis independence. Bortezomib is typically given with dexamethasone (with or without a third agent depending on patient's age and comorbidities). Based on clinical experience and trial data from the Andromeda study in light chain amyloidosis, some experts advocate for the addition of daratumumab. HSCT appears to be a viable option for patients with renal injury, including those on dialysis. A large series showed excellent hematologic response but low rate of clinically significant kidney recovery or liberation from dialysis.

There is ongoing interest in the use of extracorporeal therapies (plasmapheresis, high-cutoff [HCO] hemodialysis) to rapidly remove FLCs. Based on data from small randomized controlled trials, some experts recommend daily plasmapheresis (along with chemotherapy), however, its use remains controversial. Two key trials have examined the role of HCO hemodialysis for FLC removal. The EuLITE trial, which randomized 90 patients with de novo MM and biopsy-confirmed cast nephropathy to receive HCO versus conventional high-flux hemodialysis, failed to demonstrate improvement in clinical outcomes with the use of HCO hemodialysis; further, HCO hemodialysis was associated with a higher risk of infectious complications, primarily pulmonary infections (31% vs. 9%). In the MYRE trial, HCO hemodialysis resulted in a significantly higher renal recovery at 6 months and 12 months (compared with conventional high-flux hemodialysis), but failed to reach significance at 3 months (primary endpoint, 41.3% vs. 33.3%, $P = .42$). HCO hemodialysis is not recommended on the basis of available data, and its availability is limited in the United States.

Light Chain Proximal Tubulopathy
Light chain proximal tubulopathy (LCPT), sometimes referred to as light chain Fanconi syndrome, is a rare pattern of kidney disease that occurs in the setting of MM and other

monoclonal gammopathies. LCPT results from proximal tubular endocytosis of pathologic monoclonal light chains with intrinsic properties that allow them to resist proteolysis, with or without crystal formation. The endocytosed light chains generate intracellular oxidative stress, activating inflammatory mediators and leading to apoptosis and proximal tubular injury. Significant clinical heterogeneity exists; patients may present with normoglycemic glycosuria, aminoaciduria, uricosuria, hyperphosphaturia (with hypophosphatemia), type II renal tubular acidosis, and slowly progressive CKD or (more rarely) AKI.

The true incidence of LCPT is unknown, as biopsies are likely underperformed in the setting of proximal tubular dysfunction in the absence of significant renal insufficiency and/or proteinuria. Further, this entity poses unique diagnostic challenges, as most patients have no prior diagnosis of paraproteinemia, crystals may not be visible on light microscopy, and light chain inclusions may be undetectable by routine immunofluorescence (necessitating antigen retrieval and contributing to missed or delayed diagnosis). A clinical diagnosis of Fanconi syndrome or pathologic diagnosis of LCPT should prompt thorough and immediate hematologic evaluation, as early treatment with clone-directed therapy and/or HSCT has been shown to improve kidney outcomes. Supportive care is essential, with potassium, phosphorus, and alkali supplementation where indicated.

Paraprotein-Mediated Glomerular Diseases

Although circulating light chains may lead to cast nephropathy with AKI and light chain-associated proximal tubular dysfunction as discussed above, they may also deposit in the glomeruli, leading to organized and nonorganized patterns of immunoglobin deposits that can be seen with electron microscopy. Clinically, these diseases feature proteinuria, NS, microscopic hematuria, hypertension, and/or deterioration of renal function. Glomerular diseases with organized deposits include AL amyloidosis, fibrillary glomerulonephritis, cryoglobulinemic glomerulonephritis, and immunotactoid glomerulonephritis. Nonorganized deposits are features of MI deposition disease (MIDD) and proliferative glomerulonephritis with monoclonal immunoglobulin deposits (PGNMID). Thrombotic microangiopathy (TMA) may also be rarely associated with monoclonal proteins as discussed below.

Thrombotic Microangiopathy in the Cancer Patient

TMA is characterized by microangiopathic hemolytic anemia from red blood cell fragmentation (noted by schistocytes, increased lactate dehydrogenase (LDH), and depressed haptoglobin), thrombocytopenia (platelet count <150,000 mm^3 or >30% reduction from baseline), and end-organ damage, including AKI. Malignancies and their therapies constitute important secondary causes of TMA. HSCT is also associated with TMA as discussed separately (see "Stem Cell Therapy-Associated Kidney Disease"). TMA may present with AKI, new or acute worsening of hypertension, proteinuria, and/or active urinary sediment. AKI is often severe and may ultimately require dialysis. Kidney histology reveals endothelial cell swelling, fibrin thrombi within capillary loops and arterioles, fragmented red blood cells, mesangiolysis, and thickened arterioles and glomerular capillaries.

Certain cancers, especially when metastatic, more frequently cause TMA compared with others—these include mucinous gastric cancers, ovarian cancers, lymphomas, and acute myeloid leukemias. Cancers associated with a monoclonal gammopathy, including plasma cell dyscrasias and B cell lymphoproliferative disorders have also been recognized as being associated with TMA. There are several possible mechanisms for TMA due to malignancy. Mucin-producing adenocarcinomas may directly injure vascular endothelium, impairing production and release of von Willebrand factor. Complement activation can also play a role in the development of cancer-related TMA. While eradication of the cancer is often associated with TMA resolution, TMA may redevelop upon recurrence of some cancers.

Cancer therapies are also relatively common causes of TMA. Drug-induced TMA more closely resembles hemolytic uremic syndrome, and a renal-limited form of TMA is

```
┌──────────────┐      ┌──────────────┐      ┌──────────────┐
│   CANCER-    │      │    DRUG-     │      │  STEM CELL   │
│ ASSOCIATED   │      │ ASSOCIATED   │      │ TRANSPLANT-  │
│     TMA      │      │     TMA      │      │ ASSOCIATED   │
│              │      │              │      │     TMA      │
└──────────────┘      └──────┬───────┘      └──────────────┘
                         ↙       ↘
```

Type I Drug-Associated TMA
- Associated with chemotherapies such as gemcitabine and mitomycin C
- Delayed onset (6–12 months)
- Cumulative risk and dose-related
- Permanent/irreversible
- Likely recurrent with re-challenge
- Arteriolar and glomerular thrombosis
- High mortality and risk of CKD/ESRD
- Therapies generally not effective

Type II Drug-Associated TMA
- Associated with anti-VEGF therapies (bevacizumab)
- Can occur at any time
- Not dose-related
- Reversible; prominent hypertension and variable proteinuria without ESRD
- May be able to re-challenge
- Glomerular thrombosis
- Excellent survival after discontinuation

Figure 19-2. Classification of Thrombotic Microangiopathies (TMA). TMA can be directly associated with cancer or with stem cell transplantation as well as with exposure to medications. Medication-associated TMA is divided into type 1 (due to more traditional chemotherapies and associated with a poor prognosis) and type 2 (associated with blockade of the vascular endothelial growth factor [VEGF] pathway and with a better prognosis).

not unusual with certain drugs. Renal-limited forms of TMA are particularly challenging to diagnose and clinicians need to have a high degree of suspicion and a low threshold for performing a diagnostic kidney biopsy. Direct vascular endothelial injury, increased platelet activation/aggregation, and alternative complement pathway disorders may play a role in drug-induced TMA. Cancer drugs may initiate TMA as a "second hit" in patients with underlying genetic defects in the alternative complement cascade, such as factor H, factor I, factor B, membrane cofactor protein, thrombomodulin, and C3 complement protein. An important category of cancer-associated TMA is due to drug-induced loss or inhibition of vascular endothelial growth factor (VEGF). Other cancer drugs that cause TMA include conventional chemotherapeutics (gemcitabine, mitomycin, cisplatin) and targeted agents (proteasome inhibitors [PIs]). Anticancer drug-induced TMA can be divided into type I (associated with conventional chemotherapies) and type II (associated with anti-VEGF therapies) (Fig. 19-2). Conventional agents (type I) cause more severe, dose-dependent TMA, which is associated with increased morbidity and mortality. For example, gemcitabine-induced TMA is a rare complication (incidence, 0.015% to 0.31%) but is associated with a high mortality rate (range, 40% to 90%). While traditional therapies such as plasma exchange have not been successful in treating gemcitabine-induced TMA, case reports and series suggest that complement inhibition with eculizumab or ravulizumab may be a reasonable choice for treatment of gemcitabine-associated TMA. Mitomycin-associated TMA also develops with increasing drug exposure. Therapy hinges upon mitomycin discontinuation and supportive care; plasmapheresis is ineffective. Cisplatin and carboplatin alone or in various cancer drug combinations have also been associated with TMA. Drug discontinuation and supportive care are the main therapies. TMA associated with VEGF pathway inhibitors (type II) is generally less severe and is associated with better kidney function recovery after drug discontinuation.

Glomerular Diseases Directly Associated With Cancer
Glomerular diseases are associated with many solid and hematologic malignancies. These glomerular lesions are thought to be paraneoplastic; however, in most cases, the

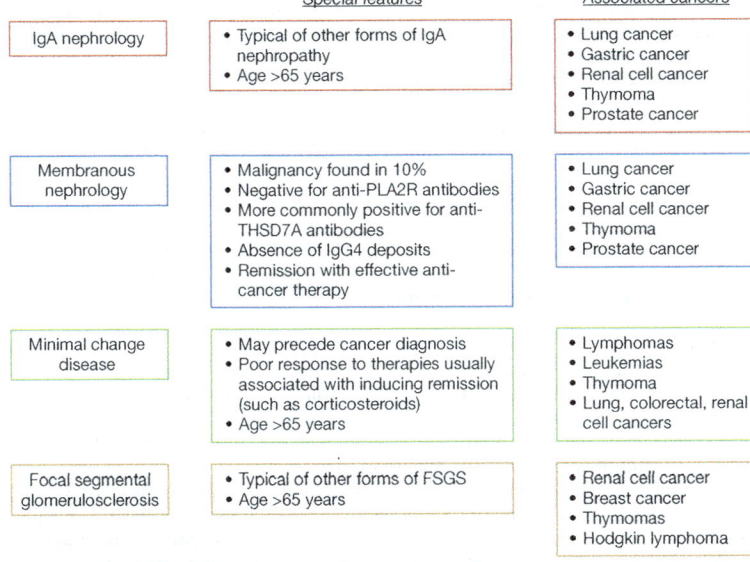

Figure 19-3. Glomerular Diseases Associated With Cancer. The most common glomerular diseases associated with cancer are IgA nephropathy, membranous nephropathy, minimal change disease, and focal segmental glomerulosclerosis (FSGS). Special features in the presentation of these diseases can give clues to an underlying malignancy. PLA2R, phospholipase A2 receptor; THSD7A, thrombospondin type 1 domain-containing 7A.

exact pathogenesis is unclear. The treatment of these cancer-associated glomerular diseases is primarily directed at the underlying malignancy as well as with immunosuppressive therapy in some circumstances. In addition, increased cancer incidence rates are seen among patients with many different types of glomerular diseases that may be related to the use of immunosuppressant drugs. Figure 19-3 summarizes common glomerular diseases (such as IgA nephropathy, membranous nephropathy [MN], minimal change disease (MCD), and focal segmental glomerulosclerosis [FSGS]) and respective cancers that have been associated with pathologies. Below we highlight glomerular diseases secondary to solid tumors, certain hematologic malignancies, and anticancer therapy. Glomerular diseases caused by paraproteins and that occur in the context of HSCT are discussed separately (see "Paraprotein-Mediated Glomerular Diseases" and "Stem Cell Therapy–Associated Kidney Disease").

MN is the most common glomerular pathology described in patients with solid tumors. In the largest systematic review of 240 patients with biopsy-proven MN, reported prevalence of malignancy was 10%. Approximately one-half of these patients had symptoms related to cancer at the time of kidney biopsy and most of these patients were diagnosed with malignancy within a year of MN diagnoses. The solid tumors most commonly associated with MN are lung and gastric cancers, followed by renal cell carcinoma (RCC), prostate cancer, and thymoma. Other cancers reported with MN are colorectal, pancreatic, esophageal, and hepatic carcinomas. Circulating autoantibodies to podocyte transmembrane glycoprotein M-type phospholipase A2 receptor (a marker for primary MN in up to 80% or more of cases) were not found in patients with cancer who had secondary MN and recent studies have shown that antibodies against thrombospondin type 1 domain-containing 7A (THSD7A) may be more likely associated with cancer-related membranous glomerulonephritis. In patients with MN, it is reasonable to perform routine age-appropriate and sex-appropriate screening for malignancy. The risk of cancer persists for >5 years from the time of kidney biopsy.

MCD has been reported in association with solid tumors like lung cancer, colorectal cancer, RCC, and thymoma and rarely in pancreatic, bladder, breast, and ovarian cancers. Of note, MCD is more strongly associated with classic Hodgkin lymphoma, and it can present around the time of diagnosis of lymphoma or preceding it by several months. A poor response to treatment of MCD with steroids, calcineurin inhibitors (CNIs), or rituximab should raise suspicion for a secondary (malignant) cause of MCD. IgA nephropathy can also be associated with cancers such as RCC and solid tumors of the respiratory tract, buccal mucosa, and nasopharynx. Crescentic or rapidly progressive glomerulonephritis has been associated with RCC, gastric cancer, and lung cancer. FSGS has also been reported with classic Hodgkin lymphoma, usually with good a response of both to chemotherapy.

Obstructive AKI

Obstruction is an important etiology of AKI in patients with cancer that may result from intratubular or extratubular causes. Intratubular obstruction may occur due to crystals composed of uric acid, xanthine, or calcium phosphate (as seen in TLS), monoclonal light chains (as seen in LCCN), or crystallization of certain drugs (i.e., *high-dose methotrexate [MTX]) as discussed separately.*

Extrarenal obstruction may result from direct tumor invasion of the urinary tract, external compression by primary or metastatic tumor, or retroperitoneal lymphadenopathy or fibrosis. Prostate, cervical, and bladder tumors account for the majority of cases of malignant urinary tract obstruction, however gastrointestinal cancers, lymphomas, and others have also been implicated. Retroperitoneal fibrosis may occur in patients with certain sarcomas, carcinoid tumors, metastatic solid tumors, lymphomas, or a history of radiation therapy. HSCT recipients are at risk for urinary tract obstruction secondary to hemorrhagic cystitis from medications or viral infections (see "Stem Cell Therapy–Associated Kidney Disease").

Clinical presentation depends on the duration and location of the obstruction; as most cases of malignant obstruction are chronic and progressive, nonspecific symptoms such as lethargy, flank discomfort, bloating, nausea, and vomiting may predominate. The diagnosis of obstructive nephropathy is typically established by imaging (i.e., kidney ultrasound), which usually demonstrates hydronephrosis/hydronephroureter in one or both kidneys. Importantly, dilation of the collecting system may be absent in patients with cancer despite the presence of malignant obstruction, the so-called "nondilated obstruction." Initial management with decompression (percutaneous nephrostomy or ureteral stenting) is typically successful, however complications such as urinary tract infection and recurrent obstruction are common, and overall survival is poor in this population.

Renal Drug Toxicities in the Cancer Patient

Traditional chemotherapies, novel targeted therapies, and evolving immunotherapies have improved survival in patients with cancer. Importantly, the kidneys play critical roles in the metabolism and excretion of many of these agents, and an understanding of the pharmacokinetics of these treatments is essential for ensuring efficacy while avoiding undue renal and systemic toxicities. Dosing may be especially challenging in patients receiving dialysis, as limited data are available with regard to drug processing and elimination. A detailed discussion of appropriate anticancer drug dosing and monitoring is beyond the scope of this chapter; the reader is referred to the recently published *International Consensus Guideline on Anticancer Drug Dosing in Kidney Dysfunction.*

Despite improvements in tolerability, nephrotoxicity remains a significant complication of anticancer treatments, with one study estimating that potentially nephrotoxic drugs were used in 80% of chemotherapy sessions. These medications may affect any segment of the nephron, with diverse manifestations ranging from subclinical increases in serum creatinine to hypertension, frank tubular injury (with associated electrolyte and acid-base disturbances), tubulointerstitial nephritis, glomerular disease, and TMA. Drug-associated TMA, as observed in patients receiving gemcitabine, mitomycin C, anti-VEGF therapies, and others, is described in detail above (see "Thrombotic Microangiopathy in the Cancer Patient"). Critically, drug discontinuation due to nephrotoxicity may limit effective tumor treatment and impact patient outcomes. Given the rapid evolution of novel agents to treat cancer, it is essential that practitioners caring for these patients keep abreast of these important kidney toxicities.

Conventional Chemotherapy

The alkylating agents cyclophosphamide and ifosfamide are well-known causes of hemorrhagic cystitis. Ifosfamide is associated with a much higher incidence of nephrotoxicity, possibly related to greater generation of chloroacetaldehyde and other tubular toxins, as well as greater uptake into proximal tubule cells through organic cation transporter 2 (OCT2), as compared with cyclophosphamide. Kidney biopsy specimens demonstrate acute tubular necrosis (ATN) and mitochondrial toxicity. Risk factors include prior nephrectomy, higher total ifosfamide dose, and coadministration with platinum-based chemotherapies. Clinically, patients present with one or more signs of proximal tubular dysfunction (aminoaciduria, tubular proteinuria, glycosuria, phosphaturia, bicarbonaturia), with or without the full Fanconi syndrome. Published data on the short and long-term kidney complications of ifosfamide exposure come largely from the pediatric literature. Limited adult data document a mean decline in eGFR of 15 mL/min/1.73 m^2 following the first ifosfamide cycle, with a slower but steady decline in eGFR thereafter. Mesna, used for the prevention of cyclophosphamide- and ifosfamide-induced hemorrhagic cystitis, is unfortunately not effective for prevention of ifosfamide nephrotoxicity.

MTX is an antimetabolite that inhibits folate metabolism and ultimately prevents the de novo synthesis of purines and pyrimidines required for DNA and RNA synthesis and the proliferation of many types of cancer cells. High-dose MTX (HD-MTX) therapy, defined as a single dose ≥ 1 g/m^2, is a well-established cause of AKI. Reported incidence of MTX-induced AKI (MTX-AKI) varies widely, with published rates of grade ≥ 2 nephrotoxicity ranging from 1.8% (osteosarcoma) to 10.7% (leukemia/lymphoma), possibly related to differences in host factors, supportive measures, and MTX doses/schedules. Patients with a history of nephrotoxicity after HD-MTX or preexisting CKD are at highest risk of MTX-AKI.

The primary mechanism of MTX-AKI is precipitation of MTX (and its metabolite 7-hydroxymethotrexate) in tubular lumens, leading to intratubular obstruction by crystals and inflammatory interstitial injury; direct cellular injury related to adenosine deaminase activity may also contribute. MTX solubility is pH-dependent, and individuals with acidic urine and low urine volumes are at greater MTX-AKI risk. Additionally, competitive inhibition of the renal tubular secretion of MTX by coadministered medications (probenecid, salicylates, sulfisoxazole, penicillins, nonsteroidal anti-inflammatory drugs) increases risk.

Critically, MTX-AKI leads to impaired MTX clearance and prolonged exposure to toxic MTX concentrations, which may exacerbate nonrenal adverse events such as myelosuppression, mucositis, dermatologic toxicity, and hepatotoxicity. While kidney function typically recovers, the systemic end-organ injury associated with delayed MTX clearance may be life-threatening, and MTX-AKI should be considered an oncologic emergency. In the setting of MTX-AKI, significant damage to renal tubule epithelial cells may have already occurred before the detection of clinically significant increases in serum creatinine concentration, underscoring the need for close monitoring for decreased urine output, an early marker of MTX-AKI.

Because acidic urine and volume depletion are major risk factors for MTX-AKI, alkalinization of the urine and aggressive hydration represent the backbone of prevention.

Discontinuation of drugs that reduce MTX excretion is also crucial. Leucovorin, an active metabolite of folic acid that allows for purine and pyrimidine synthesis in the presence of MTX, should be given to all patients receiving HD-MTX with the goal of "rescuing" nonneoplastic cells. Dosing is guided by serial MTX levels, and timing of leucovorin administration is critical to maximize MTX efficacy while avoiding excess toxicity. When delayed MTX excretion or AKI occurs despite preventive strategies, continued vigorous hydration (with close attention to urine output and cardiopulmonary status) and high-dose leucovorin are employed. Glucarpidase, a recombinant form of the bacterial carboxypeptidase G-2, enzymatically cleaves MTX into nontoxic metabolites and effectively eliminates MTX from the extracellular compartment. Fixed-dose glucarpidase should be considered for patients with 48-hour serum MTX levels >5 μmol/L with increases in serum creatinine >50% from baseline. Importantly, glucarpidase does not reduce intracellular MTX concentrations, and therefore leucovorin must still be provided. High-flux hemodialysis reduces MTX concentrations, however its utility is limited by rebound increases in plasma concentrations, among other limitations.

Cisplatin is associated with cure rates as high as 80% for testicular cancer and prolonged survival for patients with many other solid tumors. Of the platinum-based therapies, cisplatin is associated with the highest risk of AKI, which occurs in approximately 32% of patients receiving a single cisplatin dose. Risk factors include increased age, higher cisplatin dose, history of hypertension, and hypoalbuminemia. Women receiving intraperitoneal cisplatin (vs. intravenous cisplatin) are also at increased AKI risk.

The predominant form of cisplatin-mediated nephrotoxicity is acute toxic tubular injury. Accumulation of cisplatin in renal tubular cells induces DNA damage, mitochondrial damage, oxidative stress, endoplasmic reticulum stress, autophagy, and cell-cycle regulation; these lead to cell death, inflammation, and cell senescence, ultimately contributing to AKI. Cisplatin-mediated vasoconstriction may exacerbate direct cisplatin toxicity by inducing acute ischemia. AKI may be accompanied by tubulopathies, including hypomagnesemia, Fanconi-like syndrome, distal renal tubular acidosis, and renal salt wasting. Cases of cisplatin-induced TMA have also been reported, either when used alone or in combination with other chemotherapeutic agents.

Several strategies have been investigated for the prevention of cisplatin-mediated AKI, however, data from well-designed randomized trials are lacking. At this time, administration of isotonic saline remains the cornerstone of prevention. Interestingly, there is evidence that hypomagnesemia may potentiate or exacerbate AKI, and a recent small pilot randomized controlled trial suggested that magnesium-preloading was safe and effective for reducing cisplatin-induced AKI. Additional studies with regard to the potential benefits of magnesium in this context are ongoing.

While significantly less nephrotoxic than its predecessor, carboplatin has been associated with AKI in the form of ATI, AIN, and (primarily in the post-HSCT setting) TMA. Despite its more favorable side effect profile, caution should be exercised when substituting carboplatin for cisplatin, given the potential risk for inferior cancer outcomes.

Several important drugs used in the treatment of monoclonal gammopathies have been associated with AKI. In a series of 41 patients with immunoglobulin light chain amyloidosis treated with the immunomodulatory drug (IMiD) lenalidomide, 27 (66%) developed kidney dysfunction (defined as a ≥50% increase in serum creatinine); median time to kidney dysfunction was 44 days (interquartile range, 15 to 108 days). Kidney dysfunction was severe in 13 (32%) of patients, 4 of whom required dialysis. Severe kidney dysfunction tended to occur in patients who were older and had a higher incidence of renal amyloidosis, greater proteinuria, and more profound hypoalbuminemia. Because no patients in this study underwent kidney biopsy during lenalidomide treatment, a predominant histologic lesion could not be identified. Case reports have described AIN, drug reaction with eosinophilia and systemic symptoms (DRESS), Fanconi syndrome, and MCD after use of lenalidomide.

Targeted Therapies

Targeted therapies include monoclonal antibodies and small molecule agents that target specific biologic pathways active in cancer cells, reducing cell proliferation and survival. Over the past two decades, these drugs have significantly improved patient survival compared with conventional chemotherapies for certain cancers. A wide range of kidney toxicities has been identified with the use of these treatments, with varying incidences and patterns of injury based on the respective targets of these novel drugs.

PIs have revolutionized the care of patients with MM. By inhibiting the proteasome, these drugs act through multiple mechanisms to suppress tumor survival pathways and arrest tumor growth, spread, and angiogenesis. TMA has been described with the use of bortezomib, carfilzomib, and ixazomib. It has been proposed that PIs may mediate TMA through inhibition of the ubiquitination of IκB and subsequent reduction in VEGF production. In one phase 3 multicenter study comparing carfilzomib monotherapy with low-dose corticosteroids and optional cyclophosphamide for relapsed/refractory MM, grade ≥3 renal failure events occurred more commonly in the carfilzomib group (24% vs. 9%); incidence was greatest in patients with low (<30 mL/min) baseline creatinine clearance. Beyond TMA, proposed mechanisms of carfilzomib-induced AKI include prerenal injury, tumor lysis-like syndrome, and ATN.

Crizotinib, an inhibitor of the anaplastic lymphoma kinase (ALK), has been associated with both pseudo-AKI, related to reduced creatinine secretion, and true AKI. Use of non–creatinine-based assessments of kidney function, such as measurement of iothalamate clearance, may help distinguish between the two and guide drug dosing in patients receiving crizotinib who experience an increase in serum creatinine. Interestingly, crizotinib has also been linked with an increased risk for the development and progression of reversible renal cysts; the molecular mechanism behind this increased risk remains unknown.

While first approved for the treatment of metastatic melanoma, the BRAF (serine-threonine protein kinase) inhibitors vemurafenib and dabrafenib are now being used or investigated in the management of a variety of solid tumors. Like crizotinib, vemurafenib has been associated with both pseudo-AKI (reduced tubular creatinine secretion) and true AKI. Cases of true AKI have been attributed to acute tubulointerstitial injury, however biopsy data are limited in this setting. Proposed mechanisms include inhibition of the downstream MEK pathway (increasing susceptibility to ischemic tubular injury) and inhibition of ferrochelatase (leading to renal tubular epithelial cell dysfunction). Dabrafenib is considered to be less nephrotoxic than vemurafenib, however, cases of AKI have been reported. Risk of AKI is increased when dabrafenib is coadministered with the MEK inhibitor trametinib, sometimes in association with a severe febrile syndrome characterized by fever, chills, gastrointestinal symptoms, and elevated liver enzymes. Therapy for BRAF inhibitor-associated AKI is primarily supportive, with drug discontinuation leading to improvement in kidney function in the majority of cases.

VEGF is a critical mediator of tumor growth and angiogenesis, and drugs targeting the VEGF signaling pathway (VSP) are widely used in solid tumor oncology. Two primary strategies have been used to block the VSP: (1) prevention of VEGF from binding to the VEGF receptor (VEGFR) (i.e., bevacizumab, ramucirumab, aflibercept); and (2) prevention of downstream VEGF signaling by drug binding to the intracellular domain of the VEGFR (small molecular tyrosine kinase inhibitors [TKIs]) (i.e., sunitinib, sorafenib, cabozantinib, lenvatinib, among others). While crucial for the growth of many cancers, VEGF is also an essential growth factor required for maintaining glomerular endothelial cell function and the integrity of the selective barrier to filtration. Additionally, VEGF modulates local regulatory complement factors, preventing endothelial cell injury. Accordingly, interference with the VSP to target tumor growth may have various untoward effects in the kidney.

New-onset hypertension (or exacerbation of preexisting hypertension) with the use of VEGF inhibitors (VEGFis) is common, with nearly every clinical trial reporting increased blood pressure (BP) as an adverse effect and up to 80% of patients developing hypertension. In a recent meta-analysis of phase III randomized controlled trials and phase IV postmarketing studies, VEGFis were associated with a significantly higher risk of hypertension (OR, 5.28 [4.53–6.15]; number needed to harm [NNH], 6) and severe hypertension (OR, 5.59 [4.67–6.69]; NNH 17), compared with routine care. Treatment-induced hypertension is dose-dependent and correlates with the potency of VEGFR-2 inhibition, reflecting an "on-target" effect of these treatments, with some studies suggesting correlation between VEGFi-mediated hypertension and improved clinical outcomes. The molecular mechanisms underlying VEGFi-mediated hypertension are unclear, however endothelial dysfunction and increased vascular resistance (due to impaired nitric oxide signaling, reduced prostacyclin production, endothelin-1 upregulation, oxidative stress, and rarefaction) have been implicated.

Proteinuria is a dose-related side effect of VEGFis. Incidence of mild and asymptomatic proteinuria ranges from 21% to 63%, with up to 6.6% of patients developing heavy proteinuria. Patients with RCC, prior nephrectomy, diabetes, and preexisting proteinuria appear to be at highest risk. Downexpression or suppression of nephrin, a protein important for the maintenance of the glomerular slit diaphragm, may contribute to pathogenesis. Although a number of histologic lesions have been described with these drugs, TMA (bevacizumab, aflibercept) and FSGS (TKIs) are most common and are frequently associated with AKI. Importantly, TMA may be renal-limited.

Preexisting hypertension and proteinuria should be addressed in all patients prior to initiation of VEGFi therapy. Once treatment starts, BP should be monitored at least weekly during the first cycle of therapy; thereafter, patients should be encouraged to keep a home log for noticeable trends. Periodic evaluation for new-onset proteinuria (spot urine protein-to-creatinine ratios [UPCR]) is reasonable. Treatment is typically continued in the setting of hypertension and non–nephrotic-range proteinuria, however, the long-term consequences of this approach are unknown. In the context of mild–moderate proteinuria with or without hypertension, the use of ACEis/ARBs is preferred. In cases of proteinuria ≥2 g/d, hematuria, or biochemical evidence of impaired kidney function, kidney biopsy should be considered. Hypertension and proteinuria typically improve after withholding VEGFi therapy, however, the decision to continue, interrupt, or permanently discontinue VEGFi therapy is challenging and requires a multidisciplinary approach. The development of posterior reversible encephalopathy syndrome, hypertensive emergency, nephrotic-range proteinuria, and TMA are generally considered indications to discontinue the offending drug.

Immunotherapy

"Immunotherapy" includes all treatment approaches that use components or mechanisms of the patient's immune system to fight cancer cells. The older immunotherapy interferon-alpha (IFNα), which enhances innate and adaptive immune functions by various mechanisms, is a well-known cause of AKI. IFNα has been associated with high-grade proteinuria, AKI, and evidence of glomerulopathies (MCD, FSGS) on kidney biopsy. TMA has also been described with this therapy, primarily in patients with chronic myelogenous leukemia (CML). Another older immunotherapy, interleukin-2, has been associated with AKI in the context of severe capillary leak syndrome characterized by hypotension, fluid retention, oliguria, low fractional excretion of sodium, and decline in GFR (which is largely reversible with drug discontinuation).

The advent of immune checkpoint inhibitors (ICPis) has transformed the treatment landscape for patients with a wide range of cancers (i.e., melanoma, RCC, nonsmall cell lung cancer), enabling the possibility of long-term survival in patients with metastatic disease and providing new therapeutic options in earlier-stage settings. ICPis enhance the activity and proliferation of cytotoxic T lymphocytes by binding to: (1) cytotoxic T lymphocyte-associated protein 4 (CTLA-4) (ipilimumab); (2) programmed cell death protein 1 (PD-1) (nivolumab, pembrolizumab, cemiplimab, dostarlimab); or (3) programmed death ligand 1 (PD-L1) (atezolizumab, avelumab, durvalumab).

While ICPis facilitate antitumor response, augmenting T cell activation by ICPis frequently leads to immune-related adverse events (irAEs) (most commonly arthralgias, diarrhea/colitis, rash, and thyroiditis). Additionally, due to loss of immune tolerance, patients with a history of kidney transplant experience an increased risk of graft rejection and graft loss after ICPi therapy.

AKI directly attributed to ICPi therapy (ICPi-AKI) is estimated to occur in 2% to 5% of patients. The most commonly reported pathologic lesion identified on kidney biopsy is acute tubulointerstitial nephritis (ATIN), however other lesions (i.e., pauci-immune glomerulonephritis/renal vasculitis, MCD, complement 3 [C3] glomerulonephritis, immunoglobulin A [IgA] nephropathy, lupus-like nephritis, TMA) have been described. Risk factors for ICPi-AKI include lower baseline eGFR, combination ICPi therapy, and the presence of extrarenal irAEs. Concomitant use of PPis is also associated with increased risk, potentially related to activation/reactivation of drug-specific T cells in some patients.

Patients with ATIN may present with sterile pyuria and subnephrotic proteinuria, however, neither finding is sensitive nor specific. Considerable debate remains over whether patients with suspected ICPi-mediated ATIN should undergo kidney biopsy (versus empiric treatment with glucocorticoids). Differentiating between all-cause AKI (i.e., due to hypovolemia or ATN) and AKI directly caused by ICPi therapy is critical to ensure appropriate management and avoid unnecessary immunosuppression. Accordingly, recent guidelines from the Society for Immunotherapy of Cancer state that kidney biopsy should be strongly considered when feasible, particularly when a plausible alternative etiology for AKI exists or urine studies suggest glomerular disease.

Beyond discontinuation of ICPi therapy (and PPis when safe to do so), glucocorticoid therapy is the mainstay of treatment for ICPi-induced ATIN; the majority of ATIN cases are steroid-responsive, with higher rates of response in patients initiated on glucocorticoid therapy within 14 days of ICPi-AKI presentation. Patients with steroid-refractory or relapsing ATIN may benefit from mycophenolate mofetil or infliximab, however further study is warranted. Limited data from case reports suggest potential benefit of rituximab in cases of ICPi-mediated glomerular disease and renal vasculitis.

CAR T cell therapy represents a novel use of immunotherapy for certain advanced/resistant lymphomas, acute lymphoblastic leukemia, and MM. Research is ongoing with the goal of expanding CAR therapy to other hematologic malignancies and solid tumors. Human T cells are genetically modified to express CARs, fusion proteins containing both an antigen recognition moiety (for tumor recognition) and a T cell activation domain. When infused into patients, CAR T cells target and destroy malignant cells.

Case reports of TLS after CAR T therapy exist, however AKI in this setting is more commonly associated with cytokine release syndrome (CRS). CRS is a systemic inflammatory response caused by the release of proinflammatory cytokines by infused CAR T cells. Clinically, patients present with fever, tachycardia, hypotension, and multiorgan dysfunction (i.e., seizures, altered mental status, decreased left ventricular function, hypoxia, diarrhea, hepatitis). AKI may result from cytokine-mediated vasodilation and capillary leak, intravascular volume depletion, decreased cardiac output, and/or ATN. In one recent systematic review of patients treated with CAR T therapy, pooled incidences of CRS, AKI, and AKI requiring dialysis (AKI-RRT) were 75%, 19%, and 4%, respectively. Risk of AKI-RRT correlated with more severe CRS. Risk factors for CRS-mediated AKI include prior autologous or allogeneic transplant, lower baseline eGFR, use of intravenous iodinated contrast, increasing tumor lysis markers, and the need for ICU-level care.

Aggressive supportive care, including early intervention for hypotension, is essential for all patients experiencing CRS. Hemodialysis may be required in patients who progress to ATN. Interleukin-6 receptor blockade with tocilizumab remains a core pharmacologic therapy for CRS; indications for administration vary among centers.

While corticosteroids have been used with success, some experts reserve this therapy for patients who fail to improve after tocilizumab (or patients experiencing neurotoxicity), citing concerns over reduced CAR T cell efficacy after steroid treatment.

Other Causes of AKI in the Cancer Patient

The kidney is a common site of leukemic and lymphomatous infiltration, with tumor cell infiltrates identified in approximately 34% of patients with lymphoma and 33% to 63% of patients with leukemia on autopsy. This parenchymal infiltration is usually subclinical, and AKI due to infiltration is rare in this population. Most cases of AKI occur in the context of interstitial infiltration and are thought to result from tubular compression and disruption of the renal microcirculation. Though most are asymptomatic, patients may present with flank pain and hypertension in addition to AKI. Urinalysis is usually bland, however, proteinuria and hematuria may occur when intraglomerular involvement is present. Imaging typically demonstrates bilaterally enlarged kidneys. Kidney biopsies reveal diffuse infiltration of the interstitium with malignant cells that can be identified with specific stains or immunologic markers. Prompt administration of chemotherapy may lead to rapid improvement in kidney function.

Patients with acute myelogenous leukemia, CML, and (occasionally) CLL may develop AKI secondary to leukostasis. This tends to occur at very high peripheral white blood cell counts, typically >100,000/mm^3 (hyperleukocytosis). Pathogenesis has been ascribed to the formation of leukemic thrombi leading to reduced perfusion and endothelial damage mediated by the release of proinflammatory cytokines. In the absence of newer therapies, cytoreductive chemotherapy, leukapheresis, and management of associated complications (TLS, disseminated intravascular coagulation) remain the pillars of therapy.

Lysozyme-induced nephropathy, also known as lysozymuria, is a rare complication of chronic myelomonocytic leukemia (CMML) and other forms of monocytic leukemia. In these cases, large amounts of the lytic enzyme lysozyme are produced by neoplastic cells of monocyte lineage, released into circulation, filtered by the glomerulus, and reabsorbed by proximal tubular cells. The resulting proximal tubular injury may lead to AKI, hypokalemia secondary to renal potassium wasting, and tubular proteinuria. UPEP reveals significant amounts of lysozyme; proteinuria may reach nephrotic range. Kidney biopsy specimens demonstrate ATI with abundant cytoplasmic granular inclusions that stain strongly for lysozyme on immunohistochemistry. Recognition of this rare cause of AKI may guide treatment, shifting the approach from supportive care to more aggressive treatment aimed at mitigating leukemia-associated end-organ damage.

Stem Cell Therapy–Associated Kidney Disease

HSCT is an important and possibly curative treatment for patients with hematologic malignancies as well as patients with certain solid tumors. HSCT involves the administration of chemotherapy with or without radiotherapy, followed by engraftment of stem or progenitor cells from the affected patient (autologous) or a related or unrelated donor (allogeneic). Patients receiving myeloablative autologous or allogeneic HSCT receive intensive pretransplant conditioning regimens (high-dose chemotherapy with or without total body radiation [TBI]) to eradicate the bone marrow and underlying cancer, followed by infusion and engraftment of transplanted cells. Patients not eligible for aggressive myeloablative therapy due to advanced age or comorbidities may still be candidates to receive nonmyeloablative (low-intensity) or reduced intensity conditioning (RIC) regimens with the goals of reducing systemic toxicity and providing sufficient immunosuppression to permit the engraftment of transplanted cells, which then target cancer cells (graft-versus-tumor effect). Myeloablative and nonmyeloablative allogeneic (but not autologous) HSCT recipients require posttransplant immunosuppression to prevent graft-versus-host-disease (GVHD); CNIs (i.e., tacrolimus, cyclosporine) represent a cornerstone of GVHD prophylaxis at many centers.

AKI is a frequent complication after HSCT, with reported incidence and severity varying by the type of conditioning regimen, type of transplant, and definition of AKI used. AKI is most common after myeloablative allogeneic HSCT (19% to 66%), likely reflecting the longer period of profound immunosuppression (with associated risk of sepsis) and greater risk of hepatic sinusoidal obstruction syndrome (SOS), as compared with nonmyeloablative allogeneic HSCT. Incidence of AKI is lowest after autologous HSCT (12% to 50%); this has been attributed to more rapid engraftment, the absence of GVHD, and lack of CNI exposure. Risk of needing dialysis is highest after myeloablative HSCT, approaching 20% in some studies. AKI is associated with increased nonrelapse mortality, with especially poor prognosis in critically ill HSCT recipients requiring RRT. Importantly, AKI onset and severity represent key risk factors for the development of posttransplant CKD.

Patients undergoing HSCT are exposed to multiple nephrotoxic insults in the peritransplant period (i.e., volume depletion, antimicrobials, CNIs), and AKI in this setting is often multifactorial. Selected HSCT-specific etiologies of AKI are highlighted below.

Marrow infusion syndrome occurs within 24 to 48 hours of stem/progenitor cell infusion when patients are exposed to products of red blood cell lysis (released during cryopreservation), as well as the cryoprotectant dimethyl sulfoxide, leading to intratubular pigment cast formation and toxic ATN. Due to advances in cell preservation, this complication is now infrequent. Obstructive nephropathy may occur due to severe hemorrhagic cystitis after exposure to high-dose cyclophosphamide or in the setting of viral infections (i.e., adenovirus, BK virus). Adenovirus and BK nephropathies, mediated by tubulointerstitial nephritis, have also been described.

HSCT recipients are at risk for hemodynamic AKI from CNI-mediated vasoconstriction, as well as CNI-mediated TMA. Use of CNIs for GVHD prophylaxis is typically limited to the first 3 months after transplant. However, patients who develop chronic GVHD may require long-term use with associated nephrotoxicity characterized by hypertension, tubular dysfunction, and glomerular/vascular disease. Research is ongoing regarding the use of CNI-sparing T-cell depleted HSCT, with a recent study demonstrating lower incidence of AKI as compared with conventional SCT (42% vs. 31%). When CNI-driven hemodynamic AKI does occur, dose reduction or temporary drug discontinuation may be required.

GVHD is a common complication that occurs after allogeneic HSCT when donor-derived immune cells (the graft) recognize host cells as foreign and attack recipient tissues. GVHD may present as acute GVHD, chronic GVHD, or a GVHD overlap syndrome. Frequently-targeted organs in acute GVHD include the skin, gut, and liver. Prerenal AKI commonly occurs in the setting of acute gastrointestinal GVHD due to poor oral intake and volume losses from nausea, vomiting, and diarrhea. Additionally, moderate and severe acute and chronic GVHD are correlated with intrarenal AKI and CKD, attributed to T cell and cytokine-mediated tissue and endothelial damage.

"Haplostorm" and engraftment syndrome result from endothelial cell injury and the release of proinflammatory cytokines. Patients present with fever, capillary leak, pulmonary edema, multisystem organ dysfunction, and AKI. Kidney injury occurs due to intravascular volume depletion, and possibly by a direct inflammatory effect. Haplostorm is a CRS occurring within 2 weeks of haploidentical HSCT; management of these patients is challenging, with a focus on supportive care, steroid use, and anti-interleukin 6 therapy (i.e., tocilizumab). Engraftment syndrome occurs at the time of neutrophil regeneration, is seen most commonly after autologous HSCT, and is typically treated with steroids.

Hepatic sinusoidal obstructive syndrome (SOS), previously known as veno-occlusive disease, is a potentially life-threatening complication that occurs in approximately 14% of HSCT recipients. While mild to moderate cases are self-limited, mortality in severe SOS may approach 85%. Transplant-related risk factors include prior HSCT, allogeneic HSCT, myeloablative conditioning regimens (TBI-based and busulfan-based), use of horse antithymocyte globulin, and increased serum tacrolimus level

(>5 to 10 ng/mL). Patient-related risk factors include Eastern Cooperative Oncology Group Performance Status score 2 to 4 versus 0 to 1, hepatitis C seropositivity, advanced disease status, high pre-HSCT ferritin level (≥950 ng/mL) in patients with malignant lymphoma, AKI, platelet refractoriness, and high international normalized ratio. The use of gemtuzumab ozogamicin and inotuzumab ozogamicin, novel antibody-drug conjugates sometimes administered for cancer treatment prior to HSCT, have also been implicated. Pathogenesis is driven by chemoradiation-induced hepatic sinusoidal endothelial cell injury with resulting sinusoidal thrombosis, obstruction, and portal hypertension. Clinically, patients with SOS present during the first 30 days after HSCT with oliguria, painful hepatomegaly, jaundice, and diuretic-resistant ascites, mimicking hepatorenal syndrome. As seen in hepatorenal syndrome, urine sodium concentration is low (<10 mEq/L), and urinalysis and urine sediment are bland, consistent with hemodynamic pathophysiology; ATI may occur if renal ischemia is prolonged. Though data are mixed, ursodeoxycholic acid is widely used for prevention of SOS. Based on benefits observed in randomized pediatric clinical trial data and retrospective results available in adults, the antithrombotic/fibrinolytic agent defibrotide is recommended for prophylaxis in patients at highest risk and for the treatment of established SOS.

Transplant-associated thrombotic microangiopathy (TA-TMA) is a multisystem disease associated with both AKI and (more commonly) CKD. Reported incidence of AKI ranges from 2.3% to 30% in the context of widely varying definitions and study populations. While some patients may have mild and self-limited disease, reported rates of nonrelapse mortality in patients with TA-TMA and multiorgan dysfunction syndrome reach or exceed 80%. Acute GVHD (especially grades 2 to 4) is a major risk factor for TA-TMA, with emerging data suggesting that TA-TMA may represent an "endothelial complication" of GVHD. Additional risk factors include unrelated donor type, HLA mismatch, nonmyeloablative HSCT, TBI, CNI exposure, mammalian target of rapamycin (mTOR) inhibitor use, and various infections (i.e., systemic infections, BK virus, cytomegalovirus, parvovirus B19, adenovirus). Recent studies demonstrate that complement activation and genetic susceptibility to complement dysregulation also contribute to the development of TA-TMA.

Endothelial injury is the pathologic hallmark of TA-TMA and leads to complement activation, platelet activation, small vessel thrombosis, and microangiopathic hemolytic anemia with end-organ damage. This syndrome most commonly manifests as AKI, but can also lead to bowel ischemia, diffuse alveolar hemorrhage, pulmonary hypertension, seizure, and cutaneous vasculitis. Patients typically present 4 to 12 months after HSCT with slowly rising creatinine, however, some patients may demonstrate earlier or more fulminant presentations with severe nephritic syndrome. Urinalysis shows variable proteinuria and hematuria. Kidney biopsy findings resemble those seen in other forms of TMA (see "Thrombotic Microangiopathy in the Cancer Patient").

Timely diagnosis of TA-TMA may be challenging, as classic findings of microangiopathic hemolytic anemia (particularly the presence of schistocytes on peripheral blood smear) may be delayed or absent. The recently published modified Jodele criteria have gained support amongst international experts and are summarized in Table 19-3. Using these criteria, TA-TMA is diagnosed when ≥4 of the following 7 features occur twice within 14 days: (1) anemia, defined as failure to achieve transfusion independence despite neutrophil engraftment or hemoglobin decline by ≥1 g/dL or new-onset transfusion dependence; (2) thrombocytopenia, defined as failure to achieve platelet engraftment, higher-than-expected transfusion needs, refractoriness to platelet transfusions, or ≥50% reduction in baseline platelet count after full platelet engraftment; (3) LDH exceeding the upper limit of normal (ULN); (4) schistocytes; (5) hypertension; (6) soluble C5b-9 (sC5b-9) exceeding the ULN; and proteinuria (≥1 mg/mg random urine protein-to-creatinine ratio [rUPCR]). Patients with any of the following features are at highest risk for nonrelapse mortality: elevated sC5b-9, LDH ≥2 times the ULN, rUPCR ≥1 mg/mg, multiorgan dysfunction, concurrent grade II to IV acute GVHD,

TABLE 19-3	Modified Jodele Criteria for Diagnosis of Transplant-Associated Thrombotic Microangiopathy
Biopsy-proven disease (kidney or gastrointestinal)	
or	
Clinical criteria (must meet ≥4 of the following 7 criteria within 14 days at 2 consecutive time points)	
Anemia[a]	Defined as one of the following: 1. Failure to achieve transfusion independence for pRBCs despite evidence of neutrophil engraftment 2. Hgb decline from patient's baseline by 1 g/dL 3. New onset of transfusion dependence
Thrombocytopenia	Defined as one of the following: 1. Failure to achieve platelet engraftment 2. Higher-than-expected platelet transfusion needs 3. Refractoriness to platelet transfusions 4. ≥50% reduction in baseline platelet count after full platelet engraftment
Elevated LDH	>ULN for age
Schistocytes	Present
Hypertension	>99th percentile for age (<18 yrs), or systolic BP ≥140 mmHg or diastolic BP ≥90 mmHg (≥18 yrs)
Elevated sC5b-9	≥ULN
Proteinuria	≥1 mg/mg rUPCR

AIHA, autoimmune hemolytic anemia; BP, blood pressure; Hgb, hemoglobin; LDH, lactate dehydrogenase; pRBCs, packed red blood cells; PRCA, pure red cell aplasia; rUPCR, random urine protein to creatinine ratio; sC5b-9, soluble C5b-9; ULN, upper limit of normal.

[a]Other causes of anemia, such as AIHA and PRCA, ruled out.

Adapted from Jodele S, Schoettler ML, Carreras E, Cho B, et al. Harmonizing definitions for diagnostic criteria and prognostic assessment of transplantation-associated thrombotic microangiopathy: A Report on Behalf of the European Society for Blood and Marrow Transplantation, American Society for Transplantation and Cellular Therapy, Asia-Pacific Blood and Marrow Transplantation Group, and Center for International Blood and Marrow Transplant Research. *Transplant Cell Ther.* 2023;29(3):151–163.

or infection (bacterial or viral). Per international TA-TMA working group consensus, these patients should be considered to have high-risk TA-TMA and therefore be considered for early TA-TMA directed therapy. Clinicians should maintain a high index of suspicion for TA-TMA in at-risk patients; screening protocols vary by center.

Management of patients with suspected or confirmed TA-TMA includes BP control (often with renin–angiotensin–aldosterone–inhibiting agents), transfusion support, and dialysis as indicated. All patients should be evaluated for precipitating viral infections and GVHD. In patients receiving CNIs or mTOR inhibitors for GVHD prophylaxis, replacement with an alternative agent (i.e., mycophenolate, corticosteroids, IL-2 inhibitors) may be appropriate, however, this approach has not been extensively studied. Plasma exchange has been studied with mostly negative results, but may be beneficial in selected patients (i.e., documented evidence of Factor H antibodies). Small case series in pediatric and adult patients have demonstrated response rates of up to 80% with the use of rituximab. Defibrotide has been associated with recovery from TMA in 50% of patients in small studies when used alone or in combination with other therapies. Given the key role of complement dysregulation in the pathogenesis of TA-TMA, there is significant interest in the use of the C5 inhibitor eculizumab. Data come primarily from observational studies in the pediatric population, with a recent relatively large study of 64 children with high-risk TA-TMA showing 66% 1-year post-HSCT survival compared with 16.7% in a previously reported untreated cohort. Similar benefits have now been reported in adult patients, making eculizumab a potential option in selected patients with evidence of complement dysregulation.

NS has been reported in 0.4% to 6% of patients after HSCT and is considered a late complication of HSCT with the majority of cases occurring >6 months posttransplant. Data come largely from case reports and case series, with MN and MCD reported most commonly. Posttransplant NS appears to be strongly associated with the tapering of immunosuppression and presence of GVHD, however, it remains unclear if NS is caused by GVHD or other factors. Recurrence of the patient's original malignancy (i.e., MM, lymphoma), viral infections, and medication toxicity should also be considered.

CKD is an important long-term complication of HSCT, particularly allogeneic HSCT. Reported cumulative incidence ranges from 0% to 60% (varying definitions of CKD, HSCT type, and pretransplant comorbidities). Progressive CKD leading to ESRD occurs in approximately 4% of patients. Risk factors for post-HSCT CKD include older age at time of transplantation, preexisting CKD, hypertension, acute and chronic GVHD, prior AKI, and survival more than 1 year after transplantation, among others. Albuminuria has been associated with CKD progression as well as decreased posttransplant survival. Key etiologies of CKD in this population include TMA, NS, and CNI toxicity. Kidney biopsy is likely underperformed in the post-HSCT setting and should be considered when the cause of CKD is unclear.

Chronic Kidney Disease in the Cancer Patient

Observational studies have suggested an increased incidence of cancer, especially cancers of the urogenital tract, in patients with CKD. In addition, new and more effective therapies have increased cancer survival, and these patients may develop CKD as a direct result of their malignancy and/or its treatment. This is particularly true among elderly patients with cancer as well as those with common comorbidities (hypertension and type 2 diabetes), which increase the prevalence of CKD. Therefore, CKD is a risk factor for cancer, and cancer is a risk factor for the development of CKD (bidirectional relationship). This is especially true for RCC (Fig. 19-4).

Most importantly, CKD is a recognized complication of cancer and its therapy. Once CKD develops in a patient with cancer, it may limit their ability to participate

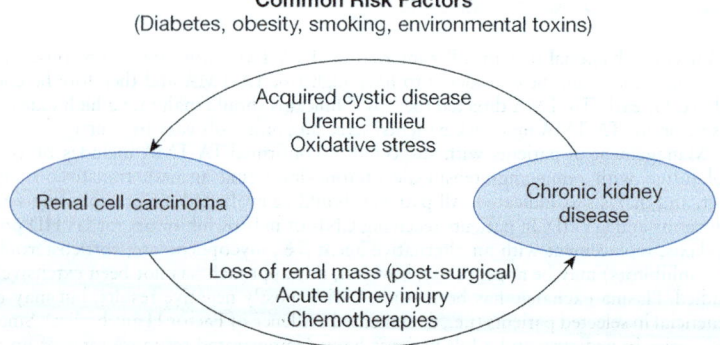

Figure 19-4. The Bidirectional Relationship Between Renal Cell Carcinoma and Chronic Kidney Disease. While chronic kidney disease can increase the risk of developing renal cell carcinoma, treatment of renal cell carcinoma often leads to chronic kidney disease.

in clinical trials, limit chemotherapy options for fear of toxicity and unknown dosing guidelines, and prevent the use of necessary computed tomography staging scans that require intravenous iodinated contrast. In this manner, CKD may increase the risk of mortality and poor outcomes in patients with concomitant cancer. However, studies have yet to quantify this effect of CKD on cancer outcomes.

The risk factors for developing CKD may be patient-specific, cancer-specific, or cancer therapy-specific. The development of AKI is an important and often overlooked etiology for CKD among patients with cancer. For example, from 10% up to 73% of patients post-HSCT develop AKI, with nearly 5% requiring RRT and up to 60% developing CKD as a direct consequence of the AKI episode. Patients with severe AKI who require RRT and who recover are at high risk for progression to CKD, as severity of AKI is a strong predictor of progression to CKD. In addition, CKD is a common complication in patients receiving antineoplastic drugs that are nephrotoxic. For example, most patients treated with cisplatin experience a small but permanent decline in eGFR; in one retrospective study of adult patients treated with cisplatin who had survived ≥5 years after the initial dose, about one in three experienced AKI, and the majority of patients who survived for at least 5 years after treatment had a permanent, small (<10 mL/min) decline in eGFR (leading to a diagnosis of CKD). Other studies have confirmed that cisplatin-associated AKI can have a negative impact on long-term renal function and patient survival. Other agents, such as those targeting the VEGF pathway, can lead to TMA or FSGS, which also result in CKD.

Another risk factor for the development of CKD includes invasive surgical procedures for the management of RCC. Postoperative AKI after radical nephrectomy is associated with a greater than fourfold higher risk of developing new-onset CKD, and nephron-sparing partial nephrectomies are associated with improved outcomes with less postoperative AKI and CKD without negatively impacting cancer outcomes.

Electrolyte and Acid–Base Disorders in the Cancer Patient

Electrolyte disturbances are common in patients with cancer and may be caused by the malignancy (i.e., as a paraneoplastic syndrome such as hypokalemia due to ectopic production of ACTH) or concurrent chemotherapy (i.e., cisplatin leading to potassium and magnesium wasting) and its side effects (vomiting and diarrhea).

Hyponatremia (serum sodium <135 mEq/L) is usually related to excess total body water in relation to sodium and is a common finding in patients with cancer. The presence of hyponatremia has been associated with shorter overall survival, a shorter time to treatment failure, and a lower disease control rate. Classification of hyponatremia is based on the duration of hyponatremia (acute if <48 hours, chronic if >48 hours), the volume status of the patient (hypovolemic, euvolemic, hypervolemic), and serum osmolality (hypo-osmolar, iso-osmolar). Hyponatremia can be present in up to 47% of hospitalized patients who have cancer, with a prevalence in most studies from 24% to 44%. Most cases result in mild hyponatremia, defined as a serum sodium level ranging from 130 to 134 mEq/L, and may have minimal clinical significance. Hyponatremia can also be a marker of occult neoplasms and should prompt a consideration for cancer screening in appropriate patients. Almost two-thirds of cases of hyponatremia in patients with cancer are present at hospital admission, and one-third are diagnosed in an outpatient setting. Common etiologies for hyponatremia in patients with cancer are listed in Table 19-4 and include the syndrome of inappropriate antidiuresis (SIADH), individual cancer treatments, reduced water excretion from kidney failure, decreased circulating volume (heart failure, cirrhosis, or hypoalbuminemia), and hypovolemia (often from chemotherapy-induced nausea, vomiting, or diarrhea). SIADH is the most common etiology in patients with cancer, accounting for one-third of all cases of hyponatremia, and should be promptly recognized by its characteristic features (see Table 19-5).

Commonly, the etiology of hyponatremia in patients with cancer is multifactorial. This can complicate the assessment and evaluation of hyponatremia in patients who have cancer compared to those who do not. For instance, patients may have SIADH related to small

TABLE 19-4	Etiologies of Hyponatremia in the Patient With Cancer

Anticancer therapies
- Chemotherapies (such as vincristine, cisplatin, vinblastine, cyclophosphamide)
- Immune checkpoint therapies (such as ipilimumab, nivolumab, pembrolizumab)

Ectopic (paraneoplastic) production of vasopression (SIADH)
- Small cell lung cancer; hematologic malignancies (i.e., Hodgkin disease, non-Hodgkin disease, chronic lymphocytic leukemia, multiple myeloma); cancers of the head and neck, brain (primary and metastatic), skin (i.e., melanoma), gastrointestinal system (i.e., esophageal, gastric, pancreatic, colon), gynecologic system, breast, prostate, bladder; sarcomas; thymomas; adrenal malignancies

Vasopressin secretion in response to stimuli
- Nausea, vomiting, pain

Volume depletion (due to nausea, vomiting, diarrhea, poor intake)

Other medications (such as antiseizure or opioids)

Salt wasting (due to cisplatin)

Pseudohyponatremia due to paraproteins

Comorbidities such as heart failure or cirrhosis

cell lung cancer along with volume depletion due to vomiting associated with chemotherapy. Regardless of the etiology, hyponatremia is associated with unfavorable cancer treatment outcomes and increased length of hospital stay, and it is an independent predictor of morbidity (falls, encephalopathy, increased risk of osteoporosis, and fractures) as well as mortality. Early clinical manifestations of hyponatremia are often nonspecific and include headache, malaise, and nausea, and can be mistaken for other diagnoses. As the severity of hyponatremia increases, more prominent symptoms, such as vomiting, ataxia, confusion, respiratory arrest, and seizure, can occur and may be life threatening.

The initial evaluation of patients with hyponatremia requires assessment of the patient's volume status along with urine and serum osmolality, with simultaneous urine and serum sodium concentrations. Ideally, this evaluation should be sent before initiation of treatment unless there are imminent, life-threatening symptoms, a scenario that should be emergently managed with a 100-mL bolus of 3% sodium chloride infused intravenously over 10 minutes (repeated up to a maximum of 400 mL as needed for persistent symptoms). This protocol generally raises the serum sodium

TABLE 19-5	Features of the Syndrome of Inappropriate Diuretic Hormone Secretion (SIADH)

- Urinary sodium typically >20–30 mEq/L and reflects dietary intake
- Serum osmolality <275 mOsm/kg water
- Urine osmolality >100 mOsm/kg water
- Euvolemic on physical examination
- Normal renal, cardiac, and hepatic function
- No recent diuretic use
- Normal thyroid and adrenal function

approximately 5 mEq/L which is often enough to reverse cerebral edema and improve life-threatening symptoms.

In less symptomatic patients, an assessment should include several key questions that will help guide treatment; what is the severity of symptoms and what is the duration of hyponatremia? In acute hyponatremia, defined as the onset of hyponatremia in <48 hours, rapid correction of serum sodium to normal levels can occur without the risk of complications, such as osmotic demyelination syndrome (ODS). For patients with hyponatremia duration >48 hours or if the duration is not known (chronic hyponatremia), the rate of correction should not exceed 4 to 8 mEq/L per day for those patients without risk factors for ODS. Alcoholism, malnutrition, hypokalemia, liver disease, and severe hyponatremia (defined as <110 mEq/L or mmol/L) are all considered significant risk factors for the development of ODS after correction of hyponatremia and should alert the clinician to lowering the rate of correction to no more than 4 to 6 mEq/L in 24 hours.

The underlying cause of the hyponatremia should be addressed if possible. For patients with hypovolemia, intravenous hydration with isotonic fluids, such as 0.9% normal saline, should be provided. It is important to avoid hypotonic fluids as they can exacerbate the hyponatremia. For patients with hypervolemic hyponatremia, fluid and salt restriction should be instituted and loop diuretics utilized as needed. For patients with SIADH, fluid restriction (500 mL/d below the 24-hour urine volume) and salt loading with either a high-sodium diet or sodium chloride tablets is an option, often along with a loop diuretic to lower urine concentrating ability. Predictors of the likely failure of fluid restriction in SIADH are a 24-hour urine volume <1,500 mL/d, a urine osmolality of >500 mOsm/kg water, the sum of the urine sodium and potassium concentrations exceeding the serum sodium concentration, and failure of serum sodium to rise by 2 mEq/L with a 1-L/d fluid restriction. It is important to recognize that long-term fluid restriction is problematic in patients with cancer and may be poorly tolerated and lead to worsening nutritional status. Other treatment options for SIADH include vasopressin 2 receptor antagonists, such as tolvaptan, or oral urea. There are only a few clinical studies, mostly observational studies with small patient numbers, that have assessed tolvaptan use in oncology patients with SIADH. Most studies showed that oral tolvaptan was effective and safe for patients with SIADH, and this approach allows for more liberal fluid intakes. Urea has also been shown to be effective, but tolerability and palatability may be issues. Additional information regarding the evaluation and management of hyponatremia may be found in Chapter 3: "The Patient With Hyponatremia or Hypernatremia" of this text.

Hypernatremia (serum sodium concentration >145 mEq/L) has an approximate prevalence rate of 2.6% among hospitalized patients with cancer. Similar to patients without cancer, hypernatremia is an independent risk factor for mortality. It results from increased free water loss or inadequate water repletion. Early symptoms may be notable for confusion, lethargy, irritability, polyuria, and weakness, with more severe symptoms marked by hyperthermia, seizure, delirium, coma, and death. Symptoms are both dependent on the degree of hypernatremia and the time course of its development. An initial evaluation for hypernatremia includes a detailed history and physical examination, including volume assessment and vital signs, urinary and serum osmolality, and sodium levels. Hypernatremia raises the serum osmolality above 295 mOsm/kg and, when associated with high urinary osmolality (usually higher than the serum osmolality) often indicates inadequate fluid intake. The presence of a low urinary osmolality (usually less than the serum osmolality and closer to 100 mOsm/kg) is diagnostic of nephrogenic or central diabetes insipidus and can be confirmed with a water deprivation test. However, a water-deprivation test is not needed when a random serum arginine vasopressin level is <1.0 pg/mL with the absence of a posterior pituitary bright spot on brain magnetic resonance imaging. In some cases, hypernatremia is also associated with excessive solute loss seen with azotemia, corticosteroid use, or post-AKI. Treatment is centered on therapy of the underlying etiology and the administration of oral water or hypotonic intravenous solutions, such as 0.45% saline or 5% dextrose, to reduce hyperosmolality. The exact amount of fluid administered depends on the free water deficit and should be calculated using a free water deficit equation (% total body water [as a fraction] × weight [kg] × [current Na/ideal Na − 1]). The rate of correction of hypernatremia typically should not exceed 0.5 mmol/L/h, although a recent observational study did not find any evidence that more rapid correction of hypernatremia is associated with adverse events in critically ill patients.

Hypercalcemia of malignancy is related to either osteolytic release of calcium from metastatic disease or from stimulation of osteoclast activity by release of tumor-derived endocrine factors (Fig. 19-5). Patients with mild hypercalcemia (corrected serum calcium <12 mg/dL) may be asymptomatic or complain of nonspecific symptoms such as nausea, vomiting, weakness, anorexia, polyuria, constipation, or depression. With more severe hypercalcemia, patients may present with volume depletion, confusion, renal failure, cardiac arrhythmias, or pancreatitis. Measurement of PTH-related peptide should be considered to identify cases of humoral hypercalcemia of malignancy (non–PTH-mediated) that can occur in squamous cell, renal cell, bladder, breast, and ovarian carcinomas and rarely in certain lymphomas and leukemias. SPEP and UPEP are key to identifying MM. In addition, plain bone radiographs and nuclear bone scans can identify cancer invasion of the bone which can contribute to hypercalcemia.

Medical treatment of hypercalcemia centers on aggressive volume resuscitation to promote calcium excretion through urine output. Loop diuretics are no longer recommended for the routine management of hypercalcemia except when volume overload exists. For patients who have ESRD or advanced-stage CKD with hypercalcemia, dialysis with a low-calcium dialysate along with cessation of all calcium-based medications and activated forms of vitamin D should be performed. Patients with hypercalcemia may be effectively treated with intravenous bisphosphonates and the use of subcutaneous calcitonin may result in more rapid normalization of the serum calcium. RANKL inhibitors, such as denosumab, may be considered as an alternative therapy to bisphosphonates especially for patients with moderate-to-severe CKD and those with ESRD. When using denosumab, it is critically important that patients have normal levels of vitamin D because, in the setting of vitamin D deficiency, the use of denosumab can lead to severe hypocalcemia. In specific circumstances, corticosteroids are useful in the treatment of hypercalcemia associated with lymphomas.

Hypocalcemia is defined as corrected total blood calcium <8.5 mg/dL or ionized blood calcium <4.6 mg/dL. Although most patients are asymptomatic from hypocalcemia, some patients experience muscle cramps, confusion, numbness, and tingling in the lips and fingers. The primary cause of hypocalcemia in patients with cancer is sequestered calcium from excessive uptake by bone-forming osteoblastic metastases (see Fig. 19-5). Hypocalcemia can occur in approximately 30% of patients with advanced prostate cancer who have proven bone metastases. The characteristic electrocardiogram finding of hypocalcemia is prolongation of the QTc interval because of lengthening of the ST segment, which is directly proportional to the degree of hypocalcemia. This finding should prompt emergent treatment with an intravenous infusion of 10% calcium gluconate 2 grams over 2 hours. Treatment with intravenous calcium is also necessary when the corrected calcium is <7.5 mg/dL or if the patient has signs or symptoms of hypocalcemia. Hypocalcemia may also be caused by hypoparathyroidism after surgery for head and neck or thyroid cancer and may result in severe and prolonged postoperative hypocalcemia. These patients are often initially managed with continuous intravenous calcium infusions, with the rate of infusion adjusted depending upon subsequent calcium levels and patient symptoms. Simultaneously, enteral calcium supplements together with an activated form of vitamin D (calcitriol) should be provided.

Hypokalemia is defined as a serum potassium level <3.5 mEq/L and is common in patients who have cancer. The causes of hypokalemia are grouped into cancer-related

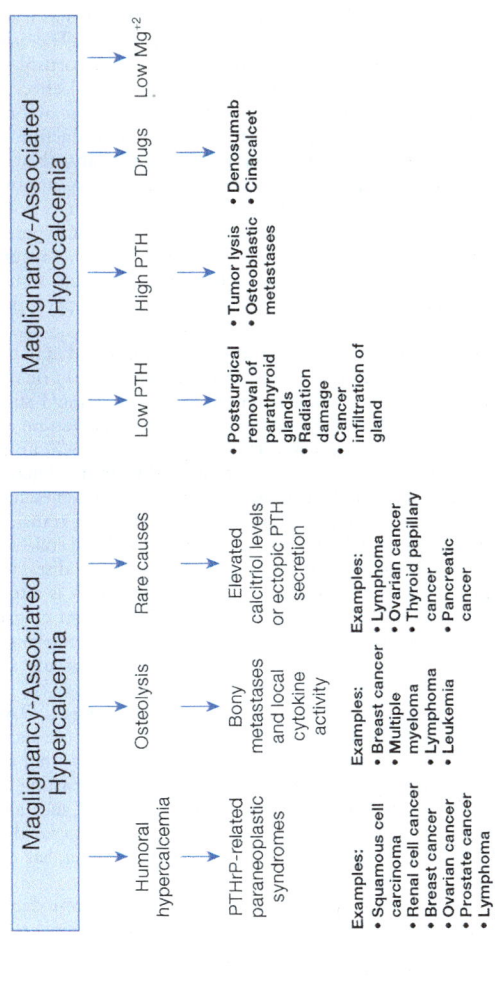

Figure 19-5. Etiologies of Malignancy-Associated Hypercalcemia and Hypocalcemia. Mg^{+2}, magnesium; PTH, parathyroid hormone; PTHrP, parathyroid hormone–related peptide.

or chemotherapy-related hypokalemia and can be broadly categorized further into four categories: (1) inadequate dietary potassium intake (anorexia, nausea, mucositis, surgery, or tumor-induced dysphagia/odynophagia); (2) increased extrarenal potassium losses (vomiting and diarrhea from chemotherapy use or gastrointestinal neuroendocrine tumors); (3) increased renal losses (diuretic use, Fanconi syndrome from chemotherapy use [cisplatin, ifosfamide, and lenalidomide]), hypomagnesemia (cetuximab use or platinum compounds), or from excess ACTH production by tumor cells (squamous cell cancers, thyroid medullary cancer, neuroendocrine tumors); and (4) redistribution of potassium into cells (high cell-turnover states, such as with leukemia, certain lymphomas, and the use of hematopoietic growth factors). The mechanism of paraneoplastic ACTH-induced hypokalemia is through excessive cortisol secretion by the adrenal gland, which produces a significant mineralocorticoid effect and can be treated with a mineralocorticoid receptor antagonist, such as spironolactone or eplerenone. Another cancer-related cause of hypokalemia is through production of lysozyme by various leukemias, resulting in tubular injury and failure to reabsorb urinary potassium. The mainstay of treatment involves intravenous or oral potassium, an increase in dietary potassium intake, avoidance of medications known to promote potassium loss (such as loop or thiazide diuretics), and co-correction of concurrent hypomagnesemia. Ultimate therapy requires either removal of the offending chemotherapeutic agent or treatment of the malignancy. In some cases, such as with cisplatin, some degree of potassium wasting may be permanent and require ongoing therapy with potassium supplementation.

Hypomagnesemia is commonly seen in patients with cancer and may be caused by diminished dietary intake or renal magnesium wasting. A fractional urinary excretion of magnesium >15% or a 24-hour urine magnesium level >24 mg/d suggests renal magnesium wasting. Levels below this suggest inadequate magnesium intake and/or gastrointestinal losses. Hypomagnesemia may be present in 4.4% up to 5.4% of patients taking antiepidermal growth factor receptor (EGFR) monoclonal antibodies, such as panitumumab and cetuximab. The mechanism of hypomagnesemia may rest between the interaction of anti-EGFR monoclonal antibody with transient receptor potential cation channel, subfamily M, member 6 (TRPM6) in distal collecting tubules, preventing TRPM6 from inserting into the apical membrane of the distal tubular cells and blocking absorption of magnesium from the tubular lumen. It is interesting that the presence of hypomagnesemia may serve as a marker for clinical efficacy of these agents. Most patients with hypomagnesemia are asymptomatic, and signs and symptoms such as weakness, muscle spasm, or ventricular arrhythmia usually do not arise until the serum magnesium concentration falls below 1.2 mg/dL.

Hypophosphatemia, defined as a serum phosphate level <2.5 mg/dL (0.81 mmol/L), can be secondary to several etiologies in patients with advanced cancer, such as malnutrition (poor phosphate intake in diet), persistent diarrhea or high-output stomas after gastrointestinal diversion surgery, or chemotherapy causing renal wasting from a Fanconi syndrome or proximal tubulopathy. Chemotherapeutic agents, such as ifosfamide and the TKIs (i.e., imatinib, dasatinib, sunitinib), have all been associated with hypophosphatemia. Dabrafenib, a BRAF inhibitor utilized for melanoma, has an incidence of hypophosphatemia in 7% of patients.

A rare cause of hypophosphatemia in patients with cancer is tumor-induced osteomalacia, a rare paraneoplastic syndrome characterized by hypophosphatemia resulting from decreased tubular phosphate reabsorption, with a low or inappropriately normal level of active vitamin D. Constitutive release of fibroblast growth factor-23 (FGF-23) from primary tumors was identified as responsible for hypophosphatemia during tumor-induced osteomalacia, such as with the rare benign phosphaturic mesenchymal tumor, mixed connective tissue variant, and can lead to profound hypophosphatemia, requiring surgical resection of tumor or use of a new anti-FGF-23 monoclonal antibody (burosumab). Another cause of hypophosphatemia is tumor genesis syndrome, a state of high cell-turnover states such as leukemia and lymphoma.

Summary
Onconephrology is relatively new and rapidly growing subspecialty of nephrology that recognizes the unique and critical renal diseases that are seen in patients with cancer. These diseases can be acute or chronic and affect every aspect of renal structures (vascular, interstitium, glomerulus, tubules) and function (acid–base and electrolyte disorders, changes in GFR). Increasingly, multidisciplinary teams are required to provide effective care for patients that minimizes the impact of kidney disease on cancer-treatment outcomes.

SUGGESTED READINGS

Abdel-Qadir H, Ethier J-L, Lee DS, Thavendiranathan P, Amir E. Cardiovascular toxicity of angiogenesis inhibitors in treatment of malignancy: a systematic review and meta-analysis. *Cancer Treat Rev*. 2017;53:120–127.

Abramson MH, Gutgarts V, Zheng J, et al. Acute kidney injury in the modern era of allogeneic hematopoietic stem cell transplantation. *Clin J Am Soc Nephrol*. 2021;16(9):1318–1327.

Abudayyeh A, Wanchoo R. Kidney disease following hematopoietic stem cell transplantation. *Adv Chronic Kidney Dis*. 2022;29(2):103–115.e1.

Adrogue HJ, Madias NE. Hypernatremia. *N Engl J Med*. 2000;342(20):1493–1499.

Ando M, Ohashi K, Akiyama H, et al. Chronic kidney disease in long-term survivors of myeloablative allogeneic haematopoietic cell transplantation: prevalence and risk factors. *Nephrol Dial Transplant*. 2010;25(1):278–282.

Barcos M, Lane W, Gomez GA, et al. An autopsy study of 1206 acute and chronic leukemias (1958 to 1982). *Cancer*. 1987;60(4):827–837.

Beck LH Jr. PLA2R and THSD7A: disparate paths to the same disease? *J Am Soc Nephrol*. 2017;28(9):2579–2589.

Bewersdorf JP, Zeidan AM. Hyperleukocytosis and leukostasis in acute myeloid leukemia: can a better understanding of the underlying molecular pathophysiology lead to novel treatments? *Cells*. 2020;9(10):2310.

Beyar-Katz O, Davila EK, Zuckerman T, et al. Adult nephrotic syndrome after hematopoietic stem cell transplantation: renal pathology is the best predictor of response to therapy. *Biol Blood Marrow Transplant*. 2016;22(6):975–981.

Body J-J, Niepel D, Tonini G. Hypercalcaemia and hypocalcaemia: finding the balance. *Support Care Cancer*. 2017;25(5):1639–1649.

Brahmer JR, Abu-Sbeih H, Ascierto PA, et al. Society for Immunotherapy of Cancer (SITC) clinical practice guideline on immune checkpoint inhibitor-related adverse events. *J Immunother Cancer*. 2021;9(6):e002435.

Brudno JN, Kochenderfer JN. Toxicities of chimeric antigen receptor T cells: recognition and management. *Blood*. 2016;127(26):3321–3330.

Cairo MS, Coiffier B, Reiter A, Younes A; TLS Expert Panel. Recommendations for the evaluation of risk and prophylaxis of tumour lysis syndrome (TLS) in adults and children with malignant diseases: an expert TLS panel consensus. *Br J Haematol*. 2010;149(4):578–586.

Chauhan K, Pattharanitima P, Patel N, et al. Rate of correction of hypernatremia and health outcomes in critically ill patients. *Clin J Am Soc Nephrol*. 2019;14:656–663.

Chen Y-J, Abila B, Kamel YM. CAR-T: what is next? *Cancers (Basel)*. 2023;15(3):663.

Chitale SV, Scott-Barrett S, Ho ETS, Burgess NA. The management of ureteric obstruction secondary to malignant pelvic disease. *Clin Radiol*. 2002;57(12):1118–1121.

Christ-Crain M, Bichet DG, Fenske WK, et al. Diabetes insipidus. *Nat Rev Dis Primers*. 2019;5:54.

Christiansen CF, Johansen MB, Langeberg WJ, Fryzek JP, Sorensen HT. Incidence of acute kidney injury in cancer patients: a Danish population-based cohort study. *Eur J Intern Med*. 2011;22(4):399–406.

Coppell JA, Richardson PG, Soiffer R, et al. Hepatic veno-occlusive disease following stem cell transplantation: incidence, clinical course, and outcome. *Biol Blood Marrow Transplant*. 2010;16(2):157–168.

Corbacioglu S, Jabbour EJ, Mohty M. Risk factors for development of and progression of hepatic veno-occlusive disease/sinusoidal obstruction syndrome. *Biol Blood Marrow Transplant*. 2019;25(7):1271–1280.

Dimopoulos MA, Sonneveld P, Leung N, et al. International myeloma working group recommendations for the diagnosis and management of myeloma-related renal impairment. *J Clin Oncol*. 2016;34(13):1544–1557.

Durani U, Shah ND, Go RS. In-hospital outcomes of tumor lysis syndrome: a population-based study using the national inpatient sample. *Oncologist*. 2017;22(12):1506–1509.

Edate S, Albanese A. Management of electrolyte and fluid disorders after brain surgery for pituitary/suprasellar tumours. *Horm Res Paediatr*. 2015;83(5):293–301.

Ensergueix G, Pallet N, Joly D, et al. Ifosfamide nephrotoxicity in adult patients. *Clin Kidney J*. 2019;13(4):660–665.

Farry JK, Flombaum CD, Latcha S. Long term renal toxicity of ifosfamide in adult patients–5 year data. *Eur J Cancer*. 2012;48(9):1326–1331.

Ferreira TL, da Silva TN, Canario D, Delerue MF. Hypertension and severe hypokalaemia associated with ectopic ACTH production. *BMJ Case Rep*. 2018;2018:bcr2017223406.

Glavey SV, Gertz MA, Dispenzieri A, et al. Long-term outcome of patients with multiple [corrected] myeloma-related advanced renal failure following auto-SCT. *Bone Marrow Transplant*. 2013;48(12):1543–1547.

Glezerman IG, Devlin S, Maloy M, et al. Long term renal survival in patients undergoing T-Cell depleted versus conventional hematopoietic stem cell transplants. *Bone Marrow Transplant*. 2017;52(5):733–738.

Gralla RJ, Ahmad F, Blais JD, et al. Tolvaptan use in cancer patients with hyponatremia due to the syndrome of inappropriate antidiuretic hormone: a post hoc analysis of the SALT-1 and SALT-2 trials. *Cancer Med*. 2017;6(4):723–729.

Gupta S, Gudsoorkar P, Jhaveri KD. Acute kidney injury in critically ill patients with cancer. *Clin J Am Soc Nephrol*. 2022;17(9):1385–1398.

Gupta S, Short SAP, Sise ME, et al. Acute kidney injury in patients treated with immune checkpoint inhibitors. *J Immunother Cancer*. 2021;9(10):e003467.

Hájek R, Masszi T, Petrucci MT, et al. A randomized phase III study of carfilzomib vs low-dose corticosteroids with optional cyclophosphamide in relapsed and refractory multiple myeloma (FOCUS). *Leukemia*. 2017;31(1):107–114.

Herlitz LC, Roglieri J, Resta R, Bhagat G, Markowitz GS. Light chain proximal tubulopathy. *Kidney Int*. 2009;76(7):792–797.

Hingorani S. Renal complications of hematopoietic-cell transplantation. *N Engl J Med*. 2016;374(23):2256–2267.

Holland-Bill L, Christiansen CF, Farkas DK, Donskov F, Jorgensen JOL, Sorensen HT. Diagnosis of hyponatremia and increased risk of a subsequent cancer diagnosis: results from a nationwide population-based cohort study. *Acta Oncol*. 2018;57(4):522–527.

Howard SC, McCormick J, Pui C-H, Buddington RK, Harvey RD. Preventing and managing toxicities of high-dose methotrexate. *Oncologist*. 2016;21(12):1471–1482.

Hurabielle C, Pillebout E, Stehlé T, et al. Mechanisms underpinning increased plasma creatinine levels in patients receiving vemurafenib for advanced melanoma. *PLoS One*. 2016;11(3):e0149873.

Izzedine H, El-Fekih RK, Perazella MA. The renal effects of ALK inhibitors. *Invest New Drugs*. 2016;34(5):643–649.

Izzedine H, Escudier B, Lhomme C, et al. Kidney diseases associated with anti-vascular endothelial growth factor (VEGF): an 8-year observational study at a single center. *Medicine (Baltimore)*. 2014;93(24):333–339.

Izzedine H, Massard C, Spano JP, Goldwasser F, Khayat D, Soria JC. VEGF signaling inhibition-induced proteinuria: mechanisms, significance and management. *Eur J Cancer*. 2010;46(2):439–448.

Jaguś D, Lis K, Niemczyk L, Basak GW. Kidney dysfunction after hematopoietic cell transplantation-Etiology, management, and perspectives. *Hematol Oncol Stem Cell Ther*. 2018;11(4):195–205.

Janus N, Launay-Vacher V, Byloos E, et al. Cancer and renal insufficiency: results of the BIRMA study. *Br J Cancer*. 2010;103(12):1815–1821.

Jhaveri KD. *Nephron Power*. 2015. Accessed March 24, 2020. http://www.nephronpower.com/2015/01/concept-map-glomerular-diseases-seen.html

Jhaveri KD, Sakhiya V, Fishbane S. Nephrotoxicity of the BRAF inhibitors vemurafenib and dabrafenib. *JAMA Oncol*. 2015;1(8):1133–1134.

Jhaveri KD, Shah HH, Calderon K, Campenot ES, Radhakrishnan J. Glomerular diseases seen with cancer and chemotherapy: a narrative review. *Kidney Int*. 2013;84:34–44.

Jhaveri KD, Wanchoo R, Sakhiya V, Ross DW, Fishbane S. Adverse renal effects of novel molecular oncologic targeted therapies: a narrative review. *Kidney Int Rep*. 2016;2(1):108–123.

Jodele S, Dandoy CE, Lane A, et al. Complement blockade for TA-TMA: lessons learned from a large pediatric cohort treated with eculizumab. *Blood*. 2020;135(13):1049–1057.

Jodele S, Sabulski A. Reeling in complement in transplant-associated thrombotic microangiopathy: you're going to need a bigger boat. *Am J Hematol*. 2023;98(Suppl 4):S57–S73.

Jodele S, Zhang K, Zou F, et al. The genetic fingerprint of susceptibility for transplant-associated thrombotic microangiopathy. *Blood.* 2016;127(8):989–996.

Johnson DB, Nebhan CA, Moslehi JJ, Balko JM. Immune-checkpoint inhibitors: long-term implications of toxicity. *Nat Rev Clin Oncol.* 2022;19(4):254–267.

Kanduri SR, Cheungpasitporn W, Thongprayoon C, et al. Systematic review of risk factors and incidence of acute kidney injury among patients treated with CAR-T cell therapies. *Kidney Int Rep.* 2021;6(5):1416–1422.

Kemlin D, Biard L, Kerhuel L, et al. Acute kidney injury in critically ill patients with solid tumours. *Nephrol Dial Transplant.* 2018;33(11):1997–2005.

Khan MI, Dellinger RP, Waguespack SG. Electrolyte disturbances in critically ill cancer patients: an endocrine perspective. *J Intensive Care Med.* 2018;33:147–158.

Khosla J, Yeh AC, Spitzer TR, Dey BR. Hematopoietic stem cell transplant-associated thrombotic microangiopathy: current paradigm and novel therapies. *Bone Marrow Transplant.* 2018; 53(2):129–137.

Kitchlu A, Jhaveri KD, Wadhwani S, et al. A systematic review of immune checkpoint inhibitor-associated glomerular disease. *Kidney Int Rep.* 2020;6(1):66–77.

Kitchlu A, McArthur E, Amir E, et al. Acute kidney injury in patients receiving systemic treatment for cancer: a population-based cohort study. *J Natl Cancer Inst.* 2019;111(7):727–736.

Larsen CP, Bell JM, Harris AA, Messias NC, Wang YH, Walker PD. The morphologic spectrum and clinical significance of light chain proximal tubulopathy with and without crystal formation. *Mod Pathol.* 2011;24(11):1462–1469.

Latcha S, Jaimes EA, Patil S, Glezerman IG, Mehta S, Flombaum CD. Long-term renal outcomes after cisplatin treatment. *Clin J Am Soc Nephrol.* 2016;11(7):1173–1179.

Launay-Vacher V. Epidemiology of chronic kidney disease in cancer patients: lessons from the IRMA Study Group. *Semin Nephrol.* 2010;30(6):548–556.

Launay-Vacher V, Izzedine H, Rey J-B, et al. Incidence of renal insufficiency in cancer patients and evaluation of information available on the use of anticancer drugs in renally impaired patients. *Med Sci Monit.* 2004;10(5):CR209–CR212.

Launay-Vacher V, Janus N, Deray G. Renal insufficiency and cancer treatments. *ESMO Open.* 2016;1(4):e000091.

Launay-Vacher V, Oudard S, Janus N, et al; Renal Insufficiency and Cancer Medications (IRMA) Study Group. Prevalence of renal insufficiency in cancer patients and implications for anticancer drug management: the renal insufficiency and anticancer medications (IRMA) study. *Cancer.* 2007;110(6):1376–1384.

Lefaucheur C, Stengel B, Nochy D, et al. Membranous nephropathy and cancer: epidemiologic evidence and determinants of high-risk cancer association. *Kidney Int.* 2006;70:1510–1517.

Leung N, Bridoux F, Batuman V, et al. The evaluation of monoclonal gammopathy of renal significance: a consensus report of the International Kidney and Monoclonal Gammopathy Research Group. *Nat Rev Nephrol.* 2019;15(1):45–59.

Leung N, Bridoux F, Nasr SH. Monoclonal gammopathy of renal significance. *N Engl J Med.* 2021;384(20):1931–1941.

Leung N, Rajkumar SV. Multiple myeloma with acute light chain cast nephropathy. *Blood Cancer J.* 2023;13(1):46.

Li L, Lau WL, Rhee CM, et al. Risk of chronic kidney disease after cancer nephrectomy. *Nat Rev Nephrol.* 2014;10:135–145.

Liborio AB, Abreu KLS, Silva GB Jr, et al. Predicting hospital mortality in critically ill cancer patients according to acute kidney injury severity. *Oncology.* 2011;80(3–4):160–166.

Lodhi A, Kumar A, Saqlain MU, Suneja M. Thrombotic microangiopathy associated with proteasome inhibitors. *Clin Kidney J.* 2015;8(5):632–636.

Maitland ML, Bakris GL, Black HR, et al; Cardiovascular Toxicities Panel, Convened by the Angiogenesis Task Force of the National Cancer Institute Investigational Drug Steering Committee. Initial assessment, surveillance, and management of blood pressure in patients receiving vascular endothelial growth factor signaling pathway inhibitors. *J Natl Cancer Inst.* 2010;102(9):596–604.

Malard F, Holler E, Sandmaier BM, Huang H, Mohty M. Acute graft-versus-host disease. *Nat Rev Dis Primers.* 2023;9(1):27.

Malina M, Roumenina LT, Seeman T, et al. Genetics of hemolytic uremic syndromes. *Presse Med.* 2012;41(3 Pt 2):e105–e114.

Mohty M, Malard F, Abecasis M, et al. Prophylactic, preemptive, and curative treatment for sinusoidal obstruction syndrome/veno-occlusive disease in adult patients: a position statement from an international expert group. *Bone Marrow Transplant.* 2020;55(3):485–495.

Moreau P, Richardson PG, Cavo M, et al. Proteasome inhibitors in multiple myeloma: 10 years later. *Blood*. 2012;120(5):947–959.

Motwani SS, Herlitz L, Monga D, Jhaveri KD, Lam AQ; American Society of Nephrology Onco-Nephrology Forum. Paraprotein-related kidney disease: glomerular diseases associated with paraproteinemias. *Clin J Am Soc Nephrol*. 2016;11(12):2260–2272.

Na SY, Sung JY, Chang JH, et al. Chronic kidney disease in cancer patients: an independent predictor of cancer-specific mortality. *Am J Nephrol*. 2011;33:121–130.

Pabla N, Dong Z. Cisplatin nephrotoxicity: mechanisms and renoprotective strategies. *Kidney Int*. 2008;73(9):994–1007.

Perazella MA. Drug-induced acute kidney injury: diverse mechanisms of tubular injury. *Curr Opin Crit Care*. 2019;25(6):550–557.

Perazella MA. Pharmacology behind common drug nephrotoxicities. *Clin J Am Soc Nephrol*. 2018;13(12):1897–1908.

Perazella MA, Shirali AC. Nephrotoxicity of cancer immunotherapies: past, present and future. *J Am Soc Nephrol*. 2018;29(8):2039–2052.

Rajkumar SV, Dimopoulos MA, Palumbo A, et al. International Myeloma Working Group updated criteria for the diagnosis of multiple myeloma. *Lancet Oncol*. 2014;15(12):e538–e548.

Rashidi A, Wanchoo R, Izzedine H. How I manage hypertension and proteinuria associated with VEGF inhibitor. *Clin J Am Soc Nephrol*. 2023;18(1):121–123.

Renaghan AD, Jaimes EA, Malyszko J, Perazella MA, Sprangers B, Rosner MH. Acute kidney injury and CKD associated with hematopoietic stem cell transplantation. *Clin J Am Soc Nephrol*. 2020;15:289–297.

Renaghan AD, Kennedy C, Magee CC. Kidney disease in liver, cardiac, lung, and hematopoietic stem cell transplantation. In: Johnson RJ, Floege J, Tonelli M, eds. *Comprehensive Clinical Nephrology*. 7th ed. Elsevier; 2024:799–808

Richmond J, Sherman RS, Diamond HD, Craver LF. Renal lesions associated with malignant lymphomas. *Am J Med*. 1962;32:184–207.

Rosner MH, Dalkin AC. Electrolyte disorders associated with cancer. *Adv Chronic Kidney Dis*. 2014;21:7–17.

Rosner MH, Dalkin AC. Onco-nephrology: the pathophysiology and treatment of malignancy-associated hypercalcemia. *Clin J Am Soc Nephrol*. 2012;7(10):1722–1729.

Rosner MH, Perazella MA. Acute kidney injury in patients with cancer. *N Engl J Med*. 2017;376(18):1770–1781.

Rosner MH, Perazella MA. Acute kidney injury in the patient with cancer. *Kidney Res Clin Pract*. 2019;38(3):295–308.

Sanders PW. Mechanisms of light chain injury along the tubular nephron. *J Am Soc Nephrol*. 2012;23(11):1777–1781.

Sandhu G, Adattini J, Armstrong Gordon E, O'Neill N; On behalf of the ADDIKD Guideline Working Group. *International Consensus Guideline on Anticancer Drug Dosing in kidney Dysfunction*. eviQ, Cancer Institute NSW; 2022. St Leonards, Australia.

Santoriello D, Andal LM, Cox R, D'Agati VD, Markowitz GS. Lysozyme-induced nephropathy. *Kidney Int Rep*. 2016;2(1):84–88.

Schoettler ML, Carreras E, Cho B, et al. Harmonizing definitions for diagnostic criteria and prognostic assessment of transplantation-associated thrombotic microangiopathy: a report on behalf of the European society for blood and marrow transplantation, American Society for Transplantation and Cellular Therapy, Asia-Pacific Blood and Marrow Transplantation Group, and Center for International Blood and Marrow Transplant Research. *Transplant Cell Ther*. 2023;29(3):151–163.

Shimada M, Johnson RJ, May WS Jr, et al. A novel role for uric acid in acute kidney injury associated with tumour lysis syndrome. *Nephrol Dial Transplant*. 2009;24(10):2960–2964.

Sorensen JB, Andersen MK, Hansen HH. Syndrome of inappropriate secretion of antidiuretic hormone (SIADH) in malignant disease. *J Intern Med*. 1995;238(2):97–110.

Specter R, Sanchorawala V, Seldin DC, et al. Kidney dysfunction during lenalidomide treatment for AL amyloidosis. *Nephrol Dial Transplant*. 2011;26(3):881–886.

Srinivasan R, Balow JE, Sabnis S, et al. Nephrotic syndrome: an under-recognised immune-mediated complication of non-myeloablative allogeneic haematopoietic cell transplantation. *Br J Haematol*. 2005;131(1):74–79.

Stokes MB, Valeri AM, Herlitz L, et al. Light chain proximal tubulopathy: clinical and pathologic characteristics in the modern treatment era. *J Am Soc Nephrol*. 2016;27(5):1555–1565.

Suppadungsuk S, Phitakwatchara W, Reungwetwattana T, et al. Preloading magnesium attenuates cisplatin-associated nephrotoxicity: pilot randomized controlled trial (PRAGMATIC study). *ESMO Open*. 2022;7(1):100351.

Tang C, Livingston MJ, Safirstein R, Dong Z. Cisplatin nephrotoxicity: new insights and therapeutic implications. *Nat Rev Nephrol*. 2023;19(1):53–72.

Thomas MH, Chisholm GD. Retroperitoneal fibrosis associated with malignant disease. *Br J Cancer*. 1973;28(5):453–458.

Törnroth T, Heiro M, Marcussen N, Franssila K. Lymphomas diagnosed by percutaneous kidney biopsy. *Am J Kidney Dis*. 2003;42(5):960–971.

Truong H, Leung N. Fixed-dose glucarpidase for toxic methotrexate levels and acute kidney injury in adult lymphoma patients: case series. *Clin Lymphoma Myeloma Leuk*. 2021;21(6):e497–e502.

US Renal Data System (USRDS). Chapter 5: Acute kidney injury. In: USRDS, ed. *2014 USRDS Annual Data Report: Epidemiology of Kidney Disease in the United States*. Vol. 1. National Institutes of Health, National Institute of Diabetes and Digestive and Kidney Diseases. USRDS; 2014:37–45. Accessed March 24, 2020. usrds.org/2014/view/v1_05.aspx

Verbalis JG, Goldsmith SR, Greenberg A, et al. Diagnosis, evaluation, and treatment of hyponatremia: expert panel recommendations. *Am J Med*. 2013;126(10 suppl 1):S1–S42.

Walter RB, Joerger M, Pestalozzi BC. Gemcitabine-associated hemolytic uremic syndrome. *Am J Kidney Dis*. 2002;40(4):E16.

Wanchoo R, Abudayyeh A, Doshi M, et al. Renal toxicities of novel agents used for treatment of multiple myeloma. *Clin J Am Soc Nephrol*. 2017;12(1):176–189.

Wanchoo R, Bayer RL, Bassil C, Jhaveri KD. Emerging concepts in hematopoietic stem cell transplantation-associated renal thrombotic microangiopathy and prospects for new treatments. *Am J Kidney Dis*. 2018;72(6):857–865.

Wanchoo R, Jhaveri KD, Deray G, Launay-Vacher V. Renal effects of BRAF inhibitors: a systematic review by the Cancer and the Kidney International Network. *Clin Kidney J*. 2016;9(2):245–251.

Wang Q, Qi Y, Zhang D, et al. Electrolyte disorders assessment in solid tumor patients treated with anti-EGFR monoclonal antibodies: a pooled analysis of 25 randomized clinical trials. *Tumour Biol*. 2015;36(5):3471–3482.

Weitz IC. Thrombotic microangiopathy in cancer. *Thromb Res*. 2018;164(Suppl 1):S103–S105.

Widemann BC, Balis FM, Kim A, et al. Glucarpidase, leucovorin, and thymidine for high-dose methotrexate-induced renal dysfunction: clinical and pharmacologic factors affecting outcome. *J Clin Oncol*. 2010;28(25):3979–3986.

Wilson FP, Berns JS. Tumor lysis syndrome: new challenges and recent advances. *Adv Chronic Kidney Dis*. 2014;21(1):18–26.

Wong L-M, Cleeve LK, Milner AD, Pitman AG. Malignant ureteral obstruction: outcomes after intervention. Have things changed? *J Urol*. 2007;178(1):178–183; discussion 183.

Yin Z, Du J, Yu F, Xia W. Tumor-induced osteomalacia. *Osteoporos Sarcopenia*. 2018;4(4):119–127.

Yoshida T, Taguchi D, Fukuda K, et al. Incidence of hypophosphatemia in advanced cancer patients: a recent report from a single institution. *Int J Clin Oncol*. 2017;22(2):244–249.

Zirlik K, Duyster J. Anti-angiogenics: current situation and future perspectives. *Oncol Res Treat*. 2018;41(4):166–171.

20 Practical Guidelines for Drug Dosing in Patients With Impaired Kidney Function

Shehzad Rehman, Ali Olyaei

Decreased kidney function, regardless of etiology, presents significant challenges to prescribing providers. Additional considerations when selecting and dosing medications for patients with kidney dysfunction include comorbidities (hypertension, diabetes, heart disease, advanced age) and the multiple drugs used to manage those conditions. These factors highlight the critical importance of establishing baseline kidney function prior to initiating new medication regimens, as well as appropriately frequent monitoring of kidney function throughout the course of medication management. Monitoring therapeutic plasma concentration, if possible, is an important consideration. However, for many pharmacotherapeutic agents, plasma concentration cannot be monitored in the clinical setting. Thus, it is important for health care providers to understand the relationship between reduced or impaired kidney function, pharmacokinetics, and appropriate drug selection and dosing protocol for specific disease state.

Properly functioning kidneys facilitate homeostasis required for optimal cellular and metabolic functioning through regulating solute and water transport, excreting metabolic waste products, conserving nutrients, and balancing acids and bases. These functional components play integral roles in the absorption, distribution, metabolism, and especially the excretion of medications and metabolites. Chronic kidney disease (CKD) and in particular uremic state influences every organ system and every aspect of drug disposition. The physiological changes associated with CKD are not limited only to drugs with high kidney excretion; in fact, kidney disease has profound effects on the pharmacology of many drugs regardless of percentage of intact kidney eliminations. Any significant decrease in kidney function, as indicated by a glomerular filtration rate (GFR), presents therapeutic drug selection and dosing challenges. Decreased GFR is commonly seen in elderly patients and obviously in patients with acute kidney injury (AKI) and CKD.

While many prescribers realize that CKD-related decreases in kidney function and end-stage kidney disease (ESKD) significantly alter the pharmacokinetics and pharmacodynamics of many medications, there is an increased awareness that many more patients are affected by poor kidney function than previously thought. Therefore, establishing baseline kidney function, as well as systematic and ongoing assessment of kidney function on all appropriate patients throughout the therapeutic regimen is necessary in order to avoid further damage to the kidneys, as well as to achieve the desired clinical outcome for the patient.

Decreases in age-related kidney function are caused primarily by a decrease in patient size, blood flow, and subsequently GFR. With changes in kidney vasculature and profusion, the number of nephrons also decreases. The speed of this loss accelerates as the patient progresses to ESRD. The kidneys also undergo degenerative changes that decrease the ability of the kidneys to concentrate urine. In addition, the injured kidney loses its ability to adapt to various stresses; glucose, sodium, and bicarbonate are not reabsorbed as efficiently, and because of decreased rates of secretion, hyperkalemia can occur more commonly. Acid–base balance is more difficult to maintain, changes in pH and fluid load can lead to critical imbalances that can lead to and exacerbate toxicity in medications that are metabolized and eliminated via kidney processes.

Chronic Kidney Disease and Drug Pharmacokinetic
Absorption
Drug absorption in both AKI and CKD is affected by possible increases in gastric pH, gastroparesis, bowel wall edema, vomiting and diarrhea, and decreasing intestinal CYP450 activity. In general, it is difficult to assess the effect of CKD on drug absorption as many of these patients take multiple medications, many of which cannot be discontinued or withheld to study the alterations in absorption of other drugs. Medications taken by patients with impaired kidney function to manage these conditions, such as antacids, proton pump inhibitors, and H2 receptor antagonists, also impact other drug's absorption. Increased gastric pH decreases the absorption, and therefore the bioavailability of drugs that are more readily absorbed in an acidic environment. Taking antacids can also decrease drug absorption, especially of mycophenolate for the treatment of autoimmune kidney disease and fluoroquinolones for the treatment of pyelonephritis, through chelation of those components into insoluble compounds. Tacrolimus; a calcineurin inhibitor, is commonly used in transplant recipients or patients with FSGS. The pharmacokinetic profile of tacrolimus alters significantly in patients with diarrhea and requires more monitoring to avoid drug toxicities. Gastroparesis, or delayed gastric emptying, is common in diabetic patients with CKD or patients taking significant phosphate binders. These factors could increase the amount of time needed to achieve maximum drug concentrations, although this appears to only impact very short-acting medications. Also, bowel wall edema, vomiting, and diarrhea can decrease overall drug absorption in CKD patients. Lastly, kidney insufficiency is linked with decreased gastrointestinal (GI) CYP450 activity. This can drastically increase the amount of drug absorbed by significantly reducing the amount of drug metabolized via CYP450 in the GI tract.

Distribution
Drug distribution in CKD patients is affected by alterations in fluid states and changes in the extent of protein binding in plasma, which impacts therapeutic drug concentrations, and tissue binding, which affects volume of distribution. Patients with advanced kidney insufficiency are commonly uremic and have low plasma albumin levels. Acidic drugs are most significantly affected by hypoalbuminemia because of increased competition for available binding sites. This can lead to both accumulation of other medications and metabolites while also increasing levels of free drug in the plasma, which can also lead to toxicity or conversely to more drug undergoing biotransformation, resulting in decreased drug action. Fluid status and overall body composition are also significantly impacted by CKD and are important considerations when choosing and dosing drugs. Prescribers must be aware that volume of distribution will change in patients with ascites, edema, and overall hydration status, especially with hydrophilic drugs. Increased adipose tissue and decreased lean muscle mass, or patients with muscle wasting, are also common for elderly patients and CKD patients. These changes in body composition can reduce the volume of distribution, thereby increasing serum levels of hydrophilic drugs.

Metabolism
Metabolism of both renal and nonrenal metabolized drugs and metabolites is significantly slowed in patients with reduced kidney function. This can lead to accumulation of drugs, pharmacologically active agents, as well as toxic metabolites and can lead to significant adverse events. When a drug undergoes biotransformation, an active drug metabolite is a frequent by-product. These metabolites have an effect and action, and while the initial drug may be effectively excreted via urine, the still-active metabolite can easily accumulate to potentially dangerous levels, causing adverse clinical outcomes. CKD also impacts drug metabolism through impaired CYP450 activities in both Phase I and Phase II reactions, which are necessary for drugs to undergo predictable biotransformation and subsequent therapeutic outcomes.

Elimination

Drug elimination of drug and active metabolites is dependent on several aspects of kidney functioning; GFR, tubular secretion, and reabsorption. Drug elimination via glomerular filtration in CKD patients occurs in relation to the patient's level of GFR, the amount of free drug compared with the amount of drug bound to protein. CKD patients also experience decreased tubular secretion, as well as reduced medication reabsorption, which is indicated by higher levels of urine concentrations of renally eliminated drugs. Finally, it is important to review that kidney insufficiency slows the elimination of active drug metabolites, which are still biologically active, and when they reach a certain level of accumulation can cause adverse clinical outcomes. For many drugs, the kidneys are the primary route for drug elimination within the body. CKD reduces glomerular filtration and can be assessed by creatinine clearance. To calculate kidney function or adjust for drug elimination and dosing schedule, the following calculations are recommended when determining creatinine clearance for those adults with stable kidney function. Thus, during AKI, the serum creatinine or creatinine clearance will no longer reflect the true kidney or drug clearance rate. In these cases, other methods should be applied (a timed urine collection) to estimate kidney function. Finally, in oliguric patients, the creatinine clearance should be considered as less than 5 mL/min.

Cockcroft–Gault (CG) Equation

CrCl (mL/min) = [(140 − age) × Weight in kg]/(serum creatinine × 72) × (0.85 if female)

Ideal body weight (IBW) was used unless actual body weight (ABW) < IBW. If ABW was >30% of IBW, adjusted body weight was used where:

$$\text{adjusted bodyweight} = [(ABW - IBW) \times 0.4] + IBW.$$

IBW male = 50 + 2.3 × (Height in inches − 60);
IBW female = 45.5 + 2.3 × (Height in inches − 60)

For obese men and women, the equation should be modified:

$$(\text{obese men}) = \frac{(137 - \text{age}) \times [(0.285 \times \text{wgt}) + (12.1 \times \text{hgt}^2)]}{51 \times \text{SCr}}$$

$$(\text{obese women}) = \frac{(146 - \text{age}) \times [(0.287 \times \text{wgt}) + (9.74 \times \text{hgt}^2)]}{60 \times \text{SCr}}$$

wgt = patient's weight in kg
hgt = patient's height in cm

Modification of Diet in Renal Disease Re-Expressed Equation (MDRD)

eGFR MDRD = 175 × SCr − 1.154 × Age − 0.203 × (0.742 if female) × (1.21 if AA)

AA refers to African American.

Chronic Kidney Disease Epidemiology Collaboration Equation (CKD-EPI)

eGFR CKD-EPI = 141 × min(SCr/k, 1)a × max(SCr/k, 1) − 1.209 × 0.993 Age × 1.018 (if female) × 1.159 (if African American),

where k is 0.7 for females and 0.9 for males, a is −0.329 for females and −0.411 for males, min indicates the minimum of SCr/k or 1, and max indicates the maximum of SCr/k or 1.

Most clinical pharmacists and pharmaceutical manufactures use Cockcroft–Gault equation to estimate GFR for drug dosing in patients with kidney insufficiency. However, Cockcroft–Gault formula overestimates kidney function by approximately 30% of the corresponding inulin clearance test.

One of the main limitations of the newer available GFR estimation equations (MDRD, CKD-EPI, CKD-EPI 2021 with and without cystatin C) is the lack of information about drug dosing in CKD. See Table 20-1.

The eGFR (2021 CKD-EPI equations) without race coefficient is an improved method because it is adjusted for body surface area while calculating creatinine clearance. Both the Food and Drug Administration (FDA) and European Medicines Agency (EMA) are issuing a new guideline for new drug applications to determine appropriate method of kidney function assessment and drug dosing for patients with reduced kidney function. Although the result yet to be published, the preliminary information indicates the use of 2021 CKD-EPI with cystatin C when is available equations will be recommended to estimate GFR for drug dosing in CKD patients. In addition, both NKF and the American Society of Nephrology recommended using the CKD-EPI Creatinine Equation (2021) to estimate GFR when both creatine and cystatin C could be obtained.

While, for all these equations, the recognition of the limitations of these estimations is essential, it is important to standardize the global approach to kidney function assessment and use 2021 CKD-EPI with cystatin C without the race variables to provide the best possible estimates of GFR when considering for drug dosing in patients with reduced kidney function.

Drug Dosing in Patients With Chronic Kidney Disease

Selecting and dosing drugs for patients with CKD is a significant clinical challenge and requires close coordination between the patient, the prescriber, and the pharmacist. A comprehensive initial assessment of the patient, including liver function tests, serum albumin levels, allergies, degree of kidney functioning, fluid status, in addition to all medications, over the counter and prescribed, allergies and comorbidities, is paramount. The review of the patient's medication list at this time is to ensure a clinical valid reason for maintaining that therapy and to ensure that medications are not a causal agent in the patient's decreased kidney functioning. If additional drugs are needed, it is critical to choose the least nephrotoxic drug available and to work closely with the pharmacist to select the appropriate loading and maintenance doses. Finally, frequent monitoring of drug levels when available and of kidney function is critical to ensure protection of remaining kidney function (Table 20-2). There are two methods for dosage adjustment in patients with reduced kidney function: prolonged interval or reduced dose. Prolonging the dose interval is often a convenient and cost-effective method for altering the drug dose in patients with reduced kidney function. This method is particularly useful for drugs with wide therapeutic ranges and long plasma half-lives. Extended parenteral therapy can be completed without prolonged hospitalization when the dose interval can safely be lengthened to allow for home therapy. If the range between the therapeutic and toxic levels is too narrow, either potentially toxic or subtherapeutic plasma concentrations may result.

To maintain the same dose interval as for patients with normal kidney function, one may decrease the amount of each individual dose given to kidney-impaired patients. This method is effective for drugs with narrow therapeutic ranges and short plasma half-lives in patients with kidney insufficiency. In practice, a combination of the methods is often effective and convenient. The combination method uses modification of both the dose and dose interval. For drugs with particularly long half-lives in patients with impaired kidney function, give the total daily dose as a single dose each day. Similarly, divide the total daily dose in half and give twice daily. The decision to extend the dosing interval beyond a 24-hour period should be based on the necessity to maintain therapeutic peak or trough drug levels. When the peak level is most important, prolong the dose interval. However, when the minimum trough level must be maintained, modification of the individual dose or a combination of the dose and interval methods may be preferred. The following Tables 20-3 through 20-23 provide information about drug dosing in several categories in patients with CKD.

TABLE 20-1 Comparison of GFR Estimation Equations

		Year	Population = N	Ethnicity	Gender Factor	Race Factor	Age of Population	Limitation	Advantage
Cockroft–Gault	CG (mL/min) = [(140 − age) *weight*1.23/ Scr]* 0.85 (if female)	1976	239	White men	X 0.85 for female	No race	18–92	Underestimate renal function	More accurate for obese patients
MDRD	MDRD (mL/min/1.73 m²) = 30849*Scr$^{-1.154}$ *age$^{-0.203}$ *0.742 (if female) *1.212 (if Black)	1999	1,623	80% White	X 0.742 for female	X 1.21 for Black	18–70	Underestimate kidney function, race variable included	More accurate for younger and nonobese patients
CKD-EPI	CKD-EPI (mL/min/1.73 m²) = 141 (Scr/k·1)^{α*} max(Scr/k·1)$^{-1.209}$*0.993^{Age} *1.018 (if female) 1.159 (if Black)	2009	3,896	30% Black	X 1.018 for female	X 1.159 for Black	50 (15)	Limited number of minorities and older patients Race variable included	Less bias and more accrued at higher eGFR
CKD-EPI 2021	eGFR = 142* min(standardized Scr/K, 1)$α*$ max(standardized Scr/K, 1)-1.200* 0.9938 Age* 1.012 (if female)	2021	4,050	14% Black	X 1.012 for female	No Race	57.0 ± 17.4	Limited minorities with low GFR	No race variable including cystatin C is most accurate. **The recommended method for estimating GFR in adults from the National Kidney Foundation is the 2021 CKD-EPI equations.**

TABLE 20-2 Therapeutic Drug Monitoring in Patients With Chronic Kidney Disease

Drug Name	Therapeutic Range	When to Draw Sample	How Often to Draw Levels
Aminoglycosides (Conventional Dosing)	Gentamicin and tobramycin:	Trough: Immediately before dose	Check peak and trough with third dose.
Gentamicin, tobramycin amikacin	Trough: 0.5–2 mg/L	Peak: 30 min after a 30–45-min infusion	For therapy less than 72 h, levels not necessary. Repeat drug levels weekly or if renal function changes.
Amikacin:	Trough: <10 mg/L 0.5–3 mg/L		
Aminoglycosides (24-h Dosing)		Obtain random drug level 12 h after dose	After initial dose. Repeat drug level in 1 wk or if renal function changes.
Gentamicin, tobramycin, amikacin			
Carbamazepine	4–12 mcg/mL	Trough: Immediately before dosing	Check 2–4 days after the first dose or change in dose.
Cyclosporin	150–400 ng/mL	Trough: Immediately before dosing	Daily for first wk, then weekly
Digoxin	0.8–2.0 ng/mL	12 h after maintenance dose	5–7 days after first dose for patients with normal renal and hepatic function; 15–20 days in anephric patients.
Lidocaine	1–5 mcg/mL	8 h after IV infusion started or changed	
Lithium		Trough: Before AM dose at least 12 h since last dose	Acute: 0.8–1.2 mmol/L
	Chronic: 0.6–0.8 mmol/L		

(continued)

TABLE 20-2 Therapeutic Drug Monitoring in Patients With Chronic Kidney Disease *(Continued)*

Drug Name	Therapeutic Range	When to Draw Sample	How Often to Draw Levels
Phenobarbital	15–40 mcg/mL	Trough: Immediately before dosing	Check 2 wk after first dose or change in dose. Follow-up level in 1–2 mo.
Phenytoin	10–20 mcg/mL	Trough: Immediately before dosing	5–7 d after first dose or after change in dose.
Free Phenytoin	1–2 mcg/mL		
Procainamide	(A) 4–10 mcg/mL	(A) Trough: Immediately before next dose or 12–18 h after starting or changing an infusion	
NAPA (N-acetyl procainamide), a procainamide metabolite	Trough: 4 mcg/mL	(B) Draw with procainamide sample	
	Peak: 8 mcg/mL (B) 10–30 mcg/mL		
Quinidine	1–5 mcg/mL	Trough: Immediately before next dose	
Sirolimus	10–20 ng/dL	Trough: Immediately before next dose	
Tacrolimus (FK-506)	10–15 ng/mL	Trough: Immediately before next dose	Daily for first week, then weekly
Theophylline PO or aminophylline IV	15–20 mcg/mL	Trough: Immediately before next dose	
Valproic acid	40–100 mcg/mL	Trough: Immediately before next dose	Check 2–4 after first dose or change in dose
Vancomycin	Trough: 12–18 mg/L	Trough: Immediately before dose	With third dose (when initially starting therapy or after each dosage adjustment). For therapy <72 h, levels not necessary. Repeat drug levels if renal function changes.

TABLE 20-3 Alzheimer Drug Dosing in Renal Failure

Drug	Normal Dosage	% of Renal Excretion	Dosage Adjustment in Renal Failure			Comments	Hemo-dialysis	Continuous Ambulatory Peritoneal Dialysis	Continuous Venovenous Hemofiltration
			GFR >50 mL/min	GFR 10-50 mL/min	GFR <10 mL/min				
Cholinesterase Inhibitors									
Donepezil	5 mg QD	79%	No renal adjustment required			Approved for all stages. Associated with QT prolongation, bradycardia, weight loss, rare cases of neuroleptic malignant syndrome (NMS).			
Galantamine	IR: 4 mg bid ER: 8 mg QD	20–25%	10–60 mL/min: Max 16 mg/d		Not recommended	Approved for mild to moderate. CNS depression, skin reaction, bradycardia, weight loss.			
Rivastigmine	1.5 mg bid	97%	No renal adjustment required			Approved for mild to moderate. CNS depression, skin reaction, bradycardia, weight loss.			
NMDA Receptor Antagonist									
Memantine	IR: 5 mg QD ER: 7 mg QD	74%	5–29 mL/min: IR: Max 5 mg bid ER: Max 14 mg/d			Approved for moderate to severe. Dizziness, headache, weight gain.			

TABLE 20-4 Analgesic Drug Dosing in Renal Failure

Drug	Normal Dosage	% of Renal Excretion	Dosage Adjustment in Renal Failure			Comments	Hemodialysis	Continuous Ambulatory Peritoneal Dialysis	Continuous Venovenous Hemofiltration
			GFR >50 mL/min	GFR 10-50 mL/min	GFR <10 mL/min				
Narcotics and Narcotic Antagonists									
Alfentanil	Anesthetic induction 8-40 mcg/kg	Hepatic	100%	100%	100%	Titrate the dose regimen, potent short-acting analgesic widely used in anesthesia	N/A	N/A	N/A
Butorphanol	2 mg intranasally q3-4h	Hepatic	100%	75%	50%		No data	No data	N/A
Codeine	30-60 mg PO q4-6h	Hepatic	100%	75%	50%	Prodrug; converted to morphine by CYP2D6	No data	No data	Dose for GFR 10-50 mL/min
Fentanyl	Anesthetic induction (individualized)	Hepatic	100%	75%	50%	CRRT: titrate; inactive metabolites; no significant accumulation in patient with advanced CKD; don't use in opioid naive patient	N/A	N/A	N/A

Meperidine	50–100 mg q3–4h	Hepatic	100%	75%	50%	Normeperidine, an active metabolite, accumulates in ESRD and may cause seizures; protein binding is reduced in ESRD; 20–25% excreted unchanged in acidic urine; not for long-term pain	Avoid	Avoid	Avoid
Methadone	2.5–10 mg q8–12h	Hepatic	100%	100%	50–75%	Useful in advanced CKD; excreted mainly in feces	None	None	N/A
Morphine	20–25 mg q4h	Hepatic	100%	75%	50%	Increased sensitivity to drug effect in ESRD	None	No data	Dose for GFR 10–50 mL/min
Naloxone	0.4–2 mg IV	Hepatic	100%	100%	100%	Repeat q2–3min prn, call emergency ASAP	N/A	N/A	Dose for GFR 10–50 mL/min
Pentazocine	50 mg q4h	Hepatic	100%	75%	75%	Used as **anesthesia**	None	No data	Dose for GFR 10–50 mL/min
Propoxyphene	65 mg PO q6–8h	Hepatic	100%	100%	Avoid	Active metabolite norpropoxyphene accumulates in ESRD, lead to cardiotoxicity, used as pain reliever and cough suppressant; moa unknown	Avoid	Avoid	N/A

(continued)

TABLE 20-4 Analgesic Drug Dosing in Renal Failure (Continued)

Drug	Normal Dosage	% of Renal Excretion	Dosage Adjustment in Renal Failure			Comments	Hemodialysis	Continuous Ambulatory Peritoneal Dialysis	Continuous Venovenous Hemofiltration
			GFR >50 mL/min	GFR 10-50 mL/min	GFR <10 mL/min				
Sufentanil	Anesthetic induction	Hepatic	100%	100%	100%	CRRT: titrate; anesthesia; metabolize in liver and small intestine	N/A	N/A	N/A
Buprenorphine	0.3 mg IM or slow IV (over 2 min) q6h prn; additional dose of up to 0.3 mg may be given 30–60 min following initial dose	27–30% (3.7% unchanged or active metabolite)	100%	100%	100%	Ceiling effect on respiration SE; two metabolite, buprenorphine-3-glucuronide (B3G) and nor-buprenorphine, excreted mainly through feces, 10–30% in urine; B3G inactive, nor-buprenorphine is active but does not cross BBB; useful in severe CKD	No, but possible with high doses and concomitant hypoalbuminemia	N/A	N/A

Oxycodone ER	Initial dosage, 9 mg orally every 12 hours with food. Adjust dose as necessary by 25–50% every 1–2 day. max dose 288 mg/d	Metabolized extensively by the liver	CrCl <60 mL/min: Conservative approach, if a dose <9 mg use alternatives		CrCl <60 mL/min: the concentrations of oxycodone in the plasma are approximately 50% higher compared to patients with normal renal function		
Oxycodone HCl	Initial, 10 mg orally every 12 hours; titrate by 25–50% of the current dose every 1–2 day based on analgesic requirement and tolerance	Extensively metabolized via CYP3A4 and partially by CYP2D6	CrCl <60 mL/min: Initiate at lower end of dosage range (use with caution)		In patients with renal impairment, initiate conservatively and adjust based on patient response		
Hydrocodone ER	Initial: 15 mg orally every 12 h	Excreted primarily through renal route	No renal dose adjustment required	No renal dose adjustment required	No renal dose adjustment required	N/A	N/A	N/A
Hydromorphone	2–4 mg PO q4–6h prn	75%, extensively metabolized by liver	100%	CrCl 40–50: 50%; CrCl <30: 25%	CrCl <30: 25%, consider alternative	Higher risk for respiratory depression, accumulation of metabolite hydromorphone-3-glucuronide (H3G) can lead to muscle jerks and delirium symptoms; not as well tolerated in severe CKD	N/A	N/A

(continued)

TABLE 20-4 Analgesic Drug Dosing in Renal Failure (*Continued*)

Drug	Normal Dosage	% of Renal Excretion	Dosage Adjustment in Renal Failure			Comments	Hemodialysis	Continuous Ambulatory Peritoneal Dialysis	Continuous Venovenous Hemofiltration
			GFR >50 mL/min	GFR 10–50 mL/min	GFR <10 mL/min				
Non-Narcotics									
Acetaminophen	650 q4h	Hepatic	q4h	q6h	q8h	Overdose may be nephrotoxic; drug is major metabolite of phenacetin	None	None	Dose for GFR 10–50 mL/min
Acetylsalicylic acid	650 mg q4h	Hepatic (renal)	q4h	q4–6h	Avoid	Nephrotoxic in high doses; may decrease GFR when RBF is prostaglandin dependent; may add to uremic GI and hematologic symptoms; protein binding reduced in ESRD	Dose after dialysis	None	Dose for GFR 10–50 mL/min
Ibuprofen	200–400 mg q4–6h prn (max 1,200 mg/d; do not take longer than 10 day unless directed by a physician)	45–79% (1% unchanged)	100%	100% (not recommended <50 eGFR)	Avoid	All nonselective NSAIDs or COX-2-specific may cause AKI via attenuation of renal vasodilation. Diuretics, ACEi, ARB, and calcineurin inhibitors may increase risk of NSAID-induced AKI	None	None	Dose for GFR 10–50 mL/min

TABLE 20-5 Anticoagulant Drug Dosing in Renal Failure

Drug	Normal Doses			Dosage Adjustment in Renal Failure				
	Starting Dose	Maximum Dose	% of Renal Excretion	GFR >50	GFR 10–50 mL/min	GFR <10 mL/min	Comments	
Alteplase	0.9 mg/kg IV 1 min, 0.81 mg/kg as continuous infusion over 60 min	No data	100	100%	100%	tpa. Patients >100 kg LD is 9 mg IV bolus over 1 min, followed by 81 mg continuous infusion over 60 min		
Anistreplase	30 U IV over 2–5 min		No data	100%	100%	100%	1–3 h of onset of symptoms for most benefit, upper limit is 5–6 h after onset	
Aspirin	81 mg/d	325 mg/d	10%	100%	100%	100%	GI irritation and bleeding tendency, dialyzable by hemodialysis	
Apixaban	5 mg bid	27	100%	50%	50%	Only reduce dose if 2 of the 3: CrCl <30, weight <60 kg, and 80 yo		
Clopidogrel	LD 300–600 mg, Maintenance 75 mg/d	50	100%	100%	100%	100%	Not dialyzable by hemodialysis	
Dabigatran	150 mg PO q12h	80	100%	50%	no data	Avoid in P-gp inhibitor		

(continued)

TABLE 20-5 Anticoagulant Drug Dosing in Renal Failure (Continued)

	Normal Doses			Dosage Adjustment in Renal Failure			
Drug	Starting Dose	Maximum Dose	% of Renal Excretion	GFR >50	GFR 10-50 mL/min	GFR <10 mL/min	Comments
Dalteparin	2,500 units SQ/d	unknown	100	100%	no data		Not dialyzable by hemodialysis
Dipyridamole	75–100 mg QID		No data	100%	100%	100%	Not dialyzable by hemodialysis
Edoxaban	60 mg/d	50	100%	50%	avoid		Not dialyzable
Enoxaparin	1 mg/kg q12h	40	100%	100%	50%	1 mg/kg q12h for treatment of DVT; check antifactor Xa activity 4 h after second dose in patients with renal dysfunction; some evidence of drug accumulation in renal failure
Fondaparinux	2.5–10 mg/d		77%	100%	Avoid	Avoid	Contraindicated in hemodialysis
Heparin	80 U/kg load then 18 U/kg/h		None	100%	100%	100%	Half-life increases with dose
Iloprost	5 mcg q15 min		68%	100%	100%	100%	
Indobufen	100 mg q12h	200 mg q12h	<15%	100%	50%	Avoid	

Prasugrel	LD 60 mg, maintenance 5–10 mg/d	68	100%	100%	100%	100%	Avoid use in patients with active bleeding or history of stroke or transient ischemic attack	Not dialyzable
Rivaroxaban	20 mg q24h	20 mg q24h	66%	100%	100%	75%	Avoid	
Streptokinase	1,500,000 IU IV infused over 60 min		Unknown	100%	100%	100%	100%	
Sulfinpyrazone	200 mg q12h		25–50%	100%	100%	100%	Avoid	Acute renal failure; uricosuric effect at low GFR
Sulotroban	No data		52–62%	50%	30%		10%	
Ticagrelol	LD 180 mg, maintenance 90 bid	26	100%	100%	100%	100%		Not dialyzable
Ticlopidine	250 mg q12h	60	100%	100%	100%	100%	100%	Decrease CSA level and may cause severe neutropenia and thrombocytopenia
Tranexamic acid	10 mg/kg IV followed by 1 mg/kg/h infusion with 1 mg/kg added to priming solution		50%	25%	10%		If ScR is 1.6–3.3 reduce maintenance to 1.5 mg/kg/h. If ScR is 3.3–6.6 reduce to 1 mg/kg h. If ScR is >6.6 then maintenance 0.5 mg/kg/h	
Urokinase	4,400 U/kg load; then 4,400 U/kg qh		No data	No data	No data	No data	No data	
Warfarin	5 mg/d	92%	100%	100%	100%	100%	Monitor INR very closely; start at 5 mg/d. 1 mg vitamin K IV over 30 min or 2.5–5 mg PO can be used to normalize INR	

TABLE 20-6 Antidepressant Drug Dosing in Renal Failure

Drug	Normal Doses Starting Dose	Maximum Dose	% of Renal Excretion	Dosage Adjustment in Renal Failure GFR >60 mL/min	GFR 30-60 mL/min	GFR <30 mL/min	Comments	Hemo-dialysis	Continuous Ambulatory Peritoneal Dialysis	Continuous Venovenous Hemofiltration
SSRIs: 1st line, serotonin syndrome risk (antidote: cyproheptadine)										
Fluoxetine	20 mg/d	80 mg/d	2.5-5% unchanged	100%	100%	100%	Norfluoxetine is active metabolite with similar activity to parent, activating	None	No data	No data
Paroxetine	20 mg/d IR; 25 mg/d ER	50 mg/d IR; 62.5 mg/d ER	2% unchanged	100%	50%	50%	Most anticholinergic; sedating; withdrawal most likely	50%	No data	No data
Sertraline	50 mg/d	200 mg/d	0% unchanged	100%	100%	100%	Good middle start	None	No data	No data
Citalopram	20 mg/d	40 mg/d (age <60); 20 mg/d (age >60)	10%	50%	50%	Not recommended for GFR <20 mL/min	Low DDIs; QTc prolongation	No data	No data	No data

SNRIs

Venlafaxine	37.5 mg/d	225 mg/d (ER), 375 mg/d (IR)	5% unchanged	75%	75%	50%	The manufacturer recommends a 25% dose reduction in patients with CrCl 10–70 mL/min (immediate release) and a 25–50% reduction with CrCl 30–89 mL/min (extended release). Highest sexual dysfunction.	50%	50%	
Duloxetine	30–60 mg/d	60–120 mg/d	70%	100%	100%	0% (avoid use)	More neuropathic	Not dialyzable	Unlikely to be dialyzable	Unlikely

Others

Trazodone	50 mg bid (IR) or 150 mg QHS (ER)	375 mg (ER), 400 mg/d (IR) (outpatient)	75%	100%	100%	100%	Neuropathic properties. Use with caution, no renal adjustments per label. Avoid in cardiac disease and seizure history.	For anxiety and insomnia. Use with caution, no renal adjustments per label.

(continued)

TABLE 20-6 Antidepressant Drug Dosing in Renal Failure (*Continued*)

Drug	Normal Doses		% of Renal Excretion	Dosage Adjustment in Renal Failure			Comments	Hemo-dialysis	Continuous Ambulatory Peritoneal Dialysis	Continuous Venovenous Hemofiltration
	Starting Dose	Maximum Dose		GFR >60 mL/min	GFR 30–60 mL/min	GFR <30 mL/min				
Amitripty-line	25–50 mg/d	150 mg/d	2% unchanged	100%	100%	100%	Neuropathic properties. Use with caution, no renal adjustments per label. Avoid in cardiac disease and seizure history.			
Nortripty-line	25 mg/d	150 mg/d	2% unchanged	100%	100%	100%	Neuropathic properties. Use with caution, no renal adjustments per label. Avoid in cardiac disease and seizure history.			

Mirtazapine	15 mg qhs	45 mg/d	75%	100%	100%	100%	For cachectic and end-of-life pts. Clearance is decreased with moderate and severe renal impairment. Use with caution.	None		
Bupropion	100 mg bid IR; 150 mg/d (12 h); 150 mg/d (24 h)	450 mg/d IR; 200 mg bid (12 h); 450 mg/d (24 h)	0.5% unchanged	Use with caution; manufacturer's labeling suggests a reduction in dose and/or frequency be considered but does not provide specific dosing recommendations.			Augmenting agent; increase seizure risk; avoid in TBI, bulimia, anorexia; abuse potential	No data	No data	No data

TABLE 20-7 Antifungal Agent Dosing in Renal Failure

Drugs	Normal Dosage	% of Renal Excretion	Dosage Adjustment in Renal Failure			Comments	Hemodialysis	Continuous Ambulatory Peritoneal Dialysis	Continuous Venovenous Hemofiltration
			GFR >50 mL/min	GFR 10–50 mL/min	GFR <10 mL/min				
Antifungal Agents									
Amphotericin B	0.5 g–1.5 mg/kg/d	<1%	No renal adjustment is required			Nephrotoxic; infusion-related reactions; give 250 cc NS before each dose	q24h	q24h	q24–36h
Amphotec	4–6 mg/kg/d	<1%	No renal adjustment is required						
Abelcet	5 mg/kg/d	<1%	No renal adjustment is required						
AmBisome	3–5 mg/kg/d	<1%	No renal adjustment is required						
Azoles and other antifungal agents: Increase CSA/FK level									
Fluconazole	200–800 mg IV q24h/q12h	70%	100%	100%	50%	QT prolongation with high dose (avoid use with terfenadine)	200 mg after dialysis	Dose for GFR <10 mL/min	Dose for GFR 10–50 mL/min
Flucytosine	37.5 mg/kg	90%	q12h	q16h	q24h	Hepatic dysfunction; marrow suppression more common in azotemic patients	Dose after dialysis	0.5–1.0 g/d	Dose for GFR 10–50 mL/min

Drug	Dose				Notes			
Griseofulvin	125–250 mg q6h	1%	100%	100%	100%		None	None
Itraconazole	200 mg q12h	35%	100%	100%	50%	Poor oral absorption	100% mg q12–24h	100 mg q12–24h	100 mg q12–24h
Ketoconazole	200–400 mg PO q24h	15%	100%	100%	100%	Hepatotoxic; requires acid to be absorbed so avoid antacid 2 h before and after dose, significant cyp450 DDI	None	None	None
Miconazole	1,200–3,600 mg/d	1%	100%	100%	100%		None	None	None
Posaconazole	200 mg q6h	1%	100%	100%	100%				
Terbinafine	250 mg PO q24h	>1%	100%	100%	100%				
Voriconazole	4–6 mg/kg q12h	1%	100%	100%	100%	Avoid IV formulation in CKD			
Caspofungin	70 mg LD; then 50 mg/d	1%	100%	100%	100%				
Micafungin	100–150 mg IV daily	1%	100%	100%	100%				
Anidulafungin	200 mg LD; then 100 mg/d	1%	100%	100%	100%		None	None	None

TABLE 20-8 Anti-Parkinson Drug Dosing in Renal Failure

Drugs	Normal Dosage	% of Renal Excretion	Dosage Adjustment in Renal Failure			Comments
			GFR >50 mL/min	GFR 10-50 mL/min	GFR <10 mL/min	
Anti-Parkinson Agents						
Carbidopa	1-tab q8h–6 tabs daily	30	100%	100%	100%	Requires careful titration of dose according to clinical response
Levodopa	25–500 mg q12h–8 g q24h	None	100%	50–100%	50–100%	Active and inactive metabolites excreted in urine; active metabolites with long $t_{1/2}$ in ESRD

TABLE 20-9 Antipsychotic Drug Dosing in Renal Failure

Drugs	Normal Dosage	% of Renal Excretion	Dosage Adjustment in Renal Failure			Comments
			GFR >50 mL/min	GFR 10–50 mL/min	GFR <10 mL/min	
Typicals or FGA: Orthostatic hypotension, EPS, and confusion can occur						
Chlorpromazine	300–800 mg q24h	Hepatic	100%	100%	100%	Orthostatic hypotension, EPS, and confusion can occur; weight gain (4–6 kg)
Promethazine	20–100 mg q24h	Hepatic	100%	100%	100%	Excessive sedation may occur in ESRD
Thioridazine	50–100 mg PO q8h; increase gradually; maximum of 800 mg/d in 2–4 divided doses	Hepatic	100%	100%	100%	BEERS—high sedation, anticholinergic effects; QT prolonging and conduction abnormalities. Low EPS; Weight gain (4–6 kg); not removed by HD and best avoided in ESRD
Trifluoperazine	1–2 mg q12h. Increase—no more than 6 mg	Hepatic	100%	100%	100%	No dose adjustments but hepatically metabolized to bioactive drug so use CI in hepatic disease; orthostatic hypotension, EPS, and confusion can occur; BEERS; avoid within 2 h of any antacid
Perphenazine	8–16 mg PO q12h, q8h, or q6h; increase–64 mg/d	Hepatic	100%	100%	100%	Caution in renal impairment; caution with CYP2D6 PM; CI in liver disease
Thiothixene	2 mg PO q8h; increase gradually–15 mg/d	Hepatic	100%	100%	100%	QT prolongation
Pimozide	1–2 mg/d in divided doses; max 10 mg/d or 0.2 mg/kg/d (whichever less)		100%	100%	100%	Used in Tourette's; QT prolongation; if dose exceeds 4 mg/d CYP2D6 genotyping should be performed, and PM should dose titrate Q 2 wk or more and max 4 mg/d
Haloperidol	1–2 mg q8–12h	Hepatic	100%	100%	100%	Used in Tourette; Hypotension, excessive sedation; dry mouth; EPS

(continued)

TABLE 20-9 Antipsychotic Drug Dosing in Renal Failure (Continued)

Drugs	Normal Dosage	% of Renal Excretion	Dosage Adjustment in Renal Failure			Comments
			GFR >50 mL/min	GFR 10–50 mL/min	GFR <10 mL/min	
Atypical or SGA						
Loxapine	10 mg PO bid increasing until sx controlled-250 mg/d in 2–4 divided doses: 12.5–50 mg IM q4–6h	Hepatic	100%	100%	100%	Do not administer drug IV; comes as IM or oral solution, capsule, or inhalation; inhalation must be administered by HCP and CI lung diseases associated with bronchospasm
Clozapine	12.5 mg PO. Increase by 25–50 mg/d–300–450 mg/d by end of 2 wks (2–3 divided doses)	Hepatic	100%	100%	100%	BEERS—sedation, anticholinergic (constipation), weight gain (4–6 kg); serious toxicity requires baseline ANC; no EPS; no dose adjustments provided but suggest dose reductions with significant renal and/or hepatic impairment
Risperidone	1–2 mg/d PO in 1–2 divided doses; 8 mg/d	Hepatic	100%	50%	50%	Label max dose up to 16 mg/d but >8 mg/d is not recommended; decreased clearance 60% in patients with RD; lacks sedation; dose-dependent EPS; risk increases >6 mg
Olanzapine	5–10 mg	Hepatic	100%	100%	100%	Potential hypotensive effects; weight gain (4–6 kg)
Quetiapine	25 mg PO bid; increase in increments of 25–50 mg/d in 2–3 divided doses on days 2 and 3; 300–400 mg/d by day 4; max 800 mg/d	Hepatic	100%	100%	100%	Hepatic and elderly dose adjustments based on IR or ER formulation; high sedation, moderate weight gain and risk for metabolic syndrome, low EPS
Paliperidone	6–12 mg PO q24h	59%	50%	75%	Avoid use	QT prolongation, tachycardia
Iloperidone	6–12 mg PO bid	Hepatic	No renal dose adjustment			Orthostatic hypotension

Lurasidone	20–160 mg PO QPM with food (> or equal 350 calories)	Hepatic	100%	50%	50%	Concomitant administration with strong CYP3A4 inducers or inhibitors is contraindicated, good choice for pregnancy
Aripiprazole	2–30 mg PO q24h	Hepatic	100%	100%	100%	Reduce dose by 50% in known CYP2D6 poor metabolizers. Reduce dose by 75% in 2D6 PMs also receiving a strong CYP3A4 inhibitor.
Ziprasidone	20–100 mg q12h	Hepatic	100%	100%	100%	No dose adjustments but extensive hepatic metabolism and renally cleared so caution with hepatic/renal impairment; QT prolongation

TABLE 20-10 Antituberculosis Drug Dosing in Renal Failure

Drugs	Normal Dosage	% of Renal Excretion	Dosage Adjustment in Renal Failure			Comments	Hemodialysis	Continuous Ambulatory Peritoneal Dialysis	Continuous Venovenous Hemofiltration
			GFR >50 mL/min	GFR 10–50 mL/min	GFR <10 mL/min				
Antituberculosis Antibiotics									
Rifampin (RIF)	300–600 mg PO q24h	20%	No renal adjustment is required			Decrease CSA/FK level; many drug interactions	None	Dose for GFR <10 mL/min	Dose for GFR <10 mL/min
Rifapentine (RPT)	5 mg/kg max: 300 mg PO QD	21–30%	100%	50–100%	50–100%		50–100% of dose, no supplementation	50–100% plus an extra 50–100% AFTER PD	
Isoniazid (INH)	(5 mg/kg) max: 300 mg PO or IM QD	75–95%	No renal adjustment is required			Hepatotoxicity	None	None	
Pyrazinamde (PZA)	1,000 mg PO QD	70%	None	25–35 mg/kg three times a week	25–35 mg/kg three times a week	Gout	25–35 mg/kg three times a week after HD, supplement if next dose not right after	None	
Ethambutol (EMB)	800–1,600 mg PO QD (weight based)	80%	None	15–25 mg/kg three times a week	15–25 mg/kg three times a week	Optic	15–25 mg/kg three times a week. No supplement	15–25 mg/kg three times a week. No supplement	

Cycloserine	10–15 mg/kg/d PO, QD, or bid	60–70%	None	500 mg three times a week OR 250 mg QD	CONTRAINDICATED (per pkg insert)	500 mg three times a week after HD, supplement if next dose not right after	Not defined
Capreomycin	10–15 mg/kg IM or IV 5–7×/wk max: 1 g/dose	52%	None	2–3 ×/wk	2–3 ×/wk	2–3 ×/wk after dialysis, consider supplement if next dose not right after	Not defined
Aminosalicylic Acid	4 PO bid-TID	80%	None	4 g PO bid	CONTRAINDICATED (per pkg insert)	4 g PO bid	Not defined
Ethionamide	15–20 mg/kg/d PO, QD, or bid	100%	None	250–500 mg QD	250–500 mg QD	250–500 mg QD, after dialysis, no supplement	Not defined
Bedaquiline	400 mg PO QD × 2 wk, then 200 mg PO 3 ×/wk	<0.001%	None	None	Not defined	Not defined	Not defined
Pretomanid	200 mg PO QD	50%	No renal dose adjustment			None	None

TABLE 20-11   Antiviral Agent Dosing in Renal Failure

Drugs	Normal Dosage	% of Renal Excretion	Dosage Adjustment in Renal Failure			Comments	Hemo-dialysis	Continuous Ambulatory Peritoneal Dialysis	Continuous Venovenous Hemofiltration
			GFR >50 mL/min	GFR 10–50 mL/min	GFR <10 mL/min				
Antiviral Agents									
Acyclovir	200–800 mg PO 5×/d	50%	100%	100%	50%	Poor absorption; neurotoxicity in ESRD; IV preparation can cause renal failure if injected rapidly (infused over 1 h), check for phlebitis and rotate infusion sites	Dose after dialysis	Dose for GFR <10 mL/min	3.5 mg/kg/d
Adefovir	10 mg q24h	45%	100%	10 mg q48h	10 mg q72h	Renal toxicity	10 mg weekly after HD	No data	No data
Amantadine	100–200 mg q12h	90%	100%	50%	q96h–7 days		None	None	Dose for GFR 10–50 mL/min
Cidofovir	5 mg/kg weekly ×2 (induction); 5 mg/kg every 2 wk	90%	Avoid in CKD	No data: avoid	No data: avoid	Dose-limiting nephrotoxicity with proteinuria, glycosuria, renal insufficiency; nephrotoxicity and renal clearance reduced with coadministration of probenecid	No data	No data	Avoid

Delavirdine	400 mg q8h	5%	No data: 100%	No data: 100%	No data: 100%		No data	No data: dose for GFR 10–50 mL/min
Didanosine	200 mg q12h (125 mg if <60 kg)	40–69%	q12h	q24h	50% q24h	Pancreatitis	Dose after dialysis	Dose for GFR <10 mL/min
Emtricitabine	200 mg q24h	86%	q24h	q48–72h	q96h			Dose for GFR <10 mL/min	No data
Entecavir	0.5 mg q24h	62%	q24h	q48–72h	q96h			Dose after dialysis	No data
Famciclovir	250–500 mg PO q8h–q12h	60%	q8h	q12h	q24h	VZV: 500 mg PO q8h HSV: 250 PO q12h Metabolized to active compound penciclovir	Dose after dialysis	No data: dose for GFR 10–50 mL/min
Foscarnet	40–80 mg IV q8h	85%	40–20 mg q8–24h according to ClCr			Nephrotoxic, neurotoxic, hypocalcemia, hypophosphatemia, hypomagnesemia, and hypokalemia	Dose after dialysis	Dose for GFR <10 mL/min	Dose for GFR 10–50 mL/min
Ganciclovir IV	5 mg/kg q12h	95%	q12h	q24h	2.5 mg/kg q24h	Granulocytopenia and thrombocytopenia	Dose after dialysis	Dose for GFR <10 mL/min	2.5 mg/kg q24h
Ganciclovir PO	1,000 mg PO q8h	95%	1,000 mg q8h	1,000 mg q12h	1,000 mg q24h	Oral ganciclovir should be used ONLY for prevention of CMV infection; always use IV ganciclovir for the treatment of CMV infection	No data: dose after dialysis	No data: dose for GFR <10 mL/min	N/A

(continued)

TABLE 20-11 Antiviral Agent Dosing in Renal Failure (Continued)

| Drugs | Normal Dosage | % of Renal Excretion | Dosage Adjustment in Renal Failure ||| Comments | Hemo-dialysis | Continuous Ambulatory Peritoneal Dialysis | Continuous Venovenous Hemofiltration |
			GFR >50 mL/min	GFR 10–50 mL/min	GFR <10 mL/min				
Indinavir	800 mg q8h	10%	No data: 100%	No data: 100%	No data: 100%	Nephrolithiasis; ARF due to crystalluria, tubulointerstitial nephritis	No data	No data: dose for GFR <10 mL/min	No data
Lamivudine	150 mg PO q12h	80%	q12h	q24h	50 mg q24h	For hepatitis B	Dose after dialysis	No data: dose for GFR <10 mL/min	Dose for GFR 10–50 mL/min
Maraviroc	300 mg q12h	20%	300 mg q12h	No data	No data	Drug interaction with CYP III-A	No data	No data	No data
Nelfinavir	750 mg q8h	No data	No data	No data	No data		No data	No data	No data
Nevirapine	200 mg q24h × 14 d	<3	No data: 100%	No data: 100%	No data: 100%	May be partially cleared by HD and PD	Dose after dialysis	No data: dose for GFR <10 mL/min	No data: dose for GFR 10–50 mL/min
Oseltamivir	75 mg q12h	99%	75q12h	75 mg/d	75 mg q48h		Dose after dialysis		
Ribavirin	500–600 mg q12h	30%	100%	100%	50%	HUS	Dose after dialysis	Dose for GFR <10 mL/min	Dose for GFR 10–50 mL/min
Rifabutin	300 mg q24h	5–10%	100%	100%	100%		None	None	No data: dose for GFR 10–50 mL/min
Rimantadine	100 mg PO q12h	25%	100%	100%	50%				

Drug	Dose	%				Comments			
Ritonavir	600 mg q12h	3.50%	No data: 100%	No data: 100%	No data: 100%	Many drug interactions	No data: none	No data: dose for GFR <10 mL/min	No data: dose for GFR 10-50 mL/min
Saquinavir	600 mg q8h	<4%	No data: 100%	No data: 100%	No data: 100%		No data: none	No data: dose for GFR <10 mL/min	No data: dose for GFR 10-50 mL/min
Stavudine	30–40 mg q12h	35–40%	100%	50% q12–24h	50% q24h		Dose for GFR <10 mL/min after dialysis	No data	No data: dose for GFR 10-50 mL/min
Telbivudine	600 mg PO daily		100%	600 mg q48h	600 mg q96 h		Dose for GFR <10 mL/min after dialysis	No data	No data: dose for GFR 10-50 mL/min
Tenofovir	300 mg q24h		100%	300 mg q48–72h	300 mg q96h	Nephrotoxic	Dose for GFR <10 mL/min after dialysis	No data	No data: dose for GFR 10-50 mL/min
Valacyclovir	500–1,000 mg q8h	50%	100%	50%	25%	TTP/HUS; CNS side effects especially in elderly and patients with renal impairment, can cause dehydration	Dose after dialysis	Dose for GFR <10 mL/min	No data: dose for GFR 10-50 mL/min
Valganciclovir	900 mg PO daily or q12h		100%	50%	25%	Granulocytopenia and thrombocytopenia	Dose after dialysis	Dose for GFR <10 mL/min	450 mg/d

(*continued*)

TABLE 20-11 Antiviral Agent Dosing in Renal Failure (Continued)

Drugs	Normal Dosage	% of Renal Excretion	Dosage Adjustment in Renal Failure			Comments	Hemo-dialysis	Continuous Ambulatory Peritoneal Dialysis	Continuous Venovenous Hemofiltration
			GFR >50 mL/min	GFR 10–50 mL/min	GFR <10 mL/min				
Vidarabine	15 mg/kg infusion q24h	50%	100%	100%	75%		Infuse after dialysis	Dose for GFR <10 mL/min	Dose for GFR 10–50 mL/min
Zanamivir	2 puffs q12h × 5 day	1%	100%	100%	100%	Bioavailability from inhalation and systemic exposure to drug is low	None	None	No data
Zalcitabine	0.75 mg q8h	75%	100%	q12h	q24h		No data: dose after dialysis	No data	No data: dose for GFR 10–50 mL/min
Zidovudine	200 mg q8h, 300 mg q12h	8%–25%	100%	100%	100 mg q8h	Enormous interpatient variation; metabolite renally excreted	Dose for GFR <10 mL/min	Dose for GFR <10 mL/min	100 mg q8h

TABLE 20-12 Corticosteroid Drug Dosing in Renal Failure

Corticosteroids	Normal Dosage	% of Renal Excretion	Dosage Adjustment in Renal Failure			Comments
			GFR >50 mL/min	GFR 10–50 mL/min	GFR <10 mL/min	
Betamethasone	0.5–9.0 mg q24h	5	100%	100%	100%	Extensively metabolized by liver, kidney excretes inactive metabolites/minimally excreted unchanged. May aggravate azotemia, Na⁺ retention, glucose intolerance, and hypertension
Budesonide	64 mcg–9 mg q24h	60	100%	100%	100%	
Cortisone	25–300 mg q24h	1	100%	100%	100%	
Dexamethasone	0.75–9.0 mg q24h	10	100%	100%	100%	
Fludrocortisone	0.05–0.2 mg q24h	No data	100%	100%	100%	
Hydrocortisone	20–500 mg q24h	1	100%	100%	100%	
Methylprednisolone	4–60 mg q24h	<10	100%	100%	100%	
Prednisolone	5–60 mg q24h	No data	100%	100%	100%	
Prednisone	5–60 mg q24h	No data	100%	100%	100%	
Triamcinolone	60 mg q24h	40–75	100%	100%	100%	

TABLE 20-13 Gastrointestinal Agent Dosing in Renal Failure

Drug	Normal Doses		% of Renal Excretion	Dosage Adjustment in Renal Failure			Comments
	Starting Dose	Maximum Dose		GFR >50 mL/min	GFR 10–50 mL/min	GFR <10 mL/min	
Antiulcer agents							
Cimetidine	300 mg PO q8h	800 mg PO q12h	60%	100%	75%	25%	Multiple drug–drug interactions; beta-blockers, sulfonylurea, theophylline, warfarin, and so on
Famotidine	20 mg PO q12h	40 mg PO q12h	70%	100%	75%	25%	Headache, fatigue, thrombocytopenia, alopecia
Lansoprazole	15 mg PO q24h	30 mg q12h	None	100%	100%	100%	Headache, diarrhea
Nizatidine	150 mg PO q12h	300 mg PO q12h	20%	100%	75%	25%	Headache, fatigue, thrombocytopenia, alopecia
Omeprazole	20 mg PO q24h	40 mg PO q24h	None	100%	100%	100%	Headache, diarrhea
Rabeprazole	20 mg PO q24h	40 mg PO q24h	None	100%	100%	100%	Headache, diarrhea
Pantoprazole	40 mg PO q24h	80 mg PO q12h	None	100%	100%	100%	Headache, diarrhea
Ranitidine	150 mg PO q12h	300 mg PO q12h	80%	100%	75%	25%	Headache, fatigue, thrombocytopenia, alopecia
Metoclopramide	10 mg PO q8h	30 mg PO q6h	15%	100%	100%	50–75%	Increase cyclosporine/tacrolimus level; neurotoxic
Misoprostol	100 mcg PO q12h	200 mcg PO q6h		100%	100%	100%	Diarrhea, N/V, abortifacient agent
Sucralfate	1 g PO q6h	1 g PO q6h	None	100%	100%	100%	Constipation; decrease absorption of MMF

TABLE 20-14 Hyperlipidemic Agent Dosing in Renal Failure

Drugs	Normal Doses		% of Renal Excretion	Dosage Adjustment in Renal Failure			Comments	Hemo-dialysis	Continuous Ambulatory Peritoneal Dialysis	Continuous Venovenous Hemofiltration
	Starting Dose	Maximum Dose		GFR >50 mL/min	GFR 10–50 mL/min	GFR <10 mL/min				
Hyperlipidemic Agents										
Alirocumab	75 mg SubQ q2wks	150 mg SubQ q2wks	0%	100%	100%	100%				
Atorvastatin	10 mg/d	80 mg/d	<2%	100%	100%	100%	Liver dysfunction, myalgia, and rhabdomyolysis with CSA/FK	No data	No data	No data
Bezafibrate	200 mg TID OR 400 mg once (SR)		50%	100%	50%	Avoid	No data	200 mg q 3rd day. (some data says to avoid)	200 mg q 3rd day. (some data says to avoid)	no data
Cholestyramine	4 g q12h	24 g/d	None	100%	100%	100%		No data	No data	No data
Clofibrate	500 mg q12h	1,000 mg q12h	40–70%	q6–12h	q12–18h	q24–48h		No data	No data	No data
Colestipol	5 g q12h	30 g/d	None	100%	100%	100%		No data	No data	No data
Evolocumab	140 mg SubQ q2wks OR 420 mg monthly		None	100%	100%	100%				
Ezetimibe	10 mg/d		11%	100%	100%	100%			No data	

(continued)

TABLE 20-14 Hyperlipidemic Agent Dosing in Renal Failure (Continued)

Drugs	Normal Doses		% of Renal Excretion	Dosage Adjustment in Renal Failure				Hemo-dialysis	Continuous Ambulatory Peritoneal Dialysis	Continuous Venovenous Hemofiltration
	Starting Dose	Maximum Dose		GFR >50 mL/min	GFR 10–50 mL/min	GFR <10 mL/min	Comments			
Fenofibrate	48 g/d	145 g/d	60–93%	100%	100%	Avoid	CI in GFR ≤30 and dialysis	Avoid	Avoid	Avoid
Fluvastatin	20 g/d	80 g/d	5%	100%	100%	100%		No data	No data	No data
Gemfibrozil	600 q12h	600 q12h	70%	100%	75%	50%	Take 30 min before meal	No data	50%	No data
Lovastatin	20 mg/d	80 mg/d	10%	100%	100%	100%	GFR <30, use with caution and carefully consider doses >20 mg/d	No data	No data	No data
Nicotinic acid	1 g q8h	2 g q8h	60–76%	100%	100%	100%	Not 1st or 2nd line in patients with dyslipidemia	No data	No data	No data
Pitavastatin	1 mg QD	4 mg QD	15%	100%	50%	50%		50%	No data	
Pravastatin	10–40 mg/d	80 mg/d	20%	100%	100%	100%		No data	No data	No data

Probucol		500 mg q12h	<2%	100%	100%	100%	Removed from market in United States in 1995.	No data	No data	No data
Rosuvastatin	5 mg/d	40 mg/d	<5%	100%	100%	Initial: 5 mg QD. max 10 mg/d	GFR <30: max 10 mg/d			
Simvastatin	5–20 mg/d	80 mg/d	13%	100%	100%	100%		No data	No data	No data

TABLE 20-15 Hypoglycemic Agent Dosing in Renal Failure

Drugs	Normal Doses – Starting Dose	Normal Doses – Maximum Dose	% of Renal Excretion	Dosage Adjustment in Renal Failure – GFR >50 mL/min	Dosage Adjustment in Renal Failure – GFR 10–50 mL/min	Dosage Adjustment in Renal Failure – GFR <10 mL/min	Comments	Hemodialysis	CAPD	Continuous Venovenous Hemofiltration
Hypoglycemic Agents: Avoid all oral hypoglycemic agents on CRRT											
Acarbose	25 mg q8h	100 mg q8h	35%	100%	50%	Avoid	Abdominal pain, N/V, and flatulence	No data	No data	Avoid
Acetohexamide	250 mg q24h	1,500 mg q24h	None	Avoid	Avoid	Avoid	Diuretic effect; may falsely elevate serum creatinine; active metabolite has $t_{1/2}$ of 5–8 h in healthy subjects and is eliminated by the kidney; prolonged hypoglycemia in azotemic patients	No data	None	Avoid
Canagliflozin	100 mg q24h	300 mg qd	None	45–<60 mL/min: max × 100 mg qd	30–<45 mL/min: avoid	< 30 mL/min: contraindication	BBW: Lower limb amputation. Common SE: UTI, hypovolemia, electrolyte abnormality (hyperkalemia), risk of euglycemic ketoacidosis	Contraindicated	Contraindicated	Contraindicated
Chlorpropamide	100 mg q24h	500 mg q24h	47%	50%	Avoid	Avoid	Impairs water excretion; prolonged hypoglycemia in azotemic patients	No data	None	Avoid
Dapagliflozin	5 mg QD	10 mg QD	None	≥60 mL/min: 100%	<60 mL/min: Avoid	<30 mL/min: contraindication	No BBW. SEs (see canagliflozin)	Contraindicated	Contraindicated	Contraindicated

Dulaglutide	0.75 mg SQ weekly	1.5 mg SQ weekly	No data	100%	100%	100%	BBW: Thyroid tumors. Common SE: N/V/D, weigh loss.	No data	No data	No data
Empagliflozin	10 mg QD	25 mg QD	None	≥45 mL/min: 100%	< 45 mL/min: avoid	<30 mL/min: contraindication	No BBW. SEs (see cana- and empa-have ASCVD benefits, HF, DKD	Contraindicated	Contraindicated	Contraindicated
Exenatide	IM: 5 mcg SQ bid. ER: 2 mg SQ weekly	IM: 10 mcg SQ bid	No data	100%	30–50 mL/min: caution, start 5 mcg and increase caution	<30 mL/min: avoid	BBW: Thyroid C cells tumors (Bydureon: ER). Common SE: N/V/D, hypoglycemia. Last 30 days after opening	No data	No data	No data
Glibornuride	12.5 mg q24h	100 mg q14h	No data	No data	No data	No data		No data	No data	Avoid
Gliclazide	80 mg q24h	320 mg q24h	<20%	50–100%	Avoid	Avoid		No data	No data	Avoid
Glipizide	5 mg q24h.	20 mg q12h	5%	100%	50%	50%		No data	No data	Avoid
Glyburide	2.5 mg q24h	10 mg q12h	50%	100%	50%	Avoid		None	None	Avoid
Liraglutide	0.6 mg SQ QD	1.8 mg SQ QD	6%	100%	100%	Avoid	BBW: Increase risk of thyroid cancer. Also use in weight loss. SE: N/V/D, hypoglycemia. Lira-, sema-: ASCVD benefits	No data	No data	No data
Lixisenatide	10 mcg SQ QD	20 mcg QD	No data	100%	15–30 mL/ min: close monitoring	<15 mL/min: avoid	SE: GI symptoms	No data	No data	No data
Metformin	500 mg q12h	2,550 mg/d (q12h or q8h)	95%	100%	Avoid	Avoid	Lactic acidosis	No data	No data	Avoid

(continued)

TABLE 20-15 Hypoglycemic Agent Dosing in Renal Failure (Continued)

Drugs	Normal Doses		% of Renal Excretion	Dosage Adjustment in Renal Failure			Comments	Hemodialysis	CAPD	Continuous Venovenous Hemofiltration
	Starting Dose	Maximum Dose		GFR >50 mL/min	GFR 10-50 mL/min	GFR <10 mL/min				
Pioglitazone	15-30 mg q24h	45 mg q24h	15-30%	100%	100%	100%	Contraindicated in HF NYHA III-IV. Caution in impaired hepatic function or injury, can lead to liver failure. Associated with weight gain. Multiple drug interactions.	None	None	NA
Pramlintide	15 mcg	60 mcg daily	No data	100%	No data	No data				
Repaglinide	0.5-1 mg	4 mg q8h								
Rosiglitazone	4 mg q24h	8 mg q24h	64%	100%	100%	100%	Increases LDL. Contraindicated in HF, NYHA III-IV. Associated with weight gain. Caution in patients with hepatic impairment or injury, rosiglitazone can induce liver failure.	None	None	NA
Semaglutide	PO: 3-7 mg QD. SQ: 0.25-0.5 mg weekly	PO: 14 mg QD. SQ: 1 mg weekly	3%	100%	100%	100%	BBW: Thyroid C cells tumor. Common SE: GI upset	No data	no data	no data
Sitagliptin	25 mg	100 mg	79%	100%	50%	25%				

Tolazamide	100 mg q24h	250 mg q24h	7%	100%	100%	100%	May impair water excretion	Avoid	Avoid	Avoid
Tolbutamide	1 g q24h	2 g q24h	None	100%	100%	100%		None	None	Avoid
Insulin Agents: Dosage guided by blood glucose levels										
Insulin regular	4–6 units or 0.1 units/kg or 10% of basal dose	Titrate to desired BG range	Largely via urine	100%	75% or normal dose	50% or normal dose	Caution for hypoglycemia. Caution for hypokalemia. Renal excretion of insulin decreases with azotemia. Risk of hypoglycemia increases with hepatic and renal impairment.	N/A	N/A	Dose for GFR 10–50 mL/min
Lispro insulin	4–5 units or 10% of basal dose	Titrate to desired BG range	Largely via urine	100%	More frequent dose adjustments and monitoring may be needed	More frequent dose adjustments and monitoring may be needed	Caution for hypoglycemia. Caution for hypokalemia. Risk of hypoglycemia increases with hepatic and renal impairment.	N/A	N/A	N/A
Insulin glargine	10 units or 0.1 to 0.2 units/kg/d	Titrate to desired BG range	Largely via urine	100%	More frequent dose adjustments and monitoring may be needed	More frequent dose adjustments and monitoring may be needed	Caution for hypoglycemia, caution for hypokalemia. Risk of hypoglycemia increases with hepatic and renal impairment.	N/A	N/A	N/A

TABLE 20-16 Mood Stabilizer Drug Dosing in Renal Failure

Drugs	Normal Doses		% of Renal Excretion	Dosage Adjustment in Renal Failure		Comments	Hemodialysis	Continuous Ambulatory Peritoneal Dialysis	Continuous Venovenous Hemofiltration
	Starting Dose	Maximum Dose		CrCl 30–89 mL/min	CrCl < 30				
Mood Stabilizers									
Lithium	150–900 mg/d divided TID	900–1,800 mg/d	89–98%	Initiate at low dose and titrate slowly	Avoid use	Avoid in pregnancy (Category D) Therapeutic range: 0.6–1.2 mEq/L (trough level)	No data	No data	No data

TABLE 20-17 Neurologic Drug Dosing in Renal Failure

Drugs	Normal Doses - Starting Dose	Normal Doses - Maximum Dose	% of Renal Excretion	Dosage Adjustment in Renal Failure - GFR >50 mL/min	GFR 10-50 mL/min	GFR <10 mL/min	Comments	Hemodialysis	Continuous Ambulatory Peritoneal Dialysis	Continuous Venovenous Hemofiltration
Anticonvulsants										
Carbamazepine	200 mg bid	1,200 mg/d	72% (3% unchanged)	100%	100%	Moderate to severe renal impairment, carbamazepine should generally not be used	Plasma concentration: 4-12 mcg/mL, myelosuppression, CYP3A4 inducer, fluid retention	N/A	N/A	N/A
Clonazepam	0.5 mg q8h	20 mg/d	Less than 2%	100%	100%	100%	No renal dose adjustments	None	No data	N/A
Ethosuximide	500 mg/d	1.5 g/d	10-20%	100%	100%	100%, no renal dose adjustments but renal function abnormalities have been reported; use caution in patients with renal disease and monitoring recommended	Plasma concentration: 40-100 mg/L, headache	No data	No data	No data
Felbamate	400 mg/q8h	1,200 mg/q8h	90%	100%	50%	25%	Anorexia, vomiting, insomnia, nausea	Dose after dialysis	No data	No data

(continued)

TABLE 20-17 Neurologic Drug Dosing in Renal Failure (Continued)

Drugs	Normal Doses		% of Renal Excretion	Dosage Adjustment in Renal Failure			Comments	Hemodialysis	Continuous Ambulatory Peritoneal Dialysis	Continuous Venovenous Hemofiltration
	Starting Dose	Maximum Dose		GFR >50 mL/min	GFR 10–50 mL/min	GFR <10 mL/min				
Gabapentin	300 mg q8h	2,400 mg/d	76–81%	100%	CrCl 30–59 mL/min: 400–1,400 mg/d given in 2 divided doses	CrCl 15–29 mL/min: 200–700 mg/d QD CrCl 15 mL/min: 100–300 mg/d QD CrCl <15 mL/min: reduce daily dose in proportion to CrCl	Fewer CNS side effects than to other agents	After 4-h session, give supplemental dose of 125 mg for maintenance daily dose of 100 mg	No data	No data
Lamotrigine	25–50 mg/d	500 mg/d	94%	100%	100%	100%, reduced maintenance dose may be effective	Autoinduction, major drug–drug interaction with valproate	No data	No data	No data
Levetiracetam	500 mg q12h	1,500 mg q12h	66%	100%	50%	50%		500–1,000 mg Q24 and 250–500 mg after dialysis	No data	1,000 mg Q12

Oxcarbazepine	300 mg q12h	2,400 mg/d	More than 95%, less than 1% unchanged	100%	100%	CrCl <30 mL/min: Extended release initially 300 mg/d may increase at 300–450 mg/d increments	Less effect on P450 compared with carbamazepine	Use immediate release instead of extended release	No data	No data
Phenobarbital	50–100 mg PO bid-TID	Adjust to maintain therapeutic serum concentration	21%	100%	100%	100%	Plasma concentration: 10–40 mg/L, no renal dose adjustments	No data	No data	No data
Phenytoin	100 mg q8	600 mg/d	excreted in urine after reabsorption from intestinal tract	100%	100%	100%	Plasma concentration: 10–20 mcg/mL, nystagmus, check free phenytoin level	No data	No data	No data
Primidone	100 mg QD-TID	2,000 mg/d	1%	100%	100%	100%	Plasma concentration: 5–20	1/3 dose following hemodialysis	No data	No data
Sodium valproate	7.5–15 mg/kg/d; adjust for side effect and TDM		1%	100%	100%	100%	Plasma concentration: 50–150; weight gain; hepatitis; check free valproate level	None	None	None

(continued)

TABLE 20-17 Neurologic Drug Dosing in Renal Failure (Continued)

Drugs	Normal Doses		% of Renal Excretion	Dosage Adjustment in Renal Failure			Comments	Hemodialysis	Continuous Ambulatory Peritoneal Dialysis	Continuous Venovenous Hemofiltration
	Starting Dose	Maximum Dose		GFR >50 mL/min	GFR 10–50 mL/min	GFR <10 mL/min				
Tiagabine	4 mg q24h, increase 4 mg/d, titrate weekly		2%	100%	100%	100%	Total daily dose may be increased by 4–8 mg at weekly intervals until clinical response is achieved or up to 32 mg/d; total daily dose should be given in divided doses two to four times daily	None	None	Dose for GFR 10–50 mL/min
Topiramate	50 mg/d	200 mg q12h	70%	100%	50%	Avoid		No data	No data	Dose for GFR 10–50 mL/min
Trimethadione	300 mg q6–q8h	600 mg q6–q8h	None	q8h	q8–q12h	q12–q24h	Active metabolites with long half-life in ESRD; nephrotic syndrome	No data	No data	Dose for GFR 10–50 mL/min

	1 g q12h	2 g q12h	70%	100%	50%	25%	Encephalopathy with drug accumulation	No data	No data	Dose for GFR 10–50 mL/min
Vigabatrin										
Zonisamide	100 mg q24h	100–300 mg q12–q24h	30%	100%	75%	50%	Manufacturer recommends that zonisamide should not be used in patients with renal failure (estimated GFR <50 mL/min) because there has been insufficient experience concerning drug dosing and toxicity; zonisamide doses of 100–600 mg/d are effective for normal renal function; dose recommendations for renal impairment based on clearance ratios	Dose for GFR <10 mL/min	Dose for GFR <10 mL/min	Dose for GFR <10–50 mL/min

TABLE 20-18 Nonsteroidal Anti-Inflammatory Drug Dosing in Renal Failure

Drugs	Normal Dosage	% of Renal Excretion	Dosage Adjustment in Renal Failure			Comments	Hemo-dialysis	Continuous Ambulatory Peritoneal Dialysis	Continuous Venovenous Hemofiltration
			GFR >50 mL/min	GFR 10–50 mL/min	GFR <10 mL/min				
Nonsteroidal Anti-Inflammatory Drugs									
Diclofenac	25–100 mg q24h	65	100%	25–50%	Avoid	May decrease renal function; decrease platelet aggregation; nephrotic syndrome; interstitial nephritis; hyperkalemia, sodium retention KDIGO: NSAIDs not recommended in GFR 30–60 mL/min if patient at risk for AKI; avoid NSAIDs in GFR <30 Topical NSAIDs appear to be safe as systemic absorption is minimal	No data	No data	No data
Diflunisal	500–1,000 mg q12h	80–90	100%	50%	50%		50%	50%	Dose for GFR 10–50 mL/min
Etodolac	300–500 mg q12h	70	100%	100%	100%		100%	100%	Dose for GFR 10–50 mL/min
Fenoprofen	300–600 mg q6h	90	100%	100%	100%		100%	100%	Dose for GFR 10–50 mL/min
Flurbiprofen	200–300 mg q23h	20	100%	Contraindicated in GFR <30	Contraindicated in GFR <30		No data	Not removed	Dose for GFR 10–50 mL/min
Ibuprofen	200–800 mg q6–8h	45–80	100%	100%	Avoid		No data	No data	Dose for GFR 10–50 mL/min
Indomethacin	25–50 mg q8h	60	100%	Not recommended	Not recommended		No data	No data	Dose for GFR 10–50 mL/min
Ketoprofen	25–75 mg q8h	80	100%	Max 150 mg/d if GFR >25; Max 100 mg/d if GFR <25	Max 100 mg/d		No data	No data	Dose for GFR 10–50 mL/min
Ketorolac	30–60 mg load; then 15–30 mg q6h	92	100%	Max 60 mg/d	Avoid	Acute hearing loss in ESRD	None	No data	Dose for GFR 10–50 mL/min

Meclofenamic acid	50–100 q6–q8h	2–4	100%	100%	100%		None	Dose for GFR 10–50 mL/min
Mefenamic acid	250 mg q6h	<6	100%	100%	100%		None	Dose for GFR 10–50 mL/min
Nabumetone	1.0–2.0 g q24h	<1	100%	50–100%	50–100%		None	Dose for GFR 10–50 mL/min
Naproxen	500 mg q12h	<1	100%	100%	100%		None	Dose for GFR 10–50 mL/min
Oxaprozin	1,200 mg q24h	<1	100%	100%	100%		None	Dose for GFR 10–50 mL/min
Phenylbutazone	100 mg q6–q8h	1	100%	100%	100%		None	Dose for GFR 10–50 mL/min
Piroxicam	20 mg q24h	10	100%	100%	100%		None	Dose for GFR 10–50 mL/min
Sulindac	200 mg q12h	7	100%	100%	100%	Active sulfide metabolite in ESRD	None	Dose for GFR 10–50 mL/min
Tolmetin	400 mg q8h	15	100%	100%	100%		None	Dose for GFR 10–50 mL/min

TABLE 20-19 Osteoporosis Drug Dosing in Renal Failure

Drug	Normal Doses		% Of Renal Excretion	Dosage Adjustment in Renal Failure			Comments
	Starting Dose	Maximum Dose		GFR >60 mL/min	GFR 30-60 mL/min	GFR <30 mL/min	
Zoledronic acid	5 mg IV infused over 15 min once a year	39 ± 16% unchanged	No dose adjustments	CI in patients with CrCl less than 35 mL/min	Not recommended	GI upset/intolerance, jaw osteonecrosis, should be given over no less than 15 min to avoid renal failure	
Teriparatide	20 mcg SubQ once daily	Unknown	No dose adjustments	Mild to moderate- no changes	A significant increase in $t_{1/2}$ and AUC (75%) but not plasma levels with severe renal impairment	Avoid in patients with severe renal impairment, max 2 yr treatment due to risk of osteosarcoma; orthostatic hypotension; may cause hypercalcemia	
Risedronate	5 mg PO QD, 35 mg PO once weekly, or 75 mg PO 2 consecutive days for total 2 tablets per mo	50%	No dose adjustments	Less than 30 not recommended	Not recommended	Delayed release taken AFTER food; contraindicated in esophageal abnormalities (stricture, achalasia) that delay esophageal emptying, CI hypocalcemia.	
Ibandronate	150 mg orally once monthly OR 3 mg IV infused over 15-30 s every 3 mo	50-60%	No dose adjustments	<30 mL/min not recommended	Not recommended	Need to wait 60 min before eating or laying down; CI esophageal abnormalities, hypocalcemia.	Dialyzable
Abaloparatide	80 mg SQ QD, given with supplemental Ca and Vit D	N/A	No dose adjustments			Potential for hypercalcemia avoid use in preexisting hypercalcemia; orthostatic hypotension	

TABLE 20-20 Rheumatologic Drug Dosing in Renal Failure

Drugs	Normal Dosage	% of Renal Excretion	Dosage Adjustment in Renal Failure			Comments	Hemodialysis	Continuous Ambulatory Peritoneal Dialysis	Continuous Venovenous Hemofiltration
			GFR >50 mL/min	GFR 10–50 mL/min	GFR <10 mL/min				
Allopurinol	300 mg q24h	30	75%	50%	25%	Interstitial nephritis; rare xanthine stones Renal excretion of active metabolite with $t_{1/2}$ of 25 h in normal renal function; $t_{1/2}$ 1 wk in patients with ESRD; exfoliative dermatitis	1/2 dose	No data	Dose for GFR 10–50 mL/min
Auranofin	6 mg q24h	50	50%	Avoid	Avoid	Proteinuria and nephritic syndrome	None	None	None
Colchicine	Acute: 2 mg; then 0.5 mg q6h Chronic: 0.5–1.0 mg q24h	5–17	100%	50–100%	25%	Avoid prolonged use if GFR <50 mL/min	None	No data	Dose for GFR 10–50 mL/min
Gold sodium	25–50 mg	60–90	50%	Avoid	Avoid	Thiomalate proteinuria; nephritic syndrome; membranous nephritis	None	None	Avoid
Penicillamine	250–1,000 mg q24h	40	100%	Avoid	Avoid	Nephrotic syndrome	1/3 dose	No data	Dose for GFR 10–50 mL/min
Probenecid	500 mg q12h	<2	100%	Avoid	Avoid	Ineffective at decreased GFR	Avoid	No data	Avoid
Pegloticase	8 mg IV q2wk	No data	100%	100%	100%			No data	
Febuxostat	40–80 mg PO daily	3%	100%	100%	50%		No data	No data	No data

TABLE 20-21 Sedative Drug Dosing in Renal Failure

Drugs	Normal Dosage	% of Renal Excretion	Dosage Adjustment in Renal Failure			Comments
			GFR >50 mL/min	GFR 10-50 mL/min	GFR <10 mL/min	
Sedatives						
Barbiturates: May cause excessive sedation, increase osteomalacia in ESRD; charcoal hemoperfusion and HD more effective than PD for poisoning						
Pentobarbital	30 mg q6-8h	Hepatic	100%	100%	100%	
Phenobarbital	50-100 mg q8-12h	Hepatic (renal)	q8-12h	q8-12h	q12-16h	Up to 50% unchanged drug excreted with urine with alkaline diuresis.
Secobarbital	30-50 mg q6-8h	Hepatic	100%	100%	100%	
Thiopental	Anesthesia induction (individualized)	Hepatic	100%	100%	100%	
Benzodiazepines: May cause excessive sedation and encephalopathy in ESRD						
Alprazolam	0.25-5.0 mg q8h	Hepatic	100%	100%	100%	
Clorazepate	15-60 mg q24h	Hepatic (renal)	100%	100%	100%	
Chlordiazepoxide	15-100 mg q24h	Hepatic	100%	100%	50%	
Clonazepam	1.5 mg q24h	Hepatic	100%	100%	100%	Although no dose reduction is recommended, the drug has not been studied in patients with renal impairment; recommendations are based on known drug characteristics not clinical trial data
Diazepam	5-40 mg q24h	Hepatic	100%	100%	100%	Active metabolites, desmethyldiazepam, and oxazepam may accumulate in renal failure; dose should be reduced if given longer than a few days; protein binding decreases in uremia

Estazolam	1 mg qhs	Hepatic	100%	100%	100%	
Flurazepam	15–30 mg qhs	Hepatic	100%	100%	100%	
Lorazepam	1–2 mg q8–12h	Hepatic	100%	100%	100%	
Midazolam	Individualized	Hepatic	100%	100%	50%	
Oxazepam	30–120 mg q24h	Hepatic	100%	100%	100%	
Quazepam	15 mg qhs	Hepatic	No data	No data	No data	
Temazepam	30 mg qhs	Hepatic	100%	100%	100%	
Triazolam	0.25–0.50 mg qhs	Hepatic	100%	100%	100%	Protein binding correlates with α_1 acid glycoprotein concentration

Benzodiazepine Antagonist: May cause excessive sedation and encephalopathy in ESRD

Flumazenil	0.2 mg IV over 15 s	Hepatic	100%	100%	100%	

Miscellaneous Sedative Agents

Buspirone	5 mg q8h	Hepatic	100%	100%	100%	
Ethchlorvynol	500 mg qhs	Hepatic	100%	Avoid	Avoid	Removed by hemoperfusion; excessive sedation
Haloperidol	1–2 mg q8–12h	Hepatic	100%	100%	100%	Hypertension, excessive sedation
Lithium carbonate	0.9–1.2 g q24h	Renal	100%	50–75%	25–50%	Nephrotoxic; nephrogenic diabetes insipidus; nephrotic syndrome; renal tubular acidosis; interstitial fibrosis; acute toxicity when serum levels >1.2 mEq/L; serum levels should be measured periodically 12 h after dose; $t_{1/2}$ does not reflect extensive tissue accumulation; plasma levels rebound after dialysis; toxicity enhanced by volume depletion, NSAIDs, and diuretics
Meprobamate	1.2–1.6 g q24h	Hepatic (renal)	q6h	q9–12h	q12–18h	Excessive sedation: excretion enhanced by forced diuresis

TABLE 20-22 Stimulant and Nonstimulant Drug Dosing in Renal Failure

Drugs	Normal Doses		% of Renal Excretion	Dosage Adjustment in Renal Failure			Comments	Hemodialysis	Continuous Ambulatory Peritoneal Dialysis	Continuous Venovenous Hemofiltration
	Starting Dose	Maximum Dose		GFR >30 mL/min	GFR 15-30 mL/min	GFR <15 mL/min				
Stimulants										
Methylphenidate IR	5 mg bid	60 mg/d	78–98%	No data	No data	No data	Take 30 min before breakfast or lunch. Contraindications: pheochromocytoma, adrenal medulla tumor	No data	No data	No data
Dextroamphetamine/ Amphetamine IR	5 mg QAM or bid	40 mg/d	30–40% unchanged	There are no dosage adjustments provided in the manufacturer's labeling; use with caution; the potential exists for elimination of amphetamine to be inhibited resulting in prolonged exposure.			Misuse can cause sudden death and serious CV events	Dextroamphetamine is not dialyzable	No data	No data
Lisdexamfetamine	30 mg QAM	70 mg/d	96%	100%	Max dose: 50 mg/d	Max dose: 30 mg/d	Low abuse potential (if injected or snorted, there is no fast rush effect)	Max dose: 30 mg/d	No data	No data
Nonstimulants: 2nd line for ADHD when stimulant medications have failed										
Atomoxetine	40 mg/d	100 mg/d	80%	100%	100%	100%	Contraindication: MAOI use within the past 14 days. Do not open the capsule	No data	No data	No data

| Guanfacine ER | 1 mg/d | 4 mg/d (with stimulants) 7 mg/d (when used alone) | 50% | There are no specific dosage adjustments provided in the manufacturer's labeling; however, the lower end of the dosing range is recommended in patients with renal impairment. | Dose-dependent CV effects (bradycardia, hypotension, orthostasis, syncope) Causes sedation and drowsiness Do not d/c abruptly because of rebound hypertension | No data | No data | No data |

TABLE 20-23 Antithyroid Drug Dosing in Renal Failure

Drug	Normal Dosage	% of Renal Excretion	Dosage Adjustment in Renal Failure			Hemodialysis	Continuous Ambulatory Peritoneal Dialysis	Continuous Venovenous Hemofiltration
			GFR >50 mL/min	GFR 10–50 mL/min	GFR <10 mL/min			
Methimazole	5–20 mg q8h	7	100%	100%	100%	No data	No data	Dose for GFR 10–50 mL/min
Propylthiouracil	100 mg q8h	<10	100%	100%	100%	No data	No data	Dose for GFR 10–50 mL/min
Thyroid medication								
Levothyroxine	25–300 mcg QD	50%	100%	100%	100%	100%	Not dialyzable	

SUGGESTED READINGS

Cockcroft DW, Gault MH. Prediction of creatinine clearance from serum creatinine. *Nephron*. 1976;16(1):31–41.

Delgado C, Baweja M, Crews DC, et al. A unifying approach for GFR estimation: recommendations of the NKF-ASN Task Force on Reassessing the Inclusion of Race in Diagnosing Kidney Disease. *Am J Kidney Dis*. 2022;79(2):268–288.e261.

Higdon EA, Kimmons LA, Duhart BT Jr., Hudson JQ. Disagreement in estimates of kidney function for drug dosing in obese inpatients. *J Pharm Pract*. 2019;32(1):41–47.

Inker LA, Eneanya ND, Coresh J, et al. New creatinine- and cystatin C-based equations to estimate GFR without race. *N Engl J Med*. 2021;385(19):1737–1749.

Lea-Henry TN, Carland JE, Stocker SL, Sevastos J, Roberts DM. Clinical pharmacokinetics in kidney disease: fundamental principles. *Clin J Am Soc Nephrol*. 2018;13(7):1085–1095.

Levey AS, Stevens LA. Estimating GFR using the CKD Epidemiology Collaboration (CKD-EPI) creatinine equation: more accurate GFR estimates, lower CKD prevalence estimates, and better risk predictions. *Am J Kidney Dis*. 2010;55(4):622–627.

Levey AS, Stevens LA, Schmid CH, et al. A new equation to estimate glomerular filtration rate. *Ann Intern Med*. 2009;150(9):604–612.

Matzke GR, Aronoff GR, Atkinson AJ Jr., et al. Drug dosing consideration in patients with acute and chronic kidney disease-a clinical update from Kidney Disease: Improving Global Outcomes (KDIGO). *Kidney Int*. 2011;80(11):1122–1137.

Paglialunga S, Offman E, Ichhpurani N, Marbury TC, Morimoto BH. Update and trends on pharmacokinetic studies in patients with impaired renal function: practical insight into application of the FDA and EMA guidelines. *Expert Rev Clin Pharmacol*. 2017;10(3):273–283.

Roberts DM, Sevastos J, Carland JE, Stocker SL, Lea-Henry TN. Clinical pharmacokinetics in kidney disease: application to rational design of dosing regimens. *Clin J Am Soc Nephrol*. 2018;13(8):1254–1263.

Stevens LA, Nolin TD, Richardson MM, et al. Chronic Kidney Disease Epidemiology Collaboration. Comparison of drug dosing recommendations based on measured GFR and kidney function estimating equations. *Am J Kidney Dis*. 2009;54(1):33–42.

Index

Note: Page numbers followed by *f* indicate figures; those followed by *t* indicate tables.

24-hour urine collection
 calcium-containing stones and, 135
 calcium oxalate stones and, 137
 creatinine clearance (CrCl) and, 197
 nephrotic syndrome and, 174
 normal values for, 136t
 preeclampsia and, 286
 for protein and creatinine clearance, 174

A

α_2-Adrenergic receptor agonists, 291t
α agonist, 30, 318
α-hemolytic streptococci, 153
AAV. *See* ANCA-associated vasculitis
abaloparatide, 420t
abdominal compartment syndrome (ACS), 217–218
abelcet, 390t
ABG. *See* arterial blood gas
acarbose, 408t
accelerated acute rejection, 259
ACEI, 209
acetaminophen, 72, 382t
acetazolamide, 16t, 19
acetohexamide, 408t
acetohydroxamic acid, 141
acetylsalicylic acid, 382t
acid–base control, 236
acid–base disorder
 cause of, 70–76
  HAGMA, 70–71
  metabolic acidosis, 70, 71f, 71t
  metabolic alkalosis, 73–75, 74f, 74t
  NAGMA, 72–73
  respiratory acidosis, 75
  respiratory alkalosis, 75–76
 compensation for primary, 67–68, 68t
 definition, 65
 detection, 65
 HCO_3 from ABG measurement *vs.* serum total CO_2 (tCO_2), 66, 67t
 identification of
  mixed, 68–70, 69t–70t
  simple, 67–68
 kidney diseases in patients with cancer, 359–365, 360t, 363f
 laboratory evaluation of, 66
 metabolic acidosis
  cause of, 70, 71f, 71t
  and respiratory acidosis, 68t, 69
  and respiratory alkalosis, 69–70
 mixed, 68–70, 69t–70t
 pH of, 65–66
 physiology of, 65–66
 step-wise approach to clinical identification of, 70t
  acid-base environment and potassium level, 52–53
acidemia, 65, 67, 77, 81, 87
acidosis, 52, 55, 65–67, 69t
acquired immunodeficiency syndrome (AIDS), 59f, 61
acromegaly, 103
ACS. *See* abdominal compartment syndrome
Action to Control Cardiovascular Risk in Diabetes (ACCORD) BP trial, 308
action to control cardiovascular risk in diabetes (ACCORD) trial, 328
active vitamin D analogs, 88
acute bacterial prostatitis, 149, 166
acute bacterial pyelonephritis, 165–166
acute decompensated heart failure (ADHF), 209
acute falciparum malaria, 203
acute fatty liver of pregnancy, 277
acute interstitial nephritis (AIN), 202–203
 causes, 202–203
 drug-induced, 203
 evaluation of, 213–214
 infection-associated, 203
 management, 222
acute kidney injury (AKI), 194–226
 ADHF and, 209
 AKIN and RIFLE criteria for diagnosis and classification of, 194, 195t
 biomarkers of, 197–198
 BUN as marker of, 197
 cancer and, 338–339
 carboplatin with, 350
 versus CKD, 198–199
  anemia, 199
  kidney ultrasonography, 198, 198t
  old records, 198
 classifications of, 199–204
  glomerular diseases, 202–203
  intrarenal/intrinsic AKI, 201–204
  postrenal AKI, 201
  prerenal disease, 199–201
  sepsis, 204
  tubular injury, 203
  vascular disorders, 201–202

429

acute kidney injury (AKI) (*continued*)
community-acquired, 204, 204*t*
creatinine clearance in, 197
crystal-associated, 217
cystatin C as marker of, 197
definition, 194–199
due to COVID-19, 219
epidemiology of, 204–205, 204*t*
estimation of eGFR in patients with, 196–197
evaluation of, 205–217
    AIN, 213–214
    ATI, 214–217
    glomerular disease from nephritic cause, 213
    glomerular disease from nephrotic cause, 212–213
    intrinsic kidney disease, large vessel disease, 211
    intrinsic kidney disease, small vessel disease, 211–212
    postrenal AKI, 210–211
    prerenal disease, 209
in HCT, 218–219
hepatorenal syndrome, 208–209
hospital-acquired, 204*t*, 205
ICPi therapy and, 353
intrarenal/intrinsic, 201–204
ischemic, 203
isplatin-induced, 350
KDIGO Clinical Practice Guidelines for, 194, 195*t*
kidney biopsy in, 219–220
in liver disease, 219
management, 220–226
    AIN, 222
    ATI, 222
    CKRT, 224
    general principles for, 222–226
    glomerulonephritis, 221–222
    KRT, 223–226
    peritoneal dialysis, 224
    PIKRT, 224
    postrenal failure, 221
    prerenal AKI, 220–221
    supportive therapy, 223
    vasculitis, 221–222
    what to avoid, 222–223
monoclonal gammopathies with, 350
morbidity associated with, 205
mortality associated with, 205
nephrology consult for, 1–8
    additional testing, 3–4, 4*f*–6*f*
    differential diagnosis, 5*f*
    history and reviewing the patient chart, 1–2
    initial management, 8
    kidney biopsy, 6, 6*f*–7*f*
    KRT, evaluate need for urgent, 6, 8
    physical examination, 1
    urinary sediment microscopy, 2–3
nephrotoxic, 203, 215–217
postrenal, 201, 211
in pregnancy, 274–277
    acute fatty liver of pregnancy, 277
    acute pyelonephritis, 276
    causes, 274, 275*t*, 276
    incidence, 274
    management, 277
    renal cortical necrosis, 276
    TMA and, 274, 276
    urinary tract obstruction, 277
prevention of, 205
prognosis of, 226
recognition of, 194–199
serum creatinine as marker of, 194–197, 196*t*
in special clinical circumstances, 217–220
    ACS, 217–218
    acute phosphate nephropathy, 218
    COVID-19, 219
    crystal-associated AKI, 217, 218*t*
    HCT, 218–219
    kidney biopsy, 219–220
    in setting of liver disease, 219
staging criteria for, 194
TLS and, 340–342
urinary diagnostic indices, 208*t*
urinary findings in various causes of, 207*t*
urine output in, 199
Acute Kidney Injury Network (AKIN), 194, 195*t*, 272
acute myelogenous leukemia, 354
acute myocardial infarction, 246
acute pancreatitis, 82*t*
acute phosphate nephropathy, 218
acute pyelonephritis, 276
acute rejection, 259
acute renal failure. *See* acute kidney injury (AKI)
Acute Renal Failure Trial Network (ATN), 226
acute symptomatic hypocalcemia, 86–88
acute symptomatic infection, 167
acute tubular injury (ATI), 203
    evaluation of, 214–217
    management, 222
acute tubular necrosis (ATN), 349
acute tubulointerstitial nephritis (ATIN), 353
acute urethral syndrome, 148–149
    prostatitis, 148–149
    prostatodynia, 149
    urethritis, 148
    vaginitis, 148
acute uric acid nephropathy, 217
acyclovir, 398*t*
ADAMTS13, 193

Index | 431

adefovir, 398t
adenosine triphosphatase, 52
adenosine triphosphate (ATP), 100
Adequacy of PD in Mexico (ADEMEX) trial, 245
ADHF. *See* acute decompensated heart failure
ADHR. *See* autosomal dominant hypophosphatemic rickets
adrenocorticotropin (ACTH), 35
adult dominant polycystic kidney disease, 281
ADVANCE trial, 307
African American Study of Kidney Disease (AASK) trial, 310
aging
   hypertension in, 308–309
   potassium level and, 52
   pseudohypertension in, 300–301
AIDS. *See* acquired immunodeficiency syndrome
AIN. *See* acute interstitial nephritis
AKI. *See* acute kidney injury
AKIN. *See* Acute Kidney Injury Network
AL/AH amyloidosis, 343t
albumin, 9–10, 18, 28–31
   anasarca in, 30
   cefotaxime with, 30
   furosemide with, 28
   HRS with, 29–30
   patients with nephrotic syndrome to, 30
albuminuria, degree and trajectory of, 324, 325f
alcohol use disorder, 105t
aldosterone, 53–54
   antagonists, 16t
   blockade, 24–25
   escape, 14, 15f
   in healthy subject, 15f
   receptors, 24–25
   sodium-retaining effect of, 14
alemtuzumab (Campath), 252, 253t
alfentanil, 378t
alirocumab, 405t
ALK. *See* anaplastic lymphoma kinase
alkalemia, 65
alkalosis, 65
allergic interstitial nephritis, 26t
allopurinol, 421t
alogliptin, 332
alprazolam, 422t
alteplase, 383t
alzheimer drug dosing in renal failure, 377t
amantadine, 398t
amikacin, 375t
amiloride, 15, 16t

aminoglycoside nephrotoxicity, 215
aminophylline IV, 376t
aminosalicylic acid, 397t
amitriptyline, 388t
amphetamine IR, 424t
amphotec, 390t
amphotericin B, 390t
ampicillin, 162t
amyloidosis, 190–191
ANA. *See* antinuclear antibody
analgesic drug dosing in renal failure, 377t–382t
anaplastic lymphoma kinase (ALK), 351
anasarca, 30
ANCA. *See* antineutrophil cytoplasmic antibody
ANCA-associated vasculitis (AAV), 177
anemia, 12, 23, 357t
associated with CKD, 235
   on dialysis, 247
   kidney transplant and, 264–265
   medical care of kidney transplanted patient from, 264–265
angioneurotic edema, 10
angiotensin, 13
angiotensin-converting enzyme (ACE) inhibitors, 24f–25f, 178–180, 184, 188, 190–191, 263, 291t, 301, 305, 307, 308–314, 316, 318
angiotensin-converting enzyme inhibitors (ACEis), 15, 23
angiotensin II receptor blockers, 291t
angiotensin receptor blockers (ARBs), 15, 23, 24f
   in hypertension, 263
   with neprilysin inhibition, 23
anidulafungin, 391t
anistreplase, 383t
ankle edema, 11, 22
antibody therapies, 253t
anticoagulant drug, 383t–385t
anticoagulant drug dosing in renal failure, 383t–385t
anticonvulsants, 413t–417t
antidepressant drug dosing in renal failure, 386t–389t
anti–double-stranded DNA (anti-dsDNA), 174
antifungal agent dosing in renal failure, 390t–391t
antifungal agents, 390t
anti-GBM antibody, 174
anti-GBM disease, 184
   diagnosis of, 184
   overview, 184
   pathophysiology of, 184
   treatment for, 184

antigen-presenting cells (APCs), 251
Antihypertensive and Lipid-Lowering Treatment to Prevent Heart Attack Trial (ALLHAT), 305, 307
antihypertensive therapy, 233, 290
antimetabolites, 253t, 254
antineutrophil cytoplasmic antibody (ANCA), 174
antinuclear antibody (ANA), 174
anti-parkinson agents, 392t
anti-Parkinson drug dosing in renal failure, 392t
antiplatelet agents, 334
antistreptolysin titer, 174
antithymocyte globulin (ATG), 252, 253t
antithyroid drugs, 426t
antituberculosis antibiotics, 396t–397t
antituberculosis drug dosing in renal failure, 396t–397t
antiulcer agents, 404t
antiviral agent dosing in renal failure, 398t–402t
antiviral agents, 398t–402t
anuria, 199
APCs. See antigen-presenting cells
APD. See automated PD
apixaban, 383t
Appropriate Blood Pressure Control in Diabetes (ABCD) trial, 307
ARB, 209
arginine vasopressin (AVP), 35, 197, 269–270
  deficiency, 45, 50
  resistance, 45, 50
aripiprazole, 395t
arrhythmias, 114
arterial blood gas (ABG), 66
arterial portion, body fluids, 12
arterial underfilling, 12, 200
arterial/venous thrombosis, 257
arteriovenous fistula (AVF), 12, 239, 242–243
arteriovenous grafts (AVGs), 243
ascites, 27–30
aspirin, 334, 383t
asthma, magnesium in, 116
asymptomatic bacteriuria, 272–273
  clinical setting, 147
  treatment of, 161–163
    children, 162
    general population, 162–163
    miscellaneous, 162
    pregnancy, 161–162
asymptomatic hyperparathyroidism, 97–98
ATG. See antithymocyte globulin

atheroembolic disease, 211–212
  history, 211
  laboratory investigation, 212
  physical examination, 211
  urinary evaluation, 212
ATI. See acute tubular injury
ATN. See acute tubular necrosis
atomoxetine, 424t
atorvastatin, 405t
ATP. See adenosine triphosphate
auranofin, 421t
automated PD (APD), 244
autosomal dominant hypophosphatemic rickets (ADHR), 105t, 106
AVF. See arteriovenous fistula
AVGs. See arteriovenous grafts
AVP. See arginine vasopressin
azathioprine, 253t, 254
azoles, 390t
  aztreonam, 162t

B

β_2-Adrenergic receptor agonists, 291t
β-adrenergic blocker, 58, 60
β-lactams, 158–159, 160t, 162t
Bacillus Calmette–Guérin (BCG) vaccines, 262
bacteremia, 145, 147, 151, 157, 163, 167–168, 219, 243
bacteremic shock and UTI, 165
bacterial cystourethritis, 149
bacteriuria
  asymptomatic, 272–273
  biochemical tests for, 156
  significant, 144
  symptomatic, 273–274
barbiturates, 422t
basiliximab, 252, 253t
B-cell malignancies, 190
B-cells, 252
bedaquiline, 397t
belatacept, 253t, 254
benzodiazepine antagonist, 423t
benzodiazepines, 422t–423t
beriberi, 12
betamethasone, 403t
beta (β)$_2$-adrenoreceptor–mediated potassium uptake, 52
beta (β)-adrenergic–mediated release of renin, 13
beta (β)-blockers, 15, 23
bezafibrate, 405t
bioavailability of diuretic drugs, 17–18
biomarkers of AKI, 194–197–5
biopsy of kidney, 174, 272, 326–327
bisphosphonates, 95t, 96
BK polyomavirus (BKPyV), 261–262
blocking mineralocorticoid (aldosterone) receptors, 24–25

blood pressure (BP), 294
　to cardiovascular risk, 296, 297t
　classification of, 295t
　diastolic, 294–295, 295t
　measuring at home, 300t
　systolic, 294–295, 295t
　target in diabetic kidney disease, 333
blood urea nitrogen (BUN)
　as marker of AKI, 197
　as marker of GFR, 197
body fluid distribution, 9–11, 10t
　cirrhosis patient in, 9
　generalized edema and, 9–11
　inside cell, 9
　localized edema and, 11
　Starling's law of fluid movement, 9–10, 10f
　total-body phenomenon of, 11
body fluid volume regulation, 11–15
bortezomib, 351
Boui-ougi-tou, 106
BP. *See* blood pressure
budesonide, 403t
bumetanide, 16t, 21t
buprenorphine, 380t
bupropion, 389t
burns, 11
buspirone, 423t
butorphanol, 378t

C

C3 glomerulopathy (C3G), 177, 183–184
　clinical presentations of, 183
　diagnosis of, 183
　overview, 183
　pathophysiology, 183–184
　treatment of, 184
calciferol, 79, 80f
calcimimetics, 95t, 96–97
calcineurin inhibitors, 252–253, 253t, 258
calcitonin, 95t
calcitriol, 88
calcium, 77–78, 106
　distribution in blood, 79f
　homeostasis, 79f
　net intestinal absorption of, 78
　oral and intravenous formulations, 87t
　plasma-ionized, 79
　reabsorption in thick ascending limb, 129
　reabsorption of, 81f
　regulation, 78–80
　total body, 78
calcium channel blockers, 290t, 291t
calcium chelators, 82t
calcium-containing stones, 127, 130–133, 131t
　CaOx, 130

　CaP, 130
　evaluation of patient, 135
　hypercalciuria and, 130–131, 131t
　hyperoxaluria and, 131–132, 131t
　hyperuricosuria and, 131, 131t
　hypocitraturia and, 131, 131t
　low urinary volume and, 131t, 132
　major risk factors for, 130–132, 131t
　medullary sponge kidney and, 131t, 132
　obesity and, 131t, 132–133
　prevention and treatment, 137–142
　　calcium phosphate stones, 140–141
　　hypercalciuria, 139–140
　　hyperoxaluria, 140
　　hypocitraturia, 140
　　nonspecific therapeutic options for, 137–138
　　specific therapeutic options for, 138–140
　　urinary volume, 138–139
　randomized trials in calcium-containing nephrolithiasis, 139t
calcium/creatinine clearance ratio, 93
calcium levels, 236
calcium oxalate dihydrate (COD), 128
calcium oxalate monohydrate (COM), 128
calcium phosphate stones, 140–141
calcium-sensing receptor (CaSR), 111
canagliflozin, 16t, 331, 408t
cancer, kidney diseases in patients with, 338–365
　AKI and, 338–358
　CKD and, 338–340, 358–359
　electrolyte and acid–base disorders, 359–365, 360t, 363f
　estimated glomerular filtration rate, 338
　etiologies of, 340
　incidence of, 338–340
　monoclonal gammopathies (paraproteinemias), 342–345
　　AKI and, 342
　　CKD and, 342
　　definition, 342
　　glomerular diseases directly associated with cancer, 346–348, 347f
　　LCCN, 343–344, 343t
　　LCPT, 343t, 344–345
　　MM and, 342
　　obstructive AKI, 348
　　paraprotein-mediated glomerular diseases, 343t, 345
　　renal drug toxicities, 348–354
　　TMA, 343t, 345–346, 346f
　multiple myeloma and, 339
　onconephrology, 338, 339f
　other causes of, 354
　prevalence of, 338–340

cancer, kidney diseases in patients with (*continued*)
  renal drug toxicities and, 348–354
    chemotherapy, 349–350
    immunotherapy, 352–354
    targeted therapies, 351–352
  stem cell therapy–associated kidney disease, 354–358, 357*t*
  tumor lysis syndrome, 340–342
    AKI and, 340
    Cairo–Bishop criteria for, 340–341, 340*t*
    causes of, 340
    hyperuricemia and, 341
    management of, 341–342
    with significant morbidity and mortality, 340–341
    xanthine oxidase inhibitor for, 341
Candida albicans, 148
CAPD. *See* continuous ambulatory PD
capillary leak syndromes, 12, 14
capreomycin, 397*t*
carbamazepine, 375*t*, 413*t*
carbidopa, 392*t*
carbonic anhydrase inhibitors, 16*t*
carboplatin, 350
cardiac failure
  causes of, 12
  sodium and water retention and, 12
cardiac output
  to edema formation, 14
  relation with systemic arterial resistance, 12
cardiovascular disease, magnesium and, 113–114
carfilzomib, 351
CAR T cell therapy, 353–354
caspofungin, 391*t*
CaSR. *See* calcium-sensing receptor
cast nephropathy, 343*t*
catecholamines, 52
catheter-associated infections, 169–170
CCPD. *See* continuous cycling PD
CD40/CD40L pathway, 251–252
cefepime, 162*t*
ceftazidime, 162*t*
ceftriaxone, 162*t*
cellulitis, 11
central venous catheters (CVCs), 243
chemotherapy, 349–350
CHF. *See* congestive heart failure
Chlamydia trachomatis, 148
chlordiazepoxide, 422*t*
chlorothiazide, 16*t*
chlorpromazine, 393*t*
chlorpropamide, 408*t*
chlorthalidone, 16*t*
Chlorthalidone for Hypertension in Advanced CKD (CLICK) trial, 310
cholestyramine, 405*t*

cholinesterase inhibitors, 377*t*
chronic allograft damage, 260
chronic bacterial prostatitis, 149, 168
chronic hypertension, 286
Chronic Hypertension and Pregnancy (CHAP) Study, 289–290
chronic kidney disease (CKD), 125, 198, 228–237
  versus acute kidney injury (AKI), 198–199
    anemia, 199
    kidney ultrasonography, 198, 198*t*
    old records, 198
  cancer and, 338–339
  cardiovascular comorbidity, managing of, 237
  cause of, 228–229
  decreased GFR and, 228
  definition, 228–230
  diabetes mellitus and, 322–334, 329*f*, 330*t*, 331*t*
    ADA 2023 Standards of Care in, 322, 323*t*–324*t*
    additional causes of, 322
    albuminuria, degree and trajectory of, 324, 325*f*
    ASCVD risk in, 334
    beta blockers in, 333
    biopsy findings, 326–327
    blood pressure targets, 333
    calcium channel blockers in, 333
    clinical course of, 322, 324, 325*f*
    comorbid, 322
    definition, 322
    diagnosis of, 322, 324–327
    diet for patients with, 328
    DPP4 inhibitors, 330*t*, 331*t*, 332
    epidemiology of, 322, 324
    evaluating patients for other causes of, 325
    GFR, 324, 325*f*
    GLP-1 RAs, 330*t*, 331*t*, 332
    glycemic control in patients with T1DM, 328, 330*t*
    glycemic control in patients with T2DM, 331–333, 331*t*
    glycemic monitoring and targets, 327–328
    HbA1c monitoring, 327
    home blood glucose monitoring, 327
    hypertension, 333–334
    insulin, 328, 330, 332
    KDIGO 2022 Clinical Practice Guideline recommendations for pharmacologic management in patients with, 329*f*
    KDIGO Clinical Practice Guidelines for management of, 322, 323*t*–324*t*

kidney biopsy for, 325–326
lifestyle counseling for patients with, 328
loop diuretics, 333
medication classes for glycemic control in patients with, 330*t*
metformin, 330*t*, 331, 331*t*
moderate-intensity physical activity for patients with, 328
MRAs in, 333–334
pharmacologic management in, 328, 329*f*, 330–334, 330*t*, 331*t*
prevalence, 322
RAAS blockade with ACEi/ARBs, 333
SGLT-2 inhibitors, 330*t*, 331–332, 331*t*
smoking cessation and, 328
sulfonylureas, 330*t*, 331*t*, 332
T1DM, 322
T1DM *vs.* T2DM, 324, 326*t*
T2DM, 322
thiazide in, 333
TZDs, 330*t*, 331*t*, 332–333
weight loss for patients with, 328
dialysis for, 239–241
anemia and, 247
cardiovascular health and, 246
dose, 245–246
education regarding, 241
indications for initiating, 239–241, 240*t*
mineral bone disorder and, 246
nutrition and, 246–247
drug dosing in patients with, 374, 375*t*–426*t*
and drug pharmacokinetic
absorption, 371
CKD-EPI, 372, 374
Cockcroft–Gault (CG) equation, 372
distribution, 371
elimination, 372
metabolism, 371
modification of diet in renal disease re-expressed equation, 372
ESA failure in, 235
hemodialysis for, 241–244
access, 242–243
advantages, 241–242
arteriovenous fistula for, 239, 242–243
complications, 243–244
versus peritoneal dialysis, 241*t*
procedure, 241–242, 242*f*
standard dialysate solutions, comparison of, 242*t*
hypertension and, 309–310
iron deficiency in, 235

managing complications of, 235–237
acid–base control, 236
anemia, 235
mineral and bone disease, 235–236
uremic toxins, accumulation of, 237
markers of, 228
mechanism of progression, 230–231
peritoneal dialysis for, 244–245
versus hemodialysis, 241*t*
standard dialysate solutions, comparison of, 242*t*
prevalence of, 230
risk factor management recommendations and treatment options, 231–232, 232*t*
risk factors for, 230
staging of, 228–230
creatinine-based equations, 229–230
Creatinine Clearance (CrCl), 229
measurement of GFR, 228
therapeutic drug monitoring in patients with, 375*t*–376*t*
when to refer to nephrologist, 237
Chronic Kidney Disease Epidemiology Collaboration (CKD-EPI), 196
chronic kidney disease epidemiology collaboration equation (CKD-EPI), 372, 374
chronic lymphocytic leukemia (CLL), 342
chronic myelogenous leukemia (CML), 352
chronic myelomonocytic leukemia (CMML), 354
chronic noninflammatory prostatitis. *See* prostatodynia
Chronic Renal Insufficiency Cohort (CRIC), 231
cidofovir, 398*t*
cimetidine, 404*t*
cinacalcet, 95*t*
ciprofloxacin, 162*t*
cirrhosis, 11
decompensated, 11, 27–28
edema and, 11
hepatic, 12, 27–30
cisplatin, 350
cisplatin-mediated AKI, 350
citalopram, 386*t*
CKD. *See* chronic kidney disease
CKD-EPI. *See* Chronic Kidney Disease Epidemiology Collaboration
CKD-epidemiology equation (CKD-EPI), 229
CKRT. *See* continuous kidney replacement therapy
CLL. *See* chronic lymphocytic leukemia
clofibrate, 405*t*
clonazepam, 413*t*, 422*t*
clopidogrel, 383*t*

clorazepate, 422t
clozapine, 394t
CMML. *See* chronic myelomonocytic leukemia
CMV. *See* cytomegalovirus
CNNM. *See* cyclin M family of proteins
Cockcroft-Gault, 196–197, 229, 372
Cockcroft–Gault equation, 229
COD. *See* calcium oxalate dihydrate
codeine, 378t
colchicine, 421t
colestipol, 405t
collecting duct diuretics, 16, 16t
COM. *See* calcium oxalate monohydrate
combination diuretic therapy, 19, 21t
community-acquired AKI, 204, 204t
compensatory renal sodium and water retention, 14
complicated UTIs, 145
congestive heart failure (CHF), 11, 22–27
    clinical symptoms of, 22–23
    etiology of, 23
    loop diuretic in, 23–24
    treatment of, 23–27
continuous ambulatory PD (CAPD), 244
continuous cycling PD (CCPD), 244
continuous diuretic infusions, 19, 21–22, 21t
continuous kidney replacement therapy (CKRT), 224, 225t
contrast-associated AKI, 216
corticosteroid drug dosing in renal failure, 403t
corticosteroid drugs, 403t
corticosteroids, 253t, 254, 258
cortisone, 403t
costimulation, 251
COVID-19 vaccination, 262
Creatinine Clearance (CrCl), 229
creatinine serum
    clearance, 197
    excretion, 194, 196
    on factors independent of kidney, 196
    levels, 196
    as marker AKI, 194–197, 196t
    medications and other conditions that affect, 196t
CRIC. *See* Chronic Renal Insufficiency Cohort
crizotinib, 351
CRS. *See* cytokine release syndrome
cryoglobulinemia (cryoglobulinemia), 186–187
    diagnosis of, 186
    overview, 186
    pathophysiology of, 186–187
    treatment for, 187
cryoglobulins, 174

crystal-associated AKI, 217, 218t
CVCs. *See* central venous catheters
cyclic adenosine monophosphate (cAMP), 52
cyclin M family of proteins (CNNM), 109
cycloserine, 397t
cyclosporin, 253t, 375t
cyclosporine, 209, 265
cyclosporine A (CsA), 252, 254
CYP450 activities, 371
cystatin C
    as marker of AKI, 197
    as marker of GFR, 197
Cystatin C–based equations, 230
cystine stones, 134–135
    evaluation of patient, 136
    pathophysiology of, 134–135
    prevention and treatment, 141–142
    signs and symptoms of, 135
cytokine release syndrome (CRS), 353
cytomegalovirus (CMV), 261

D

dabigatran, 383t
dalteparin, 384t
dapagliflozen, 16t
dapagliflozin, 331, 408t
DBP. *See* diastolic BP
deamino-8-d-arginine vasopressin (dDAVP), 269–270
deep venous disease, 11
delavirdine, 399t
delayed graft function (DGF), 259
denosumab, 95t, 96
desensitization therapy, 252
desmopressin, 42–43, 42t
dexamethasone, 403t
dextroamphetamine, 424t
DGF. *See* delayed graft function
diabetes control and complications trial (DCCT), 328
diabetes mellitus, 10, 30, 263–264
    CKD and, 322–334, 329f, 330t, 331t
        ADA 2023 Standards of Care in, 322, 323t–324t
        additional causes of, 322
        albuminuria, degree and trajectory of, 324, 325f
        ASCVD risk in, 334
        beta blockers in, 333
        biopsy findings, 326–327
        blood pressure targets, 333
        calcium channel blockers in, 333
        clinical course of, 322, 324, 325f
        comorbid, 322
        definition, 322
        diagnosis of, 322, 324–327
        diet for patients with, 328

DPP4 inhibitors, 330*t*, 331*t*, 332
epidemiology of, 322, 324
evaluating patients for other causes of, 325
GFR, 324, 325*f*
GLP-1 RAs, 330*t*, 331*t*, 332
glycemic control in patients with T1DM, 328, 330*t*
glycemic control in patients with T2DM, 331–333, 331*t*
glycemic monitoring and targets, 327–328
HbA1c monitoring, 327
home blood glucose monitoring, 327
hypertension, 333–334
insulin, 328, 330, 332
KDIGO 2022 Clinical Practice Guideline recommendations for pharmacologic management in patients with, 329*f*
KDIGO Clinical Practice Guidelines for management of, 322, 323*t*–324*t*
kidney biopsy for, 325–326
lifestyle counseling for patients with, 328
loop diuretics, 333
medication classes for glycemic control in patients with, 330*t*
metformin, 330*t*, 331, 331*t*
moderate-intensity physical activity for patients with, 328
MRAs in, 333–334
pharmacologic management in, 328, 329*f*, 330–334, 330*t*, 331*t*
prevalence, 322
RAAS blockade with ACEi/ARBs, 333
SGLT-2 inhibitors, 330*t*, 331–332, 331*t*
smoking cessation and, 328
sulfonylureas, 330*t*, 331*t*, 332
T1DM, 322
T1DM *vs.* T2DM, 324, 326*t*
T2DM, 322
thiazide in, 333
TZDs, 330*t*, 331*t*, 332–333
weight loss for patients with, 328
and hypertension, 306, 308
hypomagnesemia and, 114
and magnesium, 114
medical care of transplanted patient from, 263–264
diabetic ketoacidosis, 105*t*
diabetic kidney disease, 322–334
ADA 2023 Standards of Care in, 322, 323*t*–324*t*
additional causes of, 322
albuminuria, degree and trajectory of, 324, 325*f*
ASCVD risk in, 334
biopsy findings, 326–327
clinical course of, 322, 324, 325*f*
comorbid, 322
definition, 322
diagnosis of, 322, 324–327
diet for patients with, 328
epidemiology of, 322, 324
evaluating patients for other causes of, 325
GFR, 324, 325*f*
glycemic monitoring and targets, 327–328
HbA1c monitoring, 327
home blood glucose monitoring, 327
KDIGO 2022 Clinical Practice Guideline
for management, 322, 323*t*–324*t*
recommendations for pharmacologic management, 329*f*
kidney biopsy for, 325–326
lifestyle counseling for patients with, 328
medication classes for glycemic control in, 330*t*
moderate-intensity physical activity for, 328
pharmacologic management in, 328, 329*f*, 330–334, 330*t*, 331*t*
beta blockers in, 333
blood pressure targets, 333
calcium channel blockers in, 333
DPP4 inhibitors, 330*t*, 331*t*, 332
GLP-1 RAs, 330*t*, 331*t*, 332
glycemic control in patients with T1DM, 328, 330*t*
glycemic control in patients with T2DM, 331–333, 331*t*
hypertension, 333–334
insulin, 328, 330, 332
loop diuretics, 333
metformin, 330*t*, 331, 331*t*
MRAs in, 333–334
RAAS blockade with ACEi/ARBs, 333
SGLT-2 inhibitors, 330*t*, 331–332, 331*t*
sulfonylureas, 330*t*, 331*t*, 332
thiazide in, 333
TZDs, 330*t*, 331*t*, 332–333
prevalence, 322, 334
smoking cessation and, 328
T1DM, 322, 328
T1DM *vs.* T2DM, 324, 326*t*
T2DM, 322, 331–333
weight loss for patients with, 328
diabetic nephropathy, 190, 280

dialysis for CKD, 239–241
  anemia and, 247
  cardiovascular health and, 246
  dose, 245–246
  education regarding, 241
  general issues related to care, 245–247
  indications for initiating, 239–241, 240t
  mineral bone disorder and, 246
  nutrition and, 246–247
dialysis in pregnancy, 284–285, 285t
diarrhea, 73
diastolic BP (DBP), 294–295, 295t
diazepam, 422t
diclofenac, 418t
didanosine, 399t
dietary and diuretic treatment of edema, 15–18
dietary intake, decreased, 105t
dietary magnesium, 109
diflunisal, 418t
DiGeorge syndrome, 82t, 83
digoxin, 375t
dihydropyridine calcium channel blockers, 263
dipeptidyl peptidase-4 (DPP4) inhibitors, 330t, 331t, 332
dipyridamole, 384t
direct-acting vasodilators, 291t
distal convoluted tubule (DCT) diuretics, 16, 16t
distension syndrome, 267
diuretic drugs, 15–18, 16t, 17t
  administered by mouth, 17
  bioavailability of, 17–18
  physiologic classification of, 16t
diuretic resistance, 18–22, 201
  causes of, 18–19
  potential escalation of, 20f
  treatment of, 19–22
diuretics, 291t
diuretic therapy, 19–21
  combination, 21t
  complications of, 26, 26t
DnaJ homolog subfamily B member 9 (DNAJB9), 191
donepezil, 377t
donor-specific antibodies (DSA), 252
dopamine, 22
DOSE trial (Diuretic Optimization Strategies Evaluation), 22
doxazosin, 12
doxercalciferol, 88
drug-induced AIN, 203
drug-related stones, 135
DSA. *See* donor-specific antibodies
dulaglutide, 409t
duloxetine, 387t
dysuria, 148

E

E. coli, 147–148
EABV. *See* effective arterial blood volume
ECF. *See* extracellular fluid
ECF potassium, 52
ECF volume status
  generalized edema patient of, 9
  kidney, role of, 11
  vascular compartment in, 9
eclampsia, magnesium in, 114–115
Eculizumab, 193
Edelman equation scenarios for hypernatremia, 44–45, 44t
edema, 9
  angioneurotic, 10
  ankle, 11, 22
  cirrhosis and, 11
  dietary and diuretic treatment of, 15–18
  ECF, excess of, 9
  and fluid permeability of capillary wall, 11
  generalized, 9–11
  localized, 11
  loop diuretic for, 17
  in nephrotic patients, 30–32
  nonpitting, 9
  periorbital areas, 11
  pitting, 9
  pulmonary, 11
  relation with permeability of capillary wall, 9
  systemic arterial vasodilation to, 14
edematous patient
  body fluid distribution, 9–11, 10t
  body fluid volume regulation, 11–15
  neurohumoral and systemic hemodynamic response, 13
  pitting edema and, 9
  sodium chloride restriction, 15
edoxaban, 384t
effective arterial blood volume (EABV), 12, 15f, 35
effective blood volume, 11
elderly patients
  hypertension in, 308–309
  pseudohypertension in, 300–301
electrolyte abnormalities, and magnesium, 114
electrolyte-free water balance, 34
empagliflozin, 16t, 331, 409t
emtricitabine, 399t
end-stage kidney disease (ESKD), 100, 228
  counts in the United States by modality, 240f
  prevalence of, 248
  risk factors for progression to, 231–232
    behavioral factors, 231
    clinical factors, 231

genetic factors, 231–232
sociodemographic and economic factors, 231
slowing progression to, 233–235
antihypertensive therapy, 233
diet for, 234
GLP-1 receptor agonists for, 234
glycemic control for, 234
mineralocorticoid antagonism for, 234
RAAS inhibition for, 233
reduction in proteinuria, 233–235
SGLT2 (sodium-glucose transport protein 2) inhibition for, 233–234
smoking cessation for, 234–235
weight loss and exercise for, 234
enoxaparin, 384t
entecavir, 399t
eosinophilic granulomatosis with polyangiitis, 175t
epidermal growth factor receptor (EGFR) inhibitors, 116
epithelial sodium channels (ENaC), 53
eplerenone, 15, 16t, 25, 333
ertugliflozin, 331
erythropoiesis stimulating agent (ESA), 235
ESA. See erythropoiesis stimulating agent
Escherichia coli, 3, 134, 145–149, 151, 153, 158–159, 162, 191, 273
ESKD. See end-stage kidney disease
estazolam, 423t
etalcalcetide, 95t
ethacrynic acid, 16t
ethambutol, 396t
ethanol intake, 305
ethchlorvynol, 423t
ethionamide, 397t
ethosuximide, 413t
etodolac, 418t
EuLITE trial, 344
everolimus, 253t, 258
evolocumab, 405t
excess interstitial fluid, total-body phenomenon of, 11
exenatide, 409t
extracellular fluid (ECF), 9, 65
extracellular potassium (K), 52
ezetimibe, 405t

F

famciclovir, 399t
familial hypocalcemia, 82t, 83
familial hypocalcuric hypercalcemia (FHH), 89–90
famotidine, 404t
Fanconi syndrome. See light chain proximal tubulopathy (LCPT)

febuxostat, 421t
felbamate, 413t
fenofibrate, 406t
fenoprofen, 418t
fentanyl, 378t
FEUN. See fractional excretion of urea nitrogen
FGF-23. See fibroblast growth factor 23
FHH. See familial hypocalcuric hypercalcemia
fibrillary glomerulonephritis, 343t
fibroblast growth factor 23 (FGF-23), 100–102, 236
FimH, 164
finerenone, 16t, 333–334
Finerenone in Reducing Cardiovascular Mortality and Morbidity in Diabetic Kidney Disease (FIGARO-DKD) trial, 334
Finerenone in Reducing Kidney Failure and Disease Progression in Diabetic Kidney Disease (FIDELIO-DKD), 334
fluconazole, 390t
flucytosine, 390t
fludrocortisone, 403t
fluid permeability of capillary wall, edema and, 11
fluid resorption, 9
fluids, in human body, 9
flumazenil, 423t
fluoroquinolones, 160, 161t, 162t, 274
fluoxetine, 386t
flurazepam, 423t
flurbiprofen, 418t
fluvastatin, 406t
focal segmental glomerulosclerosis (FSGS), 172, 347
fondaparinux, 384t
foscarnet, 82t, 399t
fosfomycin, 160
fractional excretion of sodium (FENa), 209
fractional excretion of urea nitrogen (FEUN), 215
Frequent Hemodialysis Network (FHN Daily) trial, 246
FSGS. See focal segmental glomerulosclerosis
furosemide, 16t, 21–22, 21t

G

gabapentin, 414t
gadolinium-containing chelates, 84
galantamine, 377t
gallium nitrate, 97
ganciclovir IV, 399t
ganciclovir PO, 399t
Gardnerella vaginalis, 148

gastrointestinal agent dosing in renal failure, 404t
gastrointestinal upset, 26t
gemfibrozil, 406t
generalized edema, 9–11
gentamicin, 162t, 375t
gestational hypertension, 286
GFR. *See* glomerular filtration rate
glibornuride, 409t
gliclazide, 409t
glimepiride, 332
glipizide, 332, 409t
glomerular capillary endotheliosis, 288, 288f
glomerular diseases, 202–203, 280–281
    clinical approach to glomerulonephritis based upon serum complement, 176t
    clinical assessment of, 172, 174–175, 177–178
    clinical patterns of, 172
    clinicopathologic correlation, 174–175, 177–178
    definition, 172
    directly associated with cancer, 346–348, 347f
    immunofluorescence microscopy for IgG in glomerulonephritis, 178f
    from nephritic cause, 213
    nephritic clinical presentation, 175t
    from nephrotic cause, 212–213
    nephrotic clinical presentation, 177t
    overview, 172
    pathologic diagnosis of, 175, 177–178
    primary, 173t
    supportive management of patients with, 181f
    systemic diseases and, 175t, 177t
    therapy for, 178–182
    treatment of specific, 182–191
glomerular endothelial injury, 177
glomerular filtration rate (GFR), 14, 172, 194
    BUN as marker of, 197
    in CKD patients, 194–196
    cystatin C as marker of, 197
    serum creatinine as marker of, 194–197
    and sodium and water reabsorption, 12, 14
glomerulonephritis
    clinical approach to, 176t
    histologic classification of, 174t
    immunofluorescence microscopy for IgG in, 178f
    management, 221–222
glomerulonephritis in women of childbearing, 279
GLP-1 receptor agonists, 234

glucagon-like peptide-1 receptor agonists (GLP-1 RAs), 330t, 331t, 332
    adverse effects, 332
    contraindications, 332
    indications for, 332
    kidney and cardiovascular protective effects, 332
    mechanism of action, 332
glucocorticoids, 95t
glyburide, 332, 409t
glycemic control
    in patients with T1DM, 328, 330t
    in patients with T2DM, 331–333, 331t
gold sodium, 421t
Goodpasture syndrome, 175t, 184
    diagnosis of, 184
    overview, 184
    pathophysiology of, 184
    treatment for, 184
graft-*versus*-host-disease (GVHD), 354–355
gram-negative bacteria, 152t
gram-positive bacteria, 152t
granulomatosis with polyangiitis, 175t
griseofulvin, 391t
guanfacine ER, 425t
Guyton hypothesis, 296–299, 298f
gynecomastia, 26t

H

HAGMA. *See* high anion gap metabolic acidosis
haloperidol, 393t, 423t
haplostorm, 355
HbA1c monitoring, 327
HCT. *See* hematopoietic cell transplant
heavy chain deposition disease, 343t
hematopoietic cell transplant (HCT), 218–219
hematopoietic stem cell transplantation (HSCT), 344–345, 354–355
hematuria, 281–282
hemodialysis, 95t
hemodialysis (HD) for CKD, 241–244
    access, 242–243
    advantages, 241–242
    arteriovenous fistula for, 239, 242–243
    complications, 243–244
    versus peritoneal dialysis, 241t
    procedure, 241–242, 242f
    standard dialysate solutions, comparison of, 242t
hemolysis, elevated liver enzymes, low platelet count (HELLP) syndrome, 272, 276
hemolytic uremic syndrome (HUS), 175t, 191, 193, 276
Henderson–Hasselbach equation, 66

heparin, 384t
hepatic cirrhosis, 12, 27–30
Hepatitis B virus infection, 262
Hepatitis C, 175t
Hepatitis C virus infection, 262
hepatorenal syndrome (HRS), 29–30, 208–209
herpes simplex virus, 148
HHM. *See* humoral hypercalcemia of malignancy
HIF (hypoxia-inducible transcription) stabilizers, 235
high anion gap metabolic acidosis (HAGMA), 70
high-dose MTX (HD-MTX) therapy, 349
HIV infection, 262
home blood glucose monitoring, 327
homeostasis, 33
homeostasis, magnesium, 109–111
  intestinal absorption of magnesium, 109
  renal handling, 109–111
hospital-acquired AKI, 204t, 205
HRS. *See* hepatorenal syndrome
HRS-AKI, 208–209
HSCT. *See* hematopoietic stem cell transplantation
humoral hypercalcemia of malignancy (HHM), 91–92
hungry bone syndrome (HBS), 105–106, 105t
HUS. *See* hemolytic uremic syndrome
hydralazine, 12, 290t, 291t
hydraulic permeability, of capillary, 9
hydrochlorothiazide, 16t
hydrocodone ER, 381t
hydrocortisone, 403t
hydromorphone, 381t
hyperacute rejection, 259
hypercalcemia, 26t, 88–98
  algorithm for workup of, 93f
  asymptomatic hyperparathyroidism and, 97–98
  calcium absorption from gastrointestinal tract, 90–91
  causes of, 89t
  in children, 92
  in CKD, 90
  decreased calcium excretion by kidney, 92
  diagnosis of, 92–94
  etiology, 88–92
  and FHH, 89–90
  hyperparathyroidism in, 88–89
  hyperthyroidism and, 92
  hypervitaminosis A and, 92
  immobilization and, 92
  increased 1,25-dihydroxy vitamin D production, 90–91
  initial laboratory examination for, 92–94
  Jansen-type metaphyseal chondroplasia (activating PTH1R variant), 90
  and lithium, 90
  of malignancy, 91–92
  of milk-alkali syndrome, 90
  non-PTH-mediated, 90–92
  Paget disease and, 92
  PTH-mediated, 88–90
  role of calcium resorption from bone, 91–92
  secondary and tertiary hyperparathyroidism in, 98
  signs and symptoms of, 92
  treatment of, 94–98, 95t
  vitamin D intoxication, 90
hypercalciuria
  calcium-containing stones and, 130–131, 131t
  prevention and treatment, 139–140
hypercholesterolemia, 26t
hypercoagulability, 181–182
hyperglycemia, 26t
hyperkalemia, 25–26, 26t, 57–63
  causes, 60–61, 60t
  clinical manifestations, 61
  diagnosis of, 61
  diagnostic approach to, 57–58, 59f, 60–61
  spurious, 57–58
  treatment of, 61–63, 62f
hyperlipidemia, 263
hyperlipidemic agent dosing in renal failure, 405t–407t
hyperlipidemic agents, 405t–407t
hypermagnesemia, 117, 120–122
  algorithm, 121f
  clinical manifestations of, 120
  epidemiology of, 117, 120
  etiologies, 120, 120t, 122t
    decreased excretion, 120
    increased intake, 120
    intracellular shift, 120
  oral magnesium, increased intake, 120
  other magnesium sources, increased intake, 120
  parenteral magnesium, increased intake, 120
  prevalence of, 117
  treatment of, 120–122, 121f
hypernatremia
  clinical manifestations of, 45–46
    brain adaptation to plasma hypertonicity, 45–46
    symptoms, 46
  definition, 44
  diagnosis of, 46, 47f

hypermagnesemia (*continued*)
  Edelman equation scenarios for, 44, 44*t*
  pathogenesis and etiology of, 44–45
    electrolyte-free water loss, 45
    inability to drink water, 45
    net sodium gain, 45
  therapy for, 47, 50
    other, 50
    principles, 47, 50
    water replacement, 50
hyperoxaluria
  calcium-containing stones and, 131–132, 131*t*
  prevention and treatment, 140
hyperparathyroidism
  asymptomatic, 97–98
  in hypercalcemia, 88–89
  secondary, 98
  tertiary, 98
hyperphosphatemia, 82*t*, 101–105
  CKD risk factor for, 102–103
  etiologies of, 102, 102*t*
  oral phosphorus binders and, 104–105
  pathophysiology of, 101–102
  treatment of, 103–105, 104*f*
  uncommon causes of, 103
hyperpolarization of cell membranes, 52
hypersensitivity reactions, 10
hypertension, 11, 113–114, 180, 190, 263, 294–318, 357*t*
  to cardiovascular risk, 296, 297*t*
  classification of, 294, 295*t*
  definition of, 294
  diagnostic evaluation of, 299–303, 300*t*
  epidemiology of, 294–296
  identifiable causes of, 301*t*
  malignant, 313–314, 314*f*, 315*t*
  OSA and, 303
  pathogenesis of, 296–299, 298*f*
  during pregnancy, 285–291
    antihypertensive drugs used to treat, 291*t*
    chronic hypertension, 286
    chronic hypertension with superimposed preeclampsia, 286
    gestational hypertension, 286
    guidelines for treating, 290*t*
    preeclampsia, 286–291
  secondary, 302
  symptoms, 301
  treatment of, 303–312
    DASH diet, 303, 305
    in elderly, 308–309
    goals, 303
    initial approach to, 306*f*
    lifestyle modifications, 303, 304*t*, 305

    nonpharmacologic, 303, 304*t*, 305
    in patients with cardiac disease, 308
    in patients with CKD, 309–311
    in patients with metabolic syndrome, 309
    pharmacologic, 305
    with resistant hypertension, 311–312, 311*t*, 312*f*
Hypertension in the Very Elderly Trial (HYVET), 308
Hypertension Optimal Trial (HOT), 307
hypertensive crises, 312–318
  definition of, 312–313
  due to nonmalignant hypertension with acute complications, 314
  malignant hypertension, 313–314, 314*f*, 315*t*
  of severe uncomplicated hypertension in acute care setting, 316, 317*f*, 318
  spectrum of, 313*t*
  treatment of malignant hypertension, 315–316
  treatment of other, 316
hypertensive neuroretinopathy (HNR), 302
hypertensive retinopathy, classification of, 315*t*
hyperthyroidism, 92
hypertonic saline, 22
hyperuricemia, 26*t*
  tumor lysis syndrome (TLS) and, 341
hyperuricosuria, calcium-containing stones and, 131, 131*t*
Hypervitaminosis A, 92
hypoalbuminemia, 9, 12, 14, 30–31, 172
hypocalcemia, 81–88
  acute symptomatic, 86–88
  algorithm for workup of, 85*f*
  causes of, 82*t*
    defects in vitamin D metabolism, 83–84
    DiGeorge syndrome, 82*t*, 83
    drugs and contrast agents, 84
    end-organ resistance to PTH, 82*t*, 83
    familial hypocalcemia, 82*t*, 83
    hypoparathyroidism, 82–83, 82*t*
    infiltrative disorders, 82*t*, 83
    less common, 84
    parathyroid and radical neck surgery or irradiation, 82*t*, 83
    polyglandular autoimmune syndrome type I, 82–83
    severe hypomagnesemia, 82*t*, 83
    thyroid surgery, 82*t*, 83
    transient hypoparathyroidism, 82*t*, 83
    vitamin D metabolism, defects in, 82*t*, 84
  diagnosis of, 85–86

etiology of, 81–84
familial, 82t, 83
and ionized calcium concentration, 81
management of, 86–88
    active vitamin D analogs, 88
    acute symptomatic hypocalcemia, 86–88
    calcitriol for, 88
signs and symptoms of, 84–85
hypocitraturia
    calcium-containing stones and, 131, 131t
    prevention and treatment, 140
hypoglycemic agent dosing in renal failure, 408t–411t
hypoglycemic agents, 408t–411t
hypogonadism, 265
hypokalemia, 26t, 54–57
    clinical manifestations of, 57, 58t
    diagnosis of, 54–57, 54f, 56f
    genetic disorders associated with, 57
    treatment of, 57
hypomagnesemia, 111–117
    causes of, 115t
    clinical manifestations of, 113–114
        arrhythmias, 114
        cardiovascular, 113–114
        diabetes mellitus, 114
        eclampsia, 114–115
        electrolyte abnormalities, 114
        hypertension, 113–114
        myocardial infarction, 114
        preeclampsia, 114–115
    epidemiology, 113
    etiologies of, 115–116, 115t
        chemotherapy, 116
        decreased magnesium intake, 116
        magnesium in asthma, 116
        proton pump inhibitors, 116
        renal magnesium wasting, 116
    and magnesium, 114–115
    normal magnesium levels in, 117t
    signs and symptoms of, 113–114
    treatment of, 116–117, 118f–119f
hyponatremia, 26t
    clinical manifestations of, 37–38
        biochemical severity, 38
        brain adaptation to plasma hypotonicity, 37
        duration, 37
        symptoms, 37
    definition, 33
    diagnosis of, 38, 39f, 40
    pathogenesis and etiology of, 35–37
        hypertonic hyponatremia, 35
        hypotonic hyponatremia, 35–37, 36f
        isotonic hyponatremia, 35
    in patient with cancer, 359–364, 360t
    physiologic principles, 33–35
        electrolyte-free water balance, 34
        kidney's electrolyte-free water handling, 34–35
        plasma osmolality, 33
        plasma sodium concentration, 33–34
        plasma tonicity, 33
    risk factors for overcorrection of, 41t
    therapy for, 40–44
        complications of, 40–41, 41t
        moderate/severe symptoms, 42–43
        nonsevere hyponatremia, 43–44, 43t
        principles, 40
    urine-to-plasma electrolyte ratio guides fluid restriction in, 43t
hypoparathyroidism, 82–83, 82t
hypophosphatemia, 105–108, 364
    ADHR, 106
    causes, 105–106
    dietary issues and, 106
    etiologies of, 105t
    increased kidney phosphate excretion in, 106
    medication causes, 106
    oncogenic hypophosphatemic osteomalacia, 106
    with refeeding syndrome, 105
    signs and symptoms of, 106–107
    suggested replacement amount for phosphorus levels, 108t
    treatment of, 107–108
    workup approach, 107, 107f
    XLH, 106

I

ibandronate, 420t
ibuprofen, 382t, 418t
ICPi therapy, 353
idiopathic cyclic edema, 10
IFTA. *See* interstitial fibrosis/tubular atrophy
IgA nephropathy, 182–183
    diagnosis of, 182
    overview, 182
    pathophysiology of, 182
    prevalence of, 182
    treatment of, 182–183
IgA vasculitis, 175t, 182
IHD. *See* intermittent hemodialysis
iloperidone, 394t
iloprost, 384t
immobilization, 92
immune-complex membranoproliferative GN (IC-MPGN), 183–184
    clinical presentations of, 183
    diagnosis of, 183
    overview, 183
    pathophysiology, 183–184
    treatment of, 184

immunization, 262
immunofixation, 174
immunology, kidney transplant, 250–252
   antigen-presenting cells, 251
   B-cells, 252
   MHC surface molecules, 250–251
   T-cells, 251
   T-cells and APCs interactions, 251–252
immunotactoid glomerulonephritis, 343t
immunotherapy, 352–354
immunotherapy interferon-alpha (IFNα), 352
indapamide, 16t
indinavir, 400t
indobufen, 384t
indomethacin, 418t
induction therapy, 252
infection
   Hepatitis B virus, 262
   Hepatitis C virus, 262
   HIV, 262
   immunosuppression during, 261
   kidney transplant and, 257
   in nephrotic syndrome, 182
   urinary, 262
infection-related GN, 187
   diagnosis of, 187
   overview, 187
   pathophysiology of, 187
   treatment for, 187
infection stones. *See* struvite-carbonate stones
infiltrative disorders, 82t, 83
inflammation, 11
inorganic phosphorus, 100
insulin, 52, 328, 330, 332
insulin agents, 411t
insulin glargine, 411t
insulin-like growth factor–binding protein 7 (IGFBP7), 198
insulin regular, 411t
interleukin-18 (IL-18), 198
intermittent hemodialysis (IHD), 223–224, 225t
International Consensus Guideline on Anticancer Drug Dosing in Kidney Dysfunction, 348
interstitial fibrosis/tubular atrophy (IFTA), 260
interstitial fluid, excess and its impact, 9–10, 10f
intracellular fluid, 9
intracellular potassium (K), 52
intravascular volume
   depletion, 26t
   in generalized edema, 9
intravenous normal saline, 95t

intrinsic kidney disease
   AIN, 213–214
   atheroembolic disease and, 211–212
   ATI, 214–215
   evaluation of
      large vessel disease, 211
      small vessel disease, 211–212
   glomerular disease from nephritic cause, 213
   glomerular disease from nephrotic cause, 212–213
   TMA, 212
iron deficiency in CKD, 235
ischemic AKI, 203
isoniazid, 396t
isotonic saline, 11
itraconazole, 391t
IVIG, 253t
ixazomib, 351

J

Jansen-type metaphyseal chondroplasia (activating PTH1R variant), 90
jaundice, 206, 219
Jodele criteria for diagnosis of transplant-associated thrombotic microangiopathy, 357t
jugular venous pulsation (JVP), 220
JVP. *See* jugular venous pulsation

K

kaliuresis associated with hypomagnesemia, 57
KDIGO. *See* Kidney Disease/Improving Global Outcomes
Kerley B lines, 23
ketoacidosis, 70, 71t, 72
ketoacids, 72
ketoconazole, 391t
ketoprofen, 418t
ketorolac, 418t
kidney
   beta (β)-adrenergic–mediated release of renin, 13
   biopsy, 174
   biopsy in AKI, 219–220
   electrolyte-free water handling, 34–35
      arginine vasopressin, 35
      glomerular filtration, 34
      osmolar excretion rate, 34–35
      proximal tubular fluid reabsorption, 34
      tubular dilution, 34
   hemodynamics, 14
   pelvic, 281
   role in fluid volume regulation, 11
   solitary, 281
Kidney Disease/Improving Global Outcomes (KDIGO), 28, 35, 37, 194

kidney disease in pregnancy, 272–282
  adult dominant polycystic, 281
  AKI, 274–277
  antibiotic use in pregnancy, 273–274
  asymptomatic bacteriuria, 272–273
  degree of impaired kidney function, 277
  diabetic nephropathy, 280
  glomerular disease, 280–281
  glomerulonephritis, 279
  hematuria, 281–282
  hypertension, 277–278
  lupus nephritis, 279–280
  nephrotic-range proteinuria, 280
  pelvic kidneys, 281
  prognosis, 277–278
  proteinuria, 278–279
  pyelonephritis, 273
  renal hemodynamics, 278–279
  solitary kidneys, 281
  symptomatic bacteriuria, 273–274
  tubulointerstitial disease, 281
  urolithiasis, 281–282
  VUR, 281
Kidney Disease Outcomes Quality Initiative (KDOQI), 243, 333
kidney diseases in patients with cancer, 338–365
  AKI and, 338–358
  CKD and, 338–358, 358–359
  electrolyte and acid–base disorders, 359–365, 360t, 363f
  estimated glomerular filtration rate, 338
  etiologies of, 340
  incidence of, 338–340
  monoclonal gammopathies (paraproteinemias), 342–345
    AKI and, 342
    CKD and, 342
    definition, 342
    glomerular diseases directly associated with cancer, 346–348, 347f
    LCCN, 343–344, 343t
    LCPT, 343t, 344–345
    MM and, 342
    obstructive AKI, 348
    paraprotein-mediated glomerular diseases, 343t, 345
    renal drug toxicities, 348–354
    TMA, 343t, 345–346, 346f
  multiple myeloma and, 339
  onconephrology, 338, 339f
  other causes of, 354
  prevalence of, 338–340
  renal drug toxicities and, 348–354
    chemotherapy, 349–350
    immunotherapy, 352–354
    targeted therapies, 351–352
  stem cell therapy–associated kidney disease, 354–358, 357t
  tumor lysis syndrome, 340–342
    AKI and, 340
    Cairo–Bishop criteria for, 340–341, 340t
    causes of, 340
    hyperuricemia and, 341
    management of, 341–342
    with significant morbidity and mortality, 340–341
    xanthine oxidase inhibitor for, 341
kidney failure, 228
kidney function in pregnancy, 267–272
  acid–base regulation, 268–269
  detection of AKI, 272
  examination of urine, 271
  GFR, 267–268
  kidney biopsy, 272
  renal hemodynamics, changes in, 267–268, 268t
  renal plasma flow, 267–268
  tests for, 271–272
  urinary tract, anatomic and functional changes in, 267, 269f
  volume regulation, 270
  water excretion, 269–270
kidney injury molecule-1 (Kim-1), 198
kidney replacement therapy (KRT), 223–226
kidney stone disease (KSD), 125–128
  after kidney transplantation, 142
  in Hispanics, 127
  incidence, 127–128
  in non-Hispanic Whites, 127
  prevalence, 127–128
  UTO due to, 125–128
kidney stones (KS), 127–128
  after kidney transplantation, 142
  calcium-containing, 127, 130–133
  COM in, 128
  cystine stones, 134–135
  drug-related stones, 134–135
  pathogenesis of, 128
  in pregnancy, 142
  struvite-carbonate stones, 134
  uric acid stones, 133–134
  urine of, 128
kidney transplant
  commonly used drugs in, 253t
  cross-matching, 255
  desensitization, 255–256
  desensitization therapy prior to, 252
  donor nephrectomy, 256
  epidemiology, 248
  immunology, 250–252
    antigen-presenting cells, 251
    B-cells, 252

kidney transplant (*continued*)
    MHC surface molecules, 250–251
    T-cells, 251
    T-cells and APCs interactions, 251–252
  induction therapy for, 252, 256
  maintenance therapy for, 252
  medical care of transplanted patient, 260–266
    from anemia, 264–265
    from BK polyomavirus (BKPyV), 261–262
    from bone disease, 264–265
    from cardiovascular disease, 262–264
    from CMV, 261
    from diabetes mellitus, 263–264
    from hematologic disease, 265–266
    from Hepatitis B virus infection, 262
    from Hepatitis C virus infection, 262
    from HIV infection, 262
    from hyperlipidemia, 263
    from hypertension, 263
    immunization, 262
    from immunosuppression during infection, 261
    from infectious diseases, 260–262
    from malignancy, 264
    from posttransplant bone disease, 265
    from preexisting bone disease, 264–265
    pregnancy, 266
    from PTDM, 263–264
    from PTE, 265–266
    smoking and, 264
    from urinary infections, 262
  medical complications, 258–260
    acute rejection, 259
    chronic allograft damage, 260
    DGF, 259
    recurrent disease, 259–260
  overview, 248
  patient selection for, 248–250
    organ donors, 249–250
    predictors of outcome, 250
    recipient evaluation, 248–249
  pharmacotherapy, 252–255
    agents used for induction, 252
    agents used for maintenance, 252–253
    agents used for treatment of rejection, 254–255
    alemtuzumab (Campath), 252
    antimetabolites, 254
    ATG, 252
    basiliximab, 252
    belatacept, 254
    calcineurin inhibitors, 252, 253*t*, 254
    corticosteroids, 254
    drug interactions, 255
    mTOR-Is, 254
    thymoglobulin, 252
  postoperative management, 256–258
    alternative regimens, 258
    conventional therapy, 257–258
    immediate postoperative care, 256–257
    maintenance immunosuppression, 257–258
    surgical complications, 257
  surgery, 256
  surgical complications, 257
    arterial/venous thrombosis, 257
    infections, 257
    lymphocele, 257
    obstruction, 257
    urine leak, 257
    vesicoureteral reflux, 257
    wound complications, 257
  in United States, 248
Klebsiella species, 147
KRT. *See* kidney replacement therapy
KS. *See* kidney stones
KSD. *See* kidney stone disease

L

labetalol, 290*t*
laboratory examination, for hypercalcemia, 92–94
lactate dehydrogenase (LDH), 193, 345
lactobacilli, 153
lamivudine, 400*t*
lamotrigine, 414*t*
lansoprazole, 404*t*
LCCN. *See* light chain cast nephropathy
LCPT. *See* light chain proximal tubulopathy
LDH. *See* lactate dehydrogenase
lenalidomide, 350
levetiracetam, 414*t*
levodopa, 392*t*
levofloxacin, 162*t*
levothyroxine, 426*t*
L-FABP. *See* liver fatty acid binding protein
liddle syndrome, 57
lidocaine, 375*t*
light and heavy chain deposition disease, 343*t*
light chain cast nephropathy (LCCN), 343–344, 343*t*
light chain deposition disease, 343*t*
light chain proximal tubulopathy (LCPT), 343*t*, 344–345
LIMITS-2 trial, 114
linagliptin, 332
lipid-lowering therapy, 334

liraglutide, 409*t*
lisdexamfetamine, 424*t*
lispro insulin, 411*t*
lithium, 90, 375*t*, 412*t*
lithium carbonate, 423*t*
liver fatty acid binding protein (L-FABP), 198
lixisenatide, 409*t*
localized edema, 11
loop diuretics, 16–17, 16*t*, 17*t*, 95*t*, 333
   in congestive heart failure, 23–24
   continuous infusion of, 19, 21, 21*t*
   for edema, 17
   typical doses of, 17*t*
lorazepam, 423*t*
Losartan Intervention for Endpoint Reduction in Hypertension (LIFE) trial, 308
lovastatin, 406*t*
low-grade lymphoma, 342
low urinary volume, calcium-containing stones and, 131*t*, 132
loxapine, 394*t*
lupus nephritis, 175*t*, 185–186, 279–280
   diagnosis of, 186
   overview, 185
   pathophysiology of, 186
   treatment for, 186
lurasidone, 395*t*
lymphatic obstruction, 9, 11
lymphocele, 257
lysozymuria, 354

M

macrolides, 160
magnesium
   in adults, 109
   in asthma, 116
   atomic weight of, 109
   in bone reservoir, 109
   and cardiovascular disease, 113–114
   and diabetes mellitus, 114
   dietary sources of, 109
   in distal convoluted tubule, 112*f*
   in eclampsia, 114–115
   and electrolyte abnormalities, 114
   formulations, 110*t*
   homeostasis, 109–111
   and hypermagnesemia, 117, 120–122
   and hypomagnesemia, 111–117
   intestinal absorption of, 109
   in preeclampsia, 114–115
   reabsorption, 110
   renal handling of, 109–111, 111*f*
   serum, 109
   in TALH, 111
magnesium sulfate, 290*t*
maintenance therapy, 252

major histocompatibility complex (MHC) surface molecules, 250–251
malignant hypertension, 175*t*, 313–314, 314*f*, 315*t*
   treatment of, 315–316
mammalian target of rapamycin inhibitors (mTOR-Is), 254
maraviroc, 400*t*
marrow infusion syndrome, 355
MCD. *See* minimal change disease
MDRD. *See* modification of diet in renal disease
measles–mumps–rubella (MMR) vaccine, 262
mechanical ultrafiltration, 22
meclofenamic acid, 419*t*
medical care of kidney transplanted patient, 260–266
   from anemia, 264–265
   from BK polyomavirus (BKPyV), 261–262
   from bone disease, 264–265
   from cardiovascular disease, 262–264
   from CMV, 261
   from diabetes mellitus, 263–264
   from hematologic disease, 265–266
   from Hepatitis B virus infection, 262
   from Hepatitis C virus infection, 262
   from HIV infection, 262
   from hyperlipidemia, 263
   from hypertension, 263
   immunization, 262
   from immunosuppression during infection, 261
   from infectious diseases, 260–262
   from malignancy, 264
   from posttransplant bone disease, 265
   from preexisting bone disease, 264–265
   pregnancy, 266
   from PTDM, 263–264
   from PTE, 265–266
   smoking and, 264
   from urinary infections, 262
medical complications, kidney transplant, 258–260
   acute rejection, 259
   chronic allograft damage, 260
   DGF, 259
   recurrent disease, 259–260
medullary sponge kidney, calcium-containing stones and, 131*t*, 132
mefenamic acid, 419*t*
memantine, 377*t*
membranous nephropathy (MN), 347–348
meperidine, 379*t*
meprobamate, 423*t*
metabolic alkalosis, 26*t*
metalloproteinase-2 (TIMP-2), 198
metformin, 409*t*

methadone, 379t
methicillin-resistant *Staphylococcus aureus* infection, 175t
methimazole, 426t
methylphenidate IR, 424t
methylprednisolone, 403t
metoclopramide, 404t
metolazone, 16t
MGRS. See monoclonal gammopathies of renal significance
MGUS. See monoclonal gammopathies of undetermined significance
micafungin, 391t
miconazole, 391t
microbial pathogens of kidney and bladder, 152t
microscopic polyangiitis, 175t
midazolam, 423t
MIDD. See MI deposition disease
MI deposition disease (MIDD), 345
midodrine, 29
milk-alkali syndrome, 90
mineral and bone disease, CKD and, 235–236
mineralocorticoid antagonism, 234
mineralocorticoid receptor antagonists (MRAs), 311
　for diabetic kidney disease, 333–334
　nonsteroidal, 333–334
　　cardiovascular protective effects, 334
　　kidney protective effects of, 334
　steroidal, 333
mineralocorticoids, 53–54
minimal change disease (MCD), 189–190, 346–348
　diagnosis of, 189
　overview, 189
　pathophysiology of, 189
　treatment for, 189–190
minoxidil, 12
mirtazapine, 389t
misoprostol, 404t
mitochondrial toxicity, 349
mixed cryoglobulinemia, 175t
MM. See multiple myeloma
MMF. See mycophenolate mofetil
modification of diet in renal disease (MDRD), 196, 229, 241, 271, 372
modification of diet in renal disease re-expressed equation, 372
monoclonal B cell lymphocytosis, 342
monoclonal gammopathies, 190–191
monoclonal gammopathies of renal significance (MGRS), 342
monoclonal gammopathies of undetermined significance (MGUS), 342
monoclonal immunoglobulin deposition and amyloidosis, 190–191
monoclonal immunoglobulins (MIgs), 342

mood stabilizers, 412t
morphine, 379t
MPA. See mycophenolic acid
MRA. See mineralocorticoid receptor antagonist
mTOR-Is. See mammalian target of rapamycin inhibitors
mTOR-Is sirolimus, 258
MTX, 349–350
MTX-induced AKI (MTX-AKI), 349
multiple myeloma (MM), 339
mycophenolate mofetil (MMF), 253t, 254
mycophenolic acid (MPA), 253t, 254
mycoplasma hominis, 148
myocardial infarction, 114
MYRE trial, 344

N

nabumetone, 419t
Na channel blockers, 16t
NaCl inhibitors, 16t
NAGMA. See normal anion gap metabolic acidosis
Na-K-2Cl inhibitors, 16t
naloxone, 379t
NAPA (N-acetyl procainamide), 376t
naproxen, 419t
narcotic antagonists, 378t–381t
narcotics, 378t–381t
National Health and Nutrition Examination Survey (NHANES), 128
natriuresis, 11, 16–17, 24f
Neisseria gonorrhoeae, 148
nelfinavir, 400t
nephritic glomerular disorders, 201
nephritic syndrome, 172
　anti-GBM disease, 184
　C3 glomerulopathy (C3G), 183–184
　cause of, 177
　cryoglobulinemia (cryoglobulinemia), 186–187
　features of, 172, 174
　Goodpasture syndrome, 184
　IC-MPGN, 183–184
　IgA nephropathy, 182–183
　infection-related GN, 187
　lupus nephritis, 185–186
　pauci-immune renal vasculitis, 184–185
　with systemic manifestations, 184–187
Nephrocheck, 198
nephrolithiasis, 128, 130, 133
nephrology consult for AKI, 1–8
　additional testing, 3–4, 4f–6f
　differential diagnosis, 5f
　history and reviewing the patient chart, 1–2
　initial management, 8
　kidney biopsy, 6, 6f–7f

KRT, evaluate need for urgent, 6, 8
physical examination, 1
urinary sediment microscopy, 2–3
nephritic glomerular disorders, 201
nephrotic-range proteinuria, 188–189, 280
nephrotic syndrome, 30–31, 172
  causes of, 174
  diabetic nephropathy, 190
  features of, 174
  hypercoagulability in, 181–182
  hyperlipidemia in, 181
  infection in, 182
  minimal change disease, 189–190
  monoclonal gammopathies, 190–191
  monoclonal immunoglobulin deposition and amyloidosis, 190–191
  overfill vs. underfill edema in, 31t
  pathogenesis, 30–31
  in patients with serum albumin, 31
  primary FSGS, 188–189
  primary MN, 187–188
  secondary FSGS, 190
  secondary MCD, 190
  secondary MN, 189–190
  serologic assessment for, 174
  treatment, 31–32
nephrotoxic AKI, 203, 215–217
  acute uric acid nephropathy, 217
  aminoglycoside nephrotoxicity, 215
  causes of, 215–217
  contrast-associated AKI and, 216
  rhabdomyolysis, 216–217
  vancomycin with and without concomitant piperacillin-tazobactam and, 216
neural epidermal growth factor-like 1 (NELL1), 188
neurologic drug dosing in renal failure, 413t–417t
neutrophil gelatinase–associated lipocalin (NGAL), 198
nevirapine, 400t
NFAT. *See* nuclear factor of activated T-cells
NGAL. *See* neutrophil gelatinase-associated lipocalin
NHANES. *See* National Health and Nutrition Examination Survey
nicardipine, 315–316
nicotinic acid, 406t
NIPD. *See* nocturnal intermittent PD
nitrofurantoin, 159, 161t
nizatidine, 404t
N-methyl-D-aspartate (NMDA) antagonist, 115
nocturnal intermittent PD (NIPD), 244
nonbacterial chronic prostatitis, 168
nonmelanoma skin cancers, 264

non-narcotics drugs, 382t
nonpitting edema, 9
non–PTH-mediated hypercalcemia, 90–92
  decreased calcium excretion by kidney, 92
  of milk-alkali syndrome, 90
  role of calcium resorption from bone, 91–92
nonsteroidal anti-inflammatory drugs (NSAIDs), 2, 8, 15, 18, 24–25, 29–30, 60t, 61, 190, 201, 205–209, 216, 223, 418t–419t
nonsteroidal mineralocorticoid (aldosterone) receptor antagonists, 16t
nonsteroidal MRAs, 333–334
nonstimulant drugs, 424t
nonstimulants, 424t–425t
normal anion gap metabolic acidosis (NAGMA), 72–73
  Addison disease, 73
  diarrhea, 73
  hyperalimentation, 73
  pancreatic fistula/drainage, 73
  renal tubular acidosis, 73
  spironolactone, 73
  ureteral diversion, 73
nortriptyline, 388t
NOSTONE trial, 140
nuclear factor of activated T-cells (NFAT), 254

O

obesity, calcium-containing stones and, 131–132, 131t
obstructive AKI, 348
obstructive sleep apnea (OSA), 303
ODS. *See* osmotic demyelination syndrome
ofloxacin, 162t
olanzapine, 394t
oliguria, 199
omeprazole, 404t
oncogenic hypophosphatemic osteomalacia, 106
oncogenic osteomalacia, 105t
organic cation transporter 2 (OCT2), 349
organic phosphorus, 100
orthostatic hypotension, 26t, 206
OSA. *See* obstructive sleep apnea
oseltamivir, 400t
Osler maneuver, 301
osmoles, effective/ineffective, 34t
osmotic demyelination syndrome (ODS), 40–41, 41t, 361
osmotic diuretics, 15, 16t
osteitis fibrosa, 264–265
osteoblastic metastasis, 82t
osteopenia, 265
osteoporosis, 265

osteoporosis drug dosing in in renal failure, 420t
osteoporosis drugs, 420t
overcorrection of hyponatremia, 40, 41t
oxaprozin, 419t
oxazepam, 423t
oxcarbazepine, 415t
oxycodone ER, 381t
oxycodone HCL, 381t

P

Paget disease, 12, 92
paliperidone, 394t
pamidronate, 95t, 96
pancreatitis, 26t
pantoprazole, 404t
paraprotein-mediated glomerular diseases, 343t, 345
paraprotein-related kidney diseases, 343t
parathyroid hormone (PTH), 78–80, 100–101
   end-organ resistance to, 82t
   levels, 236
paricalcitol, 88
paroxetine, 386t
pathologic postobstructive diuresis (POD), 127
patient selection, for kidney transplant, 248–250
   organ donors, 249–250
   predictors of outcome, 250
   recipient evaluation, 248–249
patiromer, 62, 62f, 63t
pauci-immune renal vasculitis, 184–185
   diagnosis of, 185
   overview, 184–185
   pathophysiology of, 185
   treatment for, 185
PCT. *See* proximal convoluted tubule
pegloticase, 421t
pelvic kidneys, 281
pelvic lymphatic obstruction, 11
penicillamine, 421t
pentazocine, 379t
pentobarbital, 422t
peripherally inserted central catheters (PICCs), 243
peritoneal dialysis, 224
peritoneal dialysis (PD) for CKD, 244–245
   versus hemodialysis, 241t
   standard dialysate solutions, comparison of, 242t
perphenazine, 393t
PGNMID. *See* proliferative glomerulonephritis with monoclonal immunoglobulin deposits
pharmacotherapy, kidney transplant, 252–255
   agents used for induction, 252
   agents used for maintenance, 252–253
   agents used for treatment of rejection, 254–255
   alemtuzumab (Campath), 252
   antimetabolites, 254
   ATG, 252
   basiliximab, 252
   belatacept, 254
   calcineurin inhibitors, 252, 253t, 254
   corticosteroids, 254
   drug interactions, 255
   mTOR-Is, 254
   thymoglobulin, 252
phenobarbita, 415t
phenobarbital, 84, 376t, 422t
phenylbutazone, 419t
phenytoin, 84, 376t, 415t
pheochromocytoma, 92
phosphate-binding agents, 105t
phosphatonin, 100
phosphorous control, 236
phosphorus
   absorption in nephron, 101f
   balance, organ regulation of, 100–101
   homeostasis, kidney role in, 100–101
   hyperphosphatemia, 101–105
      CKD risk factor for, 102–103
      etiologies of, 102, 102t
      oral phosphorus binders and, 104–105
      pathophysiology of, 101–102
      treatment of, 103–105, 104f
      uncommon causes of, 103
   hypophosphatemia, 105–108
      ADHR, 106
      causes, 105–106
      dietary issues and, 106
      etiologies of, 105t
      increased kidney phosphate excretion in, 106
      medication causes, 106
      oncogenic hypophosphatemic osteomalacia, 106
      with refeeding syndrome, 105
      signs and symptoms of, 106–107
      suggested replacement amount for phosphorus levels, 108t
      treatment of, 107–108
      workup approach, 107, 107f
      XLH, 106
   inorganic, 100
   organic, 100
   regulation, 100
PICCs. *See* peripherally inserted central catheters
PIKRT. *See* prolonged intermittent kidney replacement therapy

pioglitazone, 332–333, 410*t*
piroxicam, 419*t*
pitavastatin, 406*t*
pitting edema, 9
plasma-ionized calcium, 78
plasma osmolality (POsm), 33
plasma sodium concentration (PNa), 33–34
plasma tonicity, 33
plicamycin, 97
Pneumocystis jirovecii pneumonia, 260–261
POCUS. *See* point of care ultrasound
POD. *See* pathologic postobstructive diuresis
point of care ultrasound (POCUS), 206
polyarteritis nodosa, 175*t*
polyglandular autoimmune syndrome type I, 82–83
polyuria, 46, 48*f*, 49*f*
posaconazole, 391*t*
postoperative management, kidney transplant, 256–258
 alternative regimens, 258
 conventional therapy, 257–258
 immediate postoperative care, 256–257
 maintenance immunosuppression, 257–258
 surgical complications, 257
postrenal AKI, 201
 causes of, 201
 evaluation of, 210–211
  cystoscopy for, 211
  history, 210
  isotope renography for, 211
  kidney ultrasonography for, 210
  noncontrast computed tomography for, 211
  physical examination, 210
  retrograde pyelography for, 211
  urinalysis, 210
  urine sediment, 210
 management, 221
 risk for, 201
poststreptococcal GN, 175*t*
posttransplant bone disease, 265
posttransplant diabetes mellitus (PTDM), 263–264
posttransplant erythrocytosis (PTE), 265–266
posttransplant lymphoproliferative disorder (PTLD), 254
potassium (K), 52
 external balance, 53–54
  extrarenal, 54
  kidney, 53–54
 extracellular, 52
 internal balance, 52–53
  acid–base, 52–53
  catecholamines, 52
  insulin levels, 52
  tonicity, 53
 intracellular, 52
 physiology, 52–54
 in Western diet, 52
potassium-sparing diuretics, 15
PPIs. *See* proton pump inhibitors
pramlintide, 410*t*
prasugrel, 385*t*
pravastatin, 406*t*
prednisolone, 403*t*
prednisone, 403*t*
preeclampsia, 276, 286–291
 calcium in, 288
 chronic hypertension with superimposed, 286
 GFR in, 287
 glomerular capillary endotheliosis in, 288, 288*f*
 hypertensive patient without, 289
 increased proteinuria in, 287
 magnesium in, 114–115
 management of, 289
 pathophysiology of, 286–287, 287*f*
 prevention of, 289
 RPF in, 287
 treatment guidelines for hypertensive disorders, 289–290
 uric acid in, 288
pregnancy, 12
 acid–base regulation in, 268–269
 AKI in, 274–277
  acute fatty liver of pregnancy, 277
  acute pyelonephritis, 276
  causes, 274, 275*t*, 276
  detection of, 272
  incidence, 274
  management, 277
  renal cortical necrosis, 276
  TMA and, 274, 276
  urinary tract obstruction, 277
 aldosterone escape in, 14
 antibiotic use in, 273–274
 blood pressure in, 270
 dialysis in, 284–285, 285*t*
 hypertensive disorders of, 285–291
  antihypertensive drugs used to treat, 291*t*
  chronic hypertension, 286
  chronic hypertension with superimposed preeclampsia, 286
  gestational hypertension, 286
  guidelines for treating, 290*t*
  preeclampsia, 286–291
 kidney biopsy in, 272
 kidney disease in, 272–282
  adult dominant polycystic, 281

pregnancy (*continued*)
    AKI, 274–277
        antibiotic use in pregnancy, 273–274
        asymptomatic bacteriuria, 272–273
        degree of impaired kidney function, 277
        diabetic nephropathy, 280
        glomerular disease, 280–281
        glomerulonephritis, 279
        hematuria, 281–282
        hypertension, 277–278
        lupus nephritis, 279–280
        nephrotic-range proteinuria, 280
        pelvic kidneys, 281
        prognosis, 277–278
        proteinuria, 278–279
        pyelonephritis, 273
        renal hemodynamics, 278–279
        solitary kidneys, 281
        symptomatic bacteriuria, 273–274
        tubulointerstitial disease, 281
        urolithiasis, 281–282
        VUR, 281
    kidney function in, 267–272
        acid–base regulation, 268–269
        detection of AKI, 272
        examination of urine, 271
        GFR, 267–268
        kidney biopsy, 272
        renal hemodynamics, changes in, 267–268, 268*t*
        renal plasma flow, 267–268
        tests for, 271–272
        urinary tract, anatomic and functional changes in, 267, 269*f*
        volume regulation, 270
        water excretion, 269–270
    kidney stones (KS) in, 142
    kidney transplantation in, 282–283
    medical care of kidney transplanted patient, 266
    mineral metabolism in, 270–271
    with preexisting kidney disease, 277–278, 278*t*
    renal changes in normal, 268*t*
    ureteral dilation of, 267, 269*f*
    urinary tract infections in, 272–273
    water excretion in, 269–270
prerenal disease, 199–201
    ACEI, 209
    ADHF, 209
    ARB, 209
    causes, 199–201, 200*f*
    cyclosporine and, 209
    definition, 199–201
    evaluation of, 209
        history, 206
        physical examination, 206
        urinary findings, 206, 207*t*
        urine chemistry and indices, 208*t*
    hepatorenal syndrome, 208–209
    management, 220–221
    tacrolimus, 209
    vasomotor prerenal disease due to NSAIDs, 209
pretomanid, 397*t*
Prevention of Serious Adverse Events Following Angiography (PRESERVE) trial, 216
primary FSGS, 188–189
    diagnosis of, 188
    overview, 188
    pathophysiology of, 188–189
    treatment for, 189
primary glomerular diseases, 173*t*
primary hyperparathyroidism, 105*t*
primary MN, 187–188
    diagnosis of, 187–188
    overview, 188
    pathophysiology of, 188
    treatment for, 188
primidone, 415*t*
Proactive Intravenous Iron Therapy in Haemodialysis Patients (PIVOTAL) trial, 247
probenecid, 421*t*
probucol, 407*t*
procainamide, 376*t*
proliferative glomerulonephritis with monoclonal immunoglobulin deposits (PGNMID), 191, 343*t*, 345
prolonged intermittent kidney replacement therapy (PIKRT), 224
promethazine, 393*t*
propoxyphene, 379*t*
propylthiouracil, 426*t*
prostate-specific antigens (PSAs), 148
prostate syndromes, 148
prostatitis, 148
    acute bacterial prostatitis, 149
    chronic bacterial prostatitis, 149
    treatment of, 167–168
prostatodynia, 149
proteinuria, 18–19, 172, 174, 178–180, 230–231, 278–279, 352, 357*t*
    reduction in, 233–235
proteinuric glomerular disease
    edema, 180
    general management of, 178–182
    hypercoagulability, 181–182
    hyperlipidemia, 181
    hypertension, 180
    infection, 182
    proteinuria, 178–180
Proteus mirabilis, 147
proton pump inhibitors (PPIs), 88, 116

proximal convoluted tubule (PCT), 100–101
proximal diuretics, 15, 16t
proximal straight tubule (PST), 100–101
proximal tubular dysfunction, 349
proximal venous thrombosis, 11
PSAs. *See* prostate-specific antigens
pseudohypertension, 300–301
pseudohypoaldosteronism type 1, 61
pseudohypophosphatemia, 105t
Pseudomonas aeruginosa, 244
PST. *See* proximal straight tubule
PTDM. *See* posttransplant diabetes mellitus
PTE. *See* posttransplant erythrocytosis
PTH. *See* parathyroid hormone
PTLD. *See* posttransplant lymphoproliferative disorder
pulmonary edema, 11
pulmonary infections, 262
pyelonephritis, 144, 273
pyrazinamde, 396t

Q

quazepam, 423t
quetiapine, 394t
quinidine, 376t

R

RAAS inhibition, 233
rabeprazole, 404t
Ramipril Efficacy in Nephropathy (REIN) trial, 310
Randall plaque, 129
ranitidine, 404t
rapidly progressing glomerulonephritis (RPGN), 202
rapidly progressive glomerulonephritis (RPGN), 172
recurrent cystitis (reinfections), treatment of, 164–165
   antimicrobial strategies, 164
   emerging therapies, 165
   nonantimicrobial prophylaxis issues, 164–165
recurrent disease, 259–260
recurrent renal infections (relapses), treatment of, 166–167
   acute symptomatic infection, 167
   prognosis, 167
   prolonged, 167
   risk factors, 166–167
   suppressive therapy, 167
recurrent UTI, 144
refeeding syndrome, 105, 105t
REIN-2 trial, 310
REIN (Ramipril Efficacy in Nephropathy) trial, 103
renal calculi, 282

renal changes in normal pregnancy, 268t
renal cortical necrosis, 276
renal drug toxicities, 348–354
   chemotherapy, 349–350
   immunotherapy, 352–354
   targeted therapies, 351–352
renal failure
   alzheimer drug dosing in, 377t
   analgesic drug dosing in, 377t–382t
   anticoagulant drug dosing in, 383t–385t
   antidepressant drug dosing in, 386t–389t
   antifungal agent dosing in, 390t–391t
   anti-parkinson drug dosing in, 392t
   antipsychotic drug dosing in, 393t–395t
   antithyroid drug dosing in, 426t
   antituberculosis drug dosing in, 396t–397t
   antiviral agent dosing in, 398t–402t
   corticosteroid drug dosing in, 403t
   gastrointestinal agent dosing in, 404t
   hyperlipidemic agent dosing in, 405t–407t
   hypoglycemic agent dosing in, 408t–411t
   mood stabilizer drug dosing in, 412t
   neurologic drug dosing in, 413t–417t
   nonsteroidal anti-inflammatory drug dosing in, 418t–419t
   osteoporosis drug dosing in, 420t
   rheumatologic drug dosing in, 421t
   sedative drug dosing in, 422t–423t
   stimulant and nonstimulant drug dosing in, 424t–425t
renal hemodynamics, 278–279
renal outer medullary potassium (ROMK) channels, 80
renal plasma flow (RPF), 267–268
renal replacement therapy (RRT), 342
renal tubular acidosis (RTA), 73
renin-angiotensin-aldosterone system (RAAS) blockade, 333
renin–angiotensin system, 286
repaglinide, 410t
resistant hypertension, 311, 312f
respiratory alkalosis, 105t
rhabdomyolysis, 216–217, 217t
rheumatoid factors, 174
rheumatologic drug dosing in renal failure, 421t
rheumatologic drugs, 421t
ribavirin, 400t
rifabutin, 400t
rifampin, 396t
rifapentine, 396t
RIFLE criteria. *See* Risk, Injury, Failure, Loss, End-stage kidney disease (RIFLE) criteria

rimantadine, 400t
risedronate, 420t
Risk, Injury, Failure, Loss, End-stage kidney disease (RIFLE) criteria, 194, 195t
risperidone, 394t
ritonavir, 401t
rituximab, 253t
rivaroxaban, 385t
rivastigmine, 377t
ROMK channel, 57
rosiglitazone, 332–333, 410t
rosuvastatin, 407t
RPF. See renal plasma flow
RPGN. See rapidly progressing glomerulonephritis; rapidly progressive glomerulonephritis
RRT. See renal replacement therapy
RTA. See renal tubular acidosis

S

Saline versus Albumin Fluid Evaluation (SAFE) study, 220
salmon calcitonin, 95t
saquinavir, 401t
saxagliptin, 332
SBP. See systolic BP
SCC. See squamous cell carcinomas
schistocytes, 357t
scleroderma renal crisis, 175t
secobarbital, 422t
secondary FSGS, 190
secondary hyperparathyroidism, 98, 264–265
secondary hyperparathyroidism from deficiency of vitamin D, 105t
secondary hypertension, 302
secondary MCD, 190
secondary MN, 189–190
sedative drug dosing in renal failure, 422t–423t
sedative drugs, 422t
semaglutide, 410t
sepsis, 12, 105t, 204
sertraline, 386t
serum Anion Gap (AG), 66
serum immunofixation (SIFE), 342
serum protein electrophoresis (SPEP), 174, 342
serum sodium
  and effect of aldosterone, 14
  and mineralocorticoids, 14
  role of kidney in regulation, 11
severe uncomplicated hypertension, 316, 317f, 318
sexually transmitted disease (STD) pathogen, 149
SGLT2 (sodium-glucose transport protein 2) inhibition, 233–234

Shiga toxin, 191, 192f
short daily dialysis, 241
SIADH. See syndrome of inappropriate diuretic hormone secretion
SIFE. See serum immunofixation
significant bacteriuria, 144
simvastatin, 407t
sinusoidal obstructive syndrome (SOS), 355
sirolimus, 253t, 376t
sitagliptin, 332, 410t
SLC41A2, 109
smoking
  cessation, 234–235
  kidney transplant and, 264
smoldering MM, 342
smoldering Waldenström macroglobulinemia, 342
sodium-chloride cotransporter (NCC), 53
sodium-glucose cotransporter-2 inhibitors (SGLT2), 19, 26–27
sodium-glucose co-transporter-2 (SGLT-2) inhibitors, 330t, 331–332, 331t
  adverse effects, 332
  contraindications for initiating therapy, 332
  impact on long-term cardiovascular and kidney outcomes, 332
  mechanism of action, 331
sodium-glucose cotransporter type 2 inhibitors, 16t
sodium valproate, 415t
sodium zirconium cyclosilicate (SZC), 62, 62f, 63t
solitary kidneys, 281
sotagliflozin, 331
SPEP. See serum protein electrophoresis
spironolactone, 15, 16t, 25, 28, 333
squamous cell carcinomas (SCC), 264
Staphylococcus aureus, 243
Staphylococcus saprophyticus, 147
Starling–Frank curve of myocardial contractility, 23–24, 24f
Starling's law of fluid movement, 9–10, 10f
stavudine, 401t
stem cell therapy–associated kidney disease, 354–358, 357t
steroidal mineralocorticoid (aldosterone) receptor antagonists, 16t
steroidal MRAs, 333
steroids, 265
stimulants, 424t–425t
streptokinase, 385t
struvite-carbonate stones, 134
  evaluation of patient, 136–137
  pathophysiology, 134
  presentation, 134
  prevention and treatment, 141
  risk factors, 134

subclinical rejection, 259
sucralfate, 404t
sufentanil, 380t
sulfinpyrazone, 385t
sulfonylureas, 330t, 331t, 332
sulindac, 419t
sulotroban, 385t
supine position, accumulation of edema fluid in, 11
surgical complications, kidney transplant, 257
   arterial/venous thrombosis, 257
   infections, 257
   lymphocele, 257
   obstruction, 257
   urine leak, 257
   vesicoureteral reflux, 257
   wound complications, 257
symptomatic bacteriuria, 273–274
symptomatic UTIs, 147–148
syndrome of inappropriate antidiuresis (SIAD), 38, 40
syndrome of inappropriate diuretic hormone secretion (SIADH), 359–361, 360t
systemic arterial vasodilation, 13–14, 13f
   and aldosterone escape phenomenon, 14, 15f
   to edema, 14
   effect of, 14
systemic hemodynamic response, 13
Systolic Blood Pressure Intervention Trial (SPRINT), 233, 308–310
systolic BP (SBP), 294–295, 295t
Systolic Hypertension in the Elderly Program (SHEP) trial, 308
SZC. See sodium zirconium cyclosilicate

T

T1DM. See type 1 diabetes mellitus
T2DM. See type 2 diabetes mellitus
tacrolimus, 209, 253t, 257–258
tacrolimus (FK-506), 252, 254, 376t
Tamm–Horsfall glycoprotein, 343
Tamm–Horsfall protein, 146, 344
targeted therapies, 351–352
TA-TMA. See transplant-associated thrombotic microangiopathy
T-cell rejection, 259
T-cells and APCs interactions, 251–252
telbivudine, 401t
temazepam, 423t
tenofovir, 401t
terbinafine, 391t
teriparatide, 420t
terlipressin, dosage regimen for, 222t
tertiary hyperparathyroidism, 98
tetracyclines, 160, 161t, 274

theophylline PO, 376t
therapeutic drug monitoring in patients with chronic kidney disease, 375t–376t
thiazides, 299, 333
thiazolidinediones (TZDs), 330t, 331t, 332–333
thiopental, 422t
thioridazine, 393t
thiothixene, 393t
threshold drugs, 17
thrombocytopenia, 357t
thrombophlebitis, 11
thrombospondin type-1 domain-containing 7A (THSD7A), 188
thrombospondin type 1 domain-containing 7A (THSD7A), 348
thrombotic microangiopathies (TMA), 191–193, 192f, 212, 274, 276, 345–346, 346f
thrombotic thrombocytopenic purpura (TTP), 175t, 191–193, 192f, 193, 276
thymoglobulin, 252
thyrotoxicosis, 12
tiagabine, 416t
ticagrelol, 385t
ticlopidine, 385t
tissue-invasive infection, 262
TLS. See tumor lysis syndrome
TMA. See thrombotic microangiopathies
tobramycin amikacin, 375t
tolazamide, 411t
tolbutamide, 411t
tolmetin, 419t
tolvaptan, 22
topiramate, 416t
torsemide, 16t, 21t
total-body phenomenon of excess interstitial fluid, 11
trametinib, 351
tranexamic acid, 385t
transcapillary hydrostatic pressure, 9
transcapillary oncotic pressure, 9
transient receptor potential cation channel, subfamily M, member 6 (TRPM6), 364
transient receptor potential melastatin (TRPM), 109
Transjugular Intrahepatic Portosystemic Shunt (TIPS), 28–29, 29t
transplant-associated thrombotic microangiopathy (TA-TMA), 356–358
trauma, 11
trazodone, 387t
triamcinolone, 403t
triamterene, 15, 16t
triazolam, 423t

Trichomonas vaginalis, 148
trifluoperazine, 393*t*
trimethadione, 416*t*
trimethoprim, 160, 161*t*
trimethoprim-sulfamethoxazole, 159–160, 161*t*, 162*t*
TRPM. *See* transient receptor potential melastatin
TRPM6/7 channel, 110, 116
TTP. *See* thrombotic thrombocytopenic purpura
tubulointerstitial disease, 281
tumor lysis syndrome (TLS), 340–342
   AKI and, 340
   Cairo–Bishop criteria for, 340–341, 340*t*
   causes of, 340
   hyperuricemia and, 341
   management of, 341–342
   with significant morbidity and mortality, 340–341
   xanthine oxidase inhibitor for, 341
type 1 diabetes mellitus (T1DM), 322
type 1 HRS, 208–209
type 2 diabetes mellitus (T1DM), 322
type 2 HRS, 208–209
type II membranoproliferative glomerulonephritis (MPGN), 259–260
type I membranoproliferative glomerulonephritis (MPGN), 260

U

UAG. *See* urine anion gap
ultrafiltration, 241
ultrafiltration, mechanical, 22
Ultrafiltration in Decompensated Heart Failure with Cardiorenal Syndrome (CARRESS-HF) trial, 22
uncomplicated cystitis
   seven-day regimen for, 163–164
   short-course therapy for, 163
   symptomatic pyuria without bacteriuria, 164
   treatment of, 163–164
uncomplicated UTIs, 145
United Kingdom Prospective Diabetes Study Group (UKPDS), 305, 307
UPCR. *See* urine protein-creatinine ratio
UPEP. *See* urine protein electrophoresis
urea, 16*t*
ureaplasma urealyticum, 148
urea reduction ratio, 245*t*
uremia, 174–175
uremic toxins, accumulation of, 237
ureteral dilation of pregnancy, 267, 269*f*
ureteral diversion, 73
ureteric obstruction, 257
urethritis, 148
uric acid, 288

uric acid stones, 133–134
   etiologies of, 135
   evaluation of patient, 136
   incidence, 133
   pathophysiology of, 133
   prevention and treatment, 141
   risk factors and presentation of, 133–134
urinary catheters, recommendations for care of, 168–169
urinary infections, 262
urinary tract infections (UTIs), 127, 144–170
   acute urethral syndrome, 148–149
   anatomic location, 144
   clinical classification, 145
   clinical features, 148–149
   clinical setting, 147–148
      asymptomatic bacteriuria, 147
      symptomatic UTIs, 147–148
   complicated, 145
   definition, 144
   laboratory diagnosis of, 149–158
      approach to, 150*f*
      biochemical tests for bacteriuria, 156
      interpretation of urine cultures, 152–153
      localization of site of infection, 156–157
      microscopic examination of urine, 153–156, 154*f*, 155*f*
      urine specimens for culture, 149–152
   overview, 144
   pathogenesis of, 145–147
   in pregnancy, 272–273
   prognosis, 144
   prostatitis, 148–149
   prostatodynia, 149
   radiography and other diagnostic procedures, 157–158
   recommendations for therapy for, 166*t*
   recurrence of, 144
   risk factors for, 145–147
   symptomatic, 147–148
   treatment of, 158–170
      acute bacterial pyelonephritis, 165–166
      antimicrobial agents for, 158–160
      asymptomatic bacteriuria, 161–163
      fluoroquinolones for, 160, 161*t*, 162*t*
      and follow-up, 158
      fosfomycin for, 160
      intravenous antimicrobial agents commonly used for, 162*t*
      macrolides for, 160
      nitrofurantoin for, 159, 161*t*
      oral antimicrobial agents commonly used for, 161*t*
      principles, 158
      prostatitis, 167–168

recurrent cystitis (reinfections), 164–165
recurrent renal infections (relapses), 166–167
tetracycline for, 160, 161t
trimethoprim for, 160, 161t
trimethoprim-sulfamethoxazole for, 159–160, 161t
uncomplicated cystitis, 163–164
β-lactams for, 158–159, 161t
uncomplicated, 145
urethritis, 148
vaginitis, 148
urinary tract obstruction (UTO), 125–142
approach to imaging in patients with suspected, 126f
causes of, 125
CKD and, 125
CT scanning for diagnosis of, 125
Doppler ultrasonography for diagnosis of, 125
etiologies of, 127t
evaluation of patient, 135–137
GFR in, 127
initial presentation, 129–130
flat radiographic plate of abdomen, 129
imaging examination, 129
intravenous pyelogram (IVP), 130
laboratory evaluation, 129
likelihood of spontaneous passage, 130t
management, 130
physical examination, 129
spiral CT, 130
ultrasonographic examination of genitourinary tract, 129
intrinsic blockage, 125
kidney stone disease and, 125–128
in older adults, 125
pathologic postobstructive diuresis and, 127
prevalence of, 125
prevention and treatment, 137–142
prolonged, 125
to renal dysfunction, 125
risk factors for, 127
special patient populations, 142
types of stones, 130–135
calcium-containing stones, 130–133
cystine stones, 134–135
drug-related stones, 135
struvite-carbonate stones, 134
uric acid stones, 133–134
ultrasound for diagnosis of, 125
in younger adults, 125
urine anion gap (UAG), 73
urine leak, 257

urine protein-creatinine ratio (UPCR), 352
urine protein electrophoresis (UPEP), 94, 174, 344
urokinase, 385t
urolithiasis, 281–282
UTIs. *See* urinary tract infections
UTO. *See* urinary tract obstruction

V

vaginitis, 148
valacyclovir, 401t
valganciclovir, 401t
valproic acid, 376t
vancomycin, 162t, 216, 376t
vascular compartment, fluids content in, 9
vascular disorders, 201–202
vascular endothelial growth factor (VEGF), 286, 346
vasculitis, management of, 221–222
vasoconstrictor therapy, 29–30
vasodilating drugs, 12
vasomotor prerenal disease, 209
vasopressin antagonists, 11, 13, 27, 27t, 29–30
vas washdown, 129
VBG. *See* venous blood gas
VEGF. *See* vascular endothelial growth factor
VEGF receptor (VEGFR), 351
venlafaxine, 387t
venous blood gas (VBG), 66
venous obstruction, 11
vesicoureteral reflux, 257
vidarabine, 402t
vigabatrin, 417t
vitamin D, 79–80, 236
defects in metabolism, 83–84
deficiency, 82t
dependent rickets, 84
intoxication, 90
metabolism, 80f
secondary hyperparathyroidism from deficiency of, 105t
vitamin D–dependent rickets (VDRR), 82t
von Willebrand factor (vWF) multimers, 193
voriconazole, 391t

W

warfarin, 385t
water excretion, in pregnancy, 269–270
Western diet, potassium (K) in, 52
With-No-Lysine Kinases (WNKs), 53
wound complications, 257

X

xanthine oxidase inhibitor, 341
XLH. *See* X-linked hypophosphatemia

X-linked hypophosphatemia (XLH), 106
X-linked hypophosphatemic rickets, 105t

Z
zalcitabine, 402t
zalutumumab, 116
zanamivir, 402t
zidovudine, 402t
zinc supplements, 142
ziprasidone, 395t
zoledronate, 95t
zoledronic acid, 96, 420t
zonisamide, 417t